All your questions are about to be answered, including:

- What are the most helpful drugs to take for my condition?

- What are the most experimental drugs to take for my condition?

- How long will my disorder last?

- Do I need to restrict certain foods or alcohol to get well?

- What is the difference between a chronic disease and an allergy?

- What are some of the warning symptoms of chronic disease?

THE CONCISE
ESSENTIAL GUIDE TO PRESCRIPTION DRUGS

JAMES J. RYBACKI, PHARM. D.

HarperPaperbacks

A Division of HarperCollins*Publishers*

HarperPaperbacks
A Division of HarperCollins*Publishers*
10 East 53rd Street, New York, N.Y. 10022-5299

ISBN 0-06-100864-8

HarperCollins®, 📖 ®, and HarperPaperbacks™ are trademarks
of HarperCollins*Publishers* Inc.

An unabridged edition of this book was published in 1997 by
HarperPerennial, a division of HarperCollins*Publishers*

First printing: September 1997

Printed in the United States of America

10 9 8 7 6 5 4 3 2 1

CONTENTS

AUTHOR'S NOTE

The Concise Essential Guide to Prescription Drugs offers a wealth of information on prescription drugs, and outlines appropriate ways to save money while preserving the clinical results or outcomes that we all want. Each drug profile includes current drug knowledge on the best use of medications, to help protect you and your loved ones.

Perhaps the future will bring "smarter" medicines able to regulate beneficial effects and limit toxic ones. For now, the use of *any* medicine (prescription or nonprescription) is a benefit-to-risk decision. Every year studies show huge personal and financial expenses incurred by inappropriate medicine usage. For example, the Willcox study from Cambridge Hospital and Harvard Medical School showed that an average 6.6 million elderly Americans are prescribed *the wrong medicine*. This study of hospital records clearly tells us that more prescribing information is needed.

A primary aim of this book is to give you the power—through information—with which to ask intelligent questions. It includes important characteristics to look for whenever medicines are prescribed.

This book also aims to help you understand the drugs prescribed for you in the outpatient setting, reduce the possibility of dispensing errors, clarify self-administration, improve recognition of possible adverse drug effects, reduce the risk of drug-induced disorders, and alert you to potential drug interactions with foods, beverages, and other drugs. Use the information in this book to ask better questions when you visit your doctor.

This book profiles nearly 400 major drugs used in the United States and Canada at press time. Limitation of space prevents including all drugs currently available. The criteria used for selection: the drug is used to treat a serious or significant disease or disorder; it is recognized by experts to be among "the best choices" within its class or is a novel and clear breakthrough in available therapy; its benefits equal or exceed its risks; the safe and effective use of the drug requires special information and guidance for both the health care practitioner (doctor, dentist, pharmacist, nurse) and the consumer (patient and family); and the drug is suitable, safe, and practical for use in an outpatient setting, meaning it can be self-administered in a nonmedical environment or given with limited supervision, such as via a home intravenous service or outpatient cancer or pain center.

The Concise Essential Guide to Prescription Drugs covers a wide variety of information including recommended blood level ranges for drugs that require laboratory testing and achieve the best results with informed patient participation; tables listing drugs according to potential adverse effects on the fetus and newborn infant or major organ systems; and information to help define when common contagious diseases will appear after exposure. This quick-reference information can alert prescribers and patients to drugs that are potentially hazardous in specific situations, identify possible causes for some drug-related events, and help prevent undesired exposure to infectious diseases. In addition, it provides specific suggestions to save money and current trends in benefits (outcomes). This is, after all, *your* health care and *your* money. I fully support all efforts to get the most from your health care dollars for you and your loved ones.

No claim is made by the author or the publisher that this book provides *all* known actions, side effects, adverse effects, precautions, or potential interactions for any drug. Diligent care has been taken to ensure the accuracy of the information provided during the preparation of this work; however, new information is constantly uncovered from ongoing drug research, development, and general usage.

James Joseph Rybacki, Pharm. D.

SECTION ONE

ADVICE FOR PATIENTS

Research shows that on average more than 6.6 million elderly Americans are prescribed *the wrong medicine* every year and medication usage reviews over the past 20 years show that more than half of all patients take their prescription drugs incorrectly. One result is that more than $15 billion has been spent on hospitalizations due to medication problems, a large percentage of which is preventable. The more you know about a particular medicine, the better the results will be when you use it. The following suggestions are provided to help reduce confusion and increase the likelihood that you take the right drug for the right reason, at the right time, and in the right way.

- If you have a recurrent or chronic disorder, *learn as much as you can* about its nature and medical management. Ask your doctor and pharmacist for written information; visit your local library or bookstore for pertinent publications. My coauthor on *The Essential Guide to Prescription Drugs*, Dr. James Long, has written *The Essential Guide to Chronic Illness*, and I strongly recommend this book to you. Many national organizations also provide educational materials on specific disorders. The more you know about your disorder and how it is treated, the more likely you are to use your medicines safely and effectively.

- Share responsibility for effective health care. Think before you answer your doctor's or pharmacist's questions. It can be unnerving when you are suddenly asked, for instance, which childhood illnesses you had, or when you last had a specific vaccine. These questions are all asked for good reasons. Give each answer carefully and honestly to ensure as accurate a diagnosis of your disorder as possible—and so you receive a prescription for the best medicines for you. It is *always* acceptable to ask questions, and get an answer that *you* understand.

- Many pharmaceutical companies advertise directly to consumers on television, and in magazines and newspapers.

1

Just because they do so does not mean that their medicine is the best one for you. Let it serve as a starting point for something to talk to your doctor about, nothing more. The best information comes from scientific studies performed according to specific standards with a significant number of patients. Your doctor or pharmacist can give you unbiased, objective information regarding a drug's benefits and risks and its appropriateness for you. Every decision to use a prescription or nonprescription medicine *must* be made based on each patient's individual characteristics.

CHARACTERISTICS TO WATCH FOR WHENEVER MEDICINES ARE PRESCRIBED

- Expect to be asked about any prior drug allergies and drug-induced adverse effects. If you are not, volunteer this information.
- Whoever provides medical care for you should ask about all prescription, nonprescription, herbal, or nutriceutical products that you currently take. Many will also schedule a "brown bag" session, where they ask you to bring in all the medicines you are taking.
- Whenever a medicine is chosen, your prescriber should tell you why it is the most appropriate medicine for you, considering both price and expected clinical benefit, or outcome and effect upon your quality of life. If you ask them about the specific outcomes of one treatment versus another, they should be able to discuss this information with you.

  A recent trend has evolved to gather information and establish a database to learn which medicines offer the best long-term results in treating a given disease or condition. If asked to participate, you will be asked to sign a consent form and assigned a privacy number, so that the outcomes of a given treatment can be followed. I strongly believe in and encourage your participation.

- Every medicine has its own individual quirks, and can act differently in every person. You should be told if you should avoid certain foods, alcohol, exposure to sun, other drugs, or engaging in hazardous activities while taking the medicine. Ordinary activities can be important relative to a given medicine: common grapefruit juice can cause huge increases in blood levels and toxicity from some calcium channel blockers, for instance.

- The length of therapy or a reasonable time for a follow-up visit should be clearly explained to you. Some medicines must be withdrawn slowly, others must be given for a minimum period of time to see results. It is important for you to understand if you are taking such a medicine.

- It is not uncommon for people to be taking more than one medicine at a time. Consider asking your doctor to include both the *name of the drug* and the *disorder* for which it is taken on the prescription: Capoten (captopril) for high blood pressure. It is easy to forget which prescription treats what condition when you are taking several medicines.

- Your doctor should give you a *written summary* of the medicines prescribed whenever possible. This helps you remember everything discussed during an office visit and may also answer questions you think of later. *Never hesitate to ask questions.* Virtually all of my physician and pharmacist associates welcome questions, regardless of how busy they may be.

- Important new symptoms which may result from the prescribed drug(s) should be discussed, and you should be encouraged to call your doctor if any new symptoms occur. If such changes are noticed quickly, it may be possible to avoid serious problems.

- Many medications require blood levels or blood chemistry monitoring. The need for these tests should be clearly explained to you. Be certain to keep follow-up appointments with your doctor.

- Kidney or liver compromise, aging, and other conditions *require* dose adjustments and may even preclude the use of certain medicines. Your doctor should explain that the medication and the dose chosen is the best for you, given any such compromise or condition.

WHEN YOUR PRESCRIPTION IS FILLED

- When the bottle of medicine is handed to you, read the label carefully. *Make certain you understand how much medicine is to be taken and how often.* Take the time to ask the pharmacist to help organize the timing of your medicines on a set schedule that makes sense for you. If you have a complicated schedule, ask for a dose calendar and a daily pill organizer. Get the most from your medicines by taking them the best way possible.

Verify that both the *name of the drug* and the *disorder* are specified. If these are not present, ask your pharmacist to call your doctor for permission to add them. If you prefer that the pharmacist not include the name of the condition, that is your right, but consider writing the name of the disorder on the label yourself when you get home.

It is *always* best to deal with the same pharmacy and pharmacist whenever possible. This gives you the clear benefit of one person who knows you and your medicines well. For refills, the pharmacist should verify that the drug issued is identical to that in your original supply. The color chart in this book contains many of the medications covered in the pages that follow. If you find that the medicine is not the same as the original drug, ask your pharmacist to clarify the difference: generic drug products from different manufacturers often vary in size, shape, color, etc.

- Be especially aware that there are more than 1,000 drug names that look alike in print or sound alike in speech, for example: acetazolamide—acetohexamide, cyclosporine—cycloserine, Orinase—Ornade, Xanax—Zantac. Mistaking one drug for the other can lead to serious dispensing errors. "Sound-alike" drugs are easily confused when a prescription is given by telephone. Since each drug treats a distinctively different condition, stating the **disorder** within the prescription alerts the pharmacist and the patient to the mistake. The pharmacist should call the doctor to confirm any order that does not make sense.

- Occasionally your pharmacist attaches specific warning auxiliary labels to the prescription container. Many times these will be things your doctor has already discussed with you. Read all warning labels carefully—in addition to the main prescription label—and follow them. These are important reminders regarding the proper use of the drug: they can distinguish between eyedrops and ear drops;

identify dosage forms that should not be opened, crushed, or chewed; and provide numerous precautions to improve effectiveness.

- Your pharmacist must keep a record of all prescriptions he or she has given to you, and screen for significant interactions each time a medicine is dispensed. Ask if any interactions were found. It is also critical to discuss combining any medicines (prescription or nonprescription) with your pharmacist or doctor BEFORE you actually take two or more medicines together. Remember, many medicines that do not require a prescription today were once available by prescription only.

- Take advantage of your pharmacist's computer system, which records and analyzes each patient's drug history, to prevent serious allergic reactions. Tell your pharmacist about all drugs, herbal remedies, vitamins, and nutriceuticals you are currently taking. Although we often forget that alcohol (ethanol) is a drug, it clearly is. Remember to mention exactly how much you really drink on a daily basis.

- When you go to a new pharmacy, a complete medication history should be taken as a basis for determining critical drug interactions and medicines that duplicate the effects of prior drugs. Details on prescription, nonprescription medicines, and any herbal remedies and vitamins should be obtained.

- Your pharmacist should ask if you have any drug allergies or had any adverse drug reactions in the past. This will help predict problems if medicines in the same class or chemical family have been prescribed.

- If you know you have liver or kidney problems or other significant medical conditions, ask your pharmacist if the dose has been adjusted appropriately. He or she should give you a clear and understandable answer.

- Some pharmacists are starting to take appointments in order to provide individual attention to your questions about medicines. If you have more complicated questions or need more of your pharmacist's time, an appointment can be a great idea. When all of your questions have been answered, written profiles of each medicine should also be provided for each prescription. Like the information about

your condition, the drug information profiles can answer
questions you may think of later.

ACTING AS OUR OWN PATIENT ADVOCATE

- Learn both the generic and brand name of all drugs prescribed for you.
- If you take more than one medicine, it is a good idea for the
label of each container to include the *name of the drug* and
the *condition it treats*.
- If you do not understand the directions for using a drug,
call your doctor or pharmacist before taking it, especially if
it is provided through a home IV service.
- Follow all dosing instructions carefully. If it's hard for you
to remember to take medicines on time, ask your pharmacist for a dosing calendar or weekly medication box.
- If you take medications prescribed by more than one doctor, check the *generic names* to ensure they are not duplicate drugs, which could cause serious toxicity.
- Nonprescription drugs can interact unfavorably with prescription medications. Ask your doctor or pharmacist
before you begin taking any new over-the-counter preparations.
- Make certain all drugs you take have not reached their expiration date. Periodically clean out your medicine chest
and discard any outdated medication.

How to Use This Book

We often receive an overwhelming amount of information in a single visit to the doctor. Considering we rarely visit a doctor when we are well, any doctor visit can be stressful, especially if we receive a new diagnosis or condition that makes it very difficult to remember what we've been told. Most visits occur in a limited amount of time, so it may not be possible for your doctor to provide you with *all* the appropriate information he or she would like you to have. This book provides the kind of information you may need to supplement your doctor's direction and guidance. *Never* be afraid to ask a question. I've found that virtually all of my physician colleagues welcome questions, especially where a new medicine or diagnosis is concerned.

The first section of this book helps you appreciate the complexities of modern drug therapy and make better use of the information provided in the remaining sections.

Section Two presents specific laboratory testing required for many medications. Section Three, the heart of the book, offers detailed profiles of medicines that form the basis of effective drug therapy. Nearly 1,500 brand-name drugs widely used in the United States and Canada are given in profiles arranged alphabetically by generic name. Many of the category headings are self-explanatory, but some require additional information. Not all categories appear at every entry; they are included only when substantive information is provided.

PRESCRIPTION NEEDED

This category indicates whether a drug is a prescription or a nonprescription (over-the-counter) medicine. There is a trend in the United States toward moving a greater number of prescription medications to be available in a nonprescription formulation. As this trend continues the information in this category may quickly change. Remember, even *non*prescription drugs can still cause serious drug interactions. Use all medicines carefully.

CONTROLLED DRUG

Drugs with potential for abuse are subject to regulation in the United States under the Controlled Substances Act of 1970. The designation of a particular schedule governs the dispensing guidelines in the United States. This is why a prescription may only be given for a limited time before a follow-up appointment is needed, or why some medicines can't be refilled without a new, signed prescription each time. A description of the Controlled Drug Schedules appears on the inside cover of this book.

GENERIC

Here you'll learn whether a drug is available for purchase by the official name of the drug entity or only by a manufacturer's brand name. Generic medicines can provide excellent therapy at a lower cost. Often a concern with the use of generic drugs is the comparative composition, quality, and effectiveness of the generic versus the brand-name drug product. Technically known as "bioavailability" and "bioequivalence," these terms are discussed in greater detail in the Glossary.

BRAND NAMES

The representative list of names included helps confirm that you are looking at the correct drug profile, but does not include all currently available brand names. The list may also help you recognize your current prescription as one that caused problems for you in the past. A combination drug (a product with more than one active ingredient) is identified by

[CD] following the brand name. This listing may prevent possible toxic effects by identifying a medicine that duplicates one you already take as a single drug product.

OVERVIEW OF BENEFITS VERSUS RISKS

This category provides a quick look at the pros and cons for each drug. Capital letters emphasize the drug's principal benefits and risks, and lowercase letters indicate benefits and risks of lesser significance. At a glance you can compare weights of the two columns and make a tentative impression of whether a drug's benefits exceed its risks.

No category in this book is intended to be the primary basis for deciding whether or not to use a drug. This category in particular aims to help you be more circumspect and discriminating in the use of drugs. One of the greatest weaknesses in current drug therapy is the failure to adequately consider all the individual factors in selecting a particular medicine and its dose and frequency.

ILLNESS THIS MEDICATION TREATS

The information listed here outlines the uses currently included in FDA-approved labeling as a single drug product (when the drug is used alone). When the drug is combined with other active drugs in a tablet, capsule, or other form, a separate subheading explains its primary uses in these combination drug products. Combination drugs have been developed because some conditions have more than one cause, are characterized by a variety of symptoms, or may be treated in more than one way. When appropriate, the logic for combining certain drugs to enhance their therapeutic value is explained.

TYPICAL DOSAGE RANGE

Doses represent a carefully derived consensus by appropriate authorities and are the currently recommended standard for adults, with information on dosing in children and people over 60 years old frequently included. These doses are a guide to both effective and safe medication use, but your doctor may decide to modify this standard dosage scheme to meet your particular needs and conditions. Follow appropriate doses and dosing schedules carefully. The medicine won't do you any good if it stays in the bottle. Dosing calendars and daily pill reminder boxes are great tools to help make sense of medicine schedules. Your pharmacist can help you find a device that works best for you.

CONDITIONS REQUIRING DOSING ADJUSTMENTS

Included here are some of the most critical conditions, generally kidney and/or liver compromise, which *require* adjusted dose or frequency of a particular medicine. Awareness of this information can help you avoid toxicity and contain costs at the same time. I have seen many excellent clinicians fail to take into account the natural, age-related decline in kidney function, and routinely give doses that were higher than needed.

HOW BEST TO TAKE THIS MEDICINE

Specific guidance is given regarding the timing of oral medication and food intake, and those dosage forms of each drug that may and those that should not be altered for administration. In addition, your pharmacist can provide appropriate guidance if needed.

HOW LONG THIS MEDICINE IS USUALLY TAKEN

Many factors influence how long it takes for any drug to exert beneficial effects: the nature and severity of the symptoms being treated, the formulation and strength of the drug, the presence or absence of food in the stomach, the ability of the patient to respond, and use of other drugs at the same time. It is important to be aware of these factors to help prevent premature termination of medication when improvement may not occur as quickly as you think it should. When appropriate, limitations in the duration of use are given.

TELL YOUR DOCTOR BEFORE TAKING THIS MEDICINE IF YOU

Although we generally think of medicines as tools to help us, if given in the presence of certain conditions or other medicines they can be anything *but* helpful. In this category you'll see a veritable laundry list of information your doctor needs to know about you. The wide variety of medications available and the incredible complexity of the human body require that your doctor have the most complete information available to help you. In light of the information you provide, your doctor can weigh the benefits and the risks of prescribing certain medications for you. In some cases the appearance, or even the history, of a condition will absolutely rule out your using certain drugs (technically called an *absolute* contraindication). In other cases, called *relative* contraindications, the use of a certain drug would not be ruled out, but its use requires considering additional factors (it might aggravate an existing disease or interfere with the current treatment, for instance) in deciding the best course of treatment. It is important that you communicate all relevant information to your doctor or dentist about your past, present, and in some cases upcoming medical history. You are your own best patient advocate, but you need to share this information for your doctors to best help you.

POSSIBLE SIDE EFFECTS

This category describes the natural, expected, and usually unavoidable actions of the drug. It is important to maintain a realistic perspective that properly balances side effects and the goals of treatment. Call your doctor for guidance whenever side effects are troublesome or distressing, to make appropriate adjustments to your treatment program.

POSSIBLE ADVERSE EFFECTS

This category includes unusual, unexpected, and infrequent drug effects that are commonly referred to as adverse drug reactions. For the sake of evaluation, adverse effects are classified as mild or serious in nature. It is always wise to tell your doctor as soon as you suspect you may be having an adverse drug effect. Serious adverse reactions usually announce their development initially in the form of mild, nonthreatening symptoms.

It is important to remain alert to significant changes in your well-being when you are taking a drug known to produce a serious adverse effect. It is also possible to experience an adverse reaction that has not yet been reported. If you notice a change that starts after you begin treatment with a new medicine, call your doctor. He or she will have specific report forms or an 800 number to call to report this adverse effect. It is not possible to test medicines in all possible situations or in combination with all other medicines before they are approved by the Food and Drug Administration (FDA); new information on as-yet-undetected reactions is critical.

Following standard practice, some adverse reactions (and interactions) are listed as a precaution, because these reactions are associated with a particular class of drugs. Although the literature may not document such reactions in connection with the use of an individual drug within that class, the possibility of their occurrence must be considered. I would rather be too careful in helping advise you than not be careful enough. An informed patient is much more likely to get the best possible results from any medicine or treatment.

A word of caution is appropriate here. It is important that you recognize and understand that *in the vast majority of instances a properly selected drug has a comparatively small chance of producing serious harm.* Most of the drugs included in this book only rarely produce serious adverse effects. Knowledge that a drug is capable of causing a serious adverse reaction should not deter you from using it when it has been properly selected and its use will be carefully supervised.

POSSIBLE EFFECTS ON SEX LIFE

This aspect of drug performance has not received the professional scrutiny or public disclosure consistent with its importance. Currently available information from all reliable sources is presented for consideration. In the interest of compliance and effective management, both doctor and patient are well advised to discuss frankly the full significance of any potential effect of proposed drug therapy on all aspects of sexual expression.

CAUTION

This category provides information on certain aspects of drug action and/or drug use that require special emphasis. Occasionally these warnings relate to information provided in other categories that are of sufficient importance to warrant repetition. Many of the profiles contain specific information relating to children and those over 60.

ADVISABILITY OF USE DURING PREGNANCY OR IF BREAST-FEEDING: PREGNANCY CATEGORY

Information regarding the safe use of a particular drug during pregnancy was a major force leading to the formal petitioning of the Food and Drug Administration in 1975 to provide such guidance to the public. In some cases research data may vary from the company that makes the medicine. I've included both categories where I became aware of a difference. The FDA definitions of the five Pregnancy Categories are listed inside this book's cover. The initial category assignment is the responsibility of the manufacturer marketing the drug. This designation is then reviewed and modified by the FDA. The Pregnancy Category designations here were determined by the author after thorough review of pertinent literature and consultation with appropriate authorities. They are offered for initial guidance only.

Also included is what could be ascertained regarding the drug's effects on milk production, its presence in human milk, and possible effects on the nursing infant. Prudent recommendations are given where appropriate.

SUGGESTED PERIODIC EXAMINATIONS WHILE TAKING THIS DRUG

Your doctor may recommend specific tests while you take the drug(s) prescribed to check your reaction and the outcomes on your condition. The advisability of such examinations varies greatly from one situation to another. The selection and timing of examinations or blood tests are based on many variables, including your past and present medical history, the nature of the condition under treatment, the dosage and anticipated duration of drug use, and your doctor's observations of your response to treatment. On many occasions he or she may feel no examinations are necessary.

WHILE TAKING THIS DRUG THE FOLLOWING APPLY

This multipart category alerts you to effects ordinary foods, beverages, and tobacco smoking can have on this drug. As needed, information is also included on the possible effects on driving or other hazardous activity; exposure to sun, heat, and cold; and heavy exercise or exertion, and even special storage instructions.

Marijuana Smoking

The widespread social use of marijuana has led to inquiries about the possibility of interactions between the pharmacologically active chemicals in marijuana smoke and medicinal drugs in common use. The limited information presented in this category represents those *possible interactions* considered likely in view of the known pharmacologic effects of the principal components of marijuana and of the medicinal drug reviewed. In most instances the statements are not based on documented evidence. However, the conclusions, derived by logical inductive reasoning, represent the concurrence of authorities in this field and the typical effects of the medicine being profiled.

Other Drugs

Some of the drugs listed as possible interactants have no representative profile in this book. If you are using one of these drugs, ask your doctor or pharmacist for guidance regarding potential interactions. If you are taking the generic drug, *all* brand names under which it is marketed are possible interactants. Any brand names following the generic name of an interacting drug are given for illustration only, not to imply these particular brands have interactions that are different from others of the same generic drug. In fact, a brand-name or generic medicine will have the same interactions.

It is also critical to note that even though two medicines may interact, this is sometimes used to therapeutic benefit. A good example is combining two different medicines to help lower blood pressure. Finally, it is not possible to predict the degree of interaction from person to person. It is, however, always prudent to call your doctor or pharmacist immediately if you find that a potential combination of two medicines may interact. Be certain to call them *before* combining the medicines. Please also ask your doctor or pharmacist *before* combining any two medicines.

Driving, Hazardous Activities

In addition to driving motor vehicles, the information in this category applies to any dangerous activity, such as operating machinery, working on ladders, using power tools, and handling weapons.

Occurrence of Unrelated Illness

This category relates to those drugs that require careful regulation of daily doses to maintain a constant drug effect within critical limits. Anticoagulants, antidiabetic medication, and digitalis are examples. Emphasis is given to interim illnesses, separate from the condition being treated, which might affect the established schedule of drug use.

Discontinuation

This aspect of drug use is often overlooked when a plan of drug therapy is first discussed. For some drugs, however, it is mandatory to fully inform the patient on *when* to stop, when *not* to stop, and precisely *how* to discontinue use. Another consideration is the need to adjust the dosage schedules of other drugs taken concurrently. The doctor who is primarily responsible for your overall management must be kept informed of *all* the drugs you are taking.

SAVING MONEY WHEN USING THIS MEDICINE

This category covers new concepts in pharmacoeconomics and outcomes research. In some cases a more expensive medicine may actually cost less in the long run because it is a more effective treatment. Sometimes less expensive, narrower antibiotics may be perfectly acceptable alternatives to broadspectrum antibiotics. You can learn to ask questions and make comparisons to find the best use of your money and achieve the best results or outcomes possible.

Section Four organizes medicines into specific drug classes. This section is especially helpful if you have a documented drug allergy.

Section Five is a glossary of drug-related terms, including the preferred use of each term. People in health care have developed their own language and I think it is important that you know how to speak it.

Section Six provides tables of current drug information drawn from the profiles, rearranged to emphasize pertinent aspects of drug behavior and designed to help you obtain the best therapy.

GUIDELINES FOR SAFE AND EFFECTIVE DRUG USE

DO NOT

- pressure your doctor into prescribing medicines. A pill is NOT the answer to all medical conditions.
- take prescription drugs on your own or because your friend or neighbor says your symptoms are "just like theirs." Many factors determine the appropriate use of medicines. Unless a doctor has requested it under some special circumstance, do not offer your prescription medicines to anyone else.
- change the dose or the frequency of any drug without your doctor's advice (unless the drug appears to be causing adverse effects). Many medicines require only a certain amount—more is not better.
- continue taking a medicine you feel is causing problems. Any medicine can cause adverse effects. Call your doctor immediately.
- take *any* drug (prescription or nonprescription) while pregnant or nursing until your doctor tells you no harmful effects will occur to the mother or child. Many medicines can have disastrous consequences during pregnancy and can be passed into the milk after the child is born.
- skip laboratory appointments even after you have taken a medicine for a while. Blood levels can be critical to the outcome of therapy and the avoidance of toxic effects.

- keep secrets from your doctor about previous prescription or nonprescription drug experiences, both beneficial and undesirable. A complete medication history is critical to appropriate and effective therapy.
- take any drug in the dark. Many drug overdoses result from accidental use. Look at the medicine carefully in adequate light *before* you take it.
- avoid telling your doctor if you are having pain. Having pain and communicating it is not a sign of weakness, nor does it make you a "bad" patient. You have a right to effective and timely pain management.

DO

- know the name (and correct spelling) of the drug(s) you are taking. Have your doctor or pharmacist write the brand and generic names down for you.
- ask your pharmacist if there are any damaging interactions between the nonprescription drug you are considering and the prescription medicine(s) you already take.
- read each profile carefully *before* combining two prescription medicines. Remember that many nonprescription or over-the-counter medicines were once available by prescription only. Talk with your pharmacist or doctor *before* combining any prescription and nonprescription medicines.
- understand when to take your medicine and how much you should take. Call your doctor if you feel you must change the dose or dosing time. Your pharmacist can also help arrange a reasonable dosing schedule with you and then discuss it with your doctor.
- learn if other conditions can change how your body reacts to medicines. Ask your doctor if any new prescription you are given needs to have the dose adjusted because of any long-standing or chronic diseases or conditions you may have. Critical examples here include the normal age-related decline in kidney function and any changes in liver function you may have.
- make sure you thoroughly shake liquid suspensions to ensure that each dose contains the same amount of active medicine.

- keep medicines taken for emergency use, such as nitroglycerin, on a bedside table. It is advisable to have only one such drug for use during the night.
- use a standardized measuring device for liquid medications. All spoons are not created equal; most pharmacies sell easy-to-use medicine measurers.
- follow any doctor-prescribed diet in addition to taking your medicine. For example, a salt-restricted or salt-free diet with treatment of high blood pressure can make it possible to achieve desired drug effects with smaller drug doses
- keep your personal physician informed of all drugs prescribed by someone else. Consult him or her about nonprescription drugs you intend to take at the same time as prescribed drugs. Bringing ALL of your prescription and nonprescription medicine and nutritional supplements to the same pharmacy can also bring you the skills of one pharmacist looking at all of the medicines you take.
- tell your anesthesiologist, surgeon, and dentist of *all* drugs you are taking prior to scheduling any surgery.
- tell your doctor if you become pregnant and are taking any prescription or nonprescription drugs from any source. Keep a written record of *all* drugs (and vaccines) you take during your entire pregnancy—name, dose, dates taken, and reasons for use.
- keep a written record of *all* drugs (and vaccines) to which you develop an allergic or adverse reaction.
- keep a written record of *all* drugs (and vaccines) to which *your children* or other members of your family, especially the elderly or infirm, develop an allergic or adverse reaction. Always keep a record of all medicines you are taking. Also take the time to get the number of the nearest Poison Control Center and place it on this list, near the phone. An accidental poisoning is no time to be frantically trying to remember the medicines a person takes or finding the phone number itself.
- tell your doctor or other health care professional of all known or suspected allergies, especially to drugs. Be sure this information is included in your medical record, as

people with allergies are far more prone to drug reactions than others.

- call your doctor promptly if you think you are having an overdose, side effect, or adverse effect from a drug.
- ask if it is safe to drive a car, operate machinery, or engage in other hazardous activities while taking the drug(s) prescribed *before* you leave the doctor's office.
- ask your doctor if it is safe to drink alcoholic beverages with prescribed medicines.
- ask if any particular foods, beverages, or other drugs should be avoided.
- keep all appointments for follow-up examinations or laboratory tests to determine the effects of the drugs and the course of your illness.
- ask for clarification of any point that you find confusing or difficult to understand, in writing if necessary. You have a right to accurate and understandable information.
- throw outdated medicines away to prevent the use of drugs that have deteriorated.
- store *all* drugs out of the reach of children to prevent accidental poisoning. Take extra care to place medicines with easy-open caps out of reach if young children visit.

PREVENTING ADVERSE DRUG REACTIONS

Advances in the fields of immunology and toxicology have increased our understanding of adverse reactions to medicines; however, our ability to predict who is at greater risk is still limited. Tests for the early detection of toxicity are valuable, but they do not provide a full measure of protection.

Some adverse reactions can be predicted and prevented by identifying patients who have one or several contributing factors. These fall into 11 categories:

1. Previous Adverse Reaction to a Drug

People who have had prior adverse drug reactions are more likely to have adverse reactions to other unrelated drugs. This suggests a genetic predisposition to unusual drug responses. *You MUST tell your doctor about any prior adverse drug experiences.*

2. Allergies

People who are allergic by nature (hay fever, asthma, eczema, hives) are more likely to develop allergies to drugs. The allergic patient must be watched closely for the earliest sign of a developing hypersensitivity. Known drug allergies must be written in the medical record, and added to your drug profile at the pharmacy. Tell each clinician prescriber that you are allergic by nature and allergic to specific drugs by name *without waiting to be asked*. The doctor may then be able to avoid drugs that could provoke an allergic reaction, as well as related drugs that may produce a cross-sensitivity.

3. Contraindications

Both patient and doctor must strictly observe all known contraindications to any drug considered for therapy. *Absolute contraindications* include conditions and situations that prohibit the use of the drug for any reason. *Relative contraindications* are conditions that, in the judgment of the doctor, do not preclude the use of the drug altogether, but require special considerations to prevent the worsening of preexisting disease or the development of a new disease. Such conditions usually require dosage adjustment, additional supportive measures, and close supervision.

4. Precautions in Use

The patient should know about any special precautions to take while using the drug, such as the advisability of use during pregnancy or while nursing; exposure to the sun (or ultraviolet lamps); avoidance of extreme heat or cold or heavy physical exertion.

5. Dosing

Both the amount and how often a medicine is taken can be critical. Adhere to the prescribed dosage schedule as closely as possible. *This is most important for drugs with narrow margins of safety*. Even medications taken only once every 24 hours should be taken at the same time to ensure the most constant blood drug levels. Blood levels relate to how well the medicine works to help you. Call your doctor if you are unable to take the drug as prescribed because of nausea, vomiting, or diarrhea. Appropriate adjustments can often be made.

6. Interactions

Some drugs interact unfavorably with foods, alcohol, or other drugs to cause serious problems. *The patient must be told about all likely agents* that could alter the action of the drug. During the course of treatment, you may discover a new interaction of importance, and your doctor should be promptly told. Much of our understanding of drug interactions has developed through such "phase four" observations.

7. Warning Symptoms

Many drugs produce symptoms that are actually early warnings of a developing adverse effect, for example, severe headaches and visual disturbances *before* the onset of a stroke in women taking oral contraceptives, or acid indigestion and stomach upset *before* a bleeding peptic ulcer in a man taking oxaprozin (Daypro) for shoulder bursitis. *It is critical that the patient be familiar with such signs and symptoms.* With this knowledge, he or she can stop the drug and ask the doctor for guidance.

8. Examinations to Follow Drug Effects

Many drugs are capable of damaging vital body tissues, especially over an extended period or with high doses. An adverse effect in newly released medicines may not be discovered until the drug has been in wide use for a long time. As our knowledge of such effects accumulates, we learn which kinds of drugs are most likely to produce such tissue reactions and should be closely followed to detect tissue injury as early as possible. *The patient should cooperate fully in having periodic examinations for evidence of adverse drug effects. This often means a trip to the laboratory to have some blood taken.*

9. Advanced Age and Debility

Many vital organs do not work well with advancing age and debilitating disease. This can greatly influence the body's response to drugs. Smaller doses at longer intervals are necessary for patients who don't tolerate inherently toxic medicines well. *The effects of drugs on the elderly and severely ill are unpredictable.* These patients must be carefully watched to prevent or minimize adverse effects. The age-related decline in kidney function MUST ALWAYS be taken into account when the dose and frequency of a medicine removed by the kidneys is considered.

10. Appropriate Drug Choice

Medicine(s) selected to treat any condition should be the most appropriate available. Many adverse reactions can be prevented by good judgment and restraint. Current pharmaceutical care in drug therapy demands awareness of probable outcomes (benefits) and quality of life. *The wise patient will not demand overtreatment*, but cooperate with the doctor's attempt to balance the seriousness of the illness and the hazard of the drug.

11. Polypharmacy

The frequent practice of persons using several drugs prescribed separately by two (or more) doctors for different disorders—often without appropriate communication between patient and prescriber—may cause serious drug-drug interactions. *The patient should routinely tell each prescriber visited of all the drugs (prescription, nonprescription, or nutritional) being taken.*

DRUGS AND THE ELDERLY

Age changes body structure and function in ways that affect how medicines work and how long they stay in the body. An impaired digestive system may interfere with drug absorption. Reduced capacity of the liver and kidneys to metabolize or eliminate drugs may result in toxic drug levels. By impairing the body's ability to maintain a steady state, the aging process may increase the sensitivity of many tissues to the actions of drugs and alter the responsiveness of the nervous and circulatory systems to standard drug doses. Patients experiencing deterioration of understanding, memory, vision, or physical coordination may not always use drugs safely and effectively.

Adverse reactions to drugs occur three times more frequently in the older population. Drug treatment in the elderly must always be accompanied by the most careful consideration of the individual's health and tolerances, the selection of drugs and dosage schedules, and the possible need for assistance in treatment routines.

Guidelines for the Use of Drugs by the Elderly

- be certain that drug treatment is necessary. Many health problems of the elderly can be managed without drugs.
- avoid if possible the use of many drugs at one time.
- dosage schedules should be as uncomplicated as possible. A single daily dose of each drug is ideal, provided it is coupled with a system to ensure it is taken.
- small starting doses are usually advisable. Maintenance doses should also be determined carefully. An effective maintenance dose is often smaller for people over 60.
- avoid large tablets and capsules if other dosage forms are available. Liquid preparations are much more acceptable. Talk with your pharmacist about your preferences.
- label all drug containers with the drug name and directions for use in large, easy-to-read letters.
- ask the pharmacist to package drugs in easy-to-open containers. Remember to place these containers out of reach of children. Don't forget to place these in a locked kitchen cabinet if young children come to visit, to prevent accidental poisonings.
- identify each dose of medicine carefully in adequate light.
- to avoid taking the wrong drug or an extra dose, do not keep drugs on a bedside table, except drugs for emergency use. It is best to have only one such drug at the bedside.
- drug use by older persons may require supervision. Watch drug effects continuously in yourself or in your loved ones to ensure safe and effective use.

Drugs Best Avoided by the Elderly Because of Increased Possibility of Adverse Reactions

antacids (high
  sodium)*
barbiturates
  (pentobarbital and
  secobarbital)*

benzodiazepines
  (Valium and
  Librium)
carisoprodol
chlorpropamide

cyclandelate
cyclobenzaprine
cyclophosphamide
diethylstilbestrol
dipyridamole (except

with artificial hearts)
estrogens
indomethacin
isoxsuprine (now discontinued in the U.S.)
meprobamate
methocarbamol
monoamine oxidase inhibitors (MAOIs)*
orphenadrine
oxyphenbutazone
pentazocine
phenacetin
phenylbutazone (no longer available in the U.S.)
propoxyphene
tetracyclines*
trimethobenzamide

Drugs That Should Be Used by the Elderly in Reduced Dosages Until Full Effect Has Been Determined

anticoagulants (oral)*
antidepressants (amitriptyline may cause problems in urination)*
antidiabetic drugs*
antihistamines*
antihypertensives*
anti-inflammatory drugs*
barbiturates*
beta-blockers*
colchicine
cortisonelike drugs*
digitalis preparations*
diuretics* (all types)
ephedrine
epinephrine
haloperidol
isoetharine
nalidixic acid
narcotic drugs
prazosin
pseudoephedrine
quinidine
sleep inducers (hypnotics)*
terbutaline
thyroid preparations

Drugs That May Cause Confusion and Behavioral Disturbances in the Elderly

acyclovir
albuterol
amantadine
antidepressants*
antidiabetic drugs*
antihistamines*
anti-inflammatory drugs*
asparaginase
atropine* (and drugs containing belladonna)
barbiturates*
benzodiazepines*
beta-blockers*
carbamazepine
cimetidine
digitalis preparations*
diuretics*
ergoloid mesylates
famotidine
levodopa
meprobamate
methocarbamol
methyldopa
narcotic drugs
nizatidine
pentazocine
phenytoin
primidone
ranitidine
reserpine
sedatives
sleep inducers (hypnotics)*
thiothixene
tranquilizers (mild)*
trihexyphenidyl

Drugs That May Cause Orthostatic Hypotension in the Elderly

antidepressants*
antihypertensives*
diuretics* (all types)
phenothiazines*
sedatives
selegiline
tranquilizers (mild)*
vasodilators*

*See Drug Classes, Section Four.

Drugs That May Cause Sluggishness, Unsteadiness, and Falling in the Elderly

barbiturates*
beta-blockers*
chlordiazepoxide
clorazepate

diazepam
diphenhydramine
flurazepam
halazepam

methyldopa
prazepam
sleep inducers
  (hypnotics)*

Drugs That May Cause Constipation and/or Urine Retention in the Elderly

acebutolol
amantadine
androgens
antidepressants*
antiparkinsonism

drugs*
atropinelike drugs*
epinephrine
ergoloid mesylates
isoetharine

ketorolac
narcotic drugs
phenothiazines*
ranitidine
terbutaline

Drugs That May Cause Loss of Bladder Control (Urinary Incontinence) in the Elderly

diuretics* (all types)
sedatives
sleep inducers

(hypnotics)*
tacrine
thioridazine

tranquilizers (mild)*

Laboratory Testing of Blood Levels of Medicines

MEASURING DRUG LEVELS IN BLOOD

Having to get your blood drawn just because you are taking a particular medicine seems odd for many of us, but it's actually good medical practice. Drug level measurement in the blood to help guide therapy has increased substantially over the last 40 years. This testing is critical because of the increased potency of medicines, and the kind and amount of response varies greatly from person to person for the same dose of medicine.

For many drugs the clinical responses seen by the doctor clearly show that the drug is having the intended effect and that the dosage schedule is acceptable. However, for some drugs—especially those with narrow safety margins—toxic reactions may closely resemble the symptoms of the disorder being treated. In many instances the patient's expected response is not in keeping with the clinical condition or program of drug therapy. By measuring the blood levels of certain drugs at appropriate times the doctor can adjust dosage schedules more accurately, predict drug response more precisely, reduce the risk of toxicity, and achieve greater benefit. Some medicines require both a peak and trough level to ensure best results. The timing of the blood samples is critical. Sampling should be avoided during the 2 hours following oral administration; during this absorption period blood levels do not represent tissue levels of the drug, and the tissue levels are where antibiotics work. The peak, or highest, level of the drug can measure several things: how effectively bacteria are killed or the toxic levels within the body, for instance. The trough, or lowest, level tells how effectively the antibiotic is cleared from the body between doses. This can be important because if too much remains, toxicity can result; if too little remains, the bacteria may not be killed.

The following drugs are most suitable for therapeutic drug monitoring. If you are using any of these regularly, ask your doctor about the need for periodic measurement of drug levels in your blood. The numbers are ranges where effects are usually seen, though some people may have a therapeutic response with lower levels—in this case the level should be followed closely and left alone. Fortunately most doctors treat the patient, not the level.

Generic Name/Brand Name	Blood Level Range
acetaminophen/Tylenol, etc.	10–20 mcg/ml
amikacin/Amikin	12–25 mcg/ml (peak)
	5–10 mcg/ml (trough)
amitriptyline/Elavil, etc.	120–250 ng/ml
(combined with nortriptyline)	
amoxapine/Asendin	200–500 ng/ml
aspirin (other salicylates)	100–250 mcg/ml
carbamazepine/Tegretol	5–10 mcg/ml
chloramphenicol/Chloromycetin	10–25 mcg/ml
chlorpromazine/Thorazine	50–300 ng/ml
ciprofloxacin/Cipro	0.94–3.4 mcg/ml
clonazepam/Klonopin	10–50 ng/ml
cyclosporine/Sandimmune	100–150 ng/ml
desipramine/Norpramin, Pertofrane	150–300 ng/ml
digitoxin/Crystodigin	15–30 ng/ml
digoxin/Lanoxin	0.5–2.0 ng/ml
diltiazem/Cardizem	100–200 ng/ml
disopyramide/Norpace	2.0–4.5 mcg/ml
doxepin/Adapin, Sinequan	100–275 ng/ml
ethosuximide/Zarontin	40–100 mcg/ml
flecainide/Tambocor	0.2–1.0 mcg/ml
flucytosine/Ancobon	50–100 mcg/ml
gentamicin/Garamycin	4.0–10 mcg/ml (peak)
	less than 2 mcg/ml
	(trough)
gold salts/auranofin, etc.	1.0–2.0 mcg/ml
imipramine/Janimine, Tofranil, etc.	150–300 ng/ml
kanamycin/Kantrex	25–35 mcg/ml
lidocaine/Xylocaine, etc.	2.0–5.0 mcg/ml
lithium/Lithobid, Lithotabs, etc.	0.3–1.3 mEq/L
mephobarbital/Mebaral	1–7 mcg/ml
methotrexate/Mexate	up to 0.1 mcmol/L
methsuximide/Celontin	up to 1.0 mcg/ml

Generic Name/Brand Name	Blood Level Range
metoprolol/Lopressor	20–200 ng/ml
mexiletine/Mexitil	0.75–2.0 mcg/ml
nifedipine/Procardia	25–100 ng/ml
nortriptyline/Aventyl, Pamelor	50–150 ng/ml
combined with amitriptyline	125–250 ng/ml
phenobarbital/Luminal, etc.	10–25 mcg/ml
phenytoin/Dilantin	10–20 mcg/ml
primidone/Mysoline	6–12 mcg/ml
procainamide/Pronestyl	4–10 mcg/ml
(NAPA metabolite)	4–10mcg/ml
propranolol/Inderal	50–100 ng/ml
protriptyline/Vivactil	70–250 ng/ml
quinidine/Quinaglute, etc.	1.0–4.0 mcg/ml
(specific quinidine assay method)	
sulfadiazine/Microsulfon	100–120 mcg/ml
sulfamethoxazole/Gantanol	90–100 mcg/ml
theophylline/aminophylline, etc.	10–20 mcg/ml
thioridazine/Mellaril	50–300 ng/ml
tobramycin/Nebcin	4.0–10 mcg/ml (peak)
	less than 2 mcg/ml
	(trough)
tocainide/Tonocard	5–12 mcg/ml
trimethadione/Tridione	10–30 mcg/ml
trimethoprim/Proloprim	1–3 mcg/ml
valproic acid/Depakene	50–100 mcg/ml
vancomycin/Vancocin	30–40 mcg/ml (peak)
	5–10 mcg/ml (trough)
verapamil/Calan	50–200 ng/ml

When vancomycin is taken by mouth, blood levels are not required because oral vancomycin is NOT absorbed.

DRUG PROFILES

Medicines included in this section were chosen by considering if the medicine:
- helps treat a serious or significant disease or disorder.
- is one of the best choices in its class.
- provides greater benefit than the risk of injury, and compares favorably with other drugs available in its class.
- requires special information and guidance for both the health care practitioner and the consumer for safe and effective use.
- is suitable (safe and practical) for use in an outpatient setting. The patient can take the medicine on his or her own, or may require dosing by trained medical personnel (as in home intravenous, freestanding cancer, emergency or pain centers).

It is now possible to report serious adverse drug reactions to the Food and Drug Administration (FDA) by calling 1-800-332-1088.

ACARBOSE (a KAR boz)

Prescription Needed: Yes   **Controlled Drug:** No   **Generic:** No
Brand Names: Precose

Overview of BENEFITS versus RISKS

Possible Benefits	*Possible Risks*
EFFECTIVE LOWERING OF BLOOD SUGAR	Gas and abdominal pain (often decreases over time)
DECREASED RISK OF HIGH BLOOD PRESSURE, HEART DISEASE, AND OTHER LONG-TERM PROBLEMS CAUSED BY ELEVATED BLOOD SUGAR	Possible mild decreases in hematocrit
MAY BE COMBINED WITH A SULFONYLUREA (see Drug Classes) FOR TIGHTER SUGAR CONTROL IF NEEDED	

▷ **Illness This Medication Treats:**
(1) Used in addition (adjunctive) to diet in people with diabetes who don't need insulin injections, yet do not have acceptable control of blood sugar from a strict diet alone; (2) used as part of combination therapy when diet plus acarbose or diet and a sulfonylurea don't control the blood sugar.

▷ **Typical Dosage Range:**   (Dosage or schedule must be determined by the doctor for each individual.)
18 to 65 Years of Age: Treatment starts with 25 mg taken three times daily at the start of each meal. The dose is then increased as needed and tolerated to 50 mg three times daily taken at the start of each meal. If the dose does need to be increased, increases are made at 4- to 8-week intervals in order to make certain of the best blood sugar response and also to minimize gastrointestinal side effects. If response to the medicine is still not acceptable, patients weighing more than 132 lb (60 kg) may take doses up to 100 mg three times daily. Those weighing less than 60 kg should NOT take more than 50 mg three times daily. If any dose increase doesn't result in better blood sugar control, it is best to decrease the dose back to the prior level.

▷ **Conditions Requiring Dosing Adjustments:**
Kidney function: The blood level does increase with increasing kidney damage, but specific dose-decreasing schedules are not available.

▷ **How Best to Take This Medicine:**   Each dose should be taken after starting (after the first bite of food) breakfast, lunch, and dinner respectively. Gas (flatulence) or diarrhea are common side effects. This may be decreased by limiting sucrose in the diet. In general, diarrhea and gas decrease over time. Usually the blood sugar is checked one hour after a meal (one hour postprandial) and the medicine dose is adjusted to get the best balance of blood sugar level and side effects.

▷ **How Long This Medicine Is Usually Taken:**   The dose of this medicine MUST be individualized, and dosing changes are made at 4- to 8-week intervals. Regular use is needed to see this drug's effect in maintaining the best control of blood sugar. Since noninsulin-dependent diabetes is a chronic condition, use of acarbose will be ongoing. Periodic hemoglobin A1C (glycosylated hemoglobin) tests and physician follow-up are needed.

▷ **Tell Your Doctor Before Taking This Medicine If You:**
- ever had an allergic reaction to it.
- are in diabetic ketoacidosis.
- tend to develop intestinal obstruction or have a partial obstruction of the intestine.
- have an intestinal condition (such as megacolon or bowel obstruction) that may worsen if there is gas formation in the intestine.
- have ulceration of the colon, inflammatory bowel disease, cirrhosis of the liver, or a chronic intestinal disease that alters digestion or your ability to absorb medicines from the intestines.
- know your serum creatinine (talk with your doctor) is greater than 2 mg/dl.
- are pregnant or are breast-feeding.
- plan to have surgery under general anesthesia soon.

▷ **Possible Side Effects:**   Gas (flatulence) or diarrhea that tends to decrease over time.

▷ **Possible Adverse Effects:**
If any of the following develop, call your doctor promptly for guidance.
Some Mild Problems This Drug Can Cause
   Allergic reactions: skin rash, itching.
   Diarrhea or abdominal pain (often eases with time).
Some Serious Problems This Drug Can Cause
   Low blood sugar if combined with sulfonylureas (see Drug Class).
   Rare anemia (happened in some studies and not in others).

▷ *CAUTION*
   1. This medicine itself does not cause low blood sugar or hypoglycemia, but if it is combined with insulin or sulfonylureas, low blood sugar may result.
   2. If you develop an infection, loss of blood sugar control may occur and temporary use of insulin may be needed.
   3. This medicine is only part of a total program for managing your diabetes. A properly prescribed and followed diet and exercise plan is needed to get the best results.

4. If your serum creatinine (ask your doctor) is greater than 2 mg/dl, this medicine should NOT be taken.

Advisability of Use During Pregnancy or If Breast-Feeding:

Pregnancy Category: B. Use this drug only if clearly needed (ask your doctor). Present in breast milk in rats, probably in humans. Avoid taking this drug or stop nursing.

▷ **Overdose Symptoms:** Temporary increase in gas, abdominal discomfort, and diarrhea.

▷ **While Taking This Drug the Following Apply:**

Foods: Follow the diet your doctor has discussed with you. Tight blood sugar control can help you avoid long-term effects of diabetes.

Beverages: May be taken with milk.

Alcohol: An interaction is not expected with acarbose; however, if you are taking a sulfonylurea, alcohol may exaggerate lowering of blood sugar by the sulfonylurea and could cause a disulfiramlike reaction (see Glossary) as well.

Tobacco Smoking: Lessens the drug's effect; can worsen tight airways (bronchi) in smokers.

Other Drugs:

Acarbose may *increase* the effects of

- sulfonylureas (see Drug Classes) and result in excessive lowering of the blood sugar. This is, however, an accepted combination used to get tighter control of blood sugar.

Acarbose *taken concurrently* with

- clofibrate (Atromid-S) may result in hypoglycemia.
- digestive enzyme products that contain amylase or lipase may result in loss of blood sugar control.
- disopyramide (Norpace) may result in excessive lowering of blood sugar (hypoglycemia).
- high-dose aspirin or other salicylates and some NSAIDs (see Drug Classes) may result in hypoglycemia.
- insulin poses an increased hypoglycemia risk.
- sulfonamide antibiotics (see Drug Classes) may pose an increased risk of hypoglycemia.

The following drugs may *decrease* the effects of acarbose

- beta-blockers (see Drug Classes).
- corticosteroids (see Drug Classes).
- calcium channel blockers (see Drug Classes).
- furosemide (Lasix) and bumetanide (Bumex).
- isoniazid (INH).
- nicotinic acid.
- phenytoin (Dilantin).
- rifampin (Rifadin, others).
- thiazide diuretics (see Drug Classes).

- theophylline (Theo-Dur, others).
- thyroid hormones (see Drug Classes).

Driving, Hazardous Activities: Caution: this medicine may make you feel sleepy or lethargic.

Heavy Exercise or Exertion: Because this medicine results in a lower peak blood sugar after meals, talk with your doctor about checking your blood sugar before exercising.

▷ **Saving Money When Using This Medicine:**
- Preventing the problems that result from abnormally high blood sugar (such as high blood pressure, blindness, heart attacks, strokes, kidney problems, and nerve damage) by maintaining as normal a blood sugar level as possible is the best strategy in achieving great outcomes for diabetes.
- Ask your doctor if this medicine offers the best balance of price and outcomes for you.
- The American Diabetes Association recommends that all diabetics check their blood sugar regularly. Talk to your doctor about a machine to help you do this.

ACEBUTOLOL (a se BYU toh lohl)

Prescription Needed: Yes **Controlled Drug:** No **Generic:** No

Brand Names: Sectral

Overview of BENEFITS versus RISKS	
Possible Benefits	*Possible Risks*
EFFECTIVE ANTIHYPERTENSIVE in mild to moderate high blood pressure	CONGESTIVE HEART FAILURE in advanced heart disease
MAY DECREASE the number of deaths occurring after a heart attack	Worsening of angina in coronary heart disease (abrupt withdrawal)
	Masking of low blood sugar (hypoglycemia)
	Rare lupus erythematosus syndrome

▷ **Illness This Medication Treats:**
(1) Mild to moderate high blood pressure. May be used alone or combined with other drugs, such as diuretics. (2) Prevention of premature ventricular heartbeats.

Other (unlabeled) generally accepted uses: (1) treatment of stable angina pectoris; (2) use after a heart attack may help prolong life; (3) may have a role in easing panic attacks.

Typical Dosage Range: (Dosage or schedule must be determined by the doctor for each individual.)

18 to 65 Years of Age: Dosing starts at 400 mg daily, as a single dose in the morning or 200 mg every 12 hours. The usual maintenance dose is 400 to 800 mg every 24 hours. The total dose should not exceed 1200 mg/24 hr, taken as 600 mg twice daily.

Over 65 Years of Age: The amount taken into your body per dose increases twofold; therefore lower maintenance doses are needed. Do not take more than 800 mg per day.

Conditions Requiring Dosing Adjustments:

Liver function: Extensively changed by the liver. Caution is advised.

Kidney function: Dose must be decreased if kidneys are damaged.

How Best to Take This Medicine: May be taken with food. Capsule may be opened. Do not stop taking this medicine abruptly.

How Long This Medicine Is Usually Taken: Regular use for 5 to 11 days is needed to determine best effect. See your doctor regularly.

Tell Your Doctor Before Taking This Medicine If You:
- ever had an allergic reaction to it.
- have serious heart disease or an overactive thyroid.
- have hay fever, asthma, chronic bronchitis, emphysema, or low blood sugar.
- have impaired liver or kidney function.
- have diabetes, myasthenia gravis, or an abnormally slow heart rate.
- take digoxin, quinidine, reserpine, calcium blockers, or MAO type A inhibitor drugs.
- plan to have surgery under general anesthesia soon.

Possible Side Effects: Tiredness, cold hands or feet, slow heart rate, or light-headedness on standing.

Possible Adverse Effects:

If any of the following develop, call your doctor promptly for guidance.

Some Mild Problems This Drug Can Cause

Allergic reactions: skin rash, itching.

Headache, dizziness, abnormal dreams.

Some Serious Problems This Drug Can Cause

Mental depression, anxiety; asthma attacks in asthmatics (somewhat dose-related).

Congestive heart failure.

Positive antinuclear antibody (ANA) and lupus erythematosus.

Rare liver toxicity.

▷ **Possible Effects on Sex Life:** Impotence, decreased libido, Peyronie's disease.

▷ *CAUTION*

1. *Do not stop taking this drug suddenly* without telling your doctor. Carry a note with you at all times that states you are taking this drug.
2. Ask your doctor or pharmacist before using nasal decongestants.
3. Report the development of any tendency to emotional depression.

Advisability of Use During Pregnancy or If Breast-Feeding:

Pregnancy Category: B. Use this drug only if clearly needed (ask your doctor). Present in breast milk; avoid taking this drug or stop nursing.

▷ **Overdose Symptoms:** Slow pulse, low blood pressure, fainting, cold and sweaty skin, heart failure, weakness, possible coma, and convulsions.

▷ **While Taking This Drug the Following Apply:**

Foods: Avoid excessive salt intake.

Beverages: May be taken with milk.

Alcohol: Alcohol may lower blood pressure and also have an increased sedative effect.

Tobacco Smoking: Lessens the drug's effect; can worsen tight airways (bronchi) in smokers.

Other Drugs:

Acebutolol may *increase* the effects of

• other blood pressure drugs and lower the blood pressure too much.
• reserpine (Ser-Ap-Es) causing sedation, depression, low pulse or blood pressure.

Acebutolol *taken concurrently* with

• amiodarone (Cordarone) may lead to severe slowing of the heart Use this combination with great caution.
• clonidine (Catapres) can cause rebound high blood pressure if clonidine is stopped while acebutolol is still being taken.
• insulin requires glucose testing to avoid hypoglycemia.
• nilvadipine (Escor) may pose a rare risk of heart failure.
• oral hypoglycemic agents (see Drug Classes) may result in slowed recovery from any lowering of blood glucose.

The following drugs may *decrease* the effects of acebutolol

• indomethacin (Indocin) or any NSAIDs drugs can impair this drug's effect.

Driving, Hazardous Activities: Caution: acebutolol can make you sleepy, lethargic, or cause low blood pressure.

Exposure to Heat: Can lower blood pressure and exaggerate the drug's effects.

Exposure to Cold: Can slow blood flow and cause hypothermia in the elderly.

Heavy Exercise or Exertion: Avoid if it causes light-headedness, excessive fatigue, or muscle cramping. This drug can increase your blood pressure response to exercise.

▷ **Saving Money When Using This Medicine:**
- A follow-up check with your doctor for lupuslike reaction can avoid more complicated problems.
- Ask your doctor if this medicine offers the best balance of price and outcomes for you. Effective control of blood pressure now can help you completely avoid the life-threatening kidney, eye, heart, and nerve problems that may develop if high blood pressure goes untreated.

ACETAZOLAMIDE (a set a ZOHL a mide)

Prescription Needed: Yes   **Controlled Drug:** No   **Generic:** Yes

Brand Names: Ak-Zol, Dazamide, Diamox, Diamox Sequles, Storzolamide

---

Overview of BENEFITS versus RISKS

Possible Benefits	*Possible Risks*
DECREASED INTERNAL EYE PRESSURE in selected cases of glaucoma	Acidosis with long-term use
	Increased risk of kidney stones
CONTROL OF ABSENCE (PETIT MAL) SEIZURES	Bone weakening (with long-term use)
	Rare paralysis
TREATMENT OF PERIODIC PARALYSIS	Rare bone marrow, liver, or kidney injury
FLUID DECREASE IN CONGESTIVE HEART FAILURE OR DRUG-INDUCED EDEMA	
SYMPTOMATIC HELP IN ACUTE MOUNTAIN-CLIMBING SICKNESS	

▷ **Illness This Medication Treats:**
(1) Glaucoma and petit mal epilepsy; (2) some kinds of glaucoma; (3) familial periodic paralysis and prevention of altitude sickness; (4) short-term use in heart failure and drug-induced edema.

Other (unlabeled) generally accepted uses: (1) helps prevent uric acid kidney stones; (2) used intravenously to help remove some medicine overdoses.

▷ **Typical Dosage Range:** (Dosage or schedule must be determined by the doctor for each individual.)

18 to 65 Years of Age: For glaucoma: 250 to 1000 mg every 24 hours, in two or three doses. For epilepsy: 250 to 1000 mg every 24 hours. Diuretic use: 250 to 375 mg every 24 hours for 1 or 2 days.

Over 65 Years of Age: This drug should be used with caution in this group, and started with low doses.

▷ **Conditions Requiring Dosing Adjustments:**

Liver function: This drug can cause hepatic coma in people with liver cirrhosis; these patients should use it with extreme caution.

Kidney function: This drug needs the kidney to work. Use it with great care.

▷ **How Best to Take This Medicine:**   Best taken with food or milk. Tablet may be crushed. Diamox Sequles may be opened, but do not chew or crush contents.

▷ **How Long This Medicine Is Usually Taken:**   Treatment of glaucoma and epilepsy require long-term use. If taken to control seizures, do not stop taking it abruptly. See your doctor regularly.

▷ **Tell Your Doctor Before Taking This Medicine If You:**
- ever had an allergic reaction to it.
- have serious liver or kidney disease, glaucoma, lung disease, low platelets, or Addison's disease.
- have had an allergic reaction to any sulfa drug in the past.
- have low blood sodium or potassium.
- have gout or lupus erythematosus (LE).

▷ **Possible Side Effects:**   Drowsiness, temporary nearsightedness.

▷ **Possible Adverse Effects:**
If any of the following develop, call your doctor promptly for guidance.

Mild Problems This Drug Can Cause
Allergic reactions: skin rash, hives, drug fever.
Low appetite/nausea, fatigue, dizziness/tingling.

Serious Problems This Drug Can Cause
Allergic reactions: hemolytic anemia, spontaneous bruising.
Bone marrow depression—fatigue, fever, sore throat, bleeding.
Hepatitis and jaundice—yellow eyes/skin, dark urine, light stools.
Severe muscle weakness leading to paralysis (rare).
Weakening of the bones.

▷ **Possible Effects on Sex Life:**   Decreased libido, impotence (both rare). These effects may start after 2 weeks of use.

▷ *CAUTION*
1. Watch for loss of this drug's effect when used as a diuretic or for seizures.

2. Emotional depression may occur.
3. Increased potassium loss may occur. Ask your doctor if you need more potassium.
4. High doses in infants or children cause drowsiness and numbness.
5. Excess levels in adults over 60 may cause loss of potassium and sodium: weakness, confusion, numbness in limbs, and nausea.
6. The combined use of acetazolamide with digoxin or digitoxin may require potassium supplements.

Advisability of Use During Pregnancy or If Breast-Feeding:
Pregnancy Category: C. Avoid using this drug for first 3 months and during birth. This drug is present in breast milk; may impair milk production. Stop taking this drug or nursing if adverse effects occur.

▷ **Overdose Symptoms:**   Drowsiness, tingling, nausea, vomiting, confusion, convulsions, coma.

▷ **While Taking This Drug the Following Apply:**
Foods: Ask your doctor if you need a high-potassium diet. See Table 11, "High-Potassium Foods," Section Six.
Beverages: May be taken with milk.
Alcohol: Alcohol may decrease seizure control (smaller anticonvulsant effect).
Other Drugs:
Acetazolamide may *increase* the effects of
• amphetamines and lead to toxic levels.
• aspirin and cause toxicity.
• quinidine (Quinaglute, others).
Acetazolamide may *decrease* the effects of
• lithium (Lithobid, others).
• oral hypoglycemic agents (see Drug Classes).
Driving, Hazardous Activities: This drug may cause drowsiness or dizziness.

▷ **Saving Money When Using This Medicine:**
• Ask your doctor if this medicine offers the best balance of price and outcomes for you.
• A generic form is available and can be substituted for the brand.

ACETIC ACIDS

(Nonsteroidal Anti-Inflammatory Drugs)
Diclofenac (di KLOH fen ak)
Etodolac (e TOE do lak)
Indomethacin (in doh METH a sin)
Ketorolac (KEY tor o lak)

Nabumentone (na BYU me tohn)
Sulindac (sul IN dak)
Tolmetin (TOHL met in)

Prescription Needed: Yes **Controlled Drug:** No **Generic:**
Yes: indomethacin, sulindac, tolmetin

Brand Names: Indomethacin: Indameth, Indocin, Indocin-SR; Diclofenac: Voltaren, Cataflam, Voltaren Ophthalmic; Etodolac: Lodine; Ketorolac: Toradol, Acular; Nabumetone: Relafen; Sulindac:
Clinoril; Tolmetin: Tolectin, Tolectin DS, Tolectin 600

Overview of BENEFITS versus RISKS

Possible Benefits	*Possible Risks*
EFFECTIVE RELIEF OF MILD TO MODERATE PAIN AND INFLAMMATION	Gastrointestinal pain, ulceration, bleeding (rare)
Easy change from the IM or IV form to the oral form (ketorolac)	Rare liver or kidney damage
	Rare fluid retention
Decreased stomach (GI) problems (etodolac)	Rare bone marrow depression
	Mental depression, confusion
	Rare lung fibrosis (nabumetone)
	Rare pneumonitis (sulindac)
	Rare aseptic meningitis (diclofenac)
	Rare severe skin reaction (diclofenac, etodolac, ketorolac, and sulindac)

▷ **Illness This Medication Treats.**
  (1) All of the drugs in this class except ketorolac are approved to treat
  osteoarthritis; (2) all of the drugs in this class except ketorolac and
  etodolac are approved to relieve rheumatoid arthritis; (3) etodolac
  and ketorolac are used to treat mild to moderate pain; (4) diclofenac
  is useful in ankylosing spondylitis; (5) the sustained-release form of
  indomethacin as well as the immediate-release form of sulindac
  help symptoms of tendonitis, bursitis, and acute painful shoulder;
  (6) tolmetin eases symptoms of juvenile rheumatoid arthritis; (7)
  sulindac therapy is useful in acute gout; (8) the ophthalmic form of
  diclofenac is useful after cataract surgery; (9) the ophthalmic form
  of ketorolac is used to treat itchy eyes caused by seasonal allergies.
  Other (unlabeled) generally accepted uses: (1) diclofenac used intramuscularly is effective in acute migraine headache and kidney
  colic. The ophthalmic form is useful following cataract surgery. (2)
  Indomethacin has recently proven to be useful in reducing systemic
  reactions in kidney transplants and addressing low-grade neonatal

intraventricular hemorrhage. (3) Ketorolac has been helpful in reducing swelling after cataract surgery and in treating reflex sympathetic dystrophy by injection. (4) Sulindac is effective in treating colon polyps (Gardner's syndrome) and easing diabetic nerve pain (neuropathic pain).

▷ **Typical Dosage Range:** (Dosage or schedule must be determined by the doctor for each individual.)

Indomethacin: For arthritis and related conditions: 25 to 50 mg, two to four times daily. If needed and tolerated, dose may be increased by 25 or 50 mg per day at intervals of 1 week. For acute gout: 100 mg initially, then 50 mg three times per day until pain is relieved. Maximum daily dose is 200 mg.

Diclofenac potassium: Maximum daily dose is 200 mg.

Diclofenac sodium: 100 to 200 mg daily to start in two to five divided doses. Reduction to the minimum effective dose is advisable. Maximum daily dose is 225 mg.

Etodolac: For osteoarthritis: A starting dose of 800 to 1200 mg is taken in divided doses. The lowest effective dose is advisable, and effective treatment has been accomplished with 200 to 400 mg daily. Maximum dose is 1200 mg daily.

Ketorolac: Oral: 10 mg is used every 4 to 6 hours for short-term treatment of pain. Maximum daily dose is 40 mg orally. Ophthalmic: One drop of solution four times daily. Use for a maximum of 1 week.

Nabumentone: 1000 mg daily as a single dose. Dosage is increased as needed and tolerated to 1500 mg daily. The lowest effective daily dose is advisable. Maximum daily dose is 2000 mg.

Sulindac: Therapy is started with 150 to 200 mg twice daily, taken 12 hours apart. Maximum daily dose is 400 mg.

Tolmetin: 400 mg three times daily is started, with usual ongoing doses of 600 to 1600 mg as needed and tolerated. Total daily dose should not exceed 1600 mg for osteoarthritis or 2000 mg for rheumatoid arthritis.

Children 2 years of age or older may be given 20 mg per kilogram of body weight orally, divided into three or four doses daily. The dose may be increased as needed and tolerated to a maximum daily dose of 30 mg per kilogram of body weight.

▷ **Conditions Requiring Dosing Adjustments:**

Liver function: Nonsteroidal anti-inflammatory drugs are extensively changed in the liver. Patients with liver compromise should use this drug with caution.

Kidney function: All nonsteroidal anti-inflammatory drugs may inhibit prostaglandins and alter kidney blood flow in patients with kidney (renal) compromise. Patients with kidney compromise should use this drug with caution.

▷ **How Best to Take This Medicine:**   Take with or following food to prevent stomach irritation. Take with a full glass of water and do not lie down for 30 minutes. Regular-release tablets may be crushed, but not extended-release forms. The regular capsules may be opened for administration, but not the prolonged-action capsules. Food actually increases absorption of nabumetone.

▷ **How Long This Medicine Is Usually Taken:**   Use on a regular schedule for 1 to 2 weeks usually determines the effectiveness of this drug in relieving the discomfort of arthritis. The usual length of treatment for bursitis or tendonitis for indomethacin or sulindac is 7 to 14 days. Ketorolac is used for short-term pain treatment. Long-term use of the other agents in this class requires your doctor's supervision and periodic evaluation.

▷ **Tell Your Doctor Before Taking These Medicines If You:**
- ever had an allergic reaction to them.
- have asthma or nasal polyps caused by aspirin.
- are pregnant (avoid all NSAIDs during the last 3 months of pregnancy) or are breast-feeding.
- have active peptic ulcer disease or any form of gastrointestinal ulceration or bleeding.
- have active liver disease or impaired kidney function.
- have a bleeding disorder or a blood cell disorder.
- have porphyria (diclofenac, indomethacin).
- are allergic to aspirin or aspirin substitutes.
- have a history of epilepsy, Parkinson's disease, or mental illness (psychosis).
- have high blood pressure or a history of heart failure.
- are taking acetaminophen, aspirin or aspirin substitutes, or anticoagulants.

▷ **Possible Side Effects:**   Drowsiness, ringing in ears (may also be a sign of toxicity), fluid retention.

▷ **Possible Adverse Effects:**
If any of the following develop, call your doctor promptly for guidance.
Some Mild Problems This Drug Can Cause
Allergic reactions: skin rash, hives, itching, swelling.
Headache, dizziness, feelings of detachment.
Mouth sores, nausea, vomiting, diarrhea.
Ringing in the ears.
Temporary loss of hair (indomethacin).
Some Serious Problems This Drug Can Cause
Allergic reactions: asthma, difficult breathing, mouth irritation.
Confusion, depression.
Active peptic ulcer, with or without bleeding.

Liver damage with jaundice.

Kidney damage, bloody urine, reduced urine formation.

Rare bone marrow depression—fatigue, weakness, fever, sore throat, abnormal bleeding or bruising.

Severe skin rash (Stevens-Johnson syndrome—diclofenac, ketorolac, etodolac, sulindac).

Peripheral neuritis—numbness, pain, or weakness in extremities (indomethacin).

Rare lung fibrosis (nabumetone).

Rare pneumonitis (sulindac).

Rare aseptic meningitis (diclofenac).

▷ **Possible Effects on Sex Life:** Enlargement and tenderness of both male and female breasts (indomethacin, sulindac).

Nonmenstrual vaginal bleeding (indomethacin).

Rare impotence (diclofenac, nabumetone).

Rare uterine bleeding (etodolac, sulindac).

▷ **Possible Delayed Adverse Effects:** Mild anemia due to "silent" blood loss from the stomach (less than that caused by aspirin).

▷ *CAUTION*

1. Dosage should always be limited to the smallest amount that produces reasonable improvement.

2. These drugs may hide early indications of infection. Tell your doctor if you think you are developing an infection.

3. Indomethacin: This drug frequently impairs kidney function in infants. Fatal liver reactions have occurred in children between 6 and 12 years old; avoid the use of this drug in this age group.

4. Diclofenac, etodolac, ketorolac, nabumetone, sulindac: Safety and efficacy of these drugs for those under 12 years old are not established.

5. Tolmetin: Safety and efficacy of this drug for those under 2 years old are not established.

6. People over 60 should take small starting doses. Watch for any indications of liver or kidney toxicity, fluid retention, dizziness, confusion, impaired memory, depression, peptic ulcer, or diarrhea, often with rectal bleeding.

Advisability of Use During Pregnancy or If Breast-Feeding:

Pregnancy Category: Diclofenac, tolmetin: B. Ketorolac, nabumetone, sulindac, and etodolac: C. Indomethacin, sulindac, and tolmetin (last 3 months): D.

Indomethacin: Manufacturer recommends not taking it during pregnancy.

Diclofenac, nabumetone, sulindac, tolmetin: Adequate studies of pregnant women are not available. Avoid this drug completely during the last 3 months of pregnancy. Use it during the first 6 months only if clearly needed. Ask your doctor for guidance.

Ketorolac: Adequate studies of pregnant women are not available. Ask your doctor for guidance.

Etodolac: Adequate studies of pregnant women are not available. The manufacturer advises that this drug be avoided during pregnancy.

Present in breast milk when indomethacin, diclofenac, or ketorolac is taken. Presence in breast milk is unknown when etodolac, nabumetone, sulindac, or tolmetin is taken; avoid taking these drugs or refrain from nursing.

▷ **Overdose Symptoms:** Drowsiness, agitation, confusion, nausea, vomiting, diarrhea, disorientation, seizures, coma.

▷ **Suggested Periodic Examinations While Taking This Drug:** (at doctor's discretion)

Complete blood cell counts; liver and kidney function tests; complete eye examinations if vision is altered in any way.

▷ **While Taking This Drug the Following Apply:**

Nutritional Support: Indomethacin: Take 50 mg of vitamin C (ascorbic acid) daily.

Beverages: May be taken with milk.

Alcohol: Use with caution. Alcohol irritates the stomach lining, and when added to the irritant action of this drug in sensitive individuals, can increase the risk of stomach ulceration and/or bleeding.

Other Drugs:

Medications in this class may ***increase*** the effects of

- acetaminophen (Tylenol, etc.) and increase the risk of kidney damage; avoid prolonged use of this combination.
- anticoagulants (Coumadin, etc.) and increase the risk of bleeding; monitor prothrombin time, adjust dose accordingly.
- lithium (Lithobid, others) and cause lithium toxicity.
- cyclosporine (Sandimmune) and cause toxicity.
- methotrexate (Mexate, others).
- thrombolytics such as streptokinase or tissue plasminogen activator (TPA).

Medications in this class may ***decrease*** the effects of

- beta-blocker drugs (see Drug Classes) and reduce their antihypertensive effectiveness.
- bumetanide (Bumex).
- captopril (Capoten).
- ethacrynic acid (Edecrin).
- furosemide (Lasix).

Medications in this class ***taken concurrently*** with the following drugs may increase the risk of bleeding; avoid these combinations:

- aspirin.
- diflunisal (Dolobid).

- dipyridamole (Persantine).
- sulfinpyrazone (Anturane).
- valproic acid (Depakene).

Driving, Hazardous Activities: These drugs may cause drowsiness, dizziness, or impaired vision. Restrict your activities as necessary.

Exposure to Sun: Use caution. Several of the medicines in this class cause photosensitivity.

▷ **Saving Money When Using These Medicines:**
- The effectiveness of all of these medicines is about equal. Ask your doctor to start you on the least expensive drug in the class most appropriate for you.
- Ask for generics—they are available for several acetic acid NSAIDs.
- Ask your doctor exactly how long you will need to take this medicine to treat your condition.

ACYCLOVIR (ay SI kloh ver)

Prescription Needed: Yes (nonprescription status pending)
Controlled Drug: No **Generic:** No
Brand Name: Zovirax

Overview of BENEFITS versus RISKS

Possible Benefits	*Possible Risks*
QUICKER RECOVERY FROM INITIAL EPISODE OF GENITAL HERPES	Nausea, vomiting, diarrhea
	Nervousness, depression
PREVENTION OF RECURRENCE OF GENITAL HERPES	Joint and muscle pain

---

▷ **Illness This Medication Treats:**
(1) Genital herpes (prevention); (2) herpes simplex infections of skin, brain, eye, and rectum; (3) herpes simplex virus infections in bone marrow transplant patients (prevention); (4) infectious mononucleosis; (5) shingles; (6) pneumonia caused by the chickenpox virus.
Other (unlabeled) generally accepted use: may have a role in treating nonmalignant growths in the throat (laryngeal papillomatosis).

▷ **Typical Dosage Range:** (Dosage or schedule must be determined by the doctor for each individual.)
18 to 65 Years of Age: For initial episode of genital herpes: 200 mg/4 hr for a total of five capsules daily for 10 consecutive days (total dose of 50 capsules). For intermittent recurrence: 200 mg/4 hr for a total of five capsules daily for 5 consecutive days (total dose of 25 capsules).

Begin treatment at the earliest indication of recurrence. For prevention of frequent recurrence: 400 mg taken twice daily for up to 12 months. For the ointment form: Cover all infected areas every 3 hours for a total of six times daily for 7 consecutive days. Begin treatment at the earliest indication of infection.

Treatment of chickenpox: 20 mg per kilogram of body weight (do not exceed 800 mg) orally, four times a day for 5 days. Treatment should be started at first symptom or sign.

Over 65 Years of Age: Dosing must be adjusted for any age-related decline in kidney function.

▷ **Conditions Requiring Dosing Adjustments:**

Kidney function: The dose MUST be adjusted for compromised kidney (renal) function. A complete dose change schedule is in the package insert.

▷ **How Best to Take This Medicine:**   Can be taken with food. Capsule may be opened. Take the full course of the exact dose prescribed. Use a finger cot/rubber glove to apply the ointment.

▷ **How Long This Medicine Is Usually Taken:**   Regular schedule for 10 days will achieve the peak effect. Continual use for 6 months to 3 years may be needed to prevent recurrence of herpes eruptions.

▷ **Tell Your Doctor Before Taking This Medicine If You:**
- ever had an allergic reaction to it.
- have impaired liver or kidney function.
- think you are dehydrated and have a prescription for the capsule form.

▷ **Possible Side Effects·**   With use of capsules—none.
With use of ointment—mild pain, burning, or stinging at site of application.

▷ **Possible Adverse Effects:**
If any of the following develop, call your doctor promptly for guidance.
Mild Problems Drug Can Cause
Allergic reaction: skin rash.
Headache, dizziness, insomnia, depression, fatigue.
Nausea/vomiting, diarrhea.
Joint pain/muscle cramps.
Hair loss.
Serious Problems Drug Can Cause
Superficial thrombophlebitis, enlarged lymph glands.
Kidney problems (rare).

▷ **Possible Effects on Sex Life:**   Altered timing and pattern of menstruation.

▷ *CAUTION*

1. This drug is not a permanent cure for herpes. Watch for possible recurrence, and restart treatment at the earliest indication of active infection.
2. Avoid sexual intercourse while herpes blisters and swelling persist.
3. Tell your doctor if the frequency and severity of recurrent infections do not improve. Do not use more than the prescribed dose.
4. Safety and effectiveness of this drug for those under 12 years old are unknown.
5. Patients over 60 years old should drink 2 to 3 qt of liquids daily.

Advisability of Use During Pregnancy or If Breast-Feeding:
Pregnancy Category: C. Use only if clearly needed. Presence in breast milk is unknown. Avoid taking this drug or refrain from nursing.

▷ **Overdose Symptoms:**   Possible impairment of kidney function.

▷ **While Taking This Drug the Following Apply:**
Beverages: No problems with milk. Drink 2 qt of liquids daily.
Alcohol: Dizziness or fatigue may be worsened. Use caution.
Other Drugs:
The following drug may *increase* the effects of acyclovir

- probenecid (Benemid) may delay its elimination.

Acyclovir *taken concurrently* with

- cyclosporine (Sandimmune) may pose an increased risk of kidney toxicity.
- meperidine (Demerol) may result in increased risk of nerve problems.
- probenecid (Benemid) may delay acyclovir elimination.
- varicella vaccine (Varivax) may blunt the vaccine's effectiveness.
- zidovudine (AZT) may result in severe fatigue and lethargy.

Driving, Hazardous Activities: Use caution if dizziness or fatigue occurs.

▷ **Saving Money When Using This Medicine:**
- If you start this medicine at the FIRST sign of infection, the time you have to use the medicine will be shorter than if you delay therapy.
- If your kidneys are compromised, you may only need to take the drug (capsule form) twice a day.
- Two additional agents have been approved which have activity in genital herpes and mucocutaneous infections as well. One agent achieves blood levels nearly identical to intravenous dosing. Ask your doctor if this medicine offers the best balance of price and outcomes for you.

ALBUTEROL   (al BYU ter ohl)

Prescription Needed: Yes   **Controlled Drug:** No   **Generic:** Yes

Brand Names: Proventil (inhaler, tablets, or repetabs), Ventolin (inhaler, rotacaps, tablets)

Overview of BENEFITS versus RISKS	
Possible Benefits	*Possible Risks*
VERY EFFECTIVE RELIEF OF BRONCHOSPASM	Increased blood pressure
	Fine hand tremor
	Irregular heart rhythm and very rare fatalities (with excessive use)

▷ **Illness This Medication Treats:**
(1) Acute asthma—reduces frequency/severity of chronic asthma attacks; (2) helps prevent exercise-induced asthma in children from 4 to 11 years old.

▷ **Typical Dosage Range:** (Dosage or schedule must be determined by the doctor for each individual.)
Inhaler: Adults and children 12 years or older: Two inhalations repeated every 4 to 6 hours. One inhalation every 4 hours may work well for some. Frequent administration of a larger number of inhalations is **not** recommended. Call your doctor if the dose that worked for you before becomes less effective. Tablets: 2 to 4 mg three to four times daily, every 4 to 6 hours. **Do not exceed** eight inhalations (720 mcg) every 24 hours, or 32 mg (tablet form) every 24 hours.

▷ **Conditions Requiring Dosing Adjustments:**
Liver function: This drug should be used cautiously in lower doses for patients with liver compromise.
Coronary artery disease: Maximum starting dose should be 1 mg in order to avoid chest pain (angina).
Thyroid disease: People with underactive thyroid glands may require larger doses.

▷ **How Best to Take This Medicine:**   May be taken on empty stomach or with food or milk. Tablet may be crushed. For inhaler, follow the written instructions carefully. Do not overuse.

▷ **How Long This Medicine Is Usually Taken:**   Varies. Do not use beyond the time needed to stop episodes of asthma.

▷ **Tell Your Doctor Before Taking This Medicine If You:**
- ever had an allergic reaction to it.
- currently have an irregular heart rhythm; or you are taking, or took, any MAO inhibitor drug (see Drug Classes) within the past 2 weeks.
- have diabetes, or an overactive (hyperthyroid) thyroid gland, or any type of heart or circulatory disorder, especially high blood pressure or coronary heart disease.
- are taking any form of digitalis or any stimulant drug.

▷ **Possible Side Effects:**   Aerosol—dryness or irritation of mouth or throat, altered taste.
Tablet—nervousness, palpitation.

▷ **Possible Adverse Effects:**
If any of the following develop, call your doctor promptly for guidance.
Some Mild Problems Drug Can Cause
  Fine tremor of hands, leg cramps, nausea.
Some Serious Problems Drug Can Cause
  Rapid or irregular heart rhythm and fatalities have been reported. These outcomes were associated with a pattern of increasing use.
  Hallucinations or convulsions (with excessive doses).
  Decreased blood potassium or blood sugar.

▷ *CAUTION*
  1. If this drug is used in inhaler form with beclomethasone aerosol (Beclovent, Vanceril), an increased risk of fluorocarbon propellant toxicity may occur. It is best to use albuterol aerosol 20 to 30 minutes *before* beclomethasone aerosol.
  2. Repeated dosing or prolonged use of this drug can reduce its effectiveness and cause serious heart rhythm disturbances, including cardiac arrest.
  3. Call your doctor if your usual dose loses its effectiveness in providing relief.
  4. Safety and effectiveness of this drug for children under 12 years old are not established.
  5. Patients over 60 should avoid excessive and continual use. If acute asthma is not promptly relieved, other drugs are indicated.

Advisability of Use During Pregnancy or If Breast-Feeding:
Pregnancy Category: C. Avoid use during first 3 months if possible. Presence in breast milk is unknown; avoid taking this drug or refrain from nursing.

▷ **Overdose Symptoms:**   Nervousness, palpitation, fast heart rate, sweating, vomiting, chest and head pain.

▷ **While Taking This Drug the Following Apply:**
Beverages: Avoid drinks high in caffeine: coffee, tea, cola, chocolate.

Other Drugs:
Albuterol *taken concurrently* with
- amphetamines may worsen cardiovascular side effects.
- beta-blockers (see Drug Classes) may cause loss of benefits of both medicines.
- MAO type A inhibitors may cause excessive increase in blood pressure and undesirable heart stimulation.
- theophylline (Theo-Dur, others) may cause the theophylline to be removed more rapidly from the body than expected, and result in decreased therapeutic benefits.
- tricyclic antidepressants (see Drug Classes) may result in a severe increase in blood pressure.

Driving, Hazardous Activities: Caution: nervousness, dizziness possible.

Heavy Exercise or Exertion: Use caution. Excessive exercise can cause asthma.

▷ **Saving Money When Using This Medicine:**
- Generic forms of the tablets and inhalation solution are available.
- Both Proventil and Ventolin inhalers have historically had exactly the same ingredients. Talk with your pharmacist to see if this is still the case, and if so, ask your doctor to prescribe the least expensive brand.

ALENDRONATE (a LEN drun ate)

Prescription Needed: Yes   **Controlled Drug:** No   **Generic:** No

Brand Names: Fosamax

Overview of BENEFITS versus RISKS	
Possible Benefits	*Possible Risks*
EFFECTIVE TREATMENT OF OSTEOPOROSIS	IRRITATION OF THE ESOPHAGUS (if not taken correctly)
INCREASED BONE MASS	Minor muscle pain
DECREASED RISK OF BONE FRACTURES	
SYMPTOM RELIEF IN PAGET'S DISEASE	

▷ **Illness This Medication Treats:**
(1) Osteoporosis that may happen after menopause; (2) Paget's disease; prevents postmenopausal osteoporosis.
Other (unlabeled) generally accepted uses: (1) expected to work in the prevention and treatment of male osteoporosis; (2) some clinicians

are using this medicine to prevent osteoporosis in patients who are not candidates for estrogen replacement or who do not wish to take estrogen after a heart attack (may help prolong life); (3) may have a role (intravenous form) in easing elevated blood calcium levels seen in some patients with cancer.

▷ **Typical Dosage Range:**   (Dosage or schedule must be determined by the doctor for each individual.)

Infants and Children: Safety and efficacy of this drug are not established for this age group.

18 to 65 Years of Age: For female postmenopausal osteoporosis: 10 mg taken once daily. Osteoporosis prevention: Dose is expected to be 10 mg daily. I strongly recommend an appropriate amount of calcium and vitamin D be taken every day. Talk this over with your doctor or pharmacist. An appropriate amount of weight-bearing exercise is also ideal for healthy bones.

Paget's disease: 40 mg once a day for 6 months.

Over 65 Years of Age: Same as for 18 to 65 years of age.

▷ **Conditions Requiring Dosing Adjustments:**

Kidney function: Lower doses are needed for patients with compromised kidneys. The drug should NOT be used if creatinine clearance is less than 35 ml/min (see Glossary).

▷ **How Best to Take This Medicine:**   IT IS CRITICAL TO TAKE THIS MEDICINE ONLY WITH TAP WATER in order to get the best results. Patients should drink a full glass (6 to 8 oz of water) with this medicine and should NOT take this medicine with food or other medicines (prescription or nonprescription). It is best to wait at least half an hour before consuming coffee or other beverages or foods after taking alendronate. In order to decrease the risk of irritation of the esophagus, DO NOT lie down for at least 30 minutes after you've taken alendronate.

▷ **How Long This Medicine Is Usually Taken:**   For Paget's disease, alendronate is taken once daily for 6 months, and after that time a physician evaluation is needed. When treating osteoporosis in postmenopausal women, many physicians will obtain a bone mineral density test (DEXA is most widely used) in order to help make the decision to start treatment; then they will obtain a second test in order to help decide how successful the treatment has been and whether it should be continued. Further study is needed to identify the best strategies to use in dosing long-term alendronate therapy.

▷ **Tell Your Doctor Before Taking This Medicine If You:**
• ever had an allergic reaction to it.
• have a low blood calcium (talk with your doctor).
• have significant kidney disease.

- have esophageal disease or ulcers or inflammation of the duodenum.
- have a vitamin D deficiency or a low-calcium diet.

▷ **Possible Side Effects:** Irritation of the esophagus and potential ulceration. This effect may be worsened if patients lie down immediately after taking this medicine (see **How Best to Take This Medicine**, above).

▷ **Possible Adverse Effects:**
If any of the following develop, call your doctor promptly for guidance.
Some Mild Problems This Drug Can Cause
   Allergic reactions: rare skin rash or redness.
   Constipation or mild muscle pain.
Some Serious Problems This Drug Can Cause
   Esophageal ulceration; may be worsened if you lie down immediately after taking alendronate.
   One case report of a patient with a history of ulcers who took aspirin as well as alendronate and developed an ulcer.

▷ *CAUTION*
   1. A "Dear Doctor" letter was sent out to physicians warning of an increased occurrence of esophageal ulceration. This may have been caused by patients taking alendronate without telling their doctors. Carry a note with you at all times that states you are taking this drug.
   2. Patients taking more than 10 mg a day of alendronate should avoid aspirin and aspirin-containing compounds because of an increased potential of upper gastrointestinal irritation. Ask your doctor or pharmacist before using other NSAIDs (see Drug Classes) as well.
   3. Other causes of osteoporosis besides estrogen or aging (secondary osteoporosis) should be ruled out.
Advisability of Use During Pregnancy or If Breast-Feeding:
Pregnancy Category: C. AVOID this medicine in pregnancy. Presence in breast milk is unknown; avoid taking this drug or stop nursing.

▷ **Overdose Symptoms:** Nausea, vomiting, hypocalcemia. Heartburn, irritation of the upper gastrointestinal (GI) tract.

▷ **While Taking This Drug the Following Apply:**
Foods: Getting adequate calcium in your diet (talk with your doctor) is a good idea; however, you should wait at least half an hour after taking alendronate before taking any food or medicine.
Beverages: WATER is the only liquid this medicine should be taken with.

Alcohol: Excessive alcohol intake is actually a risk factor for osteoporosis. WATER is the only liquid alendronate should be taken with.

Tobacco Smoking: Nicotine may act to increase the elimination of estrogen.

Other Drugs:

Alendronate *taken concurrently* with

- any other medicines will decrease the therapeutic benefits of alendronate.
- antacids will decrease how much alendronate gets into your body to help you.
- aspirin or aspirin-containing compounds may pose an increased risk of upper gastrointestinal (GI) adverse effects if more than 10 mg of alendronate is taken daily. Ask your doctor or pharmacist before taking other NSAIDs (see Drug Classes).
- estrogens (various) is not recommended because of lack of specific data.
- foscarnet (Foscavir) may result in decreased blood calcium.

Heavy Exercise or Exertion: If your bone density is low, heavy aerobic exercise may not be a good idea. Talk with your doctor about an appropriate exercise program for you.

▷ **Saving Money When Using This Medicine:**

- Talk with your doctor or pharmacist about other younger members of your family and how much calcium they will need in their diets to build the strongest bones possible. This concept is called peak bone mass, and will help your children build the strongest bones possible, perhaps avoiding osteoporosis later.
- It is advisable to have bone mineral density (BMD) checked in a variety of situations. Talk with your doctor about your bone health and risk factors for osteoporosis. Please note that bone density must be coupled with other individual factors when considering treatment.
- Discuss preventive use of alendronate if you have important risk factors for osteoporosis.
- Ask your doctor if this medicine offers the best balance of price and outcomes for you. Ask when bone mineral density will be rechecked once any treatments are started (this is a great way to see exactly how effective the treatments are).

ALLOPURINOL   (al oh PURE i nohl)

Prescription Needed: Yes   **Controlled Drug:** No   **Generic:** Yes

Brand Names: Lopurin, Zurinol, Zyloprim

Overview of BENEFITS versus RISKS	
Possible Benefits	*Possible Risks*
EFFECTIVE CONTROL OF GOUT	Increased frequency of acute gout initially
CONTROLS HIGH BLOOD URIC ACID in polycythemia, leukemia, cancer, or chemotherapy	Peripheral neuritis
	Allergic reactions in skin, blood vessels, and liver
	Bone marrow depression (questionable)
	Kidney toxicity

▷ **Illness This Medication Treats:**
(1) Prevents episodes of acute gout (will not help symptoms of acute gout attacks); (2) prevents abnormal uric acid levels in people who have uric acid kidney stones or are getting chemotherapy or radiation therapy.
Other (unlabeled) generally accepted use: may be of great benefit in decreasing pain and occurrence of mouth sores in people getting 5-fluorouracil chemotherapy.

▷ **Typical Dosage Range:** (Dosage or schedule must be determined by the doctor for each individual.)
Initially 100 mg/24 hr. Increase by 100 mg/24 hr at intervals of 1 week until uric acid blood level is 6 mg/dl or less. Usual dose is 200 to 300 mg every 24 hours for mild gout, and 400 to 600 mg every 24 hours for moderate to severe gout. Daily doses of 300 mg or less may be taken as a single dose. Doses exceeding 300 mg daily should be divided into two or three equal portions; for the high uric acid levels associated with cancer, 600 to 800 mg every 24 hours, divided into three equal portions.

▷ **Conditions Requiring Dosing Adjustments:**
Liver function: Dosage adjustment for patients with liver impairment is not documented.
Kidney function: Allopurinol dosing **must** be adjusted for patients with kidney compromise. Lower doses or longer dosing intervals should be adjusted to achieve desired lab test results.

▷ **How Best to Take This Medicine:** Best taken with food or milk. Tablet may be crushed. Avoid dehydration.

▷ **How Long This Medicine Is Usually Taken:** Regular use for several months may be required to prevent attacks of acute gout. See your doctor regularly.

▷ **Tell Your Doctor Before Taking This Medicine If You:**
- ever had an allergic reaction to it.
- are having an acute attack of gout.
- have a personal or family history of hemochromatosis.
- have a history of liver or kidney disease or are on a low-protein diet.
- have had a blood-cell or bone-marrow disorder.
- have any type of convulsive disorder (epilepsy).

▷ **Possible Side Effects:** The frequency or severity of acute gout may increase during the first several weeks of drug use. See your doctor for other useful drugs to help if this occurs.

▷ **Possible Adverse Effects:**
If any of the following develop, call your doctor promptly for guidance.
Some Mild Problems Drug Can Cause
Allergic reactions: skin rash, hives, itching, drug fever.
Headache.
Nausea, diarrhea.
Loss of scalp hair.
Some Serious Problems Drug Can Cause
Allergic reactions: severe skin reactions, fever, joint pains, kidney damage.
Hepatitis—yellow eyes and skin, dark urine, light stools.
Bone marrow depression.
Seizures, peripheral neuritis.
Macular eye damage, cataract formation.
Rare bronchospasm.

▷ **Possible Effects on Sex Life:** Cause unclear: male infertility, male breast enlargement, impotence.

▷ *CAUTION*
1. Early in treatment the frequency of acute attacks of gout may increase. These subside as treatment continues.
2. This drug will not relieve the symptoms of acute gout. It should not be used to treat acute gout.
3. If 2 g or more of vitamin C is taken daily while allopurinol therapy continues, the urine will become acidic and increase the risk of kidney stones.
4. Allopurinol should not be used with thiazide diuretics (may cause allergic-type kidney damage).
5. Watch infants or children for allergic skin reactions and blood-cell disorders (tiredness, weakness or irritability). Allopurinol can increase azathioprine or mercaptopurine toxicity.

6. Patients over 60 usually need smaller drug doses.

7. People on low-protein diets may not eliminate allopurinol normally, and decreased doses may be needed.

Advisability of Use During Pregnancy or If Breast-Feeding:

Pregnancy Category: C. Avoid taking this drug during the first 3 months. Use during the last 6 months only if clearly needed. Present in breast milk; avoid taking this drug or refrain from nursing.

▷ **Overdose Symptoms:** Nausea, vomiting, or diarrhea. Usually no serious toxicity.

▷ **While Taking This Drug the Following Apply:**

Foods: Follow your doctor's advice regarding the need for a low-purine diet.

Beverages: May be taken with milk.

Other Drugs:

Allopurinol may *increase* the effects of

- azathioprine (Imuran) and mercaptopurine (Purinethol)—dosages may need to be decreased.
- oral anticoagulants (see Drug Classes) in *some* people.
- theophylline (aminophylline, Elixophyllin, Theo-Dur, etc.)

Allopurinol *taken concurrently* with

- ampicillin may increase the incidence of skin rash.
- antacids containing aluminum will blunt the therapeutic effect of allopurinol.
- captopril or other ACE inhibitors (see Drug Classes) can increase the likelihood of allergic reactions.
- cyclophosphamide (Cytoxan) may result in toxicity.
- cyclosporine (Sandimmune) may result in cyclosporine toxicity.
- tamoxifen (Nolvadex) may increase the risk of liver toxicity.
- theophylline (Theo-Dur, others) may lead to toxic theophylline levels.
- vidarabine (Vira-A) may increase the risk of nerve toxicity.

Driving, Hazardous Activities: Drowsiness may limit your abilities. Use caution.

▷ **Saving Money When Using This Medicine:**

- Several generic forms are available—buy the least expensive form of this medicine.
- Ask your doctor if this medicine offers the best combination of price and outcomes for you.
- Ask your doctor if your diet should be modified (purine restriction) if this drug is being used to help gout.
- Talk with your doctor about checking for lead poisoning (if risk factors are present).
- Your doctor may want to check the health of your heart, as gout can be a risk factor for coronary heart disease.

ALPRAZOLAM (al PRAY zoh lam)

Prescription Needed: Yes   **Controlled Drug:** Yes C-IV*
Generic: No

Brand Names: Xanax, Alprazolam Intensol

▷ **Warning:** The brand names Xanax and Zantac are similar and can be mistaken; make certain that you are taking the right drug.

Overview of BENEFITS versus RISKS

Possible Benefits	*Possible Risks*
RELIEF OF ANXIETY AND NERVOUS TENSION	Habit-forming potential with prolonged use
EFFECTIVE TREATMENT OF PANIC DISORDER	Minor impairment of mental functions with therapeutic doses
Wide margin of safety with therapeutic doses	Rare tachycardia or palpitations
May have some antidepressant activity	

▷ **Illness This Medication Treats:**
(1) Used as a mild tranquilizer for short-term relief of mild to moderate anxiety and nervous tension; (2) also used to relieve anxiety associated with depression and to prevent or relieve panic attacks.

Other (unlabeled) generally accepted uses: (1) may have a role in helping ease PMS symptoms; (2) can be used to help cancer pain when used in combination with other medicines; (3) may help decrease the loudness of the sensation of ringing in the ears in tinnitus.

▷ **Typical Dosage Range:** (Dosage or schedule must be determined by the doctor for each individual.)

For anxiety and nervous tension: 0.25 to 0.5 mg, three times daily. The maximum dose is 4 mg/24 hr, taken in divided doses.

For panic disorder: Initially 0.5 mg three times daily; increased by 1 mg every 3 to 4 days as needed. The maximum daily dosage is 10 mg.

▷ **Conditions Requiring Dosing Adjustments:**

Liver function: Starting dose: 0.25 mg for patients with advanced liver disease, with slow increases in dose to beneficial effects or intolerance.

Kidney function: Specific dosage reductions are not defined.

Obesity: Doses should be calculated on ideal rather than actual weight.

Alcoholism: Lower doses and longer times between doses are needed.

*See Controlled Drug Schedules inside this book's cover.

▷ **How Best to Take This Medicine:**   May be taken on empty stomach or with food or milk. Tablet may be crushed for administration. Do not stop taking this drug abruptly if it was taken for more than 4 weeks.

▷ **How Long This Medicine Is Usually Taken:**   Several days to several weeks. Avoid prolonged and uninterrupted use. Continual use should not exceed 8 weeks without evaluation by your doctor.

▷ **Tell Your Doctor Before Taking This Medicine If You:**
   • ever had an allergic reaction to it.
   • are pregnant, planning pregnancy, or breast-feeding.
   • have acute narrow-angle glaucoma.
   • have myasthenia gravis.
   • are allergic to benzodiazepine drugs.
   • have a history of depression or serious mental illness (psychosis).
   • have a history of alcoholism or drug abuse.
   • have impaired liver or kidney function.
   • have open angle glaucoma or a seizure disorder (epilepsy).
   • have severe chronic lung disease.

▷ **Possible Side Effects:**   Drowsiness, light-headedness.

▷ **Possible Adverse Effects:**
   If any of the following develop, call your doctor promptly for guidance.
   Some Mild Problems Drug Can Cause
      Allergic reactions: skin rash, hives.
      Headache, dizziness, drowsiness, blurred vision, dry mouth.
      Nausea, vomiting, constipation.
   Some Serious Problems Drug Can Cause
      Confusion, hallucinations, depression, agitation (paradoxical reaction).
      Low blood pressure (hypotension).
      Tachycardia or palpitations.
      May worsen respiratory depression if combined with morphine.

▷ **Possible Effects on Sex Life:**   Rare: inhibited female orgasm (5 mg/day); impaired ejaculation (3.5 mg/day); decreased libido, impaired erection (4.5 mg/day); altered timing/pattern of menstruation (0.75–4 mg/day).

▷ *CAUTION*
   1. Do NOT stop taking this medicine abruptly if it was taken continually for more than 4 weeks.
   2. Use of over-the-counter drugs containing antihistamines (allergy and cold preparations, sleep aids) can cause excessive sedation.
   3. Safety and effectiveness of this drug for patients less than 18 years old are not established.

4. Patients over 60 should be started on 0.25 mg two or three times daily, and closely watched for excessive drowsiness, dizziness, unsteadiness, and incoordination caused by low blood pressure.

Advisability of Use During Pregnancy or If Breast-Feeding:
Pregnancy Category: D. Avoid use during entire pregnancy if possible. Present in breast milk; avoid taking this drug or refrain from nursing.

▷ **Habit-Forming Potential:**   This drug can cause psychological and/or physical dependence, and this risk may increase if this medicine is used in large doses for longer periods of time.

▷ **Overdose Symptoms:**   Marked drowsiness, weakness, tremor, stupor to deep sleep or coma.

▷ **While Taking This Drug the Following Apply:**
Beverages: Do NOT drink large amounts of caffeine-containing beverages: coffee, tea, cola, chocolate. These beverages may lessen the calming benefits of alprazolam. This drug may be taken with milk.
Alcohol: Alcohol may increase the sedative effects of alprazolam. Alprazolam may increase the intoxicating effects of alcohol. Avoid alcohol completely if you find it necessary to drive or to engage in *any* hazardous activity.
Tobacco Smoking: Heavy smoking may reduce the calming action of alprazolam.
Marijuana Smoking: Occasional (once or twice weekly): Sedative effect increased mildly. Daily: Marked increase in the sedative effect of this drug.
Other Drugs:
Alprazolam may *increase* the effects of
• digoxin (Lanoxin) and cause digoxin toxicity.
Alprazolam may *decrease* the effects of
• levodopa (Sinemet, etc.), and reduce its antiparkinsonism effect.
The following drugs may *increase* the effects of alprazolam
• ethanol (alcohol).
• cimetidine (Tagamet).
• disulfiram (Antabuse).
• fluoxetine (Prozac).
• isoniazid (INH, Rifamate, etc.).
• omeprazole (Prilosec).
• oral contraceptives.
• valproic acid (Depakene).
The following drugs may *decrease* the effects of alprazolam
• carbamazepine (Tegretol).
• rifampin (Rimactane, etc.).
• theophylline (aminophylline, Theo-Dur, etc.).

Alprazolam *taken concurrently* with

- alcohol (ethanol) will worsen the decline in coordination and mental abilities.
- buspirone (BuSpar) may result in additive central nervous system (CNS) depression.
- benzodiazepines (see Drug Classes) will cause increased central nervous system (CNS) depression.
- narcotics (morphine, meperidene, and others) will cause additive central nervous system (CNS) depression and breathing (respiratory) depression.
- tricyclic antidepressants (see Drug Classes) may result in additive central nervous system (CNS) depression.

Driving, Hazardous Activities: This drug can impair alertness, judgment, coordination, and reaction time. Avoid hazardous activities accordingly.

Discontinuation: Reduce dose gradually by 1 mg/week until a total daily dose of 4 mg is reached; by 0.5 mg/week until a total daily dose of 2 mg is reached; then by 0.25 mg/week thereafter. Ask your doctor for help.

▷ **Saving Money When Using This Medicine:**
- Make use of available generic forms. Ask your doctor if this medicine offers the best combination of price and beneficial outcomes for you.
- Use this drug for the shortest time necessary (this decreases the probability of dependence or withdrawal).
- See if your community or workplace offers nondrug stress management courses to help cope with stress and anxiety.

AMANTADINE (a MAN ta deen)

Prescription Needed: Yes   **Controlled Drug:** No   **Generic:** Yes

Brand Names: Symadine, Symmetrel

Overview of BENEFITS versus RISKS	
Possible Benefits	*Possible Risks*
PARTIAL RELIEF OF RIGIDITY, TREMOR, AND IMPAIRED MOTION in parkinsonism	Skin rashes, mild to severe
	Confusion, hallucinations
	Congestive heart failure
PREVENTION AND TREATMENT OF INFECTIONS CAUSED BY INFLUENZA TYPE A VIRUSES*	Increased prostatism
	Abnormally low white blood cell counts

▷ **Illness This Medication Treats:**
  (1) All forms of parkinsonism; (2) prevention and treatment of infections caused by strains of influenza type A virus.
  Other (unlabeled) generally accepted uses: (1) can help bed-wetting (enuresis) in children; (2) may help some multiple sclerosis (MS) patients who struggle with a sense of fatigue that keeps them from living a normal life.

▷ **Typical Dosage Range:** (Dosage or schedule must be determined by the doctor for each individual.)
  Antiparkinsonism: 100 mg once or twice daily. The total daily dose should not exceed 400 mg. Antiviral (flu): 200 mg once daily, or 100 mg/12 hr.

▷ **Conditions Requiring Dosing Adjustments:**
  Kidney function: Dosing must be carefully adjusted for patients with kidney compromise, and blood levels are advised.
  Epilepsy: Doses of 200 mg per day or greater should be avoided because of increased seizure risks.

▷ **How Best to Take This Medicine:**   May be taken with or following meals. The capsule may be opened.

▷ **How Long This Medicine Is Usually Taken:**   Use up to 2 weeks usually determines the effectiveness of this drug in relieving the symptoms of parkinsonism. Long-term use (months to years) requires periodic evaluation of response—see your doctor regularly.

*This drug is NOT effective for the prevention or treatment of viral infections other than those caused by influenza type A viruses.

If you are exposed to influenza type A, continual daily dosage is needed for at least 10 days. During epidemics, this drug may be taken for 6 to 8 weeks.

▷ **Tell Your Doctor Before Taking This Medicine If You:**
- ever had an allergic reaction to it.
- have any type of seizure disorder.
- have a history of serious emotional or mental disorder.
- have a history of heart disease, especially previous heart failure.
- have impaired liver or kidney function.
- have a history of peptic ulcer disease or low white blood cell counts (leukopenia).
- have eczema or recurring eczemalike skin rashes.

▷ **Possible Side Effects:** Light-headedness, dizziness, feeling faint in upright position. Dry mouth, constipation. Reddish-blue coloration of the feet or legs.

▷ **Possible Adverse Effects:**
If any of the following develop, call your doctor promptly for guidance.
Some Mild Problems Drug Can Cause
Allergic reaction: skin rash.
Headache, nervousness, insomnia.
Unsteadiness, visual and speech disturbances.
Loss of appetite.
Some Serious Problems Drug Can Cause
Allergic reaction: severe eczemalike skin rashes.
Idiosyncratic reactions: confusion, depression, hallucinations.
Increased seizure activity, or catatonia if abruptly stopped.
Swelling of the arms, feet, or ankles.
Congestive heart failure (rare).
Aggravation of prostatism.
Abnormally low white blood cell counts: fever, sore throat, infections.

▷ *CAUTION*
1. Do not exceed a total dose of 400 mg/24 hr. Watch closely for signs of adverse effects with doses over 200 mg/24 hr.
2. This drug may lose its antiparkinsonism effect after 3 to 6 months. If this happens, see your doctor about changing the dose or drug.
3. This drug is reported to increase susceptibility to rubella (German measles).
4. Call your doctor if you develop early signs of congestive heart failure: shortness of breath, mild cough, ankle or foot swelling.
5. Safety and effectiveness of this drug for patients less than 1 year old are not established.

6. Watch patients over 60 closely for confusion, delirium, and hallucinations. Patients with prostatism may have aggravated symptoms.

7. Complete blood counts and heart, liver, and kidney function should be checked periodically while this drug is being taken.

Advisability of Use During Pregnancy or If Breast-Feeding:
Pregnancy Category: C. Avoid during the first 3 months if possible. Ask your doctor for help. Present in breast milk; avoid taking this drug or refrain from nursing.

▷ **Habit-Forming Potential:** This drug does have a potential for abuse, as it can cause euphoria, hallucinations, and feelings of detachment.

▷ **Overdose Symptoms:** Hyperactivity, confusion, hallucinations, aggression, toxic psychosis, seizures, heart rhythm disturbances, drop in blood pressure.

▷ **While Taking This Drug the Following Apply:**
Beverages: May be taken with milk.
Alcohol: May impair mental function and lower blood pressure excessively.
Other Drugs:
Amantadine may *increase* the effects of
- atropinelike drugs used to treat parkinsonism, such as benztropine (Cogentin), orphenadrine (Disipal), and trihexyphenidyl (Artane). If doses are too large, concurrent use with amantadine may cause mental confusion, delirium, hallucinations, and nightmares.
- levodopa (Dopar, Larodopa, Sinemet, etc.) and enhance therapeutic effectiveness. It may also cause acute mental disturbances.

The following drugs may *increase* the effects of amantadine
- amphetamine and amphetaminelike stimulant drugs may cause excessive stimulation and adverse behavioral effects.
- hydrochlorothiazide + triamterene may increase the level of amantadine.

Amantadine *taken concurrently* with
- co-trimoxazole, sulfamethoxazole, or trimethoprim may increase the risk of central nervous system (CNS) stimulation or arrhythmias.

Driving, Hazardous Activities: This drug may cause drowsiness, dizziness, blurred vision, or confusion. Use caution.
Exposure to Cold: Use caution. Chilling may enhance skin discoloration of the feet and legs (livedo reticularis).
Discontinuation: When used to treat parkinsonism, this drug should NOT be stopped suddenly, as it may cause an acute parkinsonian crisis. If used to treat influenza A infections, this drug should be continued for 48 hours after all symptoms are gone.

▷ **Saving Money When Using This Medicine:**
- Make use of generic forms and ask your doctor if this drug provides the best combination of price and outcome for you.
- If you are taking this medicine in order to help with a case of the flu, talk with your doctor about the benefits of getting a flu shot BEFORE next year's flu season begins (before the end of November).

AMILORIDE (a MIL oh ride)

Prescription Needed: Yes   **Controlled Drug:** No   **Generic:** Yes

Brand Names: Midamor, Moduretic [CD]

Overview of BENEFITS versus RISKS	
Possible Benefits	*Possible Risks*
EFFECTIVE DIURETIC WITHOUT LOSS OF POTASSIUM	ABNORMALLY HIGH BLOOD POTASSIUM with excessive use
	Bone marrow depression (rare)
	Rare liver toxicity
	Rare kidney failure
	Rare heart arrhythmias

▷ **Illness This Medication Treats:**
(1) Excessive fluid retention (edema); (2) high blood pressure.
Other (unlabeled) generally accepted use: may help increased urination that can happen in people who take lithium.
As Combination Drug Product [CD]: Combined with other diuretics to prevent potassium loss.

▷ **Typical Dosage Range:** (Dosage or schedule must be determined by the doctor for each individual.)
Initially 5 mg once daily, preferably in the morning. Dosage may be increased up to 15 mg daily, as needed and tolerated. Dose should not exceed 20 mg/24 hr.

▷ **Conditions Requiring Dosing Adjustments:**
Liver function: Accumulation of this drug will occur in hepatorenal (both liver and kidney compromise) syndrome. Use this drug with extreme caution.
Kidney function: Amiloride should NOT be used by patients with acute or chronic kidney failure.

▷ **How Best to Take This Medicine:**   Take when you wake up on an empty stomach. May be taken with food to reduce stomach upset. Tablet may be crushed.

▷ **How Long This Medicine Is Usually Taken:**   As needed for elimination of edema or maintenance of normal blood pressure.

▷ **Tell Your Doctor Before Taking This Medicine If You:**
- ever had an allergic reaction to it.
- know your blood potassium level is above the normal range.
- realize your kidneys are not making urine.
- have diabetes or glaucoma.
- have a history of kidney disease or impaired kidney function.
- are taking diuretics, blood pressure drugs, digitalis, or lithium.

▷ **Possible Side Effects:**   High potassium level, low sodium level, dehydration, constipation.

▷ **Possible Adverse Effects:**
If any of the following develop, call your doctor promptly for guidance.
Some Mild Problems Drug Can Cause
   Allergic reactions: skin rash, itching.
   Headache, dizziness, numbness and tingling.
   Dry mouth, nausea/vomiting, diarrhea.
   Loss of scalp hair.
Some Serious Problems Drug Can Cause
   Idiosyncratic reactions: joint and muscle pains.
   High potassium level—confusion, numbness, and tingling of lips and extremities, slow and irregular heartbeats.
   Increased internal eye pressure (of concern in glaucoma).
   Mental depression, visual disturbances, ringing in ears, tremors.
   Aplastic anemia—fatigue, fever, sore throat, abnormal bleeding.

▷ **Possible Effects on Sex Life:**   Decreased libido and impotence.

▷ *CAUTION*
   1. Do not take potassium supplements or eat more high-potassium foods.
   2. Potassium levels must be checked, especially if you are taking digitalis.
   3. Do not stop taking this drug abruptly unless your doctor said to do so.
   4. Safety and effectiveness of this drug in those younger than 12 years old are not established.
   5. Patients over 60 who use amiloride for an extended time can have excessive loss of body water and an increased tendency to abnormal blood clotting.

Advisability of Use During Pregnancy or If Breast-Feeding:

Pregnancy Category: B. Use this drug only if clearly needed. Presence in breast milk is unknown, but it is probably present; avoid taking this drug if possible.

▷ **Overdose Symptoms:** Thirst, drowsiness, fatigue, nausea, vomiting, confusion, numbness and tingling of face and extremities, irregular heart rhythm, shortness of breath.

▷ **While Taking This Drug the Following Apply:**

Foods: Avoid excessive restriction of salt and high-potassium foods.

Beverages: May be taken with milk.

Alcohol: Alcohol can exaggerate the blood pressure–lowering effect of this drug and cause orthostatic hypotension.

Other Drugs:

Amiloride may *increase* the effects of

• other blood pressure–lowering drugs. Dosage adjustments may be necessary.

Amiloride may *decrease* the effects of

• digoxin (Lanoxin, etc.), reducing its effectiveness.

Amiloride *taken concurrently* with

• ACE inhibitors (see Drug Classes) can result in abnormally high blood potassium.

• NSAIDs (see Drug Classes) may blunt the lowering of blood pressure.

• potassium supplements may result in dangerously elevated blood potassium levels.

• spironolactone (Aldactone, Aldactazide) or triamterene (Dyrenium, Dyazide) may cause a dangerous increase in blood potassium levels.

• lithium (Lithobid, others) may cause lithium to accumulate to toxic levels.

Driving, Hazardous Activities: This drug may cause drowsiness, dizziness, and orthostatic hypotension. Use caution.

Exposure to Heat: Caution is advised. Excessive perspiration can cause water, sodium, and potassium imbalance, as well as lowering of blood pressure.

Occurrence of Unrelated Illness: Call your doctor if you have an illness causing vomiting or diarrhea.

Discontinuation: With high dosage or prolonged use, stopping this drug suddenly can cause a very low potassium level. It is best to withdraw this drug gradually.

▷ **Saving Money When Using This Medicine:**

• Make use of generic forms available.

• Ask your doctor if the potency of this medicine in treating high blood pressure matches the degree of increase of your blood pressure.

AMINOPHYLLINE (am in OFF i lin)

Other Name: Theophylline ethylenediamine

Prescription Needed: Yes

Brand Names: Amesec [CD], Aminophylline, Mudrane [CD], Mudrane GG [CD], Phyllocontin, Truphylline

Overview of BENEFITS versus RISKS	
Possible Benefits	*Possible Risks*
EFFECTIVE PREVENTION AND RELIEF OF ACUTE BRONCHIAL ASTHMA	NARROW TREATMENT RANGE
MODERATELY EFFECTIVE CONTROL OF CHRONIC, RECURRENT BRONCHIAL ASTHMA	FREQUENT STOMACH DISTRESS
	Gastrointestinal bleeding
Moderately effective symptomatic relief in chronic bronchitis and emphysema	Central nervous system toxicity, seizures
	Heart rhythm disturbances

▷ **Illness This Medication Treats:**

(1) The shortness of breath and wheezing characteristic of acute bronchial asthma, and to prevent the recurrence of asthmatic episodes; (2) also useful in relieving the asthmalike symptoms associated with some types of chronic bronchitis and emphysema.

As Combination Drug Product [CD]: This drug is available in combination with several other drugs that help in the management of bronchial asthma and related conditions. Ephedrine is added to enhance bronchodilator effects; guaifenesin is added to help thin mucus secretions in the bronchial tubes; phenobarbital is added to allay anxiety that often accompanies acute asthma.

▷ **Typical Dosage Range:** (Dosage or schedule must be determined by the doctor for each individual.)

Note: Once you take aminophylline, this drug yields 79% theophylline, the active medicine. See the theophylline profile for further information.

AMITRIPTYLINE (a mee TRIP ti leen)

Prescription Needed: Yes   **Controlled Drug:** No   **Generic:** Yes

Brand Names: Amitril, Elavil, Emitrip, Endep, Etrafon [CD], Etrafon-A [CD], Etrafon Forte [CD], Limbitrol [CD], SK-amitriptyline, Triavil [CD]

Overview of BENEFITS versus RISKS	
Possible Benefits	*Possible Risks*
EFFECTIVE RELIEF OF ENDOGENOUS DEPRESSION	ADVERSE BEHAVIORAL EFFECTS: confusion, disorientation, hallucinations CONVERSION OF DEPRESSION TO MANIA in manic-depressive disorders Irregular heart rhythms Blood cell abnormalities (rare)

▷ **Illness This Medication Treats:**

Symptoms of spontaneous (endogenous) depression.

Other (unlabeled) generally accepted uses: helps treat chronic pain and other pain syndromes as an additive (adjuvant).

As Combination Drug Product [CD]: Available in combination with chlordiazepoxide to relieve anxiety that may accompany depression. Also available in combination with perphenazine, a strong tranquilizer, to relieve severe agitation that may accompany depression.

▷ **Typical Dosage Range:** (Dosage or schedule must be determined by the doctor for each individual.)

Initially 25 mg two to four times daily. Dose may be increased cautiously as needed and tolerated by 10 to 25 mg daily at intervals of 1 week. Usual maintenance dose is 50 to 100 mg every 24 hours. Total dose should not exceed 150 mg/24 hr. When the best individual dose is determined, it may be taken at bedtime.

▷ **Conditions Requiring Dosing Adjustments:**

Liver function: Use of lower doses—along with careful monitoring for adverse effects and a check of blood levels—is prudent.

Kidney function: Use with caution and frequent blood levels.

▷ **How Best to Take This Medicine:** May be taken without regard to meals. Tablet can be crushed.

▷ **How Long This Medicine Is Usually Taken:** Adequate response may require continual use for 4 to 6 weeks or longer. Long-term use should not exceed 6 months without evaluation. See your doctor.

▷ **Tell Your Doctor Before Taking This Medicine If You:**
- ever had an allergic reaction to it.
- are taking or have taken within the past 14 days any MAO type A inhibitor drug (see Drug Classes).
- have a history of liver or kidney problems, schizophrenia, blood cell disorders, sexual dysfunction, or intestinal block.
- are recovering from a recent heart attack.
- have narrow-angle glaucoma.
- have a history of diabetes, epilepsy, glaucoma, heart disease, prostate gland enlargement, or overactive thyroid.
- plan to have surgery under general anesthesia soon.

▷ **Possible Side Effects:**   Drowsiness, blurred vision, dry mouth, constipation, impaired urination.

▷ **Possible Adverse Effects:**
If any of the following develop, call your doctor promptly for guidance.
Some Mild Problems Drug Can Cause
  Allergic reactions: skin rash, hives, swelling of face or tongue, drug fever.
  Headache, dizziness, fainting, tremors.
  Confusion or nightmares.
  Peculiar taste, irritation of mouth, nausea, indigestion.
  Fluctuation of blood sugar levels.
Some Serious Problems Drug Can Cause
  Allergic reactions: hepatitis, with or without jaundice.
  Idiosyncratic reactions: neuroleptic malignant syndrome.
  Hallucinations, worsening of psychosis in schizophrenic patients.
  Abnormal heart rhythm.
  Bone marrow depression—weakness, fever, sore throat, abnormal bleeding or bruising.
  Rare bowel obstruction, severe eye movement problems.
  Peripheral neuritis—numbness, tingling, weakness.
  Parkinson-like disorders.

▷ **Possible Effects on Sex Life:**   Decreased libido, increased libido (antidepressant effect), impotence, inhibited female orgasm, inhibited ejaculation, male and female breast enlargement, milk production, swelling of testicles. These effects usually disappear within 2 to 10 days after the drug is stopped.

▷ *CAUTION*
  1. It is advisable to withhold this drug if electroconvulsive therapy (ECT) is to be used to treat your depression.
  2. Safety and effectiveness of this drug for those under 12 years old are not established.
  3. The elderly should take much lower starting doses and half the usual maintenance dose. Patients over 60 should be watched dur-

ing the first 2 weeks of treatment for confusion, agitation, forgetfulness, disorientation, delusions, difficulty urinating, and falling.

Advisability of Use During Pregnancy or If Breast-Feeding:

Pregnancy Category: D. Avoid use of this drug during first 3 months. Use during last 6 months only if clearly needed. Present in breast milk in small amounts. Watch the infant closely; stop taking this drug or nursing if adverse effects develop.

▷ **Habit-Forming Potential:** Psychological or physical dependence is rare and unexpected.

▷ **Overdose Symptoms:** Confusion, hallucinations, marked drowsiness, heart palpitations, dilated pupils, tremors, stupor, deep sleep, coma, convulsions.

▷ **While Taking This Drug the Following Apply:**

Foods: This drug may increase your appetite and cause excessive weight gain.

Beverages: May be taken with milk.

Alcohol: Avoid completely. This drug can markedly increase the intoxicating effects of alcohol and worsen depression of brain function.

Tobacco Smoking: Higher doses of amitriptyline may be necessary to get a therapeutic effect.

Other Drugs:

Amitriptyline may *increase* the effects of

- albuterol.
- antihistamines (see Drug Classes); may increase risk of urinary retention, glaucoma, or bowel obstruction.
- atropinelike drugs (see Drug Classes).
- cimetidine (Tagamet).
- disulfiram (Antabuse).
- phenytoin (Dilantin).

Amitriptyline may *decrease* the effects of

- clonidine (Catapres).
- guanethidine (Ismelin).
- guanfacine (Hytrin).
- methyldopa.

Amitriptyline *taken concurrently* with

- amphetamines can blunt the amphetamine response.
- anticoagulants (blood thinners) may increase risk of bleeding.
- carbamazepine (Tegretol) may lower amitriptyline blood levels.
- epinephrine can cause increased heart rate and blood pressure.
- ethanol (alcohol) can increase nerve toxicity.
- fluoxetine (Prozac) can cause very high levels of amitriptyline.
- flovoxamine (Luvox) can cause increased amitriptyline blood levels.
- MAO type A inhibitor drugs may cause high fever, delirium, and convulsions (see Drug Classes).

- quinidine (Quinaglute, others) can increase amitriptyline blood levels.
- thyroid preparations may impair heart rhythm and function. Ask your doctor for guidance regarding adjustment of thyroid dose.

Driving, Hazardous Activities: This drug may impair mental alertness, judgment, physical coordination, and reaction time. Avoid hazardous activities.

Exposure to Sun: This drug may cause photosensitivity.

Exposure to Heat: This drug may decrease sweating and impair the body's adaptation to hot environments, increasing the risk of heatstroke. Avoid saunas.

Exposure to Cold: The elderly should use caution and avoid conditions conducive to hypothermia.

Discontinuation: It is best to discontinue taking this drug gradually. Abrupt withdrawal after long-term use can cause headache, malaise, and nausea.

▷ **Saving Money When Using This Medicine:**

- Current data do NOT demonstrate a difference in benefit in treating depression between older or newer drugs. Ask your doctor to select the least expensive medicine that successfully treats your depression and causes the fewest side effects.
- If this medicine is being used to treat a pain syndrome, ask your doctor if evaluation at a pain center by a multispecialty team is appropriate.

AMLODIPINE   (am LOH di peen)

Prescription Needed: Yes   **Controlled Drug:** No   **Generic:** No

Brand Names: Norvasc

Controversies in Medicine: Results of several studies have indicated that medicines in this chemical family should NOT be used in some patients with extremely compromised hearts. Amlodipine (Norvasc) is the only calcium channel blocker that presently has data to show that it is SAFE, even in the most severely ill congestive heart failure patients. Amlodipine is also the only calcium channel blocker to be FDA-approved as safe for use in treating hypertension or angina in patients who also have congestive heart failure. There have been several FDA hearings on calcium channel blockers in general.

One retrospective chart review yielded data showing that there was increased risk if nifedipine immediate-release forms were used for treating conditions other than angina in those over 71. There was a caution advised, but the form of nifedipine in question was not approved for uses other than angina. A recent FDA panel found medicines in this class to be safe and effective. A study of nearly 6,000 patients at Tel Aviv Medical Center found that there was no statistically significant risk of death in patients who took calcium channel blockers versus those who did not take these medicines.

Overview of BENEFITS versus RISKS	
Possible Benefits	*Possible Risks*
EFFECTIVE PREVENTION OF BOTH MAJOR TYPES OF ANGINA	Peripheral edema in feet and ankles
EFFECTIVE TREATMENT OF HYPERTENSION	Dose-related changes in heart rhythm

▷ **Illness This Medication Treats:**
  (1) Angina pectoris due to coronary artery spasm (Prinzmetal's variant angina) not associated with exertion; (2) classical angina-of-effort (due to atherosclerotic coronary artery disease) patients who did not respond to or tolerate nitrates and beta-blocker drugs (even those with congestive heart failure); (3) mild to moderate hypertension (even those with congestive heart failure).
  Other (unlabeled) generally accepted uses: (1) may reverse or block atherosclerosis, (2) may help premature labor, (3) can help prevent migraine headaches.

▷ **Typical Dosage Range:** (Dosage or schedule must be determined by the doctor for each individual.)
  Infants and Children: Dosage not established.
  12 to 60 Years of Age: 2.5 to 10 mg daily, in a single dose.
  Over 60 Years of Age: Same as for 12 to 60 years of age.

▷ **Conditions Requiring Dosing Adjustments:**
  Liver function: People with damaged livers should be started on a daily 2.5 mg dose, and have the dose slowly increased as needed and tolerated.
  Low protein diet or starvation: If protein is low, an increased drug effect may be seen even with "normal" doses. Dose lowering may be needed until low protein is corrected.

▷ **How Best to Take This Medicine:** May be taken with or following food to reduce stomach irritation. The tablet may be crushed for administration.

▷ **How Long This Medicine Is Usually Taken:** Use on a regular schedule for 2 to 4 weeks usually determines the effectiveness of this drug in reducing the frequency and severity of angina or controlling hypertension. The smallest effective dose should be used for long-term therapy (months to years), and physician supervision and periodic evaluation is essential.

▷ **Tell Your Doctor Before Taking This Medicine If You:**
- ever had an allergic reaction to it.
- have active liver disease or have had drug-induced liver damage.
- have low blood pressure—systolic pressure below 90.
- are currently taking any form of digitalis or a beta-blocker (see Drug Classes).
- are taking any drugs that lower blood pressure.
- have a history of congestive heart failure, heart attack, left ventricle failure, aorta stenosis, muscular dystrophy, circulation problems in your hands, or stroke.
- are subject to disturbances of heart rhythm.

▷ **Possible Side Effects:** Swelling of feet and ankles, flushing and sensation of warmth. Overgrowth of the gums.

▷ **Possible Adverse Effects:**
If any of the following develop, call your doctor promptly for guidance.
Some Mild Problems Drug Can Cause
Allergic reactions: skin rash.
Headache, dizziness, fatigue, nausea, joint and muscle aches, rare eye pain or double vision.
Some Serious Problems Drug Can Cause
Allergic reactions: elevated liver enzymes.
Rare exfoliative dermatitis or erythema multiforme.
Very rare agranulocytosis.
Dose-related changes in heart rhythms.
Dyspnea—difficulty breathing.

▷ **Possible Effects on Sex Life:** Decrease in male or female sex drive. Rare swelling and tenderness of male breast tissue (gynecomastia).

▷ *CAUTION*
1. Tell all prescribers of medicine who provide care for you that you are taking this drug. Carry a card that states you take amlodipine.
2. You may use nitroglycerin and other nitrate drugs as needed to relieve acute anginal pain. If your angina attacks are becoming more frequent or intense, call your doctor promptly.
3. Safety and effectiveness of this drug for those under 12 years old are not established.
4. Low starting and ongoing (maintenance) doses are indicated for the elderly. Patients over 60 may be more susceptible to development of weakness, dizziness, fainting, and falling. Take precautions to prevent injury.

Advisability of Use During Pregnancy or If Breast-Feeding:
Pregnancy Category: C. Avoid this drug during the first 3 months. Use during the last 6 months only if clearly needed. Ask your doctor for help. Presence in breast milk is unknown; avoid taking this drug or refrain from nursing.

▷ **Overdose Symptoms:** Weakness, light-headedness, fainting, fast pulse, low blood pressure, shortness of breath, flushed and warm skin, tremors.

▷ **Suggested Periodic Examinations While Taking This Drug:** (at doctor's discretion)
Evaluations of heart function, including electrocardiograms; measurements of blood pressure in supine, sitting, and standing positions.

▷ **While Taking This Drug the Following Apply:**
Foods: Avoid excessive salt intake.
Beverages: May be taken with milk.
Alcohol: Use with caution until combined effects have been determined. Alcohol may exaggerate the drop in blood pressure experienced by some individuals.
Tobacco Smoking: Nicotine may reduce the effectiveness of this drug.
Marijuana Smoking: May possibly reduce the effectiveness of this drug; mild to moderate increase in angina; possible changes in electrocardiogram, confusing interpretation.
Other Drugs:
Amlodipine *taken concurrently* with
• adenosine (Adenocard) may cause problems with slow heart rate.
• beta-blocker drugs or digitalis preparations (see Drug Classes) may adversely affect heart rate and rhythm. Your doctor MUST monitor you closely if these drugs are taken at the same time.
• cyclosporine (Sandimmune) can cause increased blood levels of cyclosporine and may lead to toxicity.
• rifampin (Rifater, others) may result in decreased therapeutic benefit of amlodipine.
The following drug may *increase* the effects of amlodipine
• cimetidine (Tagamet).
Driving, Hazardous Activities: Usually no restrictions. This drug may cause dizziness. Restrict your activities as necessary.
Exposure to Heat: Caution is advised. Hot environments can exaggerate the blood pressure–lowering effects of this drug. Watch for light-headedness or weakness.
Heavy Exercise or Exertion: This drug may let you increase your activity without resulting angina pain. Use caution and avoid excessive exercise that could impair heart function without warning pain.

Discontinuation: Do not stop taking this drug abruptly. Ask your doctor about gradual withdrawal. Watch for possible rebound angina.

▷ **Saving Money When Using This Medicine:**
- Make sure that the potency of this medicine matches the degree of increase in your blood pressure.
- If your high blood pressure is associated with narrowing of the arteries and elevated cholesterol, ask your doctor about also taking an HMG CoA inhibitor. These medicines have been shown to actually prevent first heart attacks.
- Talk with your doctor about the benefits versus risks of taking aspirin every other day.
- Ask your doctor if this medicine offers the best combination of price and outcomes for you.

AMOXAPINE (a MOX a peen)

Prescription Needed: Yes **Controlled Drug:** No **Generic** No

Brand Names: Asendin

Overview of BENEFITS versus RISKS	
Possible Benefits	*Possible Risks*
EFFECTIVE RELIEF OF PRIMARY DEPRESSIONS: endogenous, neurotic, reactive	ADVERSE BEHAVIORAL EFFECTS: confusion, delusions, disorientation, hallucinations
Well tolerated by most persons	CONVERSION OF DEPRESSION TO MANIA in manic-depressive disorders
	Rare blood cell abnormalities
	Rare seizures or movement disorders
	Rare liver toxicity

▷ **Illness This Medication Treats:**
Symptomatic relief in all types of depression.
Other (unlabeled) generally accepted uses: may be a second-line agent in panic attacks.

▷ **Typical Dosage Range:** (Dosage or schedule must be determined by the doctor for each individual.)
Initially 50 mg two or three times daily. Dose may be increased cautiously on the third day as needed and tolerated to 100 mg three times daily. Usual maintenance dose is 200 to 300 mg every 24

hours. Total dosage should not exceed 400 mg/24 hr. When determined, the optimal requirement may be taken at bedtime as one dose, not to exceed 300 mg. Some cases of loss of benefit (tolerance) have occurred. Talk to your doctor if this medicine appears to stop working for you.

▷ **Conditions Requiring Dosing Adjustments:**
Liver function: Specific guidelines are not available for adjustment for patients with liver compromise; however, the use of lower doses and a check of blood levels is prudent.
Kidney function: The steps taken for liver compromise are prudent for patients with compromised kidneys.

▷ **How Best to Take This Medicine:** May be taken without regard to meals. Tablet may be crushed for administration.

▷ **How Long This Medicine Is Usually Taken:** Benefits may occur within 4 to 7 days in some people, but use on a regular schedule for 2 to 3 weeks usually determines this drug's effectiveness. Long-term use should not exceed 6 months without a follow-up office visit to your doctor to make certain the drug is still needed and still working.

▷ **Tell Your Doctor Before Taking This Medicine If You:**
- ever had an allergic reaction to it, or are overly sensitive to other antidepressant drugs.
- are taking or have taken within the past 14 days any MAO type A inhibitor drug (see Drug Classes).
- are recovering from a recent heart attack.
- have a history of diabetes, epilepsy, glaucoma, heart disease, paranoia, asthma, a blood cell disorder, prostate gland enlargement, schizophrenia, or overactive thyroid.
- plan to have surgery under general anesthesia soon.

▷ **Possible Side Effects:** Drowsiness, blurred vision, dry mouth, constipation, impaired urination.

▷ **Possible Adverse Effects:**
If any of the following develop, call your doctor promptly for guidance.
Some Mild Problems Drug Can Cause
Allergic reactions: skin rash, swellings, drug fever.
Insomnia, nervousness, palpitations, dizziness, tremors, fainting.
Peculiar taste, nausea, vomiting.
Some Serious Problems Drug Can Cause
Idiosyncratic reactions: neuroleptic malignant syndrome.
Behavioral effects: confusion, hallucinations, delusions.
Aggravation of paranoid psychosis and schizophrenia.
Aggravation of epilepsy (seizures).

Parkinson-like disorders.
Peripheral neuritis—numbness, weakness.
Reduced white blood cell count—fever, sore throat.
Rare hepatitis.

▷ **Possible Effects on Sex Life:** Decreased libido (150 mg/day), increased libido (antidepressant effect), inhibited ejaculation (75–150 mg/day), painful ejaculation (75 mg/day), inhibited female orgasm (100 mg/day), female breast enlargement/milk production (300 mg/day), altered menstrual timing and pattern (300 mg/day), swelling of testicles. These effects usually disappear within 2 to 10 days after the drug is stopped.

▷ *CAUTION*
1. The dose of this drug must be adjusted carefully for each individual. Laboratory tests of drug levels may be needed.
2. Watch for signs of toxicity: confusion, agitation, rapid heartbeat.
3. It is best to withhold this drug if electroconvulsive therapy is to be used.
4. Safety and effectiveness of this drug for those under 16 years old are NOT established.
5. For those 60 or older, during the first 2 weeks of treatment watch for confusion, restlessness, agitation, forgetfulness, disorientation, delusions, and hallucinations. It may be necessary to decrease the dose or stop using this drug. Unsteadiness may lead to falling and injury. This drug can worsen impaired urination often seen with prostate gland enlargement. Taking the total dose at bedtime will reduce the risk of postural hypotension.

Advisability of Use During Pregnancy or If Breast-Feeding:
Pregnancy Category: C. Avoid using this drug during first 3 months. Use during the last 6 months only if clearly needed. Present in breast milk in small amounts. Monitor the nursing infant closely and discontinue this drug or nursing if adverse effects develop.

▷ **Overdose Symptoms:** Confusion, hallucinations, marked drowsiness, tremors, dilated pupils, cold skin, stupor, coma, convulsions, rapid heartbeat, low blood pressure.

▷ **Suggested Periodic Examinations While Taking This Drug:** (at doctor's discretion)
Complete blood cell counts, periodic 24-hour blood pressure readings and electrocardiograms.

▷ **While Taking This Drug the Following Apply:**
Foods: This drug may increase your appetite and cause excessive weight gain.
Beverages: May be taken with milk.

Alcohol: Avoid completely. This drug may markedly increase the intoxicating effects of alcohol and worsen its depressant action on brain function.

Tobacco Smoking: May increase drug elimination and require higher doses.

Other Drugs:

Amoxapine may ***increase*** the effects of
- amphetamines.
- atropinelike drugs (see Drug Classes).
- oral anticoagulants (such as warfarin). Increased INR (prothrombin time) testing is needed.

Amoxapine may ***decrease*** the effects of
- clonidine (Catapres).
- guanethidine (Ismelin).
- guanfacine (Tenex).

Amoxapine ***taken concurrently*** with
- acetazolamide (Diamox) can increase blood levels of amoxapine.
- antihistamines may increase urinary retention or dry mouth.
- diphenhydramine (Benadryl) and other antihistamines may increase the risk of bowel obstruction (ileus).
- MAO type A inhibitor drugs may cause high fever, delirium, and convulsions (see Drug Classes).
- phenytoin (Dilantin) may lead to increased amoxapine blood levels and toxicity.
- quinidine (Quinaglute) may result in amoxapine toxicity.
- thyroid preparations may impair heart rhythm and function. Ask your doctor for guidance regarding adjustment of thyroid dose.

Driving, Hazardous Activities: This drug may impair mental alertness, judgment, physical coordination, and reaction time. Avoid hazardous activities.

Exposure to Sun: Use caution until your sensitivity to the sun has been determined. This drug may cause photosensitivity.

Exposure to Heat: This drug can inhibit sweating and impair the body's adaptation to hot environments, increasing the risk of heatstroke. Avoid saunas.

Exposure to Cold: The elderly should use caution and avoid conditions conducive to hypothermia.

Discontinuation: It is best to discontinue taking this drug gradually. Abrupt withdrawal after long-term use can cause headache, malaise, and nausea.

▷ **Saving Money When Using This Medicine:**
- Newer agents for depression may have fewer side effects. Talk with your doctor about other medicines if this one causes problems for you.

- Ask your doctor if you are getting adequate exercise and have an appropriate diet.
- Lower starting doses and ongoing doses are indicated in older patients.
- Ask your doctor if this drug offers the best combination of outcome and price for you.

AMOXICILLIN (a mox i SIL in)

Prescription Needed: Yes   **Controlled Drug:** No   **Generic:** Yes

Brand Names: Amoxil, Larotid, Polymox, Trimox, Utimox, Wymox

Overview of BENEFITS versus RISKS	
Possible Benefits	*Possible Risks*
EFFECTIVE TREATMENT OF INFECTIONS due to susceptible microorganisms	ALLERGIC REACTIONS, mild to severe
	Superinfections (yeast)
	Drug-induced colitis

▷ **Illness This Medication Treats:**

(1) Some genitourinary tract infections; (2) acute uncomplicated gonorrhea, male and female; (3) acute otitis media (middle ear infection); (4) helps acute bacterial infections of the sinuses and throat or skin and soft tissues.

Other (unlabeled) generally accepted uses: Treatment of: (1) bronchitis; (2) biliary tract infections; (3) Lyme disease; (4) typhoid fever; (5) gonorrheal infection of the urethra; (6) combination antibiotic treatment of duodenal ulcer disease caused by *Helicobacter pylori*.

▷ **Typical Dosage Range:** (Dosage or schedule must be determined by the doctor for each individual.)

Infants and Children: Up to 6 kg of body weight: 25 to 50 mg every 8 hours.

6 to 8 kg of body weight: 50 to 100 mg every 8 hours.

8 to 20 kg of body weight: 6.7 to 13.3 mg per kilogram of body weight every 8 hours.

20 kg of body weight and over: Same as for 12 to 60 years of age.

12 to 60 Years of Age: Usual dose: 250 to 500 mg every 8 hours. The total daily dose should not exceed 4.5 g.

For gonorrhea: 3 g, together with 1 g of probenecid, taken as a single dose.

For Lyme disease: 250 to 500 mg, three or four times a day, for 10 to 30 days; dosage and duration of treatment as appropriate for the severity of infection and the response to treatment.

Over 60 Years of Age: Dose may need to be lowered because of the age-related decline in kidney function.

▷ **Conditions Requiring Dosing Adjustments:**

Kidney function: The dosing interval **must** be adjusted for patients with renal compromise: for patients with moderate to severe kidney compromise, the usual dose should be taken every 6–12 hours. People with severe kidney problems should take the usual dose every 12–16 hours.

▷ **How Best to Take This Medicine:**   May be taken on an empty stomach or with food, milk, fruit juice, ginger ale, or other cold drinks. The capsule may be opened for administration. The oral suspension should be shaken well before measuring each dose. The chewable tablets should be chewed or crushed.

▷ **How Long This Medicine Is Usually Taken:**   For all streptococcal infections: Not less than 10 consecutive days (without interruption), to reduce the possibility of developing rheumatic fever or glomerulonephritis. For all other infections: As long as necessary to kill the infection.

▷ **Tell Your Doctor Before Taking This Medicine If You:**

- ever had an allergic reaction to it or are allergic by nature (hay fever, asthma, hives, eczema).
- are certain you are allergic to *any* form of penicillin.
- are allergic to any cephalosporin anti-infective drugs (Ancef, Ceporan, Ceporex, Kafocin, Keflex, Keflin, Kefzol, Loridine, others).
- have a history of liver or kidney disease.

▷ **Possible Side Effects:**   Superinfections, often due to yeast organisms.

▷ **Possible Adverse Effects:**

If any of the following develop, call your doctor promptly for guidance.

Some Mild Problems Drug Can Cause

Allergic reactions: skin rashes, hives, itching.

Irritations of mouth and tongue, nausea, vomiting, mild diarrhea.

Some Serious Problems Drug Can Cause

Allergic reactions: anaphylactic reaction, severe skin reactions, drug fever.

Swollen painful joints, sore throat, abnormal bleeding or bruising.

Drug-induced pseudomembranous colitis: severe abdominal pain and diarrhea.

Very rare liver or kidney toxicity.

▷ *CAUTION*

1. Take the exact dose and the full course prescribed.
2. Amoxicillin should not be used concurrently with antibiotics such as erythromycin or tetracycline.

3. A generalized rash occurs in about 90% of people who take this drug while they have mononucleosis. In infants and children amoxicillin may cause diarrhea which persists, and requires discontinuation of the medication.

4. People over 60 may have itching reactions in the genital and anal regions—call your doctor if this occurs.

5. People over 60 can have decreased kidney function and may need lower doses.

Advisability of Use During Pregnancy or If Breast-Feeding:

Pregnancy Category: B. Ask your doctor for guidance. Present in breast milk. The nursing infant may be sensitized to penicillin and may be at risk for developing diarrhea or yeast infections. Avoid taking this drug if possible or refrain from nursing.

▷ **Overdose Symptoms:**   Possible nausea, vomiting, and/or diarrhea.

▷ **Suggested Periodic Examinations While Taking This Drug:** (at doctor's discretion)
Complete blood cell counts.

▷ **While Taking This Drug the Following Apply:**
Beverages: May be taken with milk, fruit juices, or carbonated drinks.
Alcohol: No interactions expected, but alcohol can blunt the immune response.
Other Drugs:
Amoxicillin may ***decrease*** the effects of
• oral contraceptives (birth control pills) in some women, and result in unwanted pregnancy.

The following drugs may ***decrease*** the effects of amoxicillin
• antacids may reduce absorption.
• chloramphenicol (Chloromycetin).
• erythromycin (Erythrocin, E-Mycin, etc.).
• tetracyclines (Achromycin, Declomycin, Minocin, etc.; see Drug Classes).

Amoxicillin ***taken concurrently*** with
• H2-blockers (cimetidine, ranitidine, nizatidine, or famotidine) may increase the absorption of amoxicillin.
• probenecid will decrease how quickly amoxicillin will be removed from the body.

Driving, Hazardous Activities: Usually no restrictions. Be alert to the rare occurrence of dizziness and/or nausea, and restrict your activities accordingly.

Special Storage Instructions: Oral suspension and pediatric drops should be refrigerated.

Observe the Following Expiration Times: Do not take the oral suspension or drops of this drug if kept at room temperature longer than 7 days or refrigerated for 14 days.

▷ **Saving Money When Using This Medicine:**
- Generic forms are available and are recommended. Ask your doctor if this medicine offers the best combination of outcomes and price for you.
- If you have compromised kidneys, make sure your dose is decreased.
- Take this medicine exactly as prescribed. Missing a dose can give the infection a chance to come back.

AMOXICILLIN/CLAVULANATE   (a mox i SIL in/KLAV yu lan ayt)

Prescription Needed: Yes   **Controlled Drug:** No   **Generic:** No

Brand Names: Augmentin

Overview of BENEFITS versus RISKS

Possible Benefits	*Possible Risks*
EFFECTIVE TREATMENT OF INFECTIONS due to susceptible microorganisms	ALLERGIC REACTIONS, mild to severe
	Superinfections (yeast)
	Drug-induced colitis
	Rare low white blood cells

▷ **Illness This Medication Treats:**
As a Combination Drug Product [CD]: Uses currently included in FDA-approved labeling: Treats: (1) some genitourinary tract infections; (2) certain bacterial pneumonias; (3) acute bacterial otitis media (middle ear infection) and sinusitis; (4) some acute bacterial infections of the skin and soft tissues.

Other (unlabeled) generally accepted uses: treatment of: (1) bronchitis; (2) biliary tract infections; (3) chancroid; (4) cat bite.

▷ **Typical Dosage Ranges:** (Dosage or schedule must be determined by the doctor for each individual.)

Infants and Children: Up to 40 kg of body weight: 6.7 to 13.3 mg (amoxicillin) per kilogram of body weight every 8 hours.

40 kg of body weight and over: Same as for 12 to 60 years of age.

12 to 60 Years of Age: Usual dose: 250 to 500 mg (amoxicillin) every 8 hours. The total daily dose should not exceed 4.5 g.

Over 60 Years of Age: Same as for 12 to 60 years of age.

Note: These dosages refer to the amoxicillin component of this combination drug. The 250 mg regular tablet and the 250 mg chewable tablet contain different amounts of clavulanate and are not interchangeable.

▷ **Conditions Requiring Dosing Adjustments:**

Liver function: Specific guidelines do not exist regarding adjustment, and the prescriber must be aware that some accumulation of clavulanate will occur. This drug has been associated with liver problems and should be discontinued if liver enzymes are increased and jaundice (usually cholestatic) occurs.

Kidney function: Amoxicillin is primarily eliminated via the kidneys and the dose **must** be adjusted for patients with kidney compromise.

▷ **How Best to Take This Medicine:**   May be taken on an empty stomach or with food, milk, fruit juice, ginger ale, or other cold drinks. Oral suspension should be shaken well before measuring each dose. The regular tablets may be crushed before taken. The chewable tablets should be chewed or crushed.

▷ **How Long This Medicine Is Usually Taken:**   For all streptococcal infections: Not less than 10 consecutive days (without interruption), to reduce the possibility of developing rheumatic fever or glomerulonephritis. For all other infections: As long as necessary to eradicate the infection.

▷ **Tell Your Doctor Before Taking This Medicine If You:**
- ever had an allergic reaction to it.
- are certain you are allergic to *any* form of penicillin.
- are allergic to any cephalosporin anti-infective drugs (Ancef, Ceporan, Ceporex, Kafocin, Keflex, Keflin, Kefzol, Loridine, others).
- have a history of low blood counts.
- are allergic by nature (hay fever, asthma, hives, eczema).
- have a history of liver or kidney disease.

▷ **Possible Side Effects:**   Superinfections, often due to yeast organisms.

▷ **Possible Adverse Effects:**

If any of the following develop, call your doctor promptly for guidance.

Some Mild Problems Drug Can Cause

Allergic reactions: skin rashes, hives, itching.

Irritations of mouth and tongue, nausea, vomiting, mild diarrhea.

Some Serious Problems Drug Can Cause

Allergic reactions: anaphylactic reaction, severe skin reactions, drug fever.

Swollen painful joints, sore throat, abnormal bleeding or bruising.

Drug-induced pseudomembranous colitis: severe abdominal pain and diarrhea.

Rare lowering of white blood cell counts or hepatitis.

▷ *CAUTION*

1. Take the exact dose and the full course prescribed.
2. This drug should not be used concurrently with antibiotics such as erythromycin or tetracycline.
3. A generalized rash occurs in 90% of people who have mononucleosis. Amoxicillin also commonly causes diarrhea in children and infants and its use may need to be discontinued.
4. People over 60 may have an itching reaction in the genitals or anal area—call your doctor if this occurs.
5. The typical age-related decline in kidney function often means that the dose should be decreased for those over 60.

Advisability of Use During Pregnancy or If Breast-Feeding:

Pregnancy Category: B. Ask your doctor for help. Present in breast milk. The nursing infant may be sensitized to penicillin and may be at risk for developing diarrhea or yeast infections. Avoid taking this drug if possible or refrain from nursing.

▷ **Overdose Symptoms:** Possible nausea, vomiting, and/or diarrhea.

▷ **Suggested Periodic Examinations While Taking This Drug:** (at doctor's discretion)
Complete blood cell counts.

▷ **While Taking This Drug the Following Apply:**

Beverages: May be taken with milk, fruit juices, or carbonated drinks.
Other Drugs:
Amoxicillin may *decrease* the effects of
- oral contraceptives (birth control pills) in some women, and impair their effectiveness in preventing pregnancy.
The following drugs may *decrease* the effects of amoxicillin
- antacids reduce the absorption of amoxicillin.
- chloramphenicol (Chloromycetin).
- erythromycin (Erythrocin, E-Mycin, etc.).
- tetracyclines (Achromycin, Declomycin, Minocin, etc.).
Amoxicillin *taken concurrently* with
- H2-blockers (cimetidine, ranitidine, nizatidine, or famotidine) may increase amoxicillin absorption.
- probenecid will increase blood levels (can be used to benefit therapy).
Driving, Hazardous Activities: Usually no restrictions. Be alert to the rare occurrence of dizziness and/or nausea, and restrict your activities accordingly.
Special Storage Instructions: Oral suspension and pediatric drops should be refrigerated.
Observe the Following Expiration Times: Do not take the oral suspension or drops of this drug if stored longer than 7 days at room temperature or refrigerated for 14 days.

▷ **Saving Money When Using This Medicine:**
- This antibiotic contains a specific inhibitor molecule that makes it a candidate for more resistant organisms. Ask your doctor if the infection really requires this drug and the drug offers the best combination of price and outcome for you.

AMPICILLIN (am pi SIL in)

Prescription Needed: Yes   **Controlled Drug:** No   **Generic:** Yes

Brand Names: Amcill, 500 Kit [CD], Omnipen, Omnipen Pediatric Drops, Polycillin, Polycillin Pediatric Drops, Polycillin-PRB [CD], Principen, Probampacin [CD], SK-Ampicillin, Totacillin

Overview of BENEFITS versus RISKS	
Possible Benefits	*Possible Risks*
EFFECTIVE TREATMENT OF INFECTIONS due to susceptible microorganisms	ALLERGIC REACTIONS, mild to severe
	Superinfections (yeast)
	Drug-induced colitis

▷ **Illness This Medication Treats:**
(1) Certain infections of the skin and soft tissues, the respiratory tract, the gastrointestinal tract, and the genitourinary tract (including gonorrhea in females); (2) also used to treat certain types of septicemia and meningitis.

As Combination Drug Product [CD]: May be combined with probenecid (Benemid) to help maintain a therapeutic blood level.

▷ **Typical Dosage Range:** (Dosage or schedule must be determined by the doctor for each individual.)
500 to 1000 mg every 6 hours or 50 to 100 mg per kilogram of body weight per day, divided into four doses. The usual maximal dose is 6000 mg/24 hr.

▷ **Conditions Requiring Dosing Adjustments:**
Kidney function: The dose MUST be decreased for people with kidney damage.

▷ **How Best to Take This Medicine:** Best taken on an empty stomach, 1 hour before or 2 hours after eating. Capsule may be opened for administration.

▷ **How Long This Medicine Is Usually Taken:** For all streptococcal infections: Not less than 10 consecutive days (without interruption) to reduce the possibility of developing rheumatic fever or glomerulonephritis. For all other infections: As long as necessary to eradicate the infection.

▷ **Tell Your Doctor Before Taking This Medicine If You:**
- ever had an allergic reaction to it or are allergic by nature (hay fever, asthma, hives, eczema).
- are certain you are allergic to *any* form of penicillin.
- are allergic to cephalosporin antibiotics (Ancef, Ceporan, Ceporex, Kafocin, Keflex, Keflin, Kefzol, Loridine, others).
- have mononucleosis.

▷ **Possible Side Effects:** Superinfections, often due to yeast organisms or *Clostridium difficile*. Possible pseudomembranous colitis.

▷ **Possible Adverse Effects:**
If any of the following develop, call your doctor promptly for guidance.
Some Mild Problems Drug Can Cause
   Allergic reactions: skin rashes, hives, itching.
   Irritations of mouth and tongue, nausea, vomiting, mild diarrhea.
Some Serious Problems Drug Can Cause
   Allergic reactions: anaphylactic reaction, severe skin reactions, drug fever.
   Rare seizures with high blood levels.
   Swollen painful joints, sore throat, abnormal bleeding or bruising.
   Rare kidney problems (interstitial nephritis).

▷ *CAUTION*
   1. Take the exact dose and the full course prescribed.
   2. Ampicillin should not be used concurrently with antibiotics such as erythromycin or tetracycline.
   3. If ampicillin is taken by people with mononucleosis, 90% will get a generalized rash. In infants and children ampicillin also causes diarrhea, which may require the patient to stop taking the medication.
   4. Patients over 60 may have itching in the genitals and anal area—call your doctor if this happens.
   5. With increasing age there is a natural decline in kidney function. If you are over 60, the dose usually must be decreased.

Advisability of Use During Pregnancy or If Breast-Feeding:
Pregnancy Category: B. Ask your doctor for guidance. Present in breast milk in small amounts. Avoid taking this drug if possible, or refrain from nursing.

▷ **Overdose Symptoms:** Possible nausea, vomiting, and/or diarrhea.

▷ **Suggested Periodic Examinations While Taking This Drug:** (at doctor's discretion)
Complete blood cell counts.

▷ **While Taking This Drug the Following Apply:**

Beverages: May be taken with milk.

Other Drugs:

Ampicillin may **decrease** the effects of

- oral contraceptives (birth control pills) in some women, and impair their effectiveness in preventing pregnancy.

Ampicillin **taken concurrently** with

- allopurinol may increase risk of rash.
- atenolol can blunt the therapeutic benefits of atenolol.

The following drugs may **decrease** the effects of ampicillin

- antacids reduce the absorption of ampicillin.
- chloramphenicol (Chloromycetin).
- erythromycin (Erythrocin, E-Mycin, etc.).
- tetracyclines (Achromycin, Declomycin, Minocin, etc.).

Driving, Hazardous Activities: Usually no restrictions. Be alert to the rare occurrence of dizziness and/or nausea, and restrict your activities accordingly.

Special Storage Instructions: Oral suspension and pediatric drops should be refrigerated.

Observe the Following Expiration Times: Do not take the oral suspension or drops of this drug if kept more than 7 days at room temperature or refrigerated for 14 days.

▷ **Saving Money When Using This Medicine:**

- This medicine is a wonderful example of a drug that can often be used instead of one of the newer medicines, such as a quinolone (Floxin, Cipro, or Noroxin). If a newer (and usually broader spectrum) antibiotic is prescribed, ask your doctor if a narrower spectrum drug such as ampicillin can be used.
- Generic forms of this drug are available and may be substituted for the brand-name drug.

ASPIRIN* (AS pir in)

Prescription Needed: No   **Controlled Drug:** No   **Generic:** Yes

Brand Names: This is a representative list only. Alka-Seltzer Effervescent Pain Reliever & Antacid [CD], Alka-Seltzer Plus [CD], Anacin Maximum Strength [CD], A.S.A. Enseals, Aspergum, Bufferin [CD], Cama Arthritis Pain Reliever [CD], Cope [CD], Ecotrin Preparations, 8-Hour Bayer, Empirin, Excedrin [CD], Fiorinal [CD], Lortab

---

*In the United States *aspirin* is an official generic designation. In Canada *Aspirin* is the Registered Trade Mark of the Bayer Company Division of Sterling Drug Limited.

ASA [CD], Midol Caplets [CD], Norgesic [CD], Percodan [CD], Robaxisal [CD], Synalgos [CD], Synalgos-DC [CD], Talwin Compound [CD], Talwin Compound–50 [CD]

Overview of BENEFITS versus RISKS

Possible Benefits	*Possible Risks*
EFFECTIVE RELIEF OF MILD TO MODERATE PAIN and INFLAMMATION	Stomach irritation, bleeding, and/or ulceration
REDUCTION OF FEVER	Hearing loss
PREVENTION OF BLOOD CLOTS (as in heart attack, phlebitis, and stroke)	Decreased numbers of white blood cells and platelets
	Hemolytic anemia
REDUCES RISK OF HEART ATTACK	Rare liver toxicity
	Possible bronchospasm in asthmatics
PREVENTION OF SOME KINDS OF STROKE	
PREVENTION OF SOME COLON CANCERS	
REDUCES SEVERITY OF A HEART ATTACK IF ASPIRIN IS TAKEN SOON AFTER ONE STARTS	

▷ **Illness This Medication Treats:**
  (1) Mild to moderate pain; provides symptomatic relief in conditions characterized by inflammation and reduces high fever; (2) reduces the risk of recurrent heart attack; (3) prevents platelet embolism to the brain (in men); (4) reduces the risk of thromboembolism in patients recovering from a recent heart attack, in those with artificial heart valves, and in those undergoing hip surgery; (5) helps prevent stroke in patients who have transient ischemic attacks (TIAs).
  Other (unlabeled) generally accepted uses: (1) can help prevent toxemia of pregnancy when used in low doses; (2) may help decrease the risk of colon polyps or colon cancer in females (and probably men); (3) can limit the size and severity of a heart attack when it is taken immediately after symptoms start and is continued for at least 30 days thereafter.
  As Combination Drug Product [CD]: Frequently combined with other mild or strong analgesics to enhance pain relief. Also combined with antihistamines and decongestants in many cold preparations, to relieve the headache and general discomfort that often accompany respiratory infections.

▷ **Typical Dosage Range:** (Dosage or schedule must be determined by the doctor for each individual.)

Infants and Children: Up to 2 years of age: Consult your doctor.

2–4 years: 160 mg/4 hr, up to 5 doses/24 hr.

4–6 years: 240 mg/4 hr, up to 5 doses/24 hr.

6–9 years: 320 mg/4 hr, up to 5 doses/24 hr.

9–11 years: 400 mg/4 hr, up to 5 doses/24 hr.

11–12 years: 480 mg/4 hr, up to 5 doses/24 hr.

Do not exceed 5 days of continual use without consulting your doctor. Give all doses with food, milk, or a full glass of water.

Over 12 Years of Age: For pain or fever: 325 to 650 mg every 4 hours as needed. For arthritis (and related conditions): 3600 to 5400 mg daily in divided doses. For blood clot prevention: 80 to 150 mg every 24 to 48 hours.

▷ **Conditions Requiring Dosing Adjustments:**

Liver function: This drug should be avoided by patients with severe liver disease.

Kidney function: Aspirin can have an important effect on kidney function. Often in damaged kidneys, the kidneys rely on prostaglandins to work. Since this drug impairs prostaglandin biosynthesis, it should be avoided or used with caution by patients with kidney problems.

▷ **How Best to Take This Medicine:**   Take with food, milk, or a full glass of water to reduce stomach irritation. Regular tablets may be crushed and capsules opened for administration. Enteric-coated tablets, prolonged-action tablets, A.S.A. Enseals, Cama tablets, and Ecotrin tablets should not be crushed.

▷ **How Long This Medicine Is Usually Taken:**   Short-term use is recommended—3 to 5 days. Daily use should not exceed 10 days without your doctor's supervision. Use on a regular schedule for 1 week usually determines aspirin's effectiveness in relieving symptoms of chronic arthritis. Long-term use requires periodic evaluation of response and dosage adjustment in arthritis. Talk with your doctor to see if regular low-dose use makes sense for you because of your family history or present circumstances. See your doctor on a regular basis.

▷ **Tell Your Doctor Before Taking This Medicine If You:**

- ever had an allergic reaction to it.
- have any type of bleeding disorder (such as hemophilia).
- have active peptic ulcer disease.
- are in the last 3 months of pregnancy.
- have a history of angina.
- have a G6PD deficiency (talk with your doctor).
- are taking any anticoagulant drug.
- are taking oral antidiabetic drugs.
- have a history of peptic ulcer disease or gout.

- have lupus erythematosus.
- are pregnant or planning pregnancy.
- plan to have surgery of any kind soon.
- take other prescription or nonprescription medications that were not discussed when aspirin was prescribed for you.

▷ **Possible Side Effects:**   Mild drowsiness in some people.

▷ **Possible Adverse Effects:**
If any of the following develop, call your doctor promptly for guidance.

Some Mild Problems Drug Can Cause
Allergic reactions: skin rash, hives, nasal discharge, nasal polyps.
Stomach irritation, nausea, vomiting, constipation.

Serious Adverse Effects
Allergic reactions: acute anaphylactic reaction, asthma, unusual bruising due to allergic destruction of blood platelets.
Idiosyncratic reactions: hemolytic anemia.
Erosion of stomach lining, with "silent" bleeding.
Activation of peptic ulcer, with or without hemorrhage.
Bone marrow depression.
Liver damage (hepatitis with jaundice).
Kidney damage, if used in large doses or for a prolonged period of time.
May worsen angina attacks and make them occur more often.
Reye's syndrome if used during some viral illnesses in children.

▷ **Adverse Effects That May Mimic Natural Diseases or Disorders:**
Liver damage may suggest viral hepatitis.

▷ *CAUTION*
1. It is most important to understand that aspirin is a drug. Although it is one of our most useful drugs, we have an unrealistic sense of safety and lack of concern about its action in the body and its potential for adverse effects.
2. Make a point to learn the contents of all drugs you take—those prescribed by your doctor and those you purchase over-the-counter (OTC) without a prescription.
3. Do NOT take more than three tablets (975 mg) at one time, Allow at least 4 hours between doses and take no more than 10 tablets (3250 mg) in 24 hours without your doctor's supervision.
4. Remember that aspirin can cause new illnesses, complicate existing illnesses, complicate pregnancy, complicate surgery, or interact unfavorably with other drugs.
5. When your doctor asks whether you are taking any drugs, answer "yes" if you are taking aspirin. This also applies to *any* nonprescription drug you may be taking.

6. If you open the bottle and it smells like vinegar, throw the medicine away. This smell means that the aspirin has decomposed.
7. Reye's syndrome (can cause brain and liver damage in children, often fatal) can follow flu or chickenpox in children and teenagers. Although the exact cause and nature of the syndrome are not known, some reports suggest that the use of aspirin by children with these illnesses can increase the risk of developing this complication. Consult your doctor before giving aspirin to a child or teenager with chickenpox, flu, or similar infection.
8. The natural decline in kidney function can reduce tolerance for aspirin in those over 60 years old. Watch for nervous irritability, confusion, ringing in the ears, deafness, loss of appetite, nausea, and stomach irritation. Aspirin can cause excessive bleeding from the stomach in sensitive individuals. This can occur as "silent" bleeding of small amounts over an extended period of time, resulting in anemia. In addition, sudden hemorrhage can occur, even without a history of stomach ulcer. Observe stools for gray to black discoloration—an indication of stomach bleeding.

Advisability of Use During Pregnancy or If Breast-Feeding:

Pregnancy Category: C. Some studies show that regular use of aspirin is detrimental to the health of the mother and the welfare of the fetus. Talk with your doctor about any use of aspirin during pregnancy. Some toxemia of pregnancy has been helped by low doses of aspirin. Present in breast milk; avoid taking this drug or refrain from nursing.

▷ **Habit-Forming Potential:**   Use in large doses for a prolonged period of time may cause a form of psychological dependence.

▷ **Overdose Symptoms:**   Stomach distress, nausea, vomiting, ringing in the ears, dizziness, impaired hearing, sweating, stupor, fever, deep and rapid breathing, muscular twitching, delirium, hallucinations, convulsions.

▷ **Suggested Periodic Examinations While Taking This Drug:** (at doctor's discretion)
Complete blood cell counts.
Kidney function tests and urine analyses.
Liver function tests.

▷ **While Taking This Drug the Following Apply:**
Nutritional Support: Do not take large doses of vitamin C while taking aspirin on a regular basis.
Beverages: May be taken with milk.
Alcohol: No interactions expected. However, the concurrent use of alcohol and aspirin may significantly increase the possibility of erosion and ulceration of the stomach lining and may result in bleeding.

Other Drugs:

Aspirin may *increase* the effects of
- oral anticoagulants and cause abnormal bleeding. Dosage adjustment is often necessary.
- oral antidiabetic drugs and insulin, and cause hypoglycemia. Dosage adjustment is often necessary.
- heparin and cause abnormal bleeding.
- methotrexate and increase its toxic effects.
- valproic acid (Depakene).

Aspirin may *decrease* the effects of
- beta-adrenergic blockers (see Drug Classes).
- captopril (Capoten).
- furosemide (Lasix).
- other NSAIDs (see Drug Classes).
- probenecid (Benemid) and reduce its effectiveness in the treatment of gout, with aspirin doses of less than 2 g/24 hr.
- spironolactone (Aldactone) and reduce its diuretic effect.
- sulfinpyrazone (Anturane) and reduce its effectiveness in the treatment of gout, with aspirin doses of less than 2 g/24 hr.

The following drugs may *increase* the effects of aspirin
- acetazolamide (Diamox).
- cimetidine (Tagamet).
- para-aminobenzoic acid (Pabalate).
- vitamin C, taken as ascorbic acid and in large doses, may acidify the urine in some individuals and cause aspirin accumulation and toxicity.

The following drugs may *decrease* the effects of aspirin
- antacids, in regular continual use.
- cortisonelike drugs (see Drug Classes).
- urinary alkalizers (sodium bicarbonate, sodium citrate).

Aspirin *taken concurrently* with
- diltiazem (Cardizem) may result in an increased risk of bleeding.
- high blood pressure medicines may blunt their effectiveness.
- IUDs (intrauterine devices) may decrease their effectiveness.
- chickenpox (varicella) vaccine (Varivax) may result in Reye's syndrome. Avoid aspirin or other salicylates for 6 weeks following inoculation.

Discontinuation: Aspirin use should be discontinued completely at least 1 week before surgery of any kind.

▷ **Saving Money When Using This Medicine:**
- Generic forms are recommended. Ask your doctor if this drug offers the best combination of price and outcome for you.

ASTEMIZOLE (a STEM i zohl)

Prescription Needed: Yes   **Controlled Drug:** No   **Generic:** No

Brand Names: Hismanal

Overview of BENEFITS versus RISKS

Possible Benefits	*Possible Risks*
EFFECTIVE, LONG-LASTING RELIEF OF ALLERGIC RHINITIS AND ALLERGIC SKIN DISORDERS, WITH MINIMAL DROWSINESS MINOR ANTICHOLINERGIC SIDE EFFECTS	RARE HEART RHYTHM DISTURBANCES Mild fatigue (infrequent)

▷ **Illness This Medication Treats:**
(1) Allergies and related disorders: provides symptomatic relief to seasonal and perennial allergic rhinitis (hay fever), allergic conjunctivitis, and vasomotor rhinitis, and also in hives and localized swellings (angioedema) of allergic origin; (2) can help relieve vertigo.
Other (unlabeled) generally accepted uses: (1) may have a role in relieving lichen nitidus lesions; (2) can help ease some asthma symptoms.

▷ **Typical Dosage Range:** (Dosage or schedule must be determined by the doctor for each individual.)
10 mg once daily. The total daily dosage should not exceed 10 mg. Some serious heart rhythm problems have resulted from drug interactions that cause high blood levels.

▷ **Conditions Requiring Dosing Adjustments:**
Liver function: This drug should be used with caution by patients with hepatic disease.

▷ **How Best to Take This Medicine:** Take on an empty stomach, 1 hour before eating or 2 hours after eating. The tablet may be crushed.

▷ **How Long This Medicine Is Usually Taken:** Regular use for 3 days usually determines the effectiveness of this drug in relieving the symptoms of allergic rhinitis and dermatosis. Some people may need to take this drug during the entire pollen season. Antihistamines should not be taken continually (without interruption) for long-term use. Limit their use to periods that require symptomatic relief. See your doctor on a regular basis.

▷ **Tell Your Doctor Before Taking This Medicine If You:**
- ever had an allergic reaction to it.
- are currently undergoing allergy skin tests.
- are taking erythromycin, clarithromycin, itraconazole, sotalol, fluconazole, or ketoconazole.
- have a history of heart rhythm disorders.
- have impaired liver or kidney function.
- take other prescription or nonprescription medications that were not discussed when astemizole was prescribed for you.

▷ **Possible Side Effects:**   Dry nose, mouth, or throat.

▷ **Possible Adverse Effects:**
If any of the following develop, call your doctor promptly for guidance.
Some Mild Problems Drug Can Cause
Allergic reactions: skin rash, itching.
Headache, nervousness, fatigue.
Increased appetite and weight, nausea, diarrhea.
Some Serious Problems Drug Can Cause
Significant heart rhythm disorders (resulting from excessive dosage or interactions with other drugs).
Rare bronchospasm, paresthesias, or convulsions.

▷ *CAUTION*
1. Do not exceed the recommended dose; high blood levels may cause serious heart rhythm disturbances.
2. Do not take this drug with any form of erythromycin, clarithromycin, itraconazole, sotalol, fluconazole, or ketoconazole.
3. Report promptly the development of faintness, dizziness, heart palpitation, or chest pain.
4. Stop taking this drug 4 days before diagnostic skin testing procedures, to prevent false-negative results.
5. Safety and effectiveness of this drug for those under 12 years old are not established.
6. Those over 60 face an increased risk of fatigue. Smaller doses should be used, with a longer time between doses.
7. Since this medicine can have serious drug interactions, talk with your doctor or pharmacist BEFORE taking any other drugs.

Advisability of Use During Pregnancy or If Breast-Feeding:
Pregnancy Category: C. Use this drug only if clearly needed. Ask your doctor for guidance. Presence in breast milk is unknown; avoid taking this drug or refrain from nursing.

▷ **Overdose Symptoms:**   Serious heart rhythm abnormalities.

▷ **Suggested Periodic Examinations While Taking This Drug:** (at doctor's discretion)

Electrocardiograms for those with heart disorders.

▷ **While Taking This Drug the Following Apply:**

Beverages: May be taken with milk.

Other Drugs:

Astemizole *taken concurrently* with the following drugs may cause increased blood levels of astemizole and resulting heart rhythm disturbances

- azithromycin (Zithromax).
- clarithromycin (Biaxin).
- erythromycin.
- fluconazole (Diflucan).
- itraconazole (Sporonox).
- ketoconazole.
- sotalol.

Astemizole *taken concurrently* with

- sotalol may cause serious heartbeat abnormalities.

Hazardous Activities: Although this medicine has minimal potential to cause drowsiness compared to other antihistamines, use it with caution until you are certain of the effect the medicine will have on you.

Exposure to Sun: Use caution until your sensitivity has been determined. Rare cases of photosensitivity have been reported.

▷ **Saving Money When Using This Medicine:**

- Several nonsedating antihistamines are available on the market at the time of this writing. Ask your doctor to choose the least expensive one that will be most effective for you.

ATENOLOL (a TEN oh lohl)

Prescription Needed: Yes   **Controlled Drug:** No   **Generic:** No

Brand Names: Tenoretic [CD], Tenormin

Overview of BENEFITS versus RISKS	
Possible Benefits	*Possible Risks*
EFFECTIVE ANTIANGINAL DRUG in the management of effort-induced angina	CONGESTIVE HEART FAILURE in advanced heart disease
EFFECTIVE, WELL-TOLERATED ANTIHYPERTENSIVE in mild to moderate high blood pressure	Worsening of angina in coronary heart disease (abrupt withdrawal)
	Masking of low blood sugar (hypoglycemia) in drug-treated diabetes
	Provocation of bronchial asthma (with high doses)

▷ **Illness This Medication Treats:**
(1) Classic effort-induced angina pectoris; (2) mild to moderate high blood pressure. May be used alone or concurrently with other antihypertensives, such as diuretics. (3) Used following heart attacks to help decrease the risk of a second heart attack, decrease the amount of heart damage, and reduce risk of abnormal heartbeats.

▷ **Typical Dosage Range:** (Dosage or schedule must be determined by the doctor for each individual.)
Initially 50 mg once daily. Dose may be increased gradually at intervals of 7 to 10 days as needed and tolerated up to 100 mg/24 hr. The usual maintenance dose is 50 to 100 mg every 24 hours. The total dose should not exceed 100 mg/24 hr.
After a heart attack: Within 12 hours, 5 mg of this drug is given intravenously, followed by a second intravenous dose 10 minutes later. 12 hours after the second dose, 50 mg is taken orally, followed by a second dose of 50 mg 12 hours later. Oral dosing is then continued for the next 10 days.

▷ **Conditions Requiring Dosing Adjustments:**
Liver function: Unlike with many other beta-blockers, the liver is minimally involved in the elimination of this medication.
Kidney function: The dose must be decreased to a maximum of 25 mg/day for some people with kidney compromise.

▷ **How Best to Take This Medicine:** May be taken without regard to eating. Tablet may be crushed. Do not stop this drug abruptly.

▷ **How Long This Medicine Is Usually Taken:** Use on a regular schedule for 3 to 7 days usually determines the effectiveness of this drug in lowering blood pressure. Long-term use will be decided by the course of your blood pressure over time and your response to an overall treatment program (weight reduction, salt restriction, smoking cessation, etc.). See your doctor on a regular basis.

▷ **Tell Your Doctor Before Taking This Medicine If You:**
- ever had an allergic reaction to it.
- have congestive heart failure.
- have had a heart attack and have not responded to furosemide (Lasix).
- have an abnormally slow heart rate or a serious form of heart block.
- are taking, or have taken within the past 14 days, any MAO type A inhibitors (see Drug Classes).
- have had an adverse reaction to any beta-blocker drug in the past (see Drug Classes).
- have a history of serious heart disease, with or without episodes of heart failure.
- have a history of hay fever (allergic rhinitis), asthma, chronic bronchitis, or emphysema.
- have a history of hyperthyroidism.
- have a history of low blood sugar.
- have impaired liver or kidney function.
- have diabetes or myasthenia gravis.
- are currently taking any form of digitalis, quinidine, or reserpine, or any calcium blockers (see Drug Classes).
- plan to have surgery under general anesthesia soon.

▷ **Possible Side Effects:** Lethargy, fatigability, cold extremities, slow heart rate, light-headedness in upright position.

▷ **Possible Adverse Effects:**
If any of the following develop, call your doctor promptly for guidance.
Some Mild Problems Drug Can Cause
   Allergic reactions: skin rash, itching.
   Headache, dizziness, abnormal dreams.
   Indigestion, nausea, diarrhea.
   Joint and muscle discomfort, fluid retention (edema).
Some Serious Problems Drug Can Cause
   Mental depression, anxiety.
   Chest pain, shortness of breath, congestive heart failure.
   Induction of bronchial asthma (in asthmatics).
   Systemic lupus erythematosus (rare).
   Psychosis (very rare).

▷ **Possible Effects on Sex Life:** Decreased libido and impaired potency (50–100 mg/day). This beta-blocker is less likely to cause reduced erectile capacity than most other drugs of this class.

▷ *CAUTION*

1. ***Do not stop taking this drug suddenly*** without the knowledge and guidance of your doctor. Carry a note with you that states you are taking this drug.
2. Consult your doctor or pharmacist before using nasal decongestants. These can cause sudden increases in blood pressure when taken concurrently with beta-blockers.
3. Report the development of any tendency to emotional depression.
4. Safety and effectiveness of this drug for those under 12 years old are not established. If this drug must be used, low blood sugar may develop, especially if meals are skipped.
5. High blood pressure should be reduced slowly in those over 60. Small doses and frequent blood pressure checks are needed. Sudden or excessive decreases in blood pressure may lead to stroke or heart attack. Maximum daily dose in this population is 100 mg. The patient should be watched for dizziness, confusion, hallucinations, depression, or urinary frequency.
6. This drug (unlike other beta-blockers) is mainly removed by the kidneys. The dose MUST be decreased for patients with kidney disease or for those over 60.

Advisability of Use During Pregnancy or If Breast-Feeding:

Pregnancy Category: D (see Pregnancy Categories inside this book's cover). Avoid use of this drug during the first 3 months if possible. Avoid use during labor and delivery because of the possible effects on the newborn. Present in breast milk; avoid taking this drug if possible. If this drug is necessary, observe the nursing infant for slow heart rate and indications of low blood sugar.

▷ **Overdose Symptoms:** Weakness, slow pulse, low blood pressure, fainting, cold and sweaty skin, congestive heart failure, possible coma, and convulsions.

▷ **Suggested Periodic Examinations While Taking This Drug:** (at doctor's discretion)

Measurements of blood pressure, evaluation of heart function.

▷ **While Taking This Drug the Following Apply:**

Foods: Avoid excessive salt intake.

Beverages: May be taken with milk.

Alcohol: Use caution. Alcohol may exaggerate this drug's ability to lower blood pressure and increase its mild sedative effect.

Tobacco Smoking: Nicotine may reduce this drug's effectiveness in treating high blood pressure. High doses may worsen bronchial tightening caused by regular smoking.

Other Drugs:
Atenolol may *increase* the effects of
- other antihypertensive drugs and cause excessive lowering of blood pressure. Dosage adjustments may be necessary.
- reserpine (Ser-Ap-Es, etc.) and cause sedation, depression, slowing of heart rate, and lowering of blood pressure.

Atenolol *taken concurrently* with
- amiodarone (Cordarone) may cause cardiac arrest.
- ampicillin may cause greater increase in heart rate after exercise.
- calcium carbonate may decrease atenolol blood levels and lessen its therapeutic benefits.
- clonidine (Catapres) requires close monitoring for rebound high blood pressure if clonidine is withdrawn while atenolol is still being taken.
- insulin requires close monitoring to avoid undetected hypoglycemia.
- oral hypoglycemic agents (see Drug Classes) may result in prolonged low blood sugar.
- phenothiazines (see Drug Classes) may result in increased effects of both medicines and excessively low blood sugar.
- verapamil (Calan, others) may result in excessive slowing of heart rate and very low blood pressure.

The following drugs may *decrease* the effects of atenolol
- indomethacin (Indocin), and possibly other aspirin substitutes or NSAIDs, may impair atenolol's antihypertensive effect.

Driving, Hazardous Activities: Use caution until the full extent of drowsiness, lethargy, and blood pressure change has been determined.

Exposure to Heat: Caution is advised. Hot environments can lower blood pressure and exaggerate the effects of this drug.

Exposure to Cold: Caution is advised. Cold environments can enhance the circulatory deficiency in the extremities that may occur with this drug. The elderly should take precautions to prevent hypothermia.

Heavy Exercise or Exertion: It is advisable to avoid exertion that produces light-headedness, excessive fatigue, or muscle cramping. The use of this drug may intensify the hypertensive response to isometric exercise.

Occurrence of Unrelated Illness: Fever can lower blood pressure and require decreased dosing. Nausea or vomiting may interrupt the regular dosage schedule. Ask your doctor for guidance.

Discontinuation: Avoid sudden discontinuation of this drug in all situations. If possible, gradual reduction of the dose over a period of 2 to 3 weeks is recommended. Ask your doctor for specific guidance.

▷ **Saving Money When Using This Medicine:**
- Unfortunately, high blood pressure does not usually have any symptoms. Have your blood pressure checked periodically, and avoid the dangerous long-term problems of increased blood pressure by keeping your blood pressure under control.
- Ask your doctor or pharmacist about stress management programs in your community.

AURANOFIN (aw RAY noh fin)

Prescription Needed: Yes   **Controlled Drug:** No   **Generic:** No

Brand Names: Ridaura

Overview of BENEFITS versus RISKS	
Possible Benefits	*Possible Risks*
REDUCTION OF JOINT PAIN, TENDERNESS, AND SWELLING in active, severe RHEUMATOID ARTHRITIS	POSSIBLE SIGNIFICANTLY REDUCED LEVELS OF RED AND WHITE BLOOD CELLS AND BLOOD PLATELETS
Medication effective when taken by mouth	RARE LIVER DAMAGE WITH JAUNDICE
	Diarrhea, RARE ulcerative colitis
	Rare lung damage
	Skin rash
	Mouth sores

▷ **Illness This Medication Treats:**
Active, severe rheumatoid arthritis in adults, but only for those who have had an inadequate response to aspirin, aspirin substitutes, other antiarthritic drugs, and treatment programs. It is usually added to a well-established program of antiarthritic drugs of the NSAID class.

Other (unlabeled) generally accepted uses: may have a role in helping decrease the need for steroids in people with asthma.

▷ **Typical Dosage Range: (Dosage or schedule must be determined by the doctor for each individual.)**
6 mg daily, taken either as one dose every 24 hours or two doses of 3 mg each every 12 hours. If response is inadequate after 6 months of regular continual use, the dose may be increased to 9 mg daily, taken as three doses of 3 mg each. Discontinue taking this drug if response remains inadequate after 3 months of 9 mg daily.

▷ **Conditions Requiring Dosing Adjustments:**
Kidney function: Blood levels are recommended, and the dose should be decreased. Some patients benefit from 3 mg every other day.

▷ **How Best to Take This Medicine:**   Take with or following food to reduce stomach irritation. Take the capsule whole with milk or a full glass of water.

▷ **How Long This Medicine Is Usually Taken:**   Use on a regular schedule for 3 to 4 months usually determines the effectiveness of this drug in reducing the joint pain, tenderness, and swelling associated with rheumatoid arthritis. The extent of long-term use is determined by the degree of benefit and the pattern of adverse effects experienced by the individual patient. Consult your doctor regularly.

▷ **Tell Your Doctor Before Taking This Medicine If You:**
- had an allergic reaction or serious adverse effect from previous use of gold.
- have active ulcerative colitis.
- have a current blood cell or bone marrow disorder.
- have active liver or kidney disease.
- are pregnant, breast-feeding, or planning pregnancy in the near future.
- are taking penicillamine or antimalarial drugs for your arthritis.
- are allergic by nature, or have a history of allergic reactions to drugs.
- have diabetes.
- have a history of heart disease, high blood pressure, circulatory disorders, liver or kidney disease, or ulcerative colitis.
- have exfoliative dermatitis or fibrous replacement of the lung tissue (pulmonary fibrosis).

▷ **Possible Side Effects:**   Metallic taste.

▷ **Possible Adverse Effects:**
If any of the following develop, call your doctor promptly for guidance.
Some Mild Problems Drug Can Cause
  Allergic reactions: itching, skin rash.
  Sores in mouth, loss of appetite, nausea, vomiting, diarrhea.
  Headache, partial or complete hair loss.
Serious Adverse Effects
  Allergic reactions: severe skin reactions, exfoliative dermatitis.
  Fever, cough, shortness of breath, drug-induced pneumonia and lung damage.
  Liver damage with jaundice, ulcerative colitis.
  Kidney damage.

Blood cell and bone marrow toxicity—fatigue, weakness, sore throat, abnormal bleeding or bruising.

Peripheral neuritis—pain, numbness, weakness of arms and legs.

Rare pancreatitis.

▷ **Possible Effects on Sex Life:**   Possible tenderness and swelling of the male breast tissue (gynecomastia).

▷ *CAUTION*

1. Periodic examinations (blood and urine tests) are mandatory while using this drug. Keep all appointments as directed by your doctor.
2. Tell your doctor promptly of any indications of possible toxic re-actions. If there is a delay in reaching your doctor, discontinue taking this drug until you obtain medical guidance.
3. Safety and effectiveness of this drug for those under 12 years old are not established.
4. Small starting doses and close monitoring for adverse effects are indicated for those over 60 years old or for those with kidney dis-ease.

Advisability of Use During Pregnancy or If Breast-Feeding:

Pregnancy Category: C. The manufacturer does not recommend use of this drug during pregnancy. Present in breast milk; avoid taking this drug or refrain from nursing.

▷ **Overdose Symptoms:**   Nausea, vomiting, diarrhea, confusion, delir-ium, peripheral neuritis.

▷ **Suggested Periodic Examinations While Taking This Drug:** (at doctor's discretion)

Complete blood cell counts, urine analyses, liver and kidney function tests.

▷ **While Taking This Drug the Following Apply:**

Beverages: May be taken with milk.

Alcohol: Use caution. Alcohol may intensify the irritant effect of this drug on the gastrointestinal tract.

Other Drugs:

Auranofin may *increase* the effects of

- phenytoin (Dilantin) by increasing its blood level. Monitor closely for indications of phenytoin toxicity.

Auranofin *taken concurrently* with

- penicillamine may result in increased risk of bone marrow depres-sion.

Exposure to Sun: Use caution. This drug may cause photosensitivity. Avoid the sun and sunlamps if a drug-induced rash occurs.

▷ **Saving Money When Using This Medicine:**

- Ask your doctor if this medicine offers the best balance of price and outcomes for you.

AZATHIOPRINE (ay za THI oh preen)

Prescription Needed: Yes   **Controlled Drug:** No   **Generic:**
Yes

Brand Names: Imuran

Overview of BENEFITS versus RISKS

Possible Benefits	*Possible Risks*
REDUCTION OF JOINT PAIN, TENDERNESS, AND SWELLING in active, severe RHEUMATOID ARTHRITIS	UNACCEPTABLE ADVERSE EFFECTS
	REDUCED LEVELS OF WHITE BLOOD CELLS
PREVENTION OF REJECTION IN ORGAN TRANSPLANTATION	REDUCED LEVELS OF RED BLOOD CELLS AND PLATELETS
	RARE LIVER DAMAGE WITH JAUNDICE
	POSSIBLE INCREASED RISK OF MALIGNANCY

▷ **Illness This Medication Treats:**

(1) Helps prevent rejection in organ transplantation (mainly kidney transplants); (2) severe rheumatoid arthritis (in adults) that has failed to respond adequately to conventional treatment. Progression of the arthritic process may be slowed or even stopped.

Other (unlabeled) generally accepted uses: (1) treatment of lupus erythematosus, ulcerative colitis, chronic active hepatitis, and other autoimmune disorders; (2) may help prevent rejection of transplanted hearts.

▷ **Typical Dosage Range: (dosage or schedule must be determined by the doctor for each individual.)**

As immunosuppressant: 3 to 5 mg per kilogram of body weight daily, 1 to 3 days before transplantation surgery; for postoperative maintenance: 1 to 2 mg per kilogram of body weight daily. As antiarthritic: 1 mg per kilogram of body weight daily for 6 to 8 weeks; increase dose by 0.5 mg per kilogram of body weight every 4 weeks as needed and tolerated. Maximal daily dose is 2.5 mg per kilogram of body weight. Total dose may be taken once daily or divided into two equal doses taken 12 hours apart.

▷ **Conditions Requiring Dosing Adjustments:**

Liver function: No specific dosing guidelines are available; however, the drug may need to be stopped if jaundice occurs. Liver function must be watched.

Kidney function: The dose may need to be decreased by up to 50% for patients with kidney failure.

▷ **How Best to Take This Medicine:** Take with or following food to reduce stomach irritation. Tablet may be crushed.

▷ **How Long This Medicine Is Usually Taken:** Use on a regular schedule for 12 weeks usually determines the effectiveness of this drug in helping rheumatoid arthritis. Use for up to 11 years has been achieved. See your doctor regularly.

▷ **Tell Your Doctor Before Taking This Medicine If You:**
- ever had an allergic reaction to it.
- are pregnant and this drug is prescribed to treat rheumatoid arthritis, or are planning pregnancy in the near future.
- have an active or a history of blood cell or bone marrow disorder.
- are taking, or have recently taken, any form of chlorambucil (Leukeran), cyclophosphamide (Cytoxan), or melphalan (Alkeran).
- have any kind of active infection.
- have any form of cancer or blood cell disorder.
- have gout or are taking allopurinol (Zyloprim) or are taking any medicine from the ACE inhibitor class.
- have impaired liver or kidney function.
- are taking any form of gold, penicillamine, or antimalarial for arthritis.

▷ **Possible Side Effects:** Development of infection.

▷ **Possible Adverse Effects:**
If any of the following develop, call your doctor promptly for guidance.
Some Mild Problems Drug Can Cause
Allergic reaction: skin rash.
Loss of appetite, nausea, vomiting, diarrhea.
Sores on lips and in mouth.
Some Serious Problems Drug Can Cause
Allergic reactions: drug fever, joint and muscle pain.
Pancreatitis—stomach pain with nausea and vomiting.
Bone marrow depression.
Liver damage—yellow eyes and skin, dark-colored urine, light-colored stools.
Drug-induced pneumonia—cough, shortness of breath.
Development of cancer—skin cancer, reticulum-cell sarcoma, lymphoma, leukemia.

▷ **Possible Effects on Sex Life:** Reversal of male infertility that is due to the body's production of autoantibodies to sperm; this drug suppresses the formation of autoantibodies and permits normal accumulation of sperm as they are produced.

▷ **Possible Delayed Adverse Effects:** Bone marrow depression may become apparent many weeks after drug is discontinued.

▷ **Adverse Effects That May Mimic Natural Diseases or Disorders:**
    Liver damage may suggest viral hepatitis.

▷ *CAUTION*
    1. Report promptly any indications of a developing infection—fever, chills, lip or mouth sores, etc.
    2. Tell your doctor promptly if you become pregnant.
    3. Periodic blood counts are mandatory for the safe use of this drug. Report for examinations as directed.
    4. Safety and effectiveness of this drug for those under 12 years old are not established.
    5. The lowest effective dose should be used by people over 60 years old.

Advisability of Use During Pregnancy or If Breast-Feeding:
Pregnancy Category: D. Avoid using this drug completely during entire pregnancy if possible. Present in breast milk; avoid taking this drug or refrain from nursing.

▷ **Overdose Symptoms:** Immediate—nausea, vomiting, diarrhea. Delayed—lowered white blood cell and platelet counts.

▷ **Suggested Periodic Examinations While Taking This Drug:** (at doctor's discretion)
Complete blood cell counts, liver function tests.

▷ **While Taking This Drug the Following Apply:**
Beverages: May be taken with milk.
Other Drugs:
Azathioprine may ***decrease*** the effects of
• oral anticoagulants (warfarin, etc.), making it necessary to increase their dosage.
• certain muscle relaxants (gallamine, pancuronium, tubocurarine), making it necessary to increase their dosage.
The following drug may ***increase*** the effects of azathioprine
• allopurinol (Zyloprim) may increase its activity and toxicity, making it necessary to reduce its dosage.
Azathioprine ***taken concurrently*** with
• ACE inhibitors (see Drug Classes) may result in severe lowering of white blood cells or anemia.
• co-trimoxazole (Bactrim, others) may result in severe lowering of white blood cell counts.
• prednisolone will blunt prednisolone response.
Discontinuation: A gradual reduction in dosage is preferable. Consult your doctor for a withdrawal schedule.

▷ **Saving Money When Using This Medicine:**
• Generic forms are recommended.
• Ask your doctor if this medicine offers the best combination of price and outcome for you.

AZITHROMYCIN (a zith roh MY sin)

Prescription Needed: Yes   **Controlled Drug:** No   **Generic:** No

Brand Names: Zithromax

Overview of BENEFITS versus RISKS

Possible Benefits	*Possible Risks*
EFFECTIVE TREATMENT OF UPPER AND LOWER RESPIRATORY TRACT INFECTIONS DUE TO SUSCEPTIBLE MICROORGANISMS	Mild gastrointestinal symptoms
	Drug-induced colitis (rare)
	Superinfections (rare)
EFFECTIVE TREATMENT OF SKIN INFECTIONS DUE TO SUSCEPTIBLE MICROORGANISMS	
EFFECTIVE TREATMENT OF URETHRAL AND CERVICAL INFECTIONS DUE TO *CHLAMYDIA TRACHOMATIS*	

▷ **Illness This Medication Treats:**

(1) Certain upper respiratory tract infections—streptococcal pharyngitis and tonsillitis; (2) some cases of acute bronchitis and pneumonia; (3) skin (and skin structure) infections; (4) nongonococcal urethritis and cervicitis due to *Chlamydia trachomatis*; (5) AIDS-related *Mycobacterium avium-intracellulare complex*. Bacterial cultures and sensitivity testing should be performed.

Other (unlabeled) generally accepted uses: may have a role in treatment of AIDS-related toxoplasmosis infection.

▷ **Typical Dosage Range:** (Dosage or schedule must be determined by the doctor for each individual.)

Infants and Children: Dosage not established.

16 to 60 Years of Age: For pharyngitis/tonsillitis, bronchitis, pneumonia, and skin infections: 500 mg as a single dose on the first day; then 250 mg once daily on days 2 through 5 for a total dose of 1.5 g. For nongonococcal urethritis and cervicitis: A single 1 g dose.

Over 60 Years of Age: Same as for 16 to 60 years. If liver or kidney function is significantly impaired, reduce dose accordingly.

▷ **Conditions Requiring Dosing Adjustments:**

Liver function: Caution must be observed if the drug is used by patients with liver impairment; however, specific guidelines for dosage adjustment have not been developed.

Kidney function: Less than 10% of this medicine is removed by the kidneys; changes in dosing are not thought to be needed.

▷ **How Best to Take This Medicine:**   Do not take with food. Take at least 1 hour before eating or 2 hours after eating. Do not take antacids containing aluminum or magnesium with this drug. The capsule may be opened for administration. A new tablet form is expected to be available soon, which can be taken with food.

▷ **How Long This Medicine Is Usually Taken:**   Use on a regular schedule for 3 to 5 days usually determines this drug's effectiveness in controlling infections. For streptococcal throat infections: not less than 5 consecutive days (without interruption) to reduce the possibility of developing rheumatic fever or glomerulonephritis. AIDS-related uses are longer term.

▷ **Tell Your Doctor Before Taking This Medicine If You:**
  • ever had an allergic reaction to it.
  • are allergic to related drugs: clarithromycin, erythromycin, or troleandomycin.
  • have impaired liver or kidney function.
  • have a history of drug-induced colitis.

▷ **Possible Side Effects:**   Superinfections, usually due to yeast.

▷ **Possible Adverse Effects:**
If any of the following develop, call your doctor promptly for guidance.
Some Mild Problems Drug Can Cause
  Allergic reactions: skin rash.
  Headache, dizziness, drowsiness, fatigue.
  Palpitation, chest pain.
  Nausea, stomach pain, diarrhea.
Some Serious Problems Drug Can Cause
  Allergic reactions: rare angioedema (swelling of soft tissues).
  Rare drug-induced jaundice or colitis.
  Rare kidney problems or hearing loss.

▷ *CAUTION*
  1. If diarrhea develops and continues for more than 24 hours, call your doctor promptly. This could indicate the onset of drug-induced colitis.
  2. Take the full dosage prescribed to prevent the possible emergence of resistant bacterial strains.
  3. Safety and effectiveness of this drug for those under 16 years old are not established.
  4. The dose must be adjusted for those over 60 with kidney or liver problems.

Advisability of Use During Pregnancy or If Breast-Feeding:

Pregnancy Category: B. Use this drug only if clearly needed. Ask your doctor for help. Present in breast milk in small amounts. Monitor the nursing infant closely and discontinue the drug or nursing if adverse effects develop.

▷ **Overdose Symptoms:** Possible nausea, vomiting, abdominal discomfort, and diarrhea.

▷ **While Taking This Drug the Following Apply:**

Other Drugs:

Azithromycin may *increase* the effects of

- carbamazepine (Tegretol) by causing increased blood levels.
- cyclosporine (Sandimmune) and lead to toxicity.
- digoxin (Lanoxin, others).
- ergotamine or other ergot derivatives. This effect was not reported for azithromycin, but reported for other macrolide antibiotics—caution is advised.
- phenytoin (Dilantin).
- terfenadine (Seldane) may result in heart (cardiac) toxicity.
- theophylline (Theo-Dur, Theolair, etc.); monitor blood levels of theophylline if appropriate.
- warfarin (Coumadin); monitor INR (prothrombin times) if appropriate.

The following drugs may *decrease* the effects of azithromycin

- antacids containing aluminum or magnesium.

Azithromycin *taken concurrently* with

- astemizole and perhaps other nonsedating antihistamines may lead to increased blood levels of the antihistamine and adverse effects on the heart.

Driving, Hazardous Activities: This drug may cause dizziness, nausea, and/or diarrhea. Restrict your activities as necessary.

Exposure to Sun: Use caution until full effect is known. This drug can cause photosensitivity.

▷ **Saving Money When Using This Medicine:**

- Several new medicines in this class work in approximately the same way. Ask your doctor to prescribe the least expensive drug that gives the best outcomes.
- If you are taking an intravenous macrolide antibiotic in the hospital, ask your doctor if it can be changed to one taken by mouth so you can recover at home.

BECLOMETHASONE (be kloh METH a sohn)

Prescription Needed: Yes   **Controlled Drug:** No   **Generic:** No

Brand Names: Beclovent, Beconase AQ Nasal Spray, Beconase Nasal Inhaler, Vancenase AQ Nasal Spray, Vancenase Nasal Inhaler, Vanceril

---

Overview of BENEFITS versus RISKS

Possible Benefits	*Possible Risks*
EFFECTIVE RELIEF OF ALLERGIC RHINITIS	FUNGUS INFECTIONS OF THE MOUTH AND THROAT
EFFECTIVE CONTROL OF SEVERE, CHRONIC ASTHMA	Localized areas of allergic pneumonia
	Changes in the lining of the nose (mucosa)

▷ **Illness This Medication Treats:**
(1) Bronchial asthma when bronchodilators don't work and cortisone-like drugs are required for asthma control. Inhalation helps prevent the more serious adverse effects of systemic cortisone. (2) Prevention of nasal polyps once they've been removed; (3) eases seasonal and perennial rhinitis in children and adults (Vancenase AQ nasal form).

▷ **Typical Dosage Range:** (Dosage or schedule must be determined by the doctor for each individual.)
Nasal inhaler: One inhalation (42 mcg) two to four times daily. Oral inhaler: Two inhalations (84 mcg) three or four times daily. For severe asthma: 12 to 16 inhalations daily. The maximal daily dose should not exceed 20 inhalations.

▷ **Conditions Requiring Dosing Adjustments:**
Liver function: This drug should be used with caution by patients with liver compromise.

▷ **How Best to Take This Medicine:** May be used as needed without regard to eating. Rinse the mouth and throat (gargle) with water thoroughly after each inhalation.

▷ **How Long This Medicine Is Usually Taken:** Use on a regular schedule for 1 to 4 weeks usually determines the effectiveness of this drug in relieving severe, chronic allergic rhinitis and in controlling severe, chronic asthma. Long-term use must be supervised by your doctor. Consult your doctor regularly.

▷ **Tell Your Doctor Before Taking This Medicine If You:**
- ever had an allergic reaction to it.
- are experiencing severe acute asthma or status asthmaticus that requires more intense treatment for prompt relief.
- have asthma that can be controlled by noncortisone-related bronchodilators and other antiasthmatic drugs.
- have asthma that requires cortisonelike drugs infrequently for control.
- have a form of nonallergic bronchitis with asthmatic features.
- are now taking or have recently taken any cortisone-related drug (including ACTH by injection) for any reason.
- have a history of tuberculosis of the lungs.
- have chronic bronchitis or bronchiectasis or are prone to nosebleeds.
- think you may have an active infection of any kind, especially a respiratory infection or chickenpox.

▷ **Possible Side Effects:**   Fungus infections (thrush) of the mouth and throat.

▷ **Possible Adverse Effects:**
If any of the following develop, call your doctor promptly for guidance.
Some Mild Problems Drug Can Cause
  Allergic reaction: skin rash (rare).
  Dryness of mouth, hoarseness, sore throat.
  Nosebleeds.
Some Serious Problems Drug Can Cause
  Allergic reaction: allergic pneumonitis (lung inflammation).
  Bronchospasm (rare).
  Yeast infections.

▷ *CAUTION*
1. This drug should not be relied on for the immediate relief of acute asthma.
2. If you were using cortisone-related drugs for your asthma *before* transferring to this medicine, you may need to resume the former cortisone-related drug for an injury or infection of any kind, or if you require surgery. Tell your doctor of your prior use of cortisone-related drugs taken either by mouth or by injection.
3. If severe asthma returns while using this drug, notify your doctor immediately so that supportive treatment with cortisone-related drugs by mouth or injection can be provided as needed.
4. Carry a personal identification card with a notation (if applicable) that you have used cortisone-related drugs within the past year. During periods of stress it may be necessary to resume cortisone treatment in adequate dosage.

5. Wait 5 to 10 minutes after using inhaled bronchodilators such as epinephrine, isoetharine, or isoproterenol (which should be used first) before inhalation of this drug. This sequence will permit greater penetration of beclomethasone into the bronchial tubes. The delay between inhalations will also reduce the possibility of adverse effects from the inhaler propellants.

6. Safety and effectiveness of the nasal inhaler for those under 12 years old are not established. Safety and effectiveness of the oral inhaler for those under 6 years old are not established. Maximum daily dose in children 6 to 12 years old should not exceed 10 inhalations.

7. People with bronchiectasis should be watched closely for the development of lung infections.

Advisability of Use During Pregnancy or If Breast-Feeding:

Pregnancy Category: C. Avoid during the first 3 months. Use this drug infrequently and only as clearly needed during the last 6 months. Probably present in breast milk; avoid taking this drug or refrain from nursing.

▷ **Habit-Forming Potential:** With recommended dosage, a state of functional dependence is not likely to develop.

▷ **Overdose Symptoms:** Indications of cortisone excess (due to systemic absorption)—fluid retention, flushing of the face, stomach irritation, nervousness.

▷ **Suggested Periodic Examinations While Taking This Drug:** (at doctor's discretion)

Inspection of nose, mouth, and throat for evidence of fungus infection.

Assessment of the status of adrenal function in individuals who have used cortisone-related drugs over an extended period of time prior to using this drug.

Lung X ray of people with a history of tuberculosis.

▷ **While Taking This Drug the Following Apply:**

Other Drugs:

*The following drugs may **increase** the effects of beclomethasone*

• inhalant bronchodilators (epinephrine, isoetharine, isoproterenol).

• oral bronchodilators (aminophylline, ephedrine, terbutaline, theophylline, etc.).

Occurrence of Unrelated Illness: Acute infections, serious injuries, and surgical procedures can create an urgent need for additional supportive cortisone-related drugs taken by mouth and/or injection. Tell your doctor immediately in the event of new illness or injury of any kind.

Discontinuation: If the regular use of this drug has made it possible to reduce or discontinue maintenance doses of cortisonelike drugs by mouth, ***do not*** stop taking this drug abruptly. If you must stop taking this drug for any reason, call your doctor promptly. It may be necessary to resume cortisone preparations and to start other measures for satisfactory management.

Special Storage Instructions: Store at room temperature. Avoid exposure to temperatures above 120° F (49° C). Do not store or use this inhaler near heat or open flame. Protect it from light.

▷ **Saving Money When Using This Medicine:**
- Beclovent and Vanceril have inhalers which at the present contain the same active medicine, dose per use, and inactive ingredients. Ask your doctor to prescribe whichever inhaler is the least expensive.
- Ask your doctor if this medicine offers the best balance of price and outcome for you.

BENAZEPRIL (ben AY ze pril)

Prescription Needed: Yes   **Controlled Drug:** No   **Generic:** No

Brand Names: Lotensin

Overview of BENEFITS versus RISKS	
Possible Benefits	*Possible Risks*
EFFECTIVE CONTROL OF MILD TO MODERATE HIGH BLOOD PRESSURE	Headache, dizziness, fatigue
	Excessively low blood pressure
	Allergic swelling of face, tongue, throat, vocal cords

▷ **Illness This Medication Treats:**
Mild to moderate high blood pressure, either alone or concurrently with a thiazide diuretic.

▷ **Typical Dosage Range:** (Dosage or schedule must be determined by the doctor for each individual.)

Infants and Children: Dosage not established.

12 to 60 Years of Age: Dosing starts at 10 mg once daily for those not taking a diuretic; 5 mg once daily for those taking a diuretic. Usual maintenance dose is 20 to 40 mg per day taken in a single dose. If once-a-day dosing does not give stable control of blood pressure over a 24-hour period, divide the dose equally into morning and evening doses. Total daily dosage should not exceed 80 mg.

Over 60 Years of Age: Same as for 12 to 60 years of age, if kidney function is normal. If kidney function is significantly impaired, reduce dose by 50%. The total daily dose should not exceed 40 mg.

▷ **Conditions Requiring Dosing Adjustments:**
Kidney function: Some of this medicine is removed by the kidneys. For people with creatinine clearances of less than 30 ml/min, or serum creatinine concentrations of greater than 3 mg/dl, the initial dose should be 5 mg once daily.

▷ **How Best to Take This Medicine:** Take on an empty stomach or with food, at the same time each day. The tablet may be crushed for administration.

▷ **How Long This Medicine Is Usually Taken:** Use on a regular schedule for 2 to 3 weeks usually determines the effectiveness of this drug in controlling high blood pressure. Therapy may be long-term. See your doctor regularly.

▷ **Tell Your Doctor Before Taking This Medicine If You:**
- ever had an allergic reaction to it.
- are at least 6 months pregnant.
- currently have a blood cell or bone marrow disorder.
- have an abnormally high level of blood potassium.
- had an allergic reaction (or other adverse effect) on using any other ACE inhibitors.
- have a history of kidney disease or impaired kidney function, or think you are dehydrated.
- have scleroderma or systemic lupus erythematosus.
- have cerebral artery disease.
- are taking an immunosuppressant drug.
- have any form of heart disease or have renal artery stenosis.
- are taking any other antihypertensives, diuretics, nitrates, or potassium supplements.
- plan to have surgery under general anesthesia soon.

▷ **Possible Side Effects:** Dizziness, orthostatic hypotension, fainting, increased blood potassium level.

▷ **Possible Adverse Effects:**
If any of the following develop, call your doctor promptly for guidance.
Some Mild Problems Drug Can Cause
  Allergic reactions: skin rash, itching.
  Headache, fatigue, drowsiness.
  Cough.
  Nausea, vomiting, constipation.
Some Serious Problems Drug Can Cause
  Allergic reactions: swelling (angioedema) of face, tongue, and/or vocal cords; can be life-threatening.
  Impairment of kidney function.
  First-dose low blood pressure or angina and palpitations.
  Rare decreased white blood cells or hemoglobin, or psoriasis.

▷ **Possible Effects on Sex Life:**   Decreased libido, impotence. Rare enlargement and tenderness of male breast tissue.

▷ *CAUTION*

1. Talk with your doctor about the advisability of discontinuing other antihypertensive drugs (especially diuretics) for 1 week before starting this drug.
2. Call your doctor if your face or tongue becomes swollen after you start taking this medicine.
3. **Tell your doctor immediately if you become pregnant.** This drug should not be taken beyond the first 3 months of pregnancy.
4. **Report promptly** any indications of infection (fever, sore throat) and water retention (weight gain, puffiness, swollen feet or ankles).
5. Do not use a salt substitute without your doctor's knowledge and approval. (Many salt substitutes contain potassium.)
6. It is prudent to obtain blood cell counts and urine analyses **before** starting this drug.
7. Safety and effectiveness of this drug for infants and children are NOT established.
8. For people over 60 years old small doses are advisable until tolerance has been determined. Sudden and excessive lowering of blood pressure can predispose to stroke or heart attack in those with impaired brain circulation or coronary artery heart disease.

Advisability of Use During Pregnancy or If Breast-Feeding:
Pregnancy Category: D during the last 6 months of pregnancy. Avoid taking this drug completely during the last 6 months. During the first 3 months of pregnancy, use only if clearly needed (C). Ask your doctor for guidance. Present in breast milk in small amounts; avoid taking this drug or refrain from nursing.

▷ **Overdose Symptoms:**   Excessive drop in blood pressure, light-headedness, dizziness, fainting.

▷ **Possible Effects of Long-Term Use:**   Gradual increase in blood potassium level.

▷ **Suggested Periodic Examinations While Taking This Drug:**   (at doctor's discretion)
Before starting drug: complete blood cell counts; urine analysis with measurement of protein content; blood potassium level.
During use of drug: blood cell counts; measurements of blood potassium.

▷ **While Taking This Drug the Following Apply:**
Foods: Ask your doctor about salt intake.
Nutritional Support: **Do not take** potassium supplements unless directed by your doctor.

Beverages: May be taken with milk.

Alcohol: Use caution until combined effect has been determined. Alcohol may enhance the blood pressure–lowering effect of this drug.

Other Drugs:

Benazepril *taken concurrently* with

- aspirin may decrease the benefits of benazepril on heart action.
- bumetanide (Bumex) or furosemide (Lasix) may cause severe lowering of the blood pressure if you suddenly stand.
- chlorpromazine (Thorazine) may cause excessive lowering of blood pressure.
- cyclosporine (Sandimmune) may cause increased kidney toxicity.
- ketorolac (Toradol) may increase the risk of kidney toxicity.
- lithium (Lithobid, others) may lead to large increases in lithium blood levels and result in lithium toxicity.
- phenothiazines (see Drug Classes) may lead to sudden lowering of blood pressure.
- potassium preparations (K-Lyte, Slow-K, etc.) may cause increased blood levels of potassium with risk of serious heart rhythm disturbances.
- potassium-sparing diuretics—amiloride (Moduretic), spironolactone (Aldactazide), or triamterene (Dyazide)—may cause increased blood levels of potassium with risk of serious heart rhythm disturbances.

Driving, Hazardous Activities: Usually no restrictions. Be aware of possible drops in blood pressure with resultant dizziness or faintness.

Exposure to Sun: Caution is advised. A similar drug of this class can cause photosensitivity.

Exposure to Heat: Caution is advised. Avoid excessive perspiring with resultant loss of body water and drop in blood pressure.

Occurrence of Unrelated Illness: Report promptly any disorder that causes nausea, vomiting, or diarrhea. Fluid and chemical imbalances must be corrected as soon as possible.

Discontinuation: This drug may be stopped abruptly without causing a sudden increase in blood pressure. However, you should consult your doctor regarding withdrawal of this drug for any reason.

▷ **Saving Money When Using This Medicine:**
- Many drugs are available in this category. Ask your doctor if this drug offers the best combination of price and outcomes.
- Have your blood pressure checked periodically to make sure this medicine is keeping the pressure under control.
- Talk with your doctor about stress management and weight loss to further help your blood pressure.

BENZTROPINE (BENZ troh peen)

Prescription Needed: Yes   **Controlled Drug:** No   **Generic:** No

Brand Names: Cogentin

Overview of BENEFITS versus RISKS

Possible Benefits	*Possible Risks*
PARTIAL RELIEF OF SYMPTOMS OF PARKINSON'S DISEASE	Atropinelike side effects: blurred vision, dry mouth, constipation, impaired urination
RELIEF OF DRUG-INDUCED EXTRAPYRAMIDAL REACTIONS	Rare toxic psychosis
	Rare movement problems (tardive dyskinesia)

▷ **Illness This Medication Treats:**

(1) Combination therapy in all types of parkinsonism to relieve the characteristic rigidity, tremor, and sluggish movement. May be supplemented with more potent drugs such as levodopa and bromocriptine. (2) Also used to control the parkinsonian reactions that can result from certain antipsychotic drugs, such as phenothiazines and related compounds.

Other (unlabeled) generally accepted uses: can help relieve prolonged and painful erections (priapism).

▷ **Typical Dosage Range:** (Dosage or schedule must be determined by the doctor for each individual.)

For Parkinson's disease: 0.5 to 2 mg daily, taken in a single dose at bedtime. For drug induced parkinsonian reactions: 1 to 4 mg daily, in either a single dose or two to three divided doses. The total daily dose should not exceed 6 mg.

▷ **Conditions Requiring Dosing Adjustments:**

Liver function: Patients with impaired liver function should use this drug with caution.

Kidney function: Caution—decreased kidney function may lead to an increased blood level and an increased risk of adverse effects.

▷ **How Best to Take This Medicine:**   May be taken with or following food to reduce stomach irritation. Tablet may be crushed for administration.

▷ **How Long This Medicine Is Usually Taken:**   Use on a regular schedule for 2 to 4 weeks usually determines the effectiveness of this drug in relieving the symptoms of parkinsonism and determines the best dosage schedule. Long-term use (months to years) requires physician supervision and guidance.

▷ **Tell Your Doctor Before Taking This Medicine If You:**
- ever had an allergic reaction to it.
- are given a prescription for a child under 3 years old.
- you have experienced an unfavorable reaction to atropine or atropinelike drugs in the past.
- you have glaucoma or myasthenia gravis.
- you have heart disease or high blood pressure.
- you have a history of liver or kidney disease.
- you have difficulty emptying your urinary bladder, especially if due to an enlarged prostate gland.
- you are taking, or have taken within the past 2 weeks, any MAO type A inhibitors (see Drug Classes).
- you have a job that requires exposure to excessive heat or you have a history of bowel obstructions.
- you take other prescription or nonprescription medications that were not discussed when benztropine was prescribed.

▷ **Possible Side Effects:** Nervousness, blurring of vision, dryness of mouth, constipation, impaired urination (these often subside as drug use continues).

▷ **Possible Adverse Effects:**
If any of the following develop, call your doctor promptly for guidance.
Some Mild Problems Drug Can Cause
  Allergic reaction: skin rashes.
  Headache, dizziness, memory problems, drowsiness, muscle cramps.
  Nausea, vomiting.
Some Serious Problems Drug Can Cause
  Idiosyncratic reactions: abnormal behavior, delusions, hallucinations.
  Rare tardive dyskinesia, dystonia, or bowel obstruction.
  Abnormal temperature increases (hyperthermia).

▷ **Possible Effects on Sex Life:** Reversal of male impotence due to the use of fluphenazine (a phenothiazine antipsychotic drug). Male infertility (0.5 to 6 mg/day). May help treat priapism.

▷ *CAUTION*
  1. Many over-the-counter medications for allergies, colds, and coughs contain drugs that can interact unfavorably with this drug. Ask your doctor or pharmacist for guidance *before* using such preparations.
  2. This drug may aggravate tardive dyskinesia. Ask your doctor for guidance.

3. Safety and effectiveness of this drug for those under 3 years old are not established. Children are especially susceptible to the atropinelike effects of this drug.

4. For those over 60 years old, small doses are advisable until your response has been determined. You may be more susceptible to impaired thinking, confusion, nightmares, hallucinations, increased internal eye pressure (glaucoma), and impaired urination associated with prostate gland enlargement.

Advisability of Use During Pregnancy or If Breast-Feeding:

Pregnancy Category: C. Avoid use of this drug if possible, especially close to delivery; benztropine can impair the proper functioning of the infant's intestinal tract following birth. Presence in breast milk is unknown; avoid taking this drug or refrain from nursing.

▷ **Habit-Forming Potential:** None with recommended doses. At higher doses it may cause euphoria and hallucinations, creating a potential for abuse.

▷ **Overdose Symptoms:** Weakness; drowsiness; stupor; impaired vision; rapid pulse; excitement; confusion; hallucinations; dry, hot skin; skin rash; dilated pupils.

▷ **Suggested Periodic Examinations While Taking This Drug:** (at doctor's discretion)
Measurement of internal eye pressure at regular intervals.

▷ **While Taking This Drug the Following Apply:**

Alcohol: Use caution until the combined effects have been determined. Alcohol may increase the sedative effects of this drug.

Other Drugs:

Benztropine may *decrease* the effects of
- haloperidol (Haldol), reducing its effectiveness.
- phenothiazines (Thorazine, etc.), reducing their effectiveness.

Benztropine *taken concurrently* with
- amantadine (Symmetrel) may cause increased confusion and possible hallucinations.
- clozapine (Clozaril) can cause an increased risk of elevated temperatures, neurologic adverse reactions, or bowel obstruction.

The following drugs may *increase* the effects of benztropine
- antihistamines may add to the dryness of mouth and throat.
- tricyclic antidepressants (Elavil, etc.) may add to the effects on the eye and further increase internal eye pressure (dangerous in glaucoma).
- MAO type A inhibitors may intensify all effects of this drug.

Driving, Hazardous Activities: Drowsiness and dizziness may occur in some people. Avoid hazardous activities until full effects and tolerance have been determined.

Exposure to Heat: Use caution. This drug may reduce sweating, cause an increase in body temperature, and contribute to the development of heatstroke.

Heavy Exercise or Exertion: Use caution. Avoid heavy exercise or exertion in hot environments.

Discontinuation: Do not stop taking this drug abruptly. Ask your doctor for guidance in gradually reducing the dose.

▷ **Saving Money When Using This Medicine:**
- Those over 60 often benefit from smaller doses.
- Ask your doctor if this drug offers the best combination of price and outcomes for you.
- Talk with your doctor about new medicines for treating Parkinson's.

BETAXOLOL (be TAX oh lohl)

Prescription Needed: Yes   **Controlled Drug:** No   **Generic:** No

Brand Names: Betoptic, Kerlone

Overview of BENEFITS versus RISKS	
Possible Benefits	*Possible Risks*
EFFECTIVE, WELL-TOLERATED ANTIHYPERTENSIVE in mild to moderate high blood pressure	CONGESTIVE HEART FAILURE in advanced heart disease
EFFECTIVE TREATMENT OF CHRONIC, OPEN-ANGLE GLAUCOMA	Worsening of angina in coronary heart disease (abrupt withdrawal)
TREATMENT OF OCULAR HYPERTENSION	Masking of hypoglycemia in drug-treated diabetes
	Provocation of bronchial asthma (with high doses)
	Rare anemia or low blood platelets

▷ **Illness This Medication Treats:**
(1) Mild to moderate high blood pressure; (2) chronic open-angle glaucoma (eyedrops); (3) ocular hypertension.
Other (unlabeled) generally accepted uses: (1) the oral form may help decrease the risk of death by decreasing damage from a heart attack and making abnormal heartbeats less likely; (2) helps decrease frequency and severity of chest pain (angina).

▷ **Typical Dosage Range:** (Dosage or schedule must be determined by the doctor for each individual.)

Hypertension: Initially 10 mg once daily. Dose may be increased gradually at intervals of 7 to 14 days as needed and tolerated, up to 20 mg/24 hr. The usual maintenance dose is 10 to 15 mg every 24 hours. The total dose should not exceed 20 mg/24 hr.

Glaucoma: One or two drops of the 2.8 mg/ml solution or one drop of the 5.6 mg/ml.

▷ **Conditions Requiring Dosing Adjustments:**

Liver function: Use with caution, as this drug is changed in the liver.

Kidney function: 5 mg is used as a starting dose and the dose is increased as needed or tolerated by 5 mg every 2 weeks, with a lowered maximum dose.

▷ **How Best to Take This Medicine:** May be taken without regard to eating. The tablet may be crushed for administration. Do not stop this drug abruptly.

▷ **How Long This Medicine Is Usually Taken:** Use on a regular schedule for 10 to 14 days usually determines the effectiveness of this drug in lowering blood pressure. The long-term use is determined by the course of your blood pressure over time and your response to the overall treatment program (weight reduction, salt restriction, smoking cessation, etc.). See your doctor on a regular basis.

▷ **Tell Your Doctor Before Taking This Medicine If You:**

- ever had an allergic reaction to it.
- have congestive heart failure or narrowing of the blood vessels in your arms or legs (peripheral vascular disease).
- have an abnormally slow heart rate or a serious form of heart block.
- are taking, or have taken within the past 14 days, any MAO type A inhibitor.
- have had an adverse reaction to any beta-blocker drug in the past (see Drug Classes).
- have a history of serious heart disease, with or without episodes of heart failure.
- have a history of hay fever (allergic rhinitis), asthma, chronic bronchitis, or emphysema—these may cause serious breathing problems.
- have a history of overactive thyroid function.
- have a history of hypoglycemia.
- have impaired liver or kidney function.
- have diabetes or myasthenia gravis.
- are currently taking any form of digitalis, quinidine, or reserpine, or any calcium blockers (see Drug Classes).
- plan to have surgery under general anesthesia soon.

▷ **Possible Side Effects:**   Lethargy, fatigability, cold extremities, slow heart rate, light-headedness in upright position.

▷ **Possible Adverse Effects:**
If any of the following develop, call your doctor promptly for guidance.
Some Mild Problems Drug Can Cause
   Allergic reactions: skin rash, itching.
   Headache, dizziness, insomnia, abnormal dreams.
   Nausea, diarrhea.
   Trouble breathing.
   Joint and muscle discomfort, fluid retention (edema).
Some Serious Problems Drug Can Cause
   Mental depression.
   Chest pain, congestive heart failure.
   Rare lowering of the blood platelets or anemia.
   Rare problems walking (intermittent claudication).
   Rare myocardial infarction.
   Can cause bronchial asthma (in asthmatics).

▷ **Possible Effects on Sex Life:**   Decreased libido, impotence.
Altered menstrual patterns.

▷ *CAUTION*
   1. ***Do not stop taking this drug suddenly*** without the knowledge and guidance of your doctor. Carry a note with you that states you are taking this drug.
   2. Ask your doctor or pharmacist before using nasal decongestants, which are usually present in over-the-counter cold preparations and nose drops. These can cause sudden increases in blood pressure when taken concurrently with beta-blockers.
   3. Report the development of any tendency to emotional depression.
   4. Safety and effectiveness of this drug for those under 12 years old are not established. However, if this drug is used, observe for the development of hypoglycemia, especially if meals are skipped.
   5. High blood pressure in people over 60 should be reduced without creating the risks associated with excessively low blood pressure. Treatment should be started with 5 mg daily and blood pressure should be checked often. Sudden, rapid, and excessive reduction of blood pressure can predispose to stroke or heart attack. Total daily dose should not exceed 10 to 15 mg. Observe for dizziness, unsteadiness, tendency to fall, confusion, hallucinations, depression, or urinary frequency. This age group is more prone to develop very slow heart rates and hypothermia.

Advisability of Use During Pregnancy or If Breast-Feeding:
Pregnancy Category: C. Avoid use of this drug during the first 3 months if possible. Avoid use during labor and delivery because of the possi-

ble effects on the newborn infant. Present in breast milk; avoid taking this drug if possible. If this drug is necessary, observe the nursing infant for slow heart rate and indications of low blood sugar.

▷ **Overdose Symptoms:** Weakness, slow pulse, low blood pressure, fainting, cold and sweaty skin, congestive heart failure, possible coma and convulsions.

▷ **Possible Effects of Long-Term Use:** Reduced heart reserve and eventual heart failure in susceptible individuals with advanced heart disease.

▷ **Suggested Periodic Examinations While Taking This Drug:** (at doctor's discretion)

Measurements of blood pressure, evaluation of heart function.

▷ **While Taking This Drug the Following Apply:**

Foods: Avoid excessive salt intake.

Beverages: May be taken with milk.

Alcohol: Use with caution. Alcohol may exaggerate this drug's ability to lower blood pressure and increase its mild sedative effect.

Tobacco Smoking: Nicotine may reduce this drug's effectiveness in treating high blood pressure. In addition, high doses may worsen the bronchial tube constriction caused by regular smoking.

Other Drugs:

Betaxolol may *increase* the effects of

• other antihypertensive drugs and cause excessive lowering of blood pressure. Dosage adjustments may be necessary.

• reserpine (Ser-Ap-Es, etc.) and cause sedation, depression, slowing of heart rate, and lowering of blood pressure (light-headedness, fainting).

• verapamil and increase the risk of congestive heart failure.

Betaxolol *taken concurrently* with

• amiodarone (Cordarone) may result in very slow heart rate and arrest.

• calcium channel blockers (see Drug Classes) may cause severe lowering of the blood pressure.

• clonidine (Catapres) requires close monitoring for rebound high blood pressure if clonidine is withdrawn while betaxolol is still being taken.

• fluvoxamine (Luvox) may cause excessive slowing of the heart and very low blood pressure.

• insulin requires close monitoring to avoid undetected hypoglycemia.

• oral hypoglycemic agents (see Drug Classes) may prolong any recovery from low blood sugars.

• phenothiazines (see Drug Classes) may cause additive blood pressure–lowering effects.

The following drugs may *decrease* the effects of betaxolol
- indomethacin (Indocin), and possibly other aspirin substitutes (NSAIDs), may impair betaxolol's antihypertensive effect.

Driving, Hazardous Activities: Use caution until the full extent of drowsiness, lethargy, and blood pressure change has been determined.

Exposure to Heat: Caution is advised. Hot environments can lower blood pressure and exaggerate the effects of this drug.

Exposure to Cold: Caution is advised. Cold environments can enhance the circulatory deficiency in the extremities that may occur with this drug. The elderly should take precautions to prevent hypothermia.

Heavy Exercise or Exertion: It is advisable to avoid exertion that produces light-headedness, excessive fatigue, or muscle cramping. The use of this drug may intensify the hypertensive response to isometric exercise.

Occurrence of Unrelated Illness: Fever can lower blood pressure and require lower doses. Illnesses that cause nausea or vomiting may interrupt the regular dosage schedule. Ask your doctor for help.

Discontinuation: Avoid sudden discontinuation of this drug in all situations. If possible, gradual reduction of the dose over a period of 2 to 3 weeks is recommended. Ask your doctor for help.

▷ **Saving Money When Using This Medicine:**
- Many medications are in this class. Ask your doctor to prescribe the one that offers the best combination of price and outcome for you.
- Ask your doctor about stress management and weight reduction to further lower your blood pressure.
- If your increased blood pressure is associated with increased cholesterol and narrowing of the arteries, talk with your doctor about HMG CoA reductase medicines.

BITOLTEROL   (bi TOHL ter ohl)

Prescription Needed: Yes   **Controlled Drug:** No   **Generic:** No

Brand Names: Tornalate

Overview of BENEFITS versus RISKS	
Possible Benefits	*Possible Risks*
EFFECTIVE PREVENTION AND RELIEF OF ASTHMA for 5–8 hours	Fine hand tremor or nervousness
	Throat irritation
	Irregular heart rhythm (with excessive use)

▷ **Illness This Medication Treats:**
(1) Relieves acute bronchial asthma and reduces the frequency and severity of chronic, recurrent asthmatic attacks; (2) may help asthmatics who require steroids to use lower doses.

Other (unlabeled) generally accepted uses: (1) may be helpful in patients with chronic obstructive lung disease (COPD); (2) can help prevent exercise-induced asthma.

▷ **Typical Dosage Range:** (Dosage or schedule must be determined by the doctor for each individual.)
For acute bronchospasm: Two inhalations at intervals of 1 to 3 minutes, followed by a third inhalation in 3 to 4 minutes if needed. For prevention of bronchospasm: 2 inhalations/8 hr.

▷ **Conditions Requiring Dosing Adjustments:**
Liver function: Patients with severe liver compromise should use this drug with caution.
Kidney function: A significant amount of this medication is eliminated by the kidneys; however, specific guidelines for adjustment of dose or intervals are not available.

▷ **How Best to Take This Medicine:** May be used without regard to eating. Follow written directions carefully. *Do not overuse.* This drug will start to work in 5 to 15 minutes after it is inhaled—give it this much time before you add other drugs.

▷ **How Long This Medicine Is Usually Taken:** According to individual requirements. Do not use beyond the time necessary to terminate episodes of acute asthma. Ask your doctor for guidance regarding duration of use for preventing asthma attacks.

▷ **Tell Your Doctor Before Taking This Medicine If You:**
• ever had an allergic reaction to it.
• currently have an irregular heart rhythm.

- are taking, or have taken within the past 2 weeks, any MAO type A inhibitors.
- have any type of heart or circulatory disorder, especially high blood pressure or coronary heart disease.
- have diabetes, epilepsy, or an overactive thyroid gland.
- are pregnant and near your delivery date.
- are taking any form of digitalis or any stimulant drug.

▷ **Possible Side Effects:**   Dryness or irritation of mouth or throat.

▷ **Possible Adverse Effects:**
If any of the following develop, call your doctor promptly for guidance.
Some Mild Problems Drug Can Cause
  Headache, dizziness, nervousness, fine hand tremor.
  Nausea.
Some Serious Problems Drug Can Cause
  Rapid/irregular heart rhythm or increased blood pressure can occur with excessive use.
  Rare paradoxical bronchospasm.

▷ *CAUTION*
  1. The combination of bitolterol inhalation with beclomethasone aerosol (Beclovent, Vanceril) may increase the risk of toxicity due to fluorocarbon propellants. It is advisable to use the bitolterol aerosol 20 to 30 minutes *before* the beclomethasone aerosol. This will reduce the risk of toxicity and enhance the penetration of beclomethasone.
  2. The excessive or prolonged use of this drug by inhalation can reduce its effectiveness and cause serious heart rhythm disturbances.
  3. Safety and effectiveness of this drug for children under 12 years old are not established.
  4. Those over 60 should avoid excessive and continual use. If acute asthma is not relieved promptly, other drugs will have to be tried. Watch for development of nervousness, palpitations, irregular heart rhythm, and muscle tremors.

Advisability of Use During Pregnancy or If Breast-Feeding:
Pregnancy Category: C. Avoid using during first 3 months if possible. Presence in breast milk is unknown; avoid taking this drug or refrain from nursing.

▷ **Overdose Symptoms:**   Nervousness, palpitation, rapid heart rate, sweating, headache, tremor, vomiting, chest pain.

▷ **Possible Effects of Long-Term Use:**   Loss of effectiveness.

▷ **Suggested Periodic Examinations While Taking This Drug:** (at doctor's discretion)

Blood pressure measurements, evaluation of heart status.

▷ **While Taking This Drug the Following Apply:**

Beverages: Avoid excessive use of coffee, tea, cola, chocolate, or caffeine.

Other Drugs:

Bitolterol *taken concurrently* with

- MAO type A inhibitors may cause excessive increase in blood pressure and undesirable heart stimulation.

Driving, Hazardous Activities: Use caution if nervousness or dizziness occurs.

Heavy Exercise or Exertion: Use caution. Excessive exercise can induce asthma in sensitive individuals.

▷ **Saving Money When Using This Medicine:**

- Ask your doctor if this medicine offers the best combination of price and outcome for you.
- If you still require steroids, ask your doctor about calcium supplements and periodical checking of bone mineral density.

BROMOCRIPTINE (broh moh KRIP teen)

Prescription Needed: Yes   **Controlled Drug:** No   **Generic:** No

Brand Names: Parlodel

Overview of BENEFITS versus RISKS

Possible Benefits	*Possible Risks*
PARTIAL RELIEF OF SYMPTOMS OF PARKINSON'S DISEASE	ABNORMAL INVOLUNTARY MOVEMENTS AND ALTERED BEHAVIOR
CORRECTION OF INFERTILITY AND ABSENT MENSTRUATION in women with high prolactin levels	Raynaud's phenomenon Low blood pressure

---

▷ **Illness This Medication Treats:**

(1) Parkinson's disease. Often used in conjunction with levodopa when it is found that levodopa is losing its effectiveness, or the patient cannot tolerate the adverse effects of levodopa and dosage adjustment or withdrawal is necessary. (2) Treats disorders due to excessive production of prolactin by the pituitary gland, such as absent menstruation, infertility, or inappropriate milk production.

Other (unlabeled) generally accepted uses: may help growth return to normal in children having abnormal skeletal growth.

▷ **Typical Dosage Range:** (Dosage or schedule must be determined by the doctor for each individual.)

For Parkinson's disease: Initially 1.25 to 2.5 mg once daily; for maintenance, 2.5 to 100 mg daily in divided doses. Increase dose by no more than 2.5 to 5 mg on alternate days. The usual dosage range is 10 to 40 mg daily. Do not exceed 300 mg daily. For absent menstruation and infertility: Initially 1.25 to 2.5 mg daily; for maintenance, 2.5 mg two or three times a day, up to 15 mg/day.

▷ **Conditions Requiring Dosing Adjustments:**

Liver function: The dose should be decreased or the dosing interval lengthened for patients with liver compromise; however, specific guidelines are not available.

Kidney function: Patients with severe kidney failure should use this drug with caution.

▷ **How Best to Take This Medicine:**   Take with food or milk. Open capsule or crush tablet to take.

▷ **How Long This Medicine Is Usually Taken:**   Regular use for 3 to 4 months usually determines the effectiveness of this drug for treating Parkinson's disease. Treatment for 4 to 12 weeks restores fertility and normal menstruation in most women; however, treatment may be necessary for 6 to 12 months. Long-term use (up to 3 years or more) must be under physician supervision and guidance. See your doctor regularly.

▷ **Tell Your Doctor Before Taking This Medicine If You:**
- ever had an allergic reaction to it.
- have had a serious adverse effect from any ergot preparation.
- have severe coronary artery disease or peripheral vascular disease.
- are pregnant.
- have constitutionally low blood pressure.
- are taking any antihypertensive drugs or phenothiazines.
- have coronary artery disease, especially after a heart attack.
- have an ulcer or a history of mental illness.
- have a history of heart rhythm abnormalities.
- have impaired liver function.
- have a seizure disorder.

▷ **Possible Side Effects:**   Fatigue, light-headedness, orthostatic hypotension.

▷ **Possible Adverse Effects:**

If any of the following develop, call your doctor promptly for guidance.

Some Mild Problems Drug Can Cause

Allergic reaction: skin rash.

Headache, drowsiness, fainting, nervousness, nightmares.

Nasal congestion, dry mouth, loss of appetite, nausea, vomiting, constipation, diarrhea.

Some Serious Problems Drug Can Cause

Abnormal movements, confusion, hallucinations, visual disturbances, depression, seizures.

Swelling of feet and ankles (edema).

Loss of urinary bladder control.

Indications of ergotism: numbness and tingling of fingers, cold hands.

Vomiting blood, bloody or black stools—stomach bleeding.

Retroperitoneal fibrosis, worsening of mania in manic patients.

Very rare blood vessel spasms and risk of heart attack.

Lung changes with long-term use (pulmonary fibrosis).

▷ **Possible Effects on Sex Life:**   Rare occurrence of impotence. However, this drug can correct impotence and reduced libido when these conditions are due to increased blood levels of prolactin.

▷ *CAUTION*

1. During treatment of parkinsonism, avoid excessive and hurried activity as improvement occurs; this will reduce the risk of falls and injury.
2. Neurologic and psychiatric disturbances due to this drug may last for 2 to 6 weeks after it is stopped.
3. During treatment to reduce the blood level of prolactin and restore normal menstruation and fertility, it is mandatory that you use a barrier method of contraception to prevent pregnancy. Oral contraceptives should not be used while taking bromocriptine.
4. If pregnancy occurs, notify your doctor immediately.
5. Safety and effectiveness of this drug for those under 15 years old are not established.
6. For those over 60, the test dose should be 1.25 mg. Watch closely for any tendency to light-headedness or faintness when attempting to stand after this first dose. You may be more susceptible to impaired thinking, confusion, agitation, nightmares, hallucinations, nausea, or vomiting. Close monitoring and careful dosage adjustments are mandatory.

Advisability of Use During Pregnancy or If Breast-Feeding:

Pregnancy Category: C. Controversy exists regarding the use of this medicine during pregnancy. Talk with your doctor about the benefits versus potential risks of use. Bromocriptine prevents the production of milk and makes nursing impossible.

▷ **Overdose Symptoms:**   Weakness, low blood pressure, nausea, vomiting, diarrhea, confusion, agitation, hallucinations, loss of consciousness.

▷ **Suggested Periodic Examinations While Taking This Drug:** (at doctor's discretion)

Blood pressure measurements; CAT scan of the pituitary gland for enlargement due to tumor; pregnancy test; blood tests for anemia; evaluation of heart, lung, and liver functions.

▷ **While Taking This Drug the Following Apply:**

Beverages: May be taken with milk.

Alcohol: Use caution until the combined effects have been determined. Alcohol can exaggerate the blood pressure–lowering effects and sedative effects of this drug.

Other Drugs:

Bromocriptine *taken concurrently* with

- antihypertensive drugs (and other drugs that can lower blood pressure) requires careful monitoring for excessive drops in pressure. Dosage adjustments may be necessary.
- erythromycins (see Drug Classes) may result in bromocriptine toxicity.
- phenylpropanolamine (watch for this in nonprescription products) can result in bromocriptine toxicity.

The following drugs may *decrease* the effects of bromocriptine

- phenothiazines. Theoretically bromocriptine and phenothiazines have opposite effects on the utilization of dopamine in the brain. It is probably best to avoid the concurrent use of these drugs until the results of further studies are available.

Driving, Hazardous Activities: Be alert to the possible occurrence of orthostatic hypotension, dizziness, drowsiness, or impaired coordination.

▷ **Saving Money When Using This Medicine:**

- Dosage should be decreased for patients with liver compromise; a smaller dose may achieve the same beneficial outcome.
- Ask your doctor if this drug offers the best combination of outcome and price for you.
- Talk with your doctor about new agents for treating Parkinson's.

BUMETANIDE (byu MET a nide)

Prescription Needed: Yes   **Controlled Drug:** No   **Generic:** No

Brand Names: Bumex

Overview of BENEFITS versus RISKS

Possible Benefits	*Possible Risks*
POTENT, EFFECTIVE DIURETIC BY MOUTH OR INJECTION	ABNORMALLY LOW BLOOD POTASSIUM
	ABNORMALLY LOW BLOOD MAGNESIUM
	Rare blood disorders

▷ **Illness This Medication Treats:**

Removes excess fluid in heart failure, liver or kidney disease.

Other (unlabeled) generally accepted uses: (1) used as add-on therapy of high blood pressure; (2) eases fluid buildup in the lungs (pulmonary edema).

▷ **Typical Dosage Range:** (Dosage or schedule must be determined by the doctor for each individual.)

0.5 to 2 mg daily, usually taken in the morning as a single dose. If needed, an additional second or third dose may be taken later in the day at 4- to 5-hour intervals. The total daily dose should not exceed 10 mg. Alternate-day dosage may work for some people.

▷ **Conditions Requiring Dosing Adjustments:**

Liver function: Rapid removal of body fluid in liver failure patients can cause a coma. This drug should only be used by liver patients in a hospital, and only then used with great caution.

Kidney function: This drug is **not** recommended for use by patients with progressive kidney failure.

▷ **How Best to Take This Medicine:**   May be taken with or following food, and tablet can be crushed for administration.

▷ **How Long This Medicine Is Usually Taken:** Use on a regular schedule for 2 to 3 days usually determines the effectiveness of this drug in relieving fluid buildup (edema). Once the peak benefit is realized, intermittent use reduces the risk of sodium, potassium, magnesium, and water imbalance. Long-term use requires physician supervision.

▷ **Tell Your Doctor Before Taking This Medicine If You:**
- ever had an allergic reaction to it.
- know your kidneys are unable to produce urine
- are allergic to any form of sulfa drug.

- are pregnant or planning pregnancy.
- have impaired liver function.
- have diabetes or a tendency to diabetes.
- have a history of gout.
- have impaired hearing.
- are taking any form of cortisone, digitalis, oral antidiabetic drugs, insulin, probenecid (Benemid), indomethacin (Indocin), lithium, or drugs for high blood pressure.
- plan to have surgery under general anesthesia soon.

▷ **Possible Side Effects:**   Light-headedness on arising from sitting or lying position.

Increase in level of blood sugar, affecting control of diabetes.

Increase in level of blood uric acid, affecting control of gout.

Decrease in levels of blood potassium and sodium, resulting in muscle weakness and cramping.

▷ **Possible Adverse Effects:**

If any of the following develop, call your doctor promptly for guidance.

Some Mild Problems Drug Can Cause

    Allergic reactions: skin rashes, hives, itching.

    Headache, dizziness, vertigo, weakness, sweating, earache.

    Nausea, vomiting, stomach pain, diarrhea.

    Breast nipple tenderness, joint and muscle pains.

Some Serious Problems Drug Can Cause

    Impaired hearing, liver coma (in preexisting liver disease).

    Rare lowered white blood cells and platelets.

    Electrolyte (low magnesium, potassium, or sodium) imbalance.

    Rare pancreatitis, lung fibrosis kidney problems, eye defects, or hearing toxicity.

▷ **Possible Effects on Sex Life:**   Difficulty maintaining an erection; premature ejaculation (0.5–2 mg/day). Male breast enlargement or tenderness (gynecomastia).

▷ *CAUTION*

    1. High doses can cause excessive loss of water, sodium, and potassium, with resultant loss of appetite, nausea, weakness, confusion, and profound drop in blood pressure (circulatory collapse).

    2. If you are also taking a digitalis preparation (digitoxin, digoxin), ensure an adequate intake of high-potassium foods to prevent potassium deficiency—a potential cause of digitalis toxicity.

    3. If you are being treated for cirrhosis of the liver, do not increase your dose without talking with your doctor. Excessive dosage can alter blood chemistry significantly and cause liver coma.

    4. Safety and effectiveness of this drug for those under 18 years old are not established.

5. For those over 60, small doses are advisable. You may be more susceptible to impaired thinking, orthostatic hypotension, potassium loss, and elevation of blood sugar. Overdosage and prolonged use of this drug can cause excessive loss of body water, thickening of the blood, and an increased tendency for blood clotting, predisposing to stroke, heart attack, or thrombophlebitis.

Advisability of Use During Pregnancy or If Breast-Feeding:

Pregnancy Category: C. Should not be used during pregnancy unless a very serious complication of pregnancy occurs, for which this drug is significantly beneficial. Presence in breast milk is unknown; avoid taking this drug or refrain from nursing.

▷ **Overdose Symptoms:** Weakness, lethargy, dizziness, confusion, nausea, vomiting, muscle cramps, thirst, drowsiness progressing to deep sleep or coma, weak and rapid pulse.

▷ **Suggested Periodic Examinations While Taking This Drug:** (at doctor's discretion)

Complete blood cell counts; measurements of blood levels of sodium, potassium, chloride, sugar, uric acid; liver and kidney function tests.

▷ **While Taking This Drug the Following Apply:**

Foods: Salt restriction and a high-potassium diet may be needed; ask your doctor. (See Table 11, "High-Potassium Foods," Section Six.)

Beverages: No restrictions unless directed by your doctor. This drug may be taken with milk.

Alcohol: Use caution. Alcohol can exaggerate the blood pressure–lowering effect of this drug and cause orthostatic hypotension.

Other Drugs:

Bumetanide may *increase* the effects of

- antihypertensive drugs. Careful adjustment of dosages is necessary to prevent excessive lowering of the blood pressure.

Bumetanide *taken concurrently* with

- ACE inhibitors (see Drug Classes) may cause severe lowering of blood pressure on standing.
- aminoglycoside antibiotics (amikacin, gentamicin, kanamycin, neomycin, streptomycin, tobramycin) may increase the risk of hearing loss or ear toxicity (balance changes).
- cortisone-related drugs may cause excessive potassium loss.
- digitalis-related drugs requires very careful monitoring and dosage adjustments to prevent serious disturbances of heart rhythm.
- lithium (Lithobid, others) may increase the risk of lithium toxicity.

The following drugs may *decrease* the effects of bumetanide

- indomethacin (Indocin) or other NSAIDs (see Drug Classes) may reduce its diuretic effect.

Driving, Hazardous Activities: Use caution until the possible occurrence of dizziness, weakness, or orthostatic hypotension has been
determined.

Occurrence of Unrelated Illness: Report any vomiting or diarrhea to
your doctor promptly.

Discontinuation: It may be advisable to stop taking this drug 5 to 7
days before major surgery. Consult your doctor, surgeon, or anesthesiologist for guidance regarding dosage reduction or withdrawal.

▷ **Saving Money When Using This Medicine:**
- Several agents are available that work similarly to this drug. Ask
  your doctor if this drug offers the best combination of price and
  outcomes for you.
- Most physicians routinely check potassium, but be certain your doctor orders a blood magnesium level if you take this medicine on an
  ongoing basis. Lowered amounts of this mineral can lead to heart
  problems.

BUPROPION (byu PROH pee on)

Prescription Needed: Yes   **Controlled Drug:** No   **Generic:**
No

Brand Names: Wellbutrin, Wellbutrin SR

Overview of BENEFITS versus RISKS	
Possible Benefits	*Possible Risks*
EFFECTIVE TREATMENT OF MAJOR DEPRESSIVE DISORDERS	RARE DRUG-INDUCED SEIZURES
Different class of medicines than MAOI, tricyclic, or SSRI antidepressants	Excessive mental stimulation: excitement, anxiety, confusion, hallucinations, insomnia
	Conversion of depression to mania in manic-depressive disorders

▷ **Illness This Medication Treats:**
Major depressive disorders.
Other (unlabeled) generally accepted uses: (1) may help chronic fatigue syndrome; (2) helps decrease cocaine craving; (3) could have a
role in helping resistant low back pain.

▷ **Typical Dosage Range:** (Dosage or schedule must be determined by
the doctor for each individual.)

Infants and Children: Dosage not established for those under 18 years old.

18 to 60 Years of Age: Initially (first 3 days) 100 mg in the morning, 100 mg in the evening; total daily dose of 200 mg.

On the fourth day, if needed and tolerated, increase dose to 100 mg in the morning, at noon, and in the evening; total daily dose of 300 mg.

Continue the schedule of 100 mg, three times daily, 6 hours apart, for 3 to 4 weeks.

If well tolerated and improvement is noted, the dose may be increased cautiously (as deemed necessary) up to a maximum of 450 mg daily. Increases should not exceed 100 mg/day within a period of 3 days. No single dose should exceed 150 mg. If a daily dose of 450 mg is reached, give 150 mg in the morning, then 100 mg/4 hr for three more doses.

Determine and continue the lowest dose that maintains remission of depression.

If significant improvement does not occur after an adequate trial of 450 mg daily, this drug should be stopped.

Author's note: An extended-release form has recently been approved. Extended-release forms allow less frequent dosing (fewer times per day) and give the same—and in some cases better—results because of more constant blood levels.

Over 60 Years of Age: Same as for 18 to 60 years of age.

▷ **Conditions Requiring Dosing Adjustments:**

Liver function: Lower doses and caution in monitoring should be followed for people with compromised livers.

Kidney function: Patients with compromised kidneys should use this drug with caution.

▷ **How Best to Take This Medicine:** May be taken with food to reduce stomach irritation. It is best to swallow the tablet whole, not chewing or crushing it; this drug has a bitter taste and a numbing effect on the lining of the mouth.

▷ **How Long This Medicine Is Usually Taken:** Use on a regular schedule for 4 to 6 weeks usually determines the effectiveness of this drug in relieving the symptoms of depression. Long-term use (months to years) requires periodic physician evaluation.

▷ **Tell Your Doctor Before Taking This Medicine If You:**
- ever had an allergic reaction to it.
- have a history of anorexia nervosa or bulimia.
- have a seizure disorder of any kind.
- are taking, or have taken within the past 14 days, any MAO type A inhibitors.
- have experienced any adverse effects from antidepressants in the past.

- are pregnant or planning pregnancy.
- are currently breast-feeding.
- have a history of serious mental illness, head injury, or brain tumor.
- have a history of alcoholism or drug abuse.
- have any kind of heart disease, especially a recent heart attack.
- have impaired liver or kidney function.

▷ **Possible Side Effects:**   Nervousness, anxiety, confusion, insomnia. Weight loss of more than 5 lb. Excessive sweating.

▷ **Possible Adverse Effects:**
If any of the following develop, call your doctor promptly for guidance.
Some Mild Problems Drug Can Cause
Allergic reactions: skin rash, itching.
Headache, dizziness, blurred vision, tremor.
Indigestion, nausea and vomiting, constipation.
Some Serious Problems Drug Can Cause
Drug-induced seizures, more common with high doses.
Change of depression to mania in bipolar (manic-depressive) disorder. Psychosis in patients with psychotic predisposition.
Decreased white blood cell counts.
Rare liver toxicity.
Ringing in the ears.

▷ **Possible Effects on Sex Life:**   Impotence; however, one study found a decrease in sexual dysfunction when patients had problems with fluoxetine (Prozac) and were changed to bupropion.
Altered menstruation.

▷ *CAUTION*
1. Adhere to dosage recommendations very strictly; rapid increases in dose can precipitate seizures. Monitor closely for indications of excessive stimulation.
2. Ask your doctor or pharmacist before taking any other prescription or over-the-counter drug while taking this medicine.
3. Do not take any MAO type A inhibitors while taking this drug (see Drug Classes). If you have taken an MAO inhibitor recently, wait 2 weeks after discontinuing it before starting bupropion.
4. Safety and effectiveness of this drug for those under 18 years old are not established.
5. Age-related liver or kidney function impairment may require dose adjustment.
Advisability of Use During Pregnancy or If Breast-Feeding:
Pregnancy Category: B. Use this drug only if clearly needed. Ask your doctor for guidance. Present in breast milk; avoid taking this drug or refrain from nursing.

▷ **Habit-Forming Potential:** Remote, with use of recommended doses. Slight potential for abuse by those who abuse stimulant drugs.

▷ **Overdose Symptoms:** Headache, agitation, confusion, hallucinations, seizures, loss of consciousness.

▷ **Suggested Periodic Examinations While Taking This Drug:** (at doctor's discretion)
Liver and/or kidney function tests as appropriate.

▷ **While Taking This Drug the Following Apply:**
Beverages: May be taken with milk.
Alcohol: Avoid completely. Alcohol may predispose to seizures.
Marijuana Smoking: Avoid completely; it may induce psychotic behavior.

Other Drugs:
The following drugs **taken concurrently** with bupropion may increase the risk of major seizures
- antidepressants (tricyclic).
- clozapine (Clozaril).
- fluoxetine (Prozac).
- haloperidol (Haldol).
- lithium (Lithobid, others).
- loxapine.
- maprotiline.
- molindone.
- phenothiazines (see Drug Classes).
- thioxanthenes.
- trazodone.

Bupropion *taken concurrently* with
- carbamazepine (Tegretol) can decrease carbamazepine levels.
- levodopa can lead to increased nausea and tremor.
- phenobarbitol may result in decreased bupropion levels.
- phenytoin (Dilantin) may result in decreased phenytoin levels and loss of seizure control.

Driving, Hazardous Activities: This drug may cause dizziness, drowsiness, or seizures. Restrict your activities as necessary.
Discontinuation: Do not stop taking this drug abruptly. Ask your doctor for help.

▷ **Saving Money When Using This Medicine:**
- A large number of drugs are available that provide similar effectiveness. Ask your doctor to prescribe the drug that offers the best combination of cost and outcome.
- Talk with your doctor about available support groups in your community.

BUSPIRONE (byou SPI rohn)

Prescription Needed: Yes   **Controlled Drug:** No   **Generic:** No

Brand Names: BuSpar

```
┌─────────────────────────────────────────────────────────┐
│           Overview of BENEFITS versus RISKS             │
│     Possible Benefits            Possible Risks         │
│  EFFECTIVE RELIEF OF MILD    Mild dizziness, faintness, or │
│   TO MODERATE ANXIETY          headache (uncommon)      │
│   without significant sedation  Rare restlessness, tremor, and │
│   or risk of dependence         rigidity (with high doses) │
│                              Fast heart rate            │
└─────────────────────────────────────────────────────────┘
```

▷ **Illness This Medication Treats:**
  Mild to moderate anxiety and nervous tension. Particularly useful in the elderly, the alcoholic, and the addiction-prone individual.
  Other (unlabeled) generally accepted uses: (1) may help aggression or hyperactivity in autistics; (2) can help sexual dysfunction in people with generalized anxiety disorder.

▷ **Typical Dosage Range:** (Dosage or schedule must be determined by the doctor for each individual.)
  20 to 30 mg per day, in divided doses. Initially 5 mg 3 times/day; if needed, increase dose by 5 to 10 mg per day every 3 to 4 days, with individual doses every 6 to 8 hours. The total daily dose should not exceed 60 mg.

▷ **Conditions Requiring Dosing Adjustments:**
  Liver function: Patients with severe liver failure should use this drug with caution. Doses MUST be decreased.
  Kidney function: The dose MUST be decreased by 25 to 50% for patients with compromised kidneys.

▷ **How Best to Take This Medicine:**   May be taken without regard to food. The tablet may be crushed.

▷ **How Long This Medicine Is Usually Taken:**   Use on a regular schedule for 7 to 10 days usually determines the effectiveness of this drug in relieving anxiety and nervous tension. Avoid prolonged and uninterrupted use.

▷ **Tell Your Doctor Before Taking This Medicine If You:**
  • ever had an allergic reaction to it.
  • are taking other drugs that affect the function of the brain and nervous system: tranquilizers, sedatives, hypnotics, analgesics, narcot-

ics, antidepressants, antipsychotics, anticonvulsants, or drugs for parkinsonism.
- have impaired liver or kidney function.
- take fluoxetine (Prozac) for depression.

▷ **Possible Side Effects:** Infrequent and mild drowsiness (less than with benzodiazepines), lethargy, fatigue.

▷ **Possible Adverse Effects:**
If any of the following develop, call your doctor promptly for guidance.
Some Mild Problems Drug Can Cause
Headache, dizziness, excitement, nausea.
Some Serious Problems Drug Can Cause
Depression.
Rare movement disorders.
With high doses: restlessness, rigidity, tremors.

▷ **Possible Effects on Sex Life:** Increased or decreased libido, inhibited ejaculation, impotence, breast milk production, altered timing and pattern of menstruation (10–40 mg/day). May increase prolactin.

▷ *CAUTION*
1. Although this drug is reported to have no significant (or very mild) sedative effects and no potential for causing dependence, it should be used with caution and only when clearly needed. It has not been used by large numbers of people for long periods of time; some unexpected side effects or adverse effects may become apparent after general use for several years.
2. Safety and effectiveness of this drug for those under 18 years old are not established.
3. For those over 60, this drug should be tolerated much better than benzodiazepines and barbiturates. Watch for possible increase in dizziness and/or weakness; use caution to avoid falls.

Advisability of Use During Pregnancy or If Breast-Feeding:
Pregnancy Category: B. Use during pregnancy only when clearly needed. Until more experience has been gained from wider use, it is advisable to avoid this drug during the first 3 months of pregnancy. Present in breast milk in rats, probably also in humans; avoid taking this drug or refrain from nursing.

▷ **Habit-Forming Potential:** None demonstrated in premarketing trials.

▷ **Overdose Symptoms:** Drowsiness, nausea, dysphoria, tingling sensations (paresthesias), and chance of seizures.

▷ **While Taking This Drug the Following Apply:**

Other Drugs:

Buspirone ***taken concurrently*** with

- fluoxetine (Prozac) may increase an underlying anxiety or mental disorder. Do NOT combine these drugs.
- fluvoxamine (Luvox) may result in serious slowing of the heart (bradycardia).
- MAO inhibitors (see Drug Classes) can result in large increases in blood pressure.
- narcotics (see Opioid Drugs in Drug Classes, Section Four) may result in additive sedation and decreased breathing (respiratory depression).

Driving, Hazardous Activities: This drug may cause dizziness, faintness, or fatigue. Restrict your activities as necessary.

▷ **Saving Money When Using This Medicine:**

- A large number of medicines are available to treat depression. Ask your doctor if this medicine offers the best combination of price and outcome for you.
- Dose must be decreased by 25 to 50% for patients with kidney compromise.
- Talk with your doctor about stress management and exercise programs available in your community or through your employer.

CALCITONIN (kal si TOH nin)

Other Names: Salcatonin, thyrocalcitonin

Prescription Needed: Yes   **Controlled Drug:** No   **Generic:** No

Brand Names: Calcimar, Cibacalcin, Miacalcin Nasal

Overview of BENEFITS versus RISKS	
Possible Benefits	*Possible Risks*
PARTIAL RELIEF OF SYMPTOMS OF PAGET'S DISEASE OF BONE	Nausea (with or without vomiting)
NASAL FORM CAN INCREASE BONE MASS	Allergic skin reactions
Effective adjunctive treatment of postmenopausal osteoporosis	
Effective adjunctive treatment of abnormally high blood calcium levels (associated with malignant disease)	

▷ **Illness This Medication Treats:**
  (1) Symptomatic Paget's disease of bone (excessive bone growth of skull, spine, and long bones); (2) adjunctive treatment of post-menopausal osteoporosis, helping prevent fractures (taken concurrently with calcium and vitamin D); (3) adjunctive treatment of excessively high blood calcium levels due to malignant bone disease.

  Other (unlabeled) generally accepted uses: (1) adjunctive treatment of osteoporosis due to medicinal drugs, hormonal disorders, or immobilization; taken concurrently with calcium and vitamin D; (2) may help prevent migraines; (3) could have a role in pain after amputation (phantom limb).

▷ **Typical Dosage Range:** (Dosage or schedule must be determined by the doctor for each individual.)

  Infants and Children: Dosage not established.

  12 to 60 Years of Age: Calcitonin-Human

  For Paget's disease: Initially 500 mcg (0.5 mg) daily, injected subcutaneously; after adequate response, dose may be decreased to 250 mcg (0.25 mg) daily, or 500 mcg (0.5 mg) two or three times per week.

Calcitonin-Salmon

For Paget's disease: Initially 100 IU daily, injected subcutaneously; after adequate response, dose may be decreased to 50 IU daily, every other day, or three times per week.

For postmenopausal osteoporosis—Injection form: 100 IU daily, every other day, or three times per week, injected subcutaneously. If adverse effects are marked, reduce dose to 50 IU daily; then increase dose gradually over a period of 2 weeks.

Nasal spray: One spray daily. Alternate nostrils daily in order to avoid nasal irritation. Calcium and vitamin D replacement are strongly advised. This can help you avoid drawing on your bones for needed calcium.

For high blood calcium levels: Initially 4 IU per kilogram of body weight every 12 hours, injected subcutaneously; as needed and tolerated, increase dose to 8 IU per kilogram of body weight every 12 hours; if necessary, the dose may be increased to a maximum of 8 IU per kilogram of body weight every 6 hours.

Over 60 Years of Age: Same as for 12 to 60 years of age.

▷ **Conditions Requiring Dosing Adjustments:**

Kidney function: Calcitonin should be used with caution by patients with obstructive renal compromise, as the diuresis (loss of fluid via the kidney) may put added pressure on an already obstructed system.

▷ **How Best to Take This Medicine:**   Skin testing before full doses are used may be recommended by your doctor. This is to help protect you from severe allergic reaction to the drug. Subcutaneous (under the skin) injection is preferred for self-administration of the injection form. Your doctor will teach you the details of proper injection technique. If the injection causes nausea or flushing, the daily injection may be taken at bedtime when your stomach is empty. The nasal spray form should be activated as directed in package instructions: the head is placed upright and the tip placed firmly in the nostril. Call your doctor if your nose becomes ulcerated.

▷ **How Long This Medicine Is Usually Taken:**   Use on a regular schedule for 1 to 3 months usually determines the effectiveness of this drug in relieving the symptoms of Paget's disease. If effective, the standard course of treatment is 6 months; if response continues, the dose may be reduced during the next 6 months. Maximal response may require treatment for up to 24 months. For postmenopausal osteoporosis, bone mineral density testing is strongly recommended. This testing can *measure* the benefits of this treatment and can help your doctor decide to continue or choose another therapy. Long-term use (months to years) requires periodic physician evaluation of response and dosage adjustment.

▷ **Tell Your Doctor Before Taking This Medicine If You:**
- ever had an allergic reaction to it.
- recently fractured a bone that has not healed completely.
- are allergic by nature (history of eczema, hives, hay fever, asthma).
- have known allergies to foreign proteins.
- develop sores (ulceration) in the nose while using the nasal form.

▷ **Possible Side Effects:**   Salty or metallic taste in mouth.

▷ **Possible Adverse Effects:**
If any of the following develop, call your doctor promptly for guidance.
Some Mild Problems Drug Can Cause
Allergic reactions: skin rash, hives, itching.
Headache, dizziness, weakness.
Loss of appetite, nausea, vomiting, diarrhea.
Increased frequency of urination.
Some Serious Problems Drug Can Cause
Allergic reactions: anaphylaxis.
Lowering of blood calcium and rigidity.
Severe ulceration of the nose with the nasal spray form.

▷ *CAUTION*
1. If you are allergic by nature, it is advisable to perform a skin test (for allergic hypersensitivity) before beginning treatment with calcitonin-salmon.
2. Maintain a well-balanced diet with adequate calcium and vitamin D content.
3. Tell your doctor if bone pain persists or increases while taking this drug.
4. No specific information is available on use of this drug by infants or children.
5. For those over 60, fluid balance should be followed carefully.
6. Calcitonin should NOT be used by people with blocked kidneys.

Advisability of Use During Pregnancy or If Breast-Feeding:
Pregnancy Category: C. Use only if clearly needed. Ask your doctor for guidance. Present in breast milk; avoid taking this drug or refrain from nursing.

▷ **Overdose Symptoms:**   Nausea, vomiting.

▷ **Suggested Periodic Examinations While Taking This Drug:** (at doctor's discretion)
Measurements of blood calcium, phosphate, and alkaline phosphatase levels. Bone density tests (BMD).
Measurement of urine hydroxyproline content.

▷ **While Taking This Drug the Following Apply:**
Nutritional Support: Ensure adequate intake of calcium and vitamin D.

Alcohol: No interactions expected, but excessive alcohol use is a risk factor for osteoporosis.

Other Drugs:

Calcitonin **taken concurrently** with

- ketoprofen may inhibit calcium and uric acid distribution by calcitonin derived from pigs. Changes with other calcitonins are not defined.
- plicamycin will cause additive loss of calcium.

Heavy Exercise or Exertion: Weight-bearing exercise can help strengthen bones. Talk with your doctor about how much and what kind of exercise is best for you.

Discontinuation: Your doctor should decide when to stop taking this drug.

Special Storage Instructions: Calcitonin-human: Store at a temperature below 77° F (25° C). Do not refrigerate. Protect from light.

Calcitonin-salmon: Store in refrigerator, between 36 and 46° F (2 and 8° C). Do not freeze.

▷ **Saving Money When Using This Medicine:**

- Many new drugs are becoming available to treat osteoporosis (for example, bisphosphonates). Ask your doctor if this medicine offers the best balance of price and outcome for you.
- If your response has been good during the first 6 months, ask if your dose can be decreased for the next 6 months. Also ask about calcium and vitamin D supplements.
- Ask your doctor if bone density testing can help define the success and continued benefit of therapy of your osteoporosis.
- Make certain you have talked with your doctor about risk factors for osteoporosis that can be changed.
- If you have children, talk with your doctor about helping your children reach peak bone mass with diet and exercise. Phosphorous in soda may change calcium needs.

CAPTOPRIL (KAP toh pril)

Prescription Needed: Yes   **Controlled Drug:** No   **Generic:** No

Brand Names: Capoten, Capozide [CD]

Overview of BENEFITS versus RISKS	
Possible Benefits	*Possible Risks*
EFFECTIVE CONTROL OF MILD TO SEVERE HIGH BLOOD PRESSURE	Rare impaired white blood cell production
USEFUL ADJUNCTIVE TREATMENT FOR CONGESTIVE HEART FAILURE	Bone marrow depression (rare) Kidney damage (rare) Liver damage (rare)
MAY DECREASE RISK OF KIDNEY PROBLEMS IN DIABETICS TAKING INSULIN	
MAY REDUCE RISK OF DEATH AFTER A HEART ATTACK	

▷ **Illness This Medication Treats:**
  (1) High blood pressure; (2) prevention of death after heart attacks; (3) advanced heart failure not helped by digoxin or diuretics; (4) diabetes with kidney problems and eye damage.
Other (unlabeled) generally accepted uses: may help ease rheumatoid arthritis or Raynaud's phenomenon.

▷ **Typical Dosage Range:** (Dosage or schedule must be determined by the doctor for each individual.)
Initially 12.5 to 25 mg two or three times daily for 2 weeks. If necessary, dose may be increased to 50 mg three times daily. Usual maintenance dose is 50 to 100 mg three times daily. Total daily dose should not exceed 450 mg. Diabetic kidney problems: 50 mg twice a day in adults.

▷ **Conditions Requiring Dosing Adjustments:**
Liver function: People with liver compromise must use this drug with extreme caution and start with a lower dose.
Kidney function: The dose MUST be decreased for patients with kidney failure.

▷ **How Best to Take This Medicine:** Take on empty stomach, 1 hour before meals, at the same time each day. The tablet may be crushed.

▷ **How Long This Medicine Is Usually Taken:** Use on a regular schedule for several weeks usually determines the effectiveness of this drug in controlling high blood pressure. Long-term use may be needed. See your doctor regularly.

▷ **Tell Your Doctor Before Taking This Medicine If You:**
- ever had an allergic reaction to it.
- are in the last 6 months of pregnancy or are planning pregnancy.
- currently have a blood cell or bone marrow disorder.
- have active liver disease.
- have an abnormally high level of blood potassium.
- had an allergic reaction (or other adverse effect) using any other ACE inhibitor (see Drug Classes).
- have a history of kidney disease or impaired kidney function.
- have scleroderma or systemic lupus erythematosus.
- have any form of heart disease or renal artery stenosis.
- have diabetes.
- are taking any other antihypertensives, diuretics, nitrates, allopurinol (Zyloprim), Indocin, immunosuppressants, or potassium supplements.
- plan to have surgery under general anesthesia soon.

▷ **Possible Side Effects:** Dizziness, light-headedness, fainting (excessive drop in blood pressure). Cough. Increased blood potassium.

▷ **Possible Adverse Effects:**
If any of the following develop, call your doctor promptly for guidance.
Some Mild Problems Drug Can Cause
Allergic reactions: skin rash; swelling of face, hands, or feet; fever.
Lost or altered taste, mouth or tongue sores.
Rapid heart rate, palpitation.
Some Serious Problems Drug Can Cause
Allergic reactions: Stevens-Johnson syndrome.
Bone marrow depression.
Rare hallucinations, pancreatitis, or pericarditis.
Kidney damage—water retention (edema).
Liver damage—with or without jaundice.
Rare lupus erythematosus.

▷ **Possible Effects on Sex Life:** Decreased male libido with recommended dosage. Impotence, rare swelling and tenderness of male breast tissue (gynecomastia).

▷ *CAUTION*
1. If possible, discontinue all other antihypertensive drugs (especially diuretics) for 1 week before starting captopril.

2. **Tell your doctor immediately if you become pregnant.** This drug should not be taken beyond the first 3 months of pregnancy.

3. **Report promptly** any indications of infection (fever, sore throat) and any indications of water retention (weight gain, puffiness, swollen feet or ankles).

4. Do not use a salt substitute without your doctor's knowledge and approval (many salt substitutes contain potassium).

5. It is best to obtain blood cell counts and urine analysis **before** starting this drug.

6. Safety and effectiveness of this drug for infants and children are not established.

7. Small starting doses are advisable for those over 60. Sudden and excessive lowering of blood pressure can predispose to stroke or heart attack in those with impaired brain circulation or coronary artery heart disease.

Advisability of Use During Pregnancy or If Breast-Feeding:

Pregnancy Category: D. Avoid using this drug completely during the last 6 months. C during the first 3 months of pregnancy; use only if clearly needed. Ask your doctor for guidance. Present in breast milk in small amounts. Monitor the nursing infant closely and discontinue taking this drug or nursing if adverse effects develop.

▷ **Overdose Symptoms:** Excessive drop in blood pressure: lightheadedness, dizziness, fainting.

▷ **Suggested Periodic Examinations While Taking This Drug:** (at doctor's discretion)

Before starting drug: Complete blood cell counts; urine analysis with measurement of protein content, blood potassium level. During use of drug: Blood cell counts every 2 weeks during the first 3 months of treatment, then periodically for duration of use. Urine protein measurements every month during the first 9 months of treatment, then periodically for duration of use. Periodic measurements of blood potassium,

▷ **While Taking This Drug the Following Apply:**

Foods: Talk with your doctor about salt intake.

Nutritional Support: **Do not take** potassium supplements unless directed by your doctor.

Beverages: May be taken with milk.

Alcohol: Alcohol may further lower blood pressure. Use with caution.

Other Drugs:

Captopril *taken concurrently* with

• allopurinol (Zyloprim) may increase risk of serious skin reactions.

• azathioprine may lead to severe anemia.

• cyclosporine (Sandimmune) may result in kidney failure.

• lithium (Lithobid, others) can lead to lithium toxicity.

- loop diuretics (such as Lasix or Bumex) may lead to excessively low blood pressure on standing (postural hypotension).
- phenothiazines (see Drug Classes) may result in postural hypotension.
- potassium preparations (K-Lyte, Slow-K, etc.) may cause increased blood levels of potassium with risk of serious heart rhythm disturbances.
- potassium-sparing diuretics—amiloride (Moduretic), spironolactone (Aldactazide), triamterene (Dyazide)—may cause increased blood levels of potassium with risk of serious heart rhythm disturbances.

The following drugs may *decrease* the effects of captopril

- antacids, by decreasing captopril absorption. Separate doses by 2 hours.
- indomethacin (Indocin) or other NSAIDs (see Drug Classes).
- naloxone (Narcan).
- salicylates (aspirin, etc.).

Driving, Hazardous Activities: Usually no restrictions. Be aware of possible drops in blood pressure with resultant dizziness or faintness.

Exposure to Sun: Caution is advised. This drug can cause photosensitivity.

Exposure to Heat: Caution is advised. Avoid excessive perspiring with resultant loss of body water and drop in blood pressure.

Occurrence of Unrelated Illness: Report promptly any disorder that causes nausea, vomiting, or diarrhea. Fluid and chemical imbalances must be corrected as soon as possible.

▷ **Saving Money When Using This Medicine:**

- Many medicines are in this class. Ask your doctor if this drug offers the best combination of price and outcome for you.
- Talk with your doctor about stress management, exercise, and weight loss. Also ask about ongoing checks of kidney function.
- Have your blood pressure checked periodically to make sure this medicine is still helping you.

CARBAMAZEPINE (kar ba MAZ e peen)

Prescription Needed: Yes **Controlled Drug:** No **Generic:** Yes

Brand Names: Epitol, Tegretol, Tegretol chewable tablet

Overview of BENEFITS versus RISKS

Possible Benefits	*Possible Risks*
RELIEF OF PAIN IN TRIGEMINAL NEURALGIA	RARE BONE MARROW DEPRESSION
EFFECTIVE CONTROL OF CERTAIN TYPES OF EPILEPTIC SEIZURES	Liver damage with jaundice
Relief of pain in some rare forms of neuralgia	

▷ **Illness This Medication Treats:**

(1) Pain in true trigeminal neuralgia (tic douloureux) and glosso-pharyngeal neuralgia; (2) controls: grand mal, psychomotor or temporal lobe, and mixed seizure pattern epilepsy. Because of its potential for serious toxic effects, precise diagnosis and careful management are mandatory for proper use.

Other (unlabeled) generally accepted uses: (1) helpful in resistant schizophrenia, posttraumatic stress disorder, or bipolar (manic-depressive) disorder; (2) can help diabetic nephropathy; (3) may have a role easing pain after amputation.

▷ **Typical Dosage Range:** (Dosage or schedule must be determined by the doctor for each individual.)

Initially 200 mg/12 hr. Dose may be increased at weekly intervals by 200 mg/24 hr as needed and tolerated. Total daily dosage should not exceed 1200 mg.

▷ **Conditions Requiring Dosing Adjustments:**

Liver function: Use this drug with extreme caution and in lower doses.
Kidney function: This medication is capable of causing kidney toxicity, and should be used with caution by patients with poorly functioning kidneys

▷ **How Best to Take This Medicine:** Take at the same time each day, with or following food to reduce stomach irritation. Tablet may be crushed for administration.

▷ **How Long This Medicine Is Usually Taken:** Use on a regular schedule for 3 months usually determines the effectiveness of this drug in relieving the pain of trigeminal neuralgia. Longer periods, with dosage adjustment, may be required to determine its ability to control epileptic seizures. Careful evaluation of individual tolerance and response should be made every 3 months during long-term treatment.

▷ **Tell Your Doctor Before Taking This Medicine If You:**
- ever had an allergic reaction to it or any tricyclic antidepressant drug.
- have active liver disease.
- currently have a blood cell or bone marrow disorder.
- are currently taking, or have taken within the past 14 days, any MAO type A inhibitor.
- have taken this drug in the past.
- have a history of any kind of blood cell or bone marrow disorder, especially drug-related.
- have a history of liver or kidney disease.
- have had serious mental depression or other mental disorders.
- have had thrombophlebitis.
- have high blood pressure, heart disease, or glaucoma.
- take more than two alcoholic drinks a day.
- are pregnant or breast-feeding your baby.

▷ **Possible Side Effects:** Dry mouth and throat, constipation, impaired urination. Neuroleptic malignant syndrome.

▷ **Possible Adverse Effects:**
If any of the following develop, call your doctor promptly for guidance.
Some Mild Problems Drug Can Cause
  Allergic reactions: skin rash, hives, itching, drug fever.
  Headache, dizziness, drowsiness, blurred vision, confusion.
  Exaggerated hearing, ringing in ears.
  Loss of appetite, nausea, vomiting, diarrhea.
  Water retention (edema), frequent urination.
  Changes in skin pigmentation, hair loss.
  Aching of muscles and joints, leg cramps.
Some Serious Problems Drug Can Cause
  Allergic reactions: severe dermatitis with skin peeling, irritation, swelling of lymph glands.
  Idiosyncratic reactions: lung inflammation (pneumonitis)—shortness of breath.
  Bone marrow depression.
  Liver damage with jaundice.
  Kidney damage—reduced urine volume, uremic poisoning.
  Rare pancreatitis or pseudolymphoma.
  Mental depression and agitation.
  Hallucinations, changes in vision, speech disturbances, peripheral neuritis.
  Drug-induced meningitis or porphyria.

Vitamin D deficiency (may lead to osteoporosis).
Thrombophlebitis.

▷ **Possible Effects on Sex Life:**   Decreased libido and/or impotence, male infertility. This drug is used to control hypersexuality resulting from injury to the temporal lobe of the brain.

▷ *CAUTION*

1. Because this drug can cause serious adverse effects, it should be used only when a trial of less hazardous drugs has been ineffective.

2. *Before* the first dose is taken, pretreatment blood cell counts and liver and kidney function tests should be performed.

3. Careful periodic testing for early indications of blood cell or bone marrow toxicity is *mandatory.*

4. During periods of spontaneous remission from trigeminal neuralgia, this drug *should not be used* to prevent recurrence.

5. If you are using carbamazepine to control epileptic seizures, *do not stop taking this drug suddenly.*

6. This drug may lose up to one-third of its effectiveness if stored in humid conditions. When exposed to humidity, the tablet form hardens, resulting in poor absorption from the gastrointestinal (GI) tract and erratic control of seizures. Store in a cool, dry place; avoid bathrooms and other humidified areas.

7. Safety and effectiveness of this drug for those under 6 years old are not established. Because of the high frequency of adverse effects (up to 25%), careful testing of blood cell production and liver and kidney function must be performed regularly. This drug can reduce the effectiveness of other anticonvulsants. Blood levels of all anticonvulsants should be checked if this drug is added to the treatment program.

8. For those over 60 years old, carbamazepine can cause confusion and agitation. Watch for possible aggravation of glaucoma, coronary artery disease (angina), or prostatism.

Advisability of Use During Pregnancy or If Breast-Feeding:
Pregnancy Category: C. Avoid this drug completely during the first 3 months. Use during the last 6 months only if clearly needed. Present in breast milk; avoid taking this drug or refrain from nursing.

▷ **Overdose Symptoms:**   Dizziness, unsteadiness, drowsiness, disorientation, tremor, involuntary movements, nausea, vomiting, flushed skin, dilated pupils, stupor progressing to coma.

▷ **Suggested Periodic Examinations While Taking This Drug:** (at doctor's discretion)
Complete blood cell counts weekly during the first 3 months of treatment, and monthly thereafter until the drug is discontinued. Liver and kidney function tests. Complete eye examinations.

▷ **While Taking This Drug the Following Apply:**

Beverages: May be taken with milk.

Alcohol: Use caution. This drug may increase the sedative effect of alcohol.

Other Drugs:

Carbamazepine may *increase* the effects of

- sedatives, tranquilizers, hypnotics, and narcotics, and enhance their sedative effects.

Carbamazepine may *decrease* the effects of

- antidepressants (see Drug Classes).
- birth control pills (oral contraceptives).
- corticosteroids (see Drug Classes).
- cyclosporine (Sandimmune).
- doxycycline (Doxy-II, Vibramycin, etc.).
- felodipine (Plendil).
- haloperidol (Haldol).
- isradipine (DynaCirc).
- itraconazole (Sporanox).
- tetracyclines (see Drug Classes).
- valproic acid (Depakene, etc.).
- warfarin (Coumadin).

Carbamazepine *taken concurrently* with

- clozapine (Clozaril) may result in serious bone marrow depression.
- felbamate (Felbatol) may decrease carbamazepine levels and result in seizures.
- lithium (Lithobid, others) may cause serious neurologic disturbances: confusion, drowsiness, weakness, unsteadiness, tremors, muscle twitching.
- MAO type A inhibitors (see Drug Classes) may cause severe toxic reactions.
- phenytoin (Dilantin, etc.) may cause unpredictable fluctuations of blood levels of both drugs and impair seizure control.
- terfenadine (Seldane) may result in carbamazepine toxicity.
- theophylline (Slo-bid, Theo-Dur, etc.) may reduce the effects of both drugs.

The following drugs may *increase* the effects of carbamazepine

- cimetidine (Tagamet).
- danazol (Danocrine).
- diltiazem (Cardizem) and perhaps other calcium channel blockers.
- fluvoxamine (Luvox), and result in toxicity.
- macrolide antibiotics—erythromycin (E.E.S., E-Mycin, etc.), clarithromycin, azithromycin.
- isoniazid (INH).
- nicotinamide (nicotinic acid amide).
- propoxyphene (Darvon, Darvocet, etc.).

- rifampin (Rifamate, others).
- troleandomycin (Tao).
- verapamil (Calan, Isoptin).

Driving, Hazardous Activities: Carbamazepine causes dizziness, drowsiness, or blurred vision. Adjust your activities accordingly.

Exposure to Sun: Carbamazepine causes photosensitivity. Use caution until your sensitivity to the sun has been determined.

Heavy Exercise or Exertion: Use caution if you have coronary artery disease. This drug can intensify angina and reduce your tolerance for physical activity.

Occurrence of Unrelated Illness: Because of this drug's potential for serious adverse effects, you MUST tell each prescriber (such as doctors or dentists) who provides health care for you that you are taking carbamazepine.

Discontinuation: If carbamazepine is used to treat trigeminal neuralgia, an attempt should be made every 3 months to reduce the maintenance dose or to stop taking this drug altogether. If used to control epilepsy, this drug *must not be stopped abruptly.*

Special Storage Instructions: Store the tablet form of this drug in a cool, dry place—NOT THE BATHROOM MEDICINE CABINET. Protect it from exposure to humid conditions.

▷ **Saving Money When Using This Medicine:**
- The generic form is acceptable for use; however, DO NOT change from one form to the other. If you are stabilized on the generic, remain on it.
- If carbamazepine is used to treat trigeminal neuralgia, an attempt should be made to decrease the dose or to stop taking this drug every 3 months.
- Ask your doctor if this medicine offers the best combination of price and outcome for you.
- A new agent (gabapentin) is available for add-on therapy if your seizures are not well controlled. Talk with your doctor about this medicine.

CARTEOLOL (KAR tee oh lohl)

Prescription Needed: Yes   **Controlled Drug:** No   **Generic:** No

Brand Names: Cartrol, Ocupress, Optipress

```
┌─────────────────────────────────────────────────────────┐
│           Overview of BENEFITS versus RISKS              │
│   Possible Benefits              Possible Risks          │
│  EFFECTIVE,                  CONGESTIVE HEART            │
│    WELL-TOLERATED              FAILURE in advanced heart │
│    ANTIHYPERTENSIVE            disease                   │
│  EFFECTIVE GLAUCOMA          Worsening of angina in      │
│    TREATMENT                   coronary heart disease    │
│                                (abrupt withdrawal)       │
│                              Masking of hypoglycemia in  │
│                                drug-treated diabetes     │
│                              Provocation of asthma       │
└─────────────────────────────────────────────────────────┘
```

▷ **Illness This Medication Treats:**
   (1) Mild to moderate high blood pressure, used alone or concurrently
   with other antihypertensive drugs; (2) classical effort-induced angina; (3) lowers eye (intraocular) pressure in people with glaucoma.
   Other (unlabeled) generally accepted uses: (1) other beta-blockers
   have shown benefits in decreasing heart attacks; however, studies
   with this medicine have not been performed. (2) May help panic
   attacks.

▷ **Typical Dosage Range:** (Dosage or schedule must be determined by
   the doctor for each individual.)
   Initially 2.5 mg once daily. The dose may be increased gradually by 2.5
   mg/day at intervals of 2 weeks, as needed and tolerated, up to 10
   mg/day. For maintenance, 2.5 to 7.5 mg once daily is usually adequate. The total daily dose should not exceed 10 mg.
   Glaucoma: One drop in the affected eye or eyes two times a day.

▷ **Conditions Requiring Dosing Adjustments:**
   Liver function: The dose should be decreased for patients with severe
   liver compromise.
   Kidney function: The dose MUST be decreased or the dosing interval
   increased for patients with kidney compromise. In cases of severe
   compromise, the drug is taken every 48 to 72 hours.

▷ **How Best to Take This Medicine:**   The tablet may be crushed and
   taken without regard to eating. Do not stop taking this drug
   abruptly.

▷ **How Long This Medicine Is Usually Taken:**   Use on a regular
   schedule for 2 to 3 weeks usually determines the effectiveness of this
   drug in lowering blood pressure. Long-term use (months to years) is
   determined by your blood pressure response and your further benefit from an overall treatment program (weight reduction, salt restriction, smoking cessation, etc.). See your doctor regularly.

▷ **Tell Your Doctor Before Taking This Medicine If You:**
- ever had an allergic reaction to it.
- have congestive heart failure.
- have an abnormally slow heart rate or a serious form of heart block.
- are subject to bronchial asthma.
- have had an adverse reaction to any beta-blocker in the past.
- have a history of serious heart disease, with or without episodes of heart failure.
- have a history of hay fever (allergic rhinitis), asthma, chronic bronchitis, or emphysema.
- have a history of hyperthyroidism.
- have a history of hypoglycemia.
- have impaired liver or kidney function.
- have diabetes or myasthenia gravis.
- have impaired circulation in the extremities (Raynaud's disorder, claudication pains in legs).
- are currently taking any form of digitalis, quinidine, or reserpine, or any calcium blocker (see Drug Classes).
- plan to have surgery under general anesthesia soon.

▷ **Possible Side Effects:**   Lethargy and fatigability, cold extremities, slow heart rate, light-headedness in upright position. Tearing and irritation with eyedrop use.

▷ **Possible Adverse Effects:**
If any of the following develop, call your doctor promptly for guidance.
Some Mild Problems Drug Can Cause
Allergic reactions: skin rash.
Dizziness, nervousness, drowsiness, abnormal dreams.
Nausea, vomiting, constipation, diarrhea.
Joint and muscle discomfort, numbness of fingers or toes.
Some Serious Problems Drug Can Cause
Mental depression, anxiety.
Chest pain, irregular heartbeat, congestive heart failure.
May cause an asthma attack in asthmatics.
May hide symptoms of low blood sugar.
Aggravation of myasthenia gravis.

▷ **Possible Effects on Sex Life:**   Decreased libido, impotence.

▷ *CAUTION*
1. ***Do not stop taking this drug suddenly*** without the knowledge and guidance of your doctor. Carry a note that states you are taking this drug.
2. Consult your doctor or pharmacist before using nasal decongestants, which are usually present in over-the-counter cold prepara-

tions and nose drops. These can cause sudden increases in blood pressure when taken concurrently with beta-blockers.

3. Report the development of any tendency to emotional depression.
4. Safety and effectiveness of this drug for those under 12 years old are not established. However, if this drug is used, watch for the development of hypoglycemia, especially if meals are skipped.
5. **ALL** antihypertensives must be used carefully by those over 60. Treatment should be started with small doses, and blood pressure checked often. Sudden, rapid, and excessive reduction of blood pressure can predispose to stroke or heart attack. Watch for dizziness, unsteadiness, tendency to fall, confusion, hallucinations, depression, or urinary frequency.

Advisability of Use During Pregnancy or If Breast-Feeding:

Pregnancy Category: C. Use only if clearly needed. Ask your doctor for guidance. Present in breast milk in animals, presence is unknown in humans; avoid taking this drug or refrain from nursing.

▷ **Overdose Symptoms:**   Weakness, slow pulse, low blood pressure, fainting, cold and sweaty skin, congestive heart failure, possible coma, and convulsions.

▷ **Suggested Periodic Examinations While Taking This Drug:** (at doctor's discretion)

Measurements of blood pressure, evaluation of heart function.

▷ **While Taking This Drug the Following Apply:**

Foods: Avoid excessive salt intake.

Beverages: May be taken with milk.

Alcohol: Use caution. Alcohol may exaggerate this drug's ability to lower blood pressure and increase its mild sedative effect.

Tobacco Smoking: Nicotine may reduce carteolol's effectiveness in treating high blood pressure. In addition, high doses may worsen constriction of bronchial tubes caused by regular smoking.

Other Drugs:

Carteolol may *increase* the effects of

- other antihypertensive drugs and cause excessive lowering of the blood pressure. Dosage adjustments may be necessary.
- reserpine (Ser-Ap-Es, etc.), causing sedation, depression, slowing of the heart rate, and lowered blood pressure. This combination is best avoided.
- theophyllines (aminophylline, dyphylline, oxtriphylline, etc.).
- verapamil (Calan, Isoptin), causing excessive depression of heart function; monitor this combination closely.

Carteolol *taken concurrently* with

- amiodarone (Cordarone) may cause severe slowing of the heart and arrest.

- clonidine (Catapres) requires close monitoring for rebound high blood pressure if clonidine is withdrawn while carteolol is still being taken.
- diltiazem (Cardizem) may be helpful in patients with normal heart function, but may result in atrioventricular (AV) conduction problems.
- epinephrine (Adrenalin, etc.) may cause sudden and excessive rise in blood pressure, followed by slowing of the heart rate. Avoid the concurrent use of beta-blockers and epinephrine.
- ergot preparations (ergotamine, methysergide, etc.) may enhance ergot-induced constriction of peripheral circulation to a dangerous degree.
- fluvoxamine (Luvox) may result in dangerous heart slowing or low blood pressure.
- insulin requires close monitoring to avoid undetected hypoglycemia.
- nifedipine may result in severe lowering of blood pressure.
- oral hypoglycemic agents (see Drug Classes) may result in prolonged recovery from hypoglycemia.
- phenothiazines (see Drug Classes) may cause increased effects of both medicines.

The following drugs may *decrease* the effects of carteolol

- indomethacin (Indocin), and possibly other aspirin substitute NSAIDs (se Drug Classes), may impair carteolol's antihypertensive effect.

Driving, Hazardous Activities: Use caution until the full extent of fatigue, dizziness, and blood pressure change have been determined.

Exposure to Heat: Caution is advised. Hot environments can lower the blood pressure and exaggerate the effects of this drug.

Exposure to Cold: Caution is advised. Cold environments can enhance the circulatory deficiency in the extremities that may occur with this drug. The elderly should take precautions to prevent hypothermia.

Heavy Exercise or Exertion: Avoid exertion that produces light-headedness, excessive fatigue, or muscle cramping. This drug may intensify the hypertensive response to isometric exercise.

Occurrence of Unrelated Illness: Fever can lower blood pressure and require adjustment of dose. Illnesses that cause nausea or vomiting may interrupt the regular dosage schedule. Ask your doctor for help.

Discontinuation: Avoid sudden discontinuation of this drug in all situations. If possible, gradual reduction of dose over a period of 2 to 3 weeks is recommended. Ask your doctor for help.

▷ **Saving Money When Using This Medicine:**
- Many beta-blockers are available today. Ask your doctor if this drug provides the best combination of cost and outcomes for you.
- If you are overweight, losing those extra pounds may allow you to stop taking high blood pressure medicine altogether. Talk with your doctor about stress management and exercise programs available in your community.

CEFACLOR (SEF a klor)

Prescription Needed: Yes   **Controlled Drug:** No   **Generic:** No

Brand Names: Ceclor

Overview of BENEFITS versus RISKS

Possible Benefits	*Possible Risks*
EFFECTIVE TREATMENT OF INFECTIONS due to susceptible microorganisms	ALLERGIC REACTIONS, mild to severe Drug-induced colitis (rare) Superinfections

---

▷ **Illness This Medication Treats:**
Some infections of the skin, skin structures, and the respiratory tract (including middle ear infections and strep throat), and certain urinary tract infections.

▷ **Typical Dosage Range:** (Dosage or schedule must be determined by the doctor for each individual.)
250 to 500 mg/8 hr. Total daily dose should not exceed 4 g.
In children: 20 to 40 mg per kilogram of body weight daily, taken in divided doses every 8 hours. Maximum is 1000 mg daily.

▷ **Conditions Requiring Dosing Adjustments:**
Liver function: Elimination by the liver has not yet been identified.
Kidney function: The dose MUST be decreased by up to 50% for people with compromised kidneys.

▷ **How Best to Take This Medicine:**   May be taken on an empty stomach or with food if stomach irritation occurs. Capsule may be opened. Shake suspension well before measuring (use a calibrated dosing device) dose. Take the full course prescribed.

▷ **How Long This Medicine Is Usually Taken:** Use on a regular schedule for 3 to 5 days usually determines the effectiveness of this drug in controlling the infection under treatment. Response varies with the nature of the infection. Total treatment time varies from 1 to 4 weeks. Certain infections require the drug be taken for 10 consecutive days to prevent development of rheumatic fever. Follow your doctor's instructions regarding duration of use.

▷ **Tell Your Doctor Before Taking This Medicine If You:**
- are allergic to any cephalosporin antibiotic.
- have a history of allergy to any form of penicillin.
- have a history of regional enteritis or ulcerative colitis.
- have impaired kidney function.

▷ **Possible Side Effects:**   Superinfections.

▷ **Possible Adverse Effects:**
If any of the following develop, call your doctor promptly for guidance.

Some Mild Problems Drug Can Cause
Allergic reactions: skin rash, itching, hives.
Nausea and vomiting, mild diarrhea, sore mouth.

Some Serious Problems Drug Can Cause
Allergic reactions: drug fever, joint aches and pains, anaphylactic reaction.
Genital itching (may represent a fungus superinfection).
Severe diarrhea, which may be drug-induced colitis (rare).
Rare cholestatic jaundice.

▷ *CAUTION*
1. In management of diabetes, it should be noted that this drug can cause a false-positive test result for urine sugar when using Clinitest tablets, Benedict's solution, or Fehling's solution, but not with Tes-Tape.
2. Cefaclor is not recommended for use for infants less than 1 month old. The maximal dose in children should not exceed 1 g/24 hr
3. Dose for those over 60 must be carefully individualized and based on evaluation of kidney function. Natural changes in the skin may predispose to severe and prolonged itching reactions in the genital and anal regions. Such reactions should be reported promptly.
4. If you are allergic to penicillin, it is possible that you may also be allergic to this medicine.

Advisability of Use During Pregnancy or If Breast-Feeding:
Pregnancy Category: B. Generally considered safe. Ask your doctor for guidance. Present in breast milk in small amounts: avoid taking this drug or refrain from nursing.

▷ **Overdose Symptoms:**   Nausea, vomiting, stomach cramps, and/or diarrhea.

▷ **While Taking This Drug the Following Apply:**
Beverages: May be taken with milk.

Other Drugs:
Cefaclor *taken concurrently* with
- oral contraceptives (birth control pills) may result in failure of the contraceptive and pregnancy.
- loop diuretics may pose an increased risk of kidney toxicity.
- probenecid (Benemid) slows elimination of cefaclor, resulting in higher blood levels and prolonged effect.

Special Storage Instructions: Oral suspension should be refrigerated.
Observe the Following Expiration Times: Do not take the oral suspension of this drug if it is older than 14 days.

▷ **Saving Money When Using This Medicine:**
- Many antibiotics are available today, particularly to treat streptococcus infections. Ask your doctor if this medicine offers the best combination of price and outcomes for you—perhaps a penicillin could be used instead.

CEFADROXIL (sef a DROX il)

Prescription Needed: Yes   **Controlled Drug:** No   **Generic:** Yes

Brand Names: Duricef, Ultracef

Overview of BENEFITS versus RISKS	
Possible Benefits	*Possible Risks*
EFFECTIVE TREATMENT OF INFECTIONS due to susceptible microorganisms	ALLERGIC REACTIONS, mild to severe Drug-induced colitis (rare) Superinfections

▷ **Illness This Medication Treats:**
Certain infections of the skin, skin structures, and the upper respiratory tract (including tonsillitis and strep throat), and some urinary tract infections.

▷ **Typical Dosage Range:** (Dosage or schedule must be determined by the doctor for each individual.)
Skin infections: 500 mg/12 hr, or 1 g daily. Strep throat: 500 mg/12 hr for 10 days. Urinary tract infections: 500 mg to 1 g every 12 hours, or 1 to 2 g daily. Total daily dosage should not exceed 6 g.

▷ **Conditions Requiring Dosing Adjustments:**
Kidney function: For creatinine clearances of 10 to 50 ml/min, use the usual doses every 12 to 24 hours. For creatinine clearances less than 10 ml/min, use the usual doses taken every 24 to 48 hours.

▷ **How Best to Take This Medicine:**   May be taken on an empty stomach or with food if stomach irritation occurs. Capsule may be opened. Shake suspension well before measuring dose. Take the full course prescribed.

▷ **How Long This Medicine Is Usually Taken:**   Use on a regular schedule for 3 to 5 days usually determines the effectiveness of this drug in controlling the infection under treatment. Response varies with the nature of the infection. Total treatment time varies from 1 to 4 weeks. Certain infections require that this drug be taken for 10 consecutive days to prevent the development of rheumatic fever. Follow your doctor's instructions on how long to take it.

▷ **Tell Your Doctor Before Taking This Medicine If You:**
• are allergic to any cephalosporin antibiotic.
• have a history of allergy to any form of penicillin.
• have a history of regional enteritis or ulcerative colitis.
• have impaired kidney function.

▷ **Possible Side Effects:**   Superinfections.

▷ **Possible Adverse Effects:**
If any of the following develop, call your doctor promptly for guidance.
Some Mild Problems Drug Can Cause
Allergic reactions: skin rash, itching, localized swellings.
Headache, drowsiness, dizziness.
Nausea, vomiting, mild diarrhea, sore mouth or tongue.
Some Serious Problems Drug Can Cause
Allergic reactions: drug fever, joint aches and pains, anaphylactic reaction.
Idiosyncratic reactions: minor and temporary changes in white blood cell counts and liver function tests (infrequent).
Genital itching (may represent a fungus superinfection).
Severe diarrhea, which may be drug-induced colitis (rare).

▷ *CAUTION*
1. In management of diabetes, it should be noted that this drug can cause a false-positive test result for urine sugar when using Clinitest tablets, Benedict's solution, or Fehling's solution, but not with Tes-Tape.
2. For infants and children, dose is based upon weight, and must be determined by the doctor for each individual. Follow your doctor's instructions exactly.
3. In those over 60 years old, dose must be carefully individualized and based on evaluation of kidney function. Natural changes in the skin may predispose to severe and prolonged itching reactions

in the genital and anal regions. Such reactions should be reported promptly.

4. Dose must be decreased for best effect for patients with kidney compromise.
5. If you are allergic to penicillin, you may also be allergic to this medicine. Talk to your doctor about your allergy.

Advisability of Use During Pregnancy or If Breast-Feeding:

Pregnancy Category: B. Generally considered safe. Ask your doctor for guidance. Present in breast milk in small amounts; avoid taking this drug or refrain from nursing.

▷ **Overdose Symptoms:** Nausea, vomiting, stomach cramps and/or diarrhea.

▷ **Suggested Periodic Examinations While Taking This Drug:** (at doctor's discretion)

Complete blood cell counts. Liver and kidney function tests.

▷ **While Taking This Drug the Following Apply:**

Beverages: May be taken with milk.

Other Drugs:

Cefadroxil *taken concurrently* with

- aminoglycoside antibiotics (see Drug Classes) may increase risk of kidney toxicity.
- oral contraceptives (birth control pills) may result in LOSS OF CONTRACEPTION and pregnancy.
- probenecid (Benemid) slows the elimination of cefadroxil, resulting in higher blood levels and prolonged effect.

Driving, Hazardous Activities: Usually no restrictions. If drowsiness or dizziness occurs, restrict your activities accordingly.

Special Storage Instructions: Oral suspension should be refrigerated.

Observe the Following Expiration Times: Do not take the oral suspension of this drug if it is older than 14 days.

▷ **Saving Money When Using This Medicine:**

- Many antibiotics are available today. Ask your doctor if this medicine offers the best combination of price and outcomes for you—perhaps a penicillin could be used instead.
- A generic form of this medicine can be used instead of the more expensive brand.

CEFIXIME (sef IX eem)

Prescription Needed: Yes   **Controlled Drug:** No   **Generic:** No

Brand Names: Suprax

Overview of BENEFITS versus RISKS	
Possible Benefits	*Possible Risks*
EFFECTIVE TREATMENT OF INFECTIONS due to susceptible microorganisms	ALLERGIC REACTIONS, mild to severe Drug-induced colitis (rare) Superinfections Low white blood cells or platelets

▷ **Illness This Medication Treats:**
Certain infections of the middle ear, tonsils, throat, bronchial tubes, and urinary tract.

▷ **Typical Dosage Range:** (Dosage or schedule must be determined by the doctor for each individual.)
400 mg daily, taken as a single dose or 200 mg every 12 hours.

▷ **Conditions Requiring Dosing Adjustments:**
Liver function: Dose must be decreased for patients with severe hepatic compromise and long-term therapy.
Kidney function: The dose MUST be decreased for patients with mild to moderate kidney compromise. For patients with severe kidney failure, a single dose of 400 mg is taken every 2 days.

▷ **How Best to Take This Medicine:** May be taken on an empty stomach or with food if stomach irritation occurs. The tablet may be crushed and mixed with food (such as applesauce or ice cream) if necessary to facilitate swallowing. Take the full course prescribed.

▷ **How Long This Medicine Is Usually Taken:** Use on a regular schedule for 3 to 5 days usually determines the effectiveness of this drug in controlling the infection under treatment. Response varies with the nature of the infection. Total treatment time varies from 1 to 4 weeks. Certain infections require that this drug be taken for 10 consecutive days to prevent the development of rheumatic fever. Follow your doctor's instructions on how long to take this drug.

▷ **Tell Your Doctor Before Taking This Medicine If You:**
- are allergic to any cephalosporin antibiotic.
- have active colitis of any type.
- have a history of allergy to any form of penicillin.
- have a history of regional enteritis or ulcerative colitis.

- have a history of low blood platelets or white blood cells.
- have impaired kidney function.

▷ **Possible Side Effects:**   Superinfections: vaginitis (yeast infection).

▷ **Possible Adverse Effects:**

If any of the following develop, call your doctor promptly for guidance.

Some Mild Problems Drug Can Cause

Allergic reactions: skin rash, itching, drug fever.

Nausea, indigestion, loose stools, diarrhea, abdominal pain.

Headache, dizziness.

Some Serious Problems Drug Can Cause

Severe diarrhea, which may be drug-induced colitis (rare).

Low blood platelets or white blood cells.

Kidney toxicity.

▷ **CAUTION**

1. Otitis media should be treated with the oral suspension; this produces higher blood levels of the drug. Tablets should not be substituted for the suspension.

2. In management of diabetes, it should be noted that this drug can cause a false-positive test result for urine sugar when using Clinitest tablets, Benedict's solution, or Fehling's solution, but not with Clinistix or Tes-Tape. This drug can also cause a false-positive reaction for urine ketones with tests that use nitroprusside but not nitroferricyanide.

3. Safety and effectiveness of this drug for use by those under 6 months old have not been established. For those over 6 months old the recommended dose is 8 mg per kilogram of body weight per day of the oral suspension. This may be given as a single daily dose or 4 mg per kilogram of body weight every 12 hours.

4. For those over 60, dosage must be carefully individualized and based on evaluation of kidney function. Natural changes in the skin may predispose to severe and prolonged itching reactions in the genital and anal regions. Such reactions should be reported promptly.

5. If you are allergic to penicillin, you may also be allergic to this medicine. Talk with your doctor about your allergy.

Advisability of Use During Pregnancy or If Breast-Feeding:

Pregnancy Category: B. Generally considered safe. Ask your doctor for guidance. Presence in breast milk is unknown; avoid taking this drug or refrain from nursing.

▷ **Overdose Symptoms:**   Nausea, vomiting, stomach cramps, and/or diarrhea.

▷ **Suggested Periodic Examinations While Taking This Drug:** (at doctor's discretion)

Complete blood cell counts.

▷ **While Taking This Drug the Following Apply:**
Beverages: This drug may be taken with milk.
Other Drugs:
Cefixime *taken concurrently* with
- aminoglycoside antibiotics (see Drug Classes) may pose an increased risk of kidney toxicity.

Driving, Hazardous Activities: Usually no restrictions. Observe for the rare occurrence of dizziness.
Special Storage Instructions: Keep the oral suspension at room temperature. Do not refrigerate. Shake well before measuring dose.
Observe the Following Expiration Time: Do not take the oral suspension of this drug if it is older than 14 days.

▷ **Saving Money When Using This Medicine:**
- Many antibiotics are available today. Ask your doctor if this medicine offers the best combination of price and outcomes for you. This medicine also kills many kinds of bacteria (broad spectrum). Ask your doctor if a narrower spectrum antibiotic could be used.

CEFPROZIL (SEF pro zil)

Prescription Needed: Yes   **Controlled Drug:** No   **Generic:** No

Brand Names: Cefzil

Overview of BENEFITS versus RISKS	
Possible Benefits	*Possible Risks*
EFFECTIVE TREATMENT OF INFECTIONS due to susceptible microorganisms	ALLERGIC REACTIONS, mild to severe
	Drug-induced colitis (rare)
	Superinfections

▷ **Illness This Medication Treats:**
(1) Upper respiratory tract infections: pharyngitis, tonsillitis, otitis media (caused by susceptible organisms); (2) lower respiratory tract infections: acute bronchitis and exacerbation of chronic bronchitis (caused by susceptible organisms); (3) skin and skin structure infections (caused by susceptible organisms).

▷ **Typical Dosage Range:** (Dosage or schedule must be determined by the doctor for each individual.)
Infants and Children: For otitis media (6 months to 12 years of age): 15 mg per kilogram of body weight every 12 hours, for 10 days.
13 to 60 Years of Age: For pharyngitis or tonsillitis: 500 mg every 24 hours, for 10 days.

For acute and chronic bronchitis: 500 mg every 12 hours, for 10 days.
For skin and skin structure infections: 250 to 500 mg every 12 to 24 hours, for 10 days.

Over 60 Years of Age: Same as for 13 to 60 years of age. Dosage should be reduced for significantly decreased kidney function.

▷ **Conditions Requiring Dosing Adjustments:**

Liver function: The liver is not known to be involved in elimination of this drug. This drug has rarely caused liver damage.

Kidney function: For creatinine clearances of 30 ml/min or less (moderate kidney failure), use 50% of the usual dose at the usual dosing interval.

Phenylketonuria (PKU): The suspension has 28 mg of phenylalanine in every 5 ml. This may preclude the use of cefixime suspension by patients with PKU.

▷ **How Best to Take This Medicine:**   May be taken on an empty stomach or with food, if stomach irritation occurs. The tablet may be crushed and mixed with food (such as applesauce or ice cream) if necessary to help swallowing. Shake the oral suspension well before measuring each dose.

▷ **How Long This Medicine Is Usually Taken:**   Use on a regular schedule for 3 to 5 days usually determines the effectiveness of this drug in controlling the infection under treatment. Response varies with the nature of the infection. Total treatment time varies from 1 to 4 weeks. Certain infections require that this drug be taken for 10 consecutive days to prevent the development of rheumatic fever. Follow your doctor's instructions regarding duration of use. Make certain you take this medicine exactly as prescribed.

▷ **Tell Your Doctor Before Taking This Medicine If You:**
• are allergic to any cephalosporin antibiotic.
• have a history of allergy to any form of penicillin.
• have a history of regional enteritis or ulcerative colitis.
• have a history of clotting problems or low white blood cell counts.
• have impaired kidney function.

▷ **Possible Side Effects:**   Superinfections: vaginitis.

▷ **Possible Adverse Effects:**
If any of the following develop, call your doctor promptly for guidance.
Some Mild Problems Drug Can Cause
    Allergic reactions: skin rash, hives.
    Nausea, vomiting, mild diarrhea.
    Headache, dizziness.
Some Serious Problems Drug Can Cause
    Rare liver damage.

▷ *CAUTION*

1. In management of diabetes, it should be noted that this drug may cause a false-positive test result for urine sugar when using Clinitest tablets, Benedict's solution, or Fehling's solution, but not with Clinistix or Tes-Tape.

2. Safety and effectiveness of this drug for those under 6 months old are not established.

3. For those over 60 years old, dose must be carefully individualized and based on evaluation of kidney function. Natural changes in the skin may predispose to severe and prolonged itching reactions in the genital and anal regions. Such reactions should be reported promptly.

Advisability of Use During Pregnancy or If Breast-Feeding:
Pregnancy Category: B. Generally considered safe. Ask your doctor for guidance. Presence in breast milk is unknown; avoid taking this drug or refrain from nursing.

▷ **Overdose Symptoms:**   Nausea, vomiting, stomach cramps, and/or diarrhea.

▷ **Suggested Periodic Examinations While Taking This Drug:** (at doctor's discretion)
Complete blood cell counts.

▷ **While Taking This Drug the Following Apply:**   *Beverages:* May be taken with milk.
Other Drugs:
Cefprozil *taken concurrently* with

• aminoglycosides (see Drug Classes) may result in increased kidney toxicity.

• probenecid (Benemid) may slow the elimination of cefprozil, resulting in higher blood levels and prolonged effect.

Driving, Hazardous Activities: Usually no restrictions. Observe for the rare occurrence of dizziness.

Special Storage Instructions: Oral suspensions should be refrigerated.

Observe the Following Expiration Times: Discard unused portion after 14 days.

▷ **Saving Money When Using This Medicine:**

• Dose must be decreased for best effect for patients with kidney compromise.

• Many antibiotics are available today. Ask your doctor if this medicine offers the best combination of price and outcomes for you— perhaps a penicillin could be used instead.

• If you are allergic to penicillin, you may also be allergic to this medicine.

CEFTRIAXONE (SEF try ax own)

Prescription Needed: Yes   **Controlled Drug:** No   **Generic:** No

Brand Names: Rocephin

Overview of BENEFITS versus RISKS

Possible Benefits	*Possible Risks*
HOME IV TREATMENT OF ADVANCED LYME DISEASE (STAGE 2 OR 3)	PALPITATIONS (RARE)
	HEMATOLOGIC EFFECTS: THROMBOCYTOSIS, LEUKOPENIA, or ANEMIA
HOME IV TREATMENT OF OSTEOMYELITIS (BONE INFECTIONS)	PSEUDOMEMBRANOUS COLITIS (RARE)
Home IV treatment of other serious infections	

▷ **Illness This Medication Treats:**
   (1) Lower respiratory infections; (2) skin and skin structure infections; (3) urinary tract infections; (4) uncomplicated gonorrhea; (5) pelvic inflammatory disease; (6) bacterial septicemia; (7) bone and joint infections; (8) intra-abdominal infections; (9) meningitis; (10) surgical prophylaxis.
   Other (unlabeled) generally accepted use: intravenous treatment of late (stage 2 or 3) Lyme disease.

▷ **Typical Dosage Range:** (Dosage or schedule must be determined by the doctor for each individual.)
   Infants and Children: For neonates and children under 12 years old: For treatment of serious infections caused by susceptible organisms (other than central nervous system infections such as meningitis), 50 to 75 mg per kilogram of body weight per day given in two equal doses, 12 hours apart (not to exceed 2 g daily). Some doctors suggest neonates 1 week old or younger and those older than 1 week weighing 2 kg or less receive 50 mg per kilogram of body weight per day, and neonates older than 1 week and weighing more than 2 kg be given 50 to 75 mg per kilogram of body weight per day.
   For central nervous system infections such as meningitis, the dose for neonates and children 12 years old or younger is 100 mg per kilogram of body weight daily, divided into two equal doses taken every 12 hours. The American Academy of Pediatrics suggests 80 to 100 mg per kilogram of body weight be taken once daily or in two equal doses every 12 hours for children older than 1 month.
   12 to 60 Years of Age: The dosing of ceftriaxone for treatment of most infections is 1 to 2 g daily or in equal doses two times a day, depend-

ing on the type and severity of the infection. Children older than 12 years old can be given the adult dose. Some physicians recommend that central nervous system infections in adults may require 4 g daily, the maximum adult dosage recommended by the manufacturer.

Uncomplicated gonorrhea caused by penicillinase-producing strains of *Neisseria* gonorrhea (PPNG) or nonpenicillinase-producing strains may be treated by a single intramuscular (IM) 250 mg dose. Disseminated gonococcal infection should be treated by 1 g IV or IM once a day for 7 days. Patients with nonsepticemic gonococcal ophthalmia need a single 1 g IM dose. Acute sexually transmitted epididymitis in adults may be treated with a single 250 mg IM dose followed by 7 days of oral tetracycline or erythromycin. For treatment of acute pelvic inflammatory disease, a single 250 mg IM dose should be taken, followed by 100 mg of oral doxycycline two times a day for 10 to 14 days.

Treatment of serious arthritis, or cardiac or neurologic complications of early or late (stage 2 or 3) Lyme disease.

Arthritis: 2 g IV daily for adults. Children should be given 75 to 100 mg per kilogram of body weight per day IV.

Serious central nervous system disease: 2 g IV daily for 21 days in adults. Children can be treated with 75 to 100 mg per kilogram of body weight IV daily for 21 days.

Cardiac disease: 2 g IV/day for 21 days in adults. Children can be given 75 to 100 mg per kilogram of body weight per day IV.

Surgical prophylaxis: Although FDA-approved for surgical prophylaxis, routine use of ceftriaxone is not recommended. Other readily available agents are equally effective and much less expensive. Use for surgical prophylaxis also increases the potential for resistance to this drug, and could decrease its usefulness in treating later infections.

Over 60 Years of Age: Same as for 12 to 60 years of age.

▷ **Conditions Requiring Dosing Adjustments:**

Liver function: Patients with both liver and substantial kidney impairment should have drug levels monitored. The total daily dose should not exceed 2 g.

Kidney function: Compromise of the kidneys alone is cause for careful monitoring.

▷ **How Best to Take This Medicine:**   MUST be taken via a vein. Bring refrigerated IV solutions to room temperature before using them. Do not use any IV solutions containing particles or precipitates. Do not use outdated solutions—they will not treat your infection as effectively.

▷ **How Long This Medicine Is Usually Taken:**   Depends heavily on the type and severity of the infection. In general, therapy should be continued (except gonorrhea) for at least 48 hours after the infection has been eliminated and you are asymptomatic. For invasive infections, antibiotic therapy is usually continued for 5 to 7 days after negative bacteriologic cultures are obtained.

Gram-negative bacillary meningitis should be treated for at least 21 days.

Osteomyelitis may require 6 weeks of IV therapy, with reassessment for continued therapy when the antibiotics course is completed.

Continual use on a regular schedule for 3 weeks usually determines the effectiveness of this drug in treating Lyme disease. Serologic tests may remain positive for a significant time, even though the infection has been cured. See your doctor regularly.

▷ **Tell Your Doctor Before Taking This Medicine If You:**
- ever had an allergic reaction to it.
- have active colitis of any type.
- have a hematologic (blood) disorder such as anemia.
- have liver or kidney problems.
- have a history of regional enteritis or ulcerative colitis.
- have an allergy to any prescription or nonprescription medicine.
- have a history of gallbladder disease.
- have a blood clotting disorder.
- are allergic to penicillin.
- are pregnant or plan to become pregnant.

▷ **Possible Side Effects:**   Superinfections such as vaginitis (a vaginal yeast infection), as well as oral yeast infections, and overgrowth of nonsusceptible organisms with long-term use.

▷ **Possible Adverse Effects:**
If any of the following develop, call your doctor promptly for guidance.
Some Mild Problems Drug Can Cause
Allergic reactions: skin rash, fever, and chills.
Headache, flushing, dizziness and sweating, transient diarrhea of children and adults.
Asymptomatic gallbladder concretions of children receiving 60 to 100 mg per kilogram of body weight per day in one study.
Diarrhea, pain and induration at the injection site (intramuscular use), increased liver enzymes.
Some Serious Problems Drug Can Cause
Allergic reactions: bronchospasm, anaphylaxis, and serum sickness.
Leukopenia, neutropenia, anemia, lymphopenia, and thrombocytopenia.
Rare kidney stones, gallstones, or decreased kidney function.

▷ **Possible Delayed Adverse Effects:** Biliary symptoms may be more likely to develop with longer term high-dose therapy.

▷ *CAUTION*

1. Ceftriaxone should be used with caution by people who are allergic to penicillin, regardless of the symptoms.
2. Neonates with jaundice may be at increased risk of bilirubin encephalopathy if treated with this drug.
3. Ceftriaxone reconstituted with bacteriostatic water (with benzyl alcohol as a preservative) should not be used intramuscularly in neonates.
4. Very specific dosing schedules and ranges have been developed for children less than 12 years old.
5. Dose must be decreased for best effect for patients with kidney compromise.

Advisability of Use During Pregnancy or If Breast-Feeding:
Pregnancy Category: B. Ask your doctor for guidance. Distributed in the milk of nursing mothers; nursing mothers should use this drug with caution.

▷ **Overdose Symptoms:** This medication has a wide therapeutic index (is safe over a wide dosage range). Severe overdoses may increase the likelihood of the listed adverse effects.

▷ **Suggested Periodic Examinations While Taking This Drug:** (at doctor's discretion)
Prothrombin time, complete blood count, SGOT and SGPT, BUN creatinine, and routine urinalysis.

▷ **While Taking This Drug the Following Apply:**
Nutritional Support: Some studies have been performed with nutritional support compatibility. We recommend calling the manufacturer's scientific services division for total parenteral nutrition (TPN) formulation combinations and percent decomposition over time.
Alcohol: Severe disulfiramlike reaction (nausea, vomiting) has been rarely reported. Avoid alcohol while taking this drug.
Other Drugs:
Ceftriaxone may *increase* the effects of
• anticoagulants such as warfarin (Coumadin) or heparin.
Ceftriaxone *taken concurrently* with
• alcohol may cause a disulfiramlike reaction.
• aminoglycoside antibiotics (see Drug Classes) may increase the effectiveness of both drugs against certain bacteria. This additive or synergistic effect may provide a great therapeutic benefit against resistant organisms; it may also increase the likelihood of kidney damage.
• colistimethate may increase the renal toxicity of colistin.

- cyclosporine (Sandimmune) may increase renal toxicity and the level of cyclosporine over time.
- ethacrynic acid may increase the occurrence of renal toxicity.
- furosemide may increase renal toxicity.
- methotrexate may decrease or antagonize the antibiotic effect.

The following drugs may **decrease** the effects of ceftriaxone

- methotrexate.
- probenecid in high doses (1–2 g).

Driving, Hazardous Activities: Ceftriaxone is a rare cause of dizziness. Restrict your activities as necessary.

Special Storage Instructions: Refrigeration is the preferred storage method once the medicine is reconstituted, as the time until expiration is greatly prolonged. The medicine does not keep as long stored at room temperature.

Following reconstitution with 0.9% sodium chloride, 5% dextrose, or sterile water for injection, ceftriaxone solutions of 100 mg/ml are stable for 3 days at room temperature or 10 days in the refrigerator. Consult guidelines and specific expiration dates from your provider regarding frozen ceftriaxone.

Observe the Following Expiration Times: This medication has a large range of stability and expiration times once it has been reconstituted. Important points influencing stability are concentration of the antibiotic, solution in which it has been placed, solution used to reconstitute it, and temperature at which the medication has been stored. Because of the complexity, contact the home IV service or hospital that provided the IV solutions.

▷ **Saving Money When Using This Medicine:**

- Many antibiotics are available today. Ask your doctor if this medicine offers the best combination of price and outcomes for you—perhaps a different antibiotic could be used.
- If you are in the hospital and are given ceftriaxone, ask your doctor if the remainder of your therapy can be given by a home IV service.

CEFUROXIME   (sef yur OX eem)

Prescription Needed: Yes   **Controlled Drug:** No   **Generic:** No

Brand Names: Ceftin

Overview of BENEFITS versus RISKS

Possible Benefits

EFFECTIVE TREATMENT OF INFECTIONS due to susceptible microorganisms

Possible Risks

ALLERGIC REACTIONS, mild to severe

Drug-induced colitis (rare)

Superinfections

▷ **Illness This Medication Treats:**

Certain infections of the middle ear, tonsils, throat, bronchial tubes, urinary tract, and skin.

▷ **Typical Dosage Range:** (Dosage or schedule must be determined by the doctor for each individual.)

250 to 500 mg every 12 hours. Total daily dosage should not exceed 4 g.

▷ **Conditions Requiring Dosing Adjustments:**

Kidney function: Dosage adjustments for patients with kidney compromise for medication taken orally are not needed except in cases of severe kidney failure.

▷ **How Best to Take This Medicine:** May be taken on an empty stomach or with food if stomach irritation occurs. The tablet may be crushed and mixed with food (such as applesauce or ice cream) if necessary to facilitate swallowing. (Note: The crushed tablet has a persistent, bitter taste.) Take the full course prescribed. If you are in the hospital and taking the intravenous form with good results, ask your doctor if you can change to the oral form and leave the hospital.

▷ **How Long This Medicine Is Usually Taken:** Use on a regular schedule for 3 to 5 days usually determines the effectiveness of this drug in controlling the infection under treatment. Response varies with the nature of the infection. Total treatment time varies from 1 to 4 weeks. Certain infections require that this drug be taken for 10 consecutive days to prevent development of rheumatic fever. Follow your doctor's instructions regarding duration of use.

▷ **Tell Your Doctor Before Taking This Medicine If You:**

- are allergic to any cephalosporin antibiotic.
- have a history of allergy to any form of penicillin.
- have a history of regional enteritis or ulcerative colitis.
- have a history of low white blood cell counts.
- have impaired kidney function.

▷ **Possible Side Effects:** Superinfections: vaginitis.

▷ **Possible Adverse Effects:**

If any of the following develop, call your doctor promptly for guidance.

Some Mild Problems Drug Can Cause
   Allergic reactions: skin rash, itching.
   Nausea, vomiting, loose stools, mild diarrhea.
   Headache, dizziness.
Some Serious Problems Drug Can Cause
   Severe diarrhea, which may be drug-induced colitis (rare).
   Rare decreased low white blood cell counts.
   Rare thrombophlebitis with the intravenous form.

▷ **CAUTION**
   1. This drug can cause a false-positive test result for urine sugar when using Clinitest tablets, Benedict's solution, or Fehling's solution, but not with Clinistix or Tes-Tape.
   2. The usual dose is 125 mg every 12 hours. For middle ear infection the recommended dose for those under 2 years old is 125 mg/12 hr, and 250 mg/12 hr for those over 2 years old.
   3. For those over 60 years old the dose must be carefully individualized, based on evaluation of kidney function. Natural changes in the skin may predispose to severe and prolonged itching reactions in the genital and anal regions. Such reactions should be reported promptly.
   4. Dose must be decreased for best effect in patients with kidney compromise.
   5. If you are allergic to penicillin, you may also react to this medicine. Discuss this with your doctor.

Advisability of Use During Pregnancy or If Breast-Feeding:
Pregnancy Category: B. Generally considered safe. Ask your doctor for guidance. Present in breast milk in small amounts; avoid taking this drug or refrain from nursing.

▷ **Overdose Symptoms:**   Nausea, vomiting, stomach cramps, and/or diarrhea.

▷ **While Taking This Drug the Following Apply:**
Foods: Food enhances the absorption of this drug.
Beverages: May be taken with milk.
Other Drugs:
Cefuroxime *taken concurrently* with
   • aminoglycoside antibiotics (see Drug Classes) may pose an increased risk of kidney toxicity.
   • oral contraceptives (birth control pills) may result in loss of contraception and pregnancy.
   • probenecid (Benemid) slows the elimination of cefuroxime, resulting in higher blood levels and prolonged effect.
Driving, Hazardous Activities: Usually no restrictions. Observe for the rare occurrence of dizziness.

▷ **Saving Money When Using This Medicine:**
- Many antibiotics are available today. Ask your doctor if this medicine offers the best combination of price and outcomes for you—perhaps a penicillin could be used instead.
- If you are in a hospital and taking the intravenous form, ask if therapy could be completed by a home IV service.

CEPHALEXIN (sef a LEX in)

Prescription Needed: Yes   **Controlled Drug:** No   **Generic:** Yes

Brand Names: Cefanex, Keflet, Keflex, Keftab

Overview of BENEFITS versus RISKS	
Possible Benefits	*Possible Risks*
EFFECTIVE TREATMENT OF INFECTIONS due to susceptible microorganisms	ALLERGIC REACTIONS, mild to severe
	Drug-induced colitis (rare)
	Superinfections
	Rare hemolytic anemia

▷ **Illness This Medication Treats:**
Certain infections of the skin and skin structures, the upper respiratory tract (including middle ear infections and strep throat), the genitourinary tract, and of bones and joints.

▷ **Typical Dosage Range:** (Dosage or schedule must be determined by the doctor for each individual.)
250 to 500 mg every 6 hours. Total daily dose should not exceed 4 g.

▷ **Conditions Requiring Dosing Adjustments:**
Kidney function: For patients with moderate to severe kidney compromise take the usual dose every 6 hours. For patients with severe kidney compromise take the usual dose every 8 to 12 hours.

▷ **How Best to Take This Medicine:** May be taken on an empty stomach or with food if stomach irritation occurs. Capsule may be opened and tablet may be crushed for administration. Shake suspension well before measuring dose. Take the full course prescribed.

▷ **How Long This Medicine Is Usually Taken:** Use on a regular schedule for 3 to 5 days usually determines the effectiveness of this drug in controlling the infection under treatment. Total treatment time varies from 1 to 4 weeks. Certain infections require that this drug be taken for 10 consecutive days to prevent rheumatic fever. Follow your doctor's instructions regarding duration of use.

▷ **Tell Your Doctor Before Taking This Medicine If You:**
- are allergic to any cephalosporin antibiotic.
- have a history of allergy to any form of penicillin.
- have a history of regional enteritis or ulcerative colitis.
- have a history of blood cells disorders, especially hemolytic anemia.
- have a seizure disorder.
- have impaired kidney function.

▷ **Possible Side Effects:**   Superinfections.

▷ **Possible Adverse Effects:**
If any of the following develop, call your doctor promptly for guidance.
Some Mild Problems Drug Can Cause
   Allergic reactions: skin rash, itching.
   Headache, drowsiness, dizziness.
   Irritation of mouth, nausea, vomiting, diarrhea.
Some Serious Problems Drug Can Cause
   Allergic reactions: drug fever, joint aches and pains, anaphylactic reaction.
   Idiosyncratic reactions: minor and temporary changes in white blood cell counts and liver function tests (infrequent).
   Genital itching (may represent a fungus superinfection).
   Severe diarrhea, which may be drug-induced colitis (rare).
   Rare hemolytic anemia.

▷ *CAUTION*
1. In management of diabetes, it should be noted that this drug can cause a false-positive test result for urine sugar when using Clinitest tablets, Benedict's solution, or Fehling's solution, but not with Tes-Tape.
2. Do not use cephalexin concurrently with other antibiotics such as erythromycin or tetracyclines.
3. This drug is not recommended for use in infants less than 1 year old. Monitor allergic children closely for evidence of allergy to this drug.
4. For those over 60 years old, the dose must be carefully individualized and based on evaluation of kidney function. Natural changes in the skin may predispose to severe and prolonged itching reactions in the genital and anal regions. Such reactions should be reported promptly.
5. Dose must be decreased for best effect in patients with kidney compromise.

Advisability of Use During Pregnancy or If Breast-Feeding:
Pregnancy Category: B. Generally considered to be safe. Ask your doctor for guidance. Present in breast milk in small amounts; avoid taking this drug or refrain from nursing.

▷ **Overdose Symptoms:**   Nausea, vomiting, stomach cramps, and/or diarrhea.

▷ **Suggested Periodic Examinations While Taking This Drug:** (at doctor's discretion)
Complete blood cell counts. Liver and kidney function tests.

▷ **While Taking This Drug the Following Apply:**
Beverages: May be taken with milk.
Other Drugs:
Cephalexin *taken concurrently* with

- aminoglycoside antibiotics (see Drug Classes) may pose an increased risk of kidney toxicity.
- oral contraceptives (birth control pills) may result in loss of contraception and pregnancy.
- cholestyramine may blunt cephalexin blood levels and decrease its ability to fight infection.
- probenecid (Benemid) slows the elimination of cephalexin, resulting in higher blood levels and prolonged effect.

Driving, Hazardous Activities: Usually no restrictions. Use caution if drowsiness or dizziness occurs.
Special Storage Instructions: Oral suspension should be refrigerated.
Observe the Following Expiration Times: Do not take the oral suspension of this drug if it is older than 14 days.

▷ **Saving Money When Using This Medicine:**

- Many antibiotics are available today. Ask your doctor if this medicine offers the best combination of price and outcomes for you— perhaps a penicillin could be used instead.

CHLORAMBUCIL (klor AM byu sil)

Prescription Needed: Yes   **Controlled Drug:** No   **Generic:**
No

Brand Names: Leukeran

Overview of BENEFITS versus RISKS

Possible Benefits	*Possible Risks*
EFFECTIVE PALLIATIVE TREATMENT FOR CHRONIC LYMPHOCYTIC LEUKEMIA	BONE MARROW DEPRESSION
EFFECTIVE PALLIATIVE TREATMENT FOR HODGKIN'S DISEASE AND OTHER LYMPHOMAS	INCREASED SUSCEPTIBILITY TO INFECTIONS
Immunosuppression of nephrotic syndrome	CENTRAL NERVOUS SYSTEM TOXICITY
Immunosuppression of rheumatoid arthritis	Male and female sterility
	Drug-induced liver damage
	Drug-induced lung damage
	Development of secondary cancers

▷ **Illness This Medication Treats:**
   (1) Chronic lymphocytic leukemia; (2) Hodgkin's lymphoma and other
   malignant lymphomas.
   Other (unlabeled) generally accepted uses: may have a role in treating
   rheumatoid arthritis or nephrotic syndrome.

▷ **Typical Dosage Range:** (Dosage or schedule must be determined by
   the doctor for each individual.)
   For leukemia and lymphoma: Initially 0.1 to 0.2 mg per kilogram of
   body weight daily, or 3 to 6 mg per square meter of body surface
   daily (usually 4 to 10 mg daily) as a single dose or in divided doses.
   For immunosuppression: 0.1 to 0.2 mg per kilogram of body weight
   daily, in a single dose, for 8 to 12 weeks.

▷ **Conditions Requiring Dosing Adjustments:**
   Liver function: Chlorambucil can cause liver damage. People with
   compromised livers should use this drug with extreme caution.
   Kidney function: Chlorambucil can cause bladder inflammation in patients with compromised urine outflow.

▷ **How Best to Take This Medicine:** Take with food or milk to reduce
   stomach irritation. The tablet may be crushed for administration.
   Consult your doctor if vomiting prevents adherence to dosage
   schedule.

▷ **How Long This Medicine Is Usually Taken:** Use on a regular
   schedule for 3 to 4 weeks usually determines the effectiveness of this

drug in controlling leukemia or lymphoma; several months of treatment may be required to assess the effects of immunosuppression. Long-term use requires periodic physician evaluation.

▷ **Tell Your Doctor Before Taking This Medicine If You:**
- ever had an allergic reaction to it.
- have recently had or been exposed to chickenpox or herpes zoster (shingles).
- currently have an uncontrolled infection (chlorambucil may worsen it).
- are allergic to melphalan (Alkeran).
- are pregnant, planning pregnancy, or breast-feeding.
- currently have any bone marrow depression, a history of bone marrow depression, or a blood cell disorder.
- have a history of gout or urate kidney stones.
- have a seizure disorder of any kind.
- have a history of porphyria.
- have impaired liver or kidney function.
- have had cancer chemotherapy or radiation therapy previously.
- are currently taking prednisone or other drugs that can impair your immunity.

▷ **Possible Side Effects:** Decreased white blood cell and platelet counts.
Decreased immunity, susceptibility to infections.
Increased blood levels of uric acid, formation of urate kidney stones.

▷ **Possible Adverse Effects:**
If any of the following develop, call your doctor promptly for guidance.
Some Mild Problems Drug Can Cause
Allergic reactions: skin rash, drug fever.
Mouth and lip sores, nausea, vomiting.
Some Serious Problems Drug Can Cause
Allergic reactions: drug-induced hepatitis with jaundice.
Cataract formation with high doses.
Agitation, confusion, hallucinations, seizures, paralysis.
Peripheral neuritis.
Lung damage: cough, shortness of breath.
Bone marrow damage, aplastic anemia.
Toxic epidermal necrolysis.
Increased risk of leukemia.

▷ **Possible Effects on Sex Life:** Can inhibit reproduction: stops sperm production (male sterility); alters menstrual patterns, blocks ovulation and menstruation (female sterility).

▷ **Possible Delayed Adverse Effects:** Evidence of severe bone marrow depression may occur after the drug is stopped.
Secondary cancers (especially leukemia) have been reported.
Lung damage (pulmonary fibrosis).

▷ *CAUTION*

1. Long-term use (as for immunosuppression) of this drug in non-cancerous conditions requires extreme caution. The risks include permanent sterility, lung damage, and the development of secondary cancers. Its use is recommended only for conditions that have not responded satisfactorily to conventional use of less toxic drugs.

2. Complete necessary dental procedures before using this drug. Its bone marrow depressant effects could predispose to gum infection, excessive bleeding, and delayed healing.

3. For treating individuals with gout, allopurinol is the drug of choice to control the increased blood levels of uric acid caused by chlorambucil.

4. This drug impairs the body's immune system by decreasing its ability to produce protective antibodies. For this reason, both killed and live virus vaccines are ineffective. In addition, there is an increased risk that a live virus vaccine may actually induce infection and cause significant adverse effects. An estimated 3 months to 1 year after discontinuation of this and similar drugs are required for the immune system to recover its ability to respond appropriately to vaccination. To eliminate the risk of accidental exposure to live polio virus, persons in close contact with anyone taking this drug should not receive oral poliovirus vaccine.

5. Report immediately: onset of infection, unusual bruising or bleeding, excessive fatigue or weakness, tremors or muscle twitching, difficulty walking, loss of appetite with nausea or vomiting.

6. It is advisable to avoid pregnancy while taking this drug. A nonhormonal method of contraception is recommended. Tell your doctor promptly if you think you are pregnant.

7. Dosage schedules and treatment monitoring for infants and children should be supervised by a qualified pediatrician. Children with nephrotic syndrome may be more prone to seizures induced by this drug.

8. People over 60 may be more likely to have central nervous system toxicity.

Advisability of Use During Pregnancy or If Breast-Feeding:
Pregnancy Category: D. If possible, avoid using this drug during pregnancy, especially the first 3 months. A nonhormonal contraceptive is generally recommended during treatment with this and similar

drugs. Presence in breast milk is unknown; avoid taking this drug or refrain from nursing.

▷ **Overdose Symptoms:** Fatigue, weakness, fever, sore throat, bruising, agitation, unstable gait, seizures.

▷ **Suggested Periodic Examinations While Taking This Drug:** (at doctor's discretion)

Before drug treatment is started and *periodically* during drug use: complete blood cell counts, blood uric acid levels, liver function tests, sperm counts.

▷ **While Taking This Drug the Following Apply:**

Beverages: May be taken with milk. It is advisable to drink 2 to 3 qt of liquids daily to reduce the risk of kidney stone formation.

Alcohol: Use with caution. Avoid if platelet counts are low and there is a risk of stomach bleeding.

Marijuana Smoking: Best avoided. This could increase the risk of central nervous system toxicity.

Other Drugs:

Chlorambucil *taken concurrently* with

- aspirin may increase the risk of bruising or bleeding; the platelet-reduction effects of chlorambucil and the antiplatelet action of aspirin are additive. Avoid aspirin while taking chlorambucil.
- antidepressant or antipsychotic (neuroleptic) drugs requires careful monitoring; these drugs can lower the threshold for the occurrence of seizures and increase the risk of chlorambucil-induced seizures.
- other immunosuppressants can increase the risk of infection and the development of secondary cancers.

Driving, Hazardous Activities: This drug may cause nervous agitation, confusion, hallucinations, or seizures. Restrict your activities as necessary.

Discontinuation: Whether chlorambucil is used as an anticancer drug or immunosuppressant, many factors will determine when and how this drug should be discontinued. To obtain maximal benefit, comply as closely as possible with your doctor's guidance.

▷ **Saving Money When Using This Medicine:**

- Several drugs are available that accomplish a similar effect. Ask your doctor if this drug represents the best combination of cost and outcome for you.

CHLORAMPHENICOL (klor am FEN i kohl)

Prescription Needed: Yes   **Controlled Drug:** No   **Generic:** Yes

Brand Names: Ak-Chlor, Chloromycetin, Chloroptic, Ophthochlor

Overview of BENEFITS versus RISKS	
Possible Benefits	*Possible Risks*
VERY EFFECTIVE TREATMENT OF INFECTIONS due to susceptible microorganisms	BONE MARROW DEPRESSION APLASTIC ANEMIA Peripheral neuritis Liver damage, jaundice

▷ **Illness This Medication Treats:**

A broad spectrum of serious infections; however, because of its potential for serious toxicity (fatal aplastic anemia), its use is now reserved for life-threatening infections caused by organisms that are resistant to safer antibiotics, and infections in people who cannot take other appropriate anti-infective drugs.

Other (unlabeled) generally accepted uses: (1) used topically to help pressure sores (bedsores); (2) may be used topically to treat acne.

▷ **Typical Dosage Range:** (Dosage or schedule must be determined by the doctor for each individual.)

Ophthalmic: Chloramphenicol plus hydrocortisone is taken as two drops to the affected eye every 3 hours around the clock for 48 hours. After this the time between doses is usually increased and treatment continued until 48 hours after the eye appears normal. Intravenous: Total daily dose is 50 to 100 mg per kilogram of body weight divided into four equal doses taken 6 hours apart. Total daily dose should not exceed 500 mg for each 10 lb of body weight.

CHLOROQUINE (KLOR oh kwin)

Prescription Needed: Yes   **Controlled Drug:** No   **Generic:** Yes

Brand Names: Aralen

▷ **Warning:** The brand names Aralen and Arlidin can be mistaken for each other, leading to serious medication errors. They are very different drugs. Aralen (a purple tablet imprinted with a "W" in a square) is the generic drug chloroquine (see above). Arlidin (a white round tablet imprinted with an "A" in a shield) is the generic drug nylidrin, a vasodilator. Verify that you are taking the correct drug.

```
┌─────────────────────────────────────────────────────────┐
│           Overview of BENEFITS versus RISKS              │
│     Possible Benefits            Possible Risks          │
│  EFFECTIVE PREVENTION      INFREQUENT BUT SERIOUS         │
│    AND TREATMENT OF          DAMAGE OF CORNEAL AND        │
│    CERTAIN FORMS OF          RETINAL EYE TISSUES          │
│    MALARIA                 RARE BUT SERIOUS BONE          │
│  EFFECTIVE COMBINATION       MARROW DEPRESSION:          │
│    TREATMENT OF SOME         aplastic anemia, deficiency of │
│    FORMS OF AMEBIC           white blood cells and platelets │
│    INFECTION               Heart muscle damage (rare)    │
│                            Ear damage: hearing loss,     │
│                              ringing in ears (rare)      │
└─────────────────────────────────────────────────────────┘
```

▷ **Illness This Medication Treats:**

(1) Acute attacks of certain types of malarial infection; (2) adjunctive treatment for certain forms of amebic infection.

Other (unlabeled) generally accepted uses: (1) eases symptoms of refractory rheumatoid arthritis; (2) suppresses lupus erythematosus, (3) helps sarcoidosis; (4) eases palindromic rheumatism.

▷ **Typical Dosage Range:** (Dosage or schedule must be determined by the doctor for each individual.)

For malaria suppression: 500 mg/7 days.

For malaria treatment: Initially 1 g, followed by 500 mg in 6 to 8 hours; then 500 mg once a day on the second and third days.

For amebiasis (other than intestinal): Initially 250 mg four times daily for 2 days; then 250 mg two times daily for 2 to 3 weeks.

For rheumatoid arthritis or lupus erythematosus: 4 mg per kilogram of lean body weight daily.

▷ **Conditions Requiring Dosing Adjustments:**

Liver function: Blood levels should be obtained, and the dose adjusted appropriately.

Kidney function: For patients with severe kidney failure, 50% of the normal dose at the normal interval should be used. If therapy is to be extended, 50 to 100 mg of chloroquine base should be taken daily.

▷ **How Best to Take This Medicine:**   Take with food or milk to reduce stomach irritation. The tablet may be crushed for administration. Take full course of treatment as prescribed.

Note: For malaria prevention, begin medication 2 weeks before entering a malarious area; continue medication while in the area and for 4 weeks after leaving the area.

▷ **How Long This Medicine Is Usually Taken:**   Use on a regular schedule for 2 weeks before exposure, during period of exposure, and 4 weeks after exposure usually determines the effectiveness of this drug in preventing attacks of malaria. Regular use for up to 6 months may be required to evaluate benefits in treating rheumatoid arthritis or lupus erythematosus. The drug is often changed to hydroxychloroquine because it is potentially less toxic. Long-term use (months to years) requires periodic physician evaluation of response and dosage adjustment.

CHLOROTHIAZIDE (klor oh THI a zide)

Prescription Needed: Yes   **Controlled Drug:** No   **Generic:** Yes

Brand Names: Aldoclor [CD], Diachlor, Diupres [CD], Diurigen, Diuril, SK-Chlorothiazide

Overview of BENEFITS versus RISKS	
Possible Benefits	*Possible Risks*
EFFECTIVE, WELL-TOLERATED DIURETIC	Loss of body potassium
	Increased blood sugar
POSSIBLY EFFECTIVE IN MILD HYPERTENSION	Increased blood uric acid
	Increased blood calcium
ENHANCES EFFECTIVENESS OF OTHER ANTIHYPERTENSIVES	Blood cell disorders (rare)
Beneficial in treatment of diabetes insipidus	

See the thiazide diuretics profile for further information.

CHLORPROMAZINE (klor PROH ma zeen)

Prescription Needed: Yes   **Controlled Drug:** No   **Generic:** Yes

Brand Names: Ormazine, Promapar, Sonazine, Thora-Dex, Thorazine, Thorazine-SR

Overview of BENEFITS versus RISKS

Possible Benefits	*Possible Risks*
EFFECTIVE CONTROL OF ACUTE MENTAL DISORDERS	SERIOUS TOXIC EFFECTS ON BRAIN with long-term use
Beneficial effects on thinking, mood, and behavior	Liver damage with jaundice
Moderately effective control of nausea and vomiting	Rare blood disorders: hemolytic anemia, low white blood count
	Eye toxicity

▷ **Illness This Medication Treats:**

(1) Acute and chronic psychotic disorders such as agitated depression and schizophrenia; (2) may be used for presurgical anxiety; (3) stopping prolonged hiccups; (4) may be used for stopping vomiting caused by chemotherapy.

▷ **Typical Dosage Range:** (Dosage or schedule must be determined by the doctor for each individual.)

Initially 10 to 25 mg three or four times daily. Dose may be increased by 20 to 50 mg at 3- to 4-day intervals as needed and tolerated. Usual dosage range is 300 to 800 mg daily. Extreme range is 25 to 2000 mg daily; total daily dosage should not exceed 2000 mg.

▷ **Conditions Requiring Dosing Adjustments:**

Liver function. Patients with liver compromise should use this drug with caution and in decreased doses. This drug can also be a cause of cholestatic jaundice.

Kidney function: Blood levels of this drug are recommended if the drug is used by patients with severe renal (kidney) compromise.

▷ **How Best to Take This Medicine:** May be taken with or following meals to reduce stomach irritation. Tablets may be crushed. Prolonged-action capsules may be opened, but do not crush or chew contents.

▷ **How Long This Medicine Is Usually Taken:** Use on a regular schedule for several weeks usually determines the effectiveness of this drug in controlling psychotic disorders. If not significantly beneficial within 6 weeks, it should be stopped. Long-term use (months to years) requires periodic evaluation of response, appropriate dosage adjustment, and consideration of continued need. See your doctor regularly.

▷ **Tell Your Doctor Before Taking This Medicine If You:**
- ever had an allergic reaction to it.
- have active liver disease.
- have cancer of the breast.
- have a current blood cell or bone marrow disorder.
- are allergic or abnormally sensitive to any phenothiazine drug.
- have impaired liver or kidney function.
- have any type of seizure disorder.
- have diabetes, glaucoma, or heart disease.
- have a history of lupus erythematosus.
- are taking any drug with sedative effects.
- plan to have surgery under general or spinal anesthesia soon.

▷ **Possible Side Effects:** Drowsiness (usually during the first 2 weeks), orthostatic hypotension, blurred vision, dry mouth, nasal congestion, constipation, impaired urination.

Pink or purple coloration of urine, of no significance.

▷ **Possible Adverse Effects:**
If any of the following develop, call your doctor promptly for guidance.
Some Mild Problems Drug Can Cause
    Allergic reactions: skin rash, low-grade fever.
    Low body temperature, especially in the elderly.
    Increased appetite and weight gain.
    Weakness, insomnia, impaired day and night vision.
    Chronic constipation, fecal impaction.
Some Serious Problems Drug Can Cause
    Allergic reactions: hepatitis with jaundice, usually between second and fourth week; high fever; asthma; anaphylactic reaction.
    Idiosyncratic reactions: neuroleptic malignant syndrome.
    Depression, disorientation, seizures.
    Disturbances of heart rhythm, rapid heart rate.
    Hemolytic anemia, impaired production of white blood cells—fever, sore throat, infections.
    Parkinson-like disorders.
    Prolonged drop in blood pressure with weakness, sweating, and fainting.

▷ **Possible Effects on Sex Life:** Decreased libido and impotence (1200 mg/day); inhibited ejaculation (400 mg/day); priapism (250 mg/day); male infertility (30–800 mg/day); enlargement of male breasts, enlargement of female breasts with milk production, cessation of menstruation (30–800 mg/day).

▷ *CAUTION*
    1. Many over-the-counter medications for allergies, colds, and coughs contain drugs that can interact unfavorably with this

drug. Ask your doctor or pharmacist for guidance before using any such medications.

2. Antacids that contain aluminum and/or magnesium can prevent the absorption of this drug and reduce its effectiveness.
3. Obtain prompt evaluation of any change or disturbance of vision.
4. This drug can cause false-positive pregnancy tests.
5. Do not use this drug for infants under 6 months old, or for children of any age with symptoms suggestive of Reye's syndrome. Monitor carefully for blood cell changes.
6. For those over 60, small doses are advisable until individual response has been determined. You may be more susceptible to the development of drowsiness, lethargy, constipation, hypothermia, and orthostatic hypotension. This drug can enhance existing prostatism. You may also be more susceptible to the development of Parkinson-like reactions and/or tardive dyskinesia. These reactions must be recognized early since they may become unresponsive to treatment and irreversible.

Advisability of Use During Pregnancy or If Breast-Feeding:

Pregnancy Category: C. Limit use of this drug to small and infrequent doses only when clearly needed. Avoid during the last month because of possible adverse effects on the newborn infant. Present in breast milk in small amounts; avoid taking this drug or refrain from nursing.

▷ **Overdose Symptoms:** Marked drowsiness, weakness, tremor, agitation, unsteadiness, deep sleep, coma, convulsions.

▷ **Suggested Periodic Examinations While Taking This Drug:** (at doctor's discretion)

Complete blood cell counts, especially between the fourth and tenth weeks of treatment.

Liver function tests, electrocardiograms,

Complete eye examinations—eye structures and vision.

Careful inspection of the tongue for early evidence of fine, involuntary, wavelike movements that could indicate the beginning of tardive dyskinesia.

▷ **While Taking This Drug the Following Apply:**

Nutritional Support: A riboflavin (vitamin B-2) supplement should be taken with long-term use.

Beverages: May be taken with milk.

Alcohol: Avoid completely. Alcohol can increase the sedative action of phenothiazines and accentuate their depressant effects on brain function and blood pressure. Phenothiazines can increase the intoxicating effects of alcohol.

Tobacco Smoking: Possible reduction of drowsiness from drug.

Marijuana Smoking: Moderate increase in drowsiness; accentuation of orthostatic hypotension; increased risk of precipitating latent psychoses, confusing the interpretation of mental status and drug responses.

Other Drugs:

Chlorpromazine may *increase* the effects of

- all sedative drugs, especially meperidine (Demerol), causing excessive sedation.
- all atropinelike drugs, causing nervous system toxicity.
- zolpidem (Ambien).

Chlorpromazine may *decrease* the effects of

- guanethidine (Ismelin, Esimil), reducing its effectiveness in lowering blood pressure.
- oral hypoglycemic agents (see Drug Classes).

Chlorpromazine *taken concurrently* with

- amphetamines decreases the effects of both medicines.
- ACE inhibitors (see Drug Classes) may cause excessive lowering of blood pressure.
- lithium (Lithobid, others) may result in a decrease in lithium or chlorpromazine benefits.
- propranolol (Inderal) (and probably other beta-blockers—see Drug Classes) may cause increased effects of both drugs; monitor drug effects closely and adjust dosages as necessary.
- valproic acid may result in valproic acid toxicity.

The following drugs may *decrease* the effects of chlorpromazine

- antacids containing aluminum and/or magnesium.
- benztropine (Cogentin).
- trihexyphenidyl (Artane).

Driving, Hazardous Activities: Chlorpromazine can impair mental alertness, judgment, and physical coordination. Avoid hazardous activities.

Exposure to Sun: Use caution until your sensitivity has been determined. Some phenothiazines can cause photosensitivity.

Exposure to Heat: Use caution and avoid excessive heat as much as possible. This drug may impair body temperature regulation and increase the risk of heatstroke.

Exposure to Cold: Use caution and dress warmly. This drug can increase the risk of hypothermia in the elderly.

Discontinuation: After a period of long-term use, do not stop taking this drug suddenly. Gradual withdrawal over 2 to 3 weeks under your doctor's supervision is recommended. Do not discontinue this drug without your doctor's knowledge and approval. The relapse rate of schizophrenia after discontinuation may be 50 to 60%.

▷ **Saving Money When Using This Medicine:**
- Many medications are available today. Ask your doctor if this medicine offers the best combination of price and outcome for you.
- A new medicine called olanzapine was recently approved, which appears to offer a more favorable adverse movement effect profile. Discuss this with your doctor.

CHLORPROPAMIDE (klor PROH pa mide)

Prescription Needed: Yes **Controlled Drug:** No **Generic:** Yes

Brand Names: Diabinese, Glucamide

Overview of BENEFITS versus RISKS

Possible Benefits	*Possible Risks*
Helps regulate blood sugar in noninsulin-dependent diabetes (adjunctive to appropriate diet and weight control)	HYPOGLYCEMIA, severe and prolonged
	Allergic skin reactions (some severe)
	Water retention
	Liver damage
	Rare blood cell and bone marrow disorders

▷ **Illness This Medication Treats:**
Mild to moderate type II diabetes mellitus (adult, maturity-onset) that does not require insulin, but is not adequately controlled by diet alone.

▷ **Typical Dosage Range:** (Dosage or schedule must be determined by the doctor for each individual.)
Initially 250 mg daily with breakfast. After 5 to 7 days, dose may be increased to 500 mg daily if needed and tolerated. Total daily dosage should not exceed 750 mg.

▷ **Conditions Requiring Dosing Adjustments:**
Liver function: The dose **must** be decreased for patients with liver compromise.
Kidney function: It is prudent to change to a drug such as tolbutamide, which has no active metabolites.
Occurrence of Unrelated Illness: Acute infections, illnesses causing vomiting or diarrhea, serious injuries, and surgical procedures can interfere with diabetic control and may require the use of insulin. If any of these conditions occur, consult your doctor promptly.
Discontinuation: Only about 12% of patients remain well controlled

by this drug for more than 6 to 7 years. Because of the high incidence of secondary failures, it is best to evaluate the continued benefit of this drug every 6 months.

▷ **Saving Money When Using This Medicine:**
- Many oral hypoglycemic drugs are available. Ask your doctor if this medicine offers the best combination of price and outcome for you.
- Discuss the need for a total program of exercise, periodic blood sugar testing, aspirin use, and outcome-based symptom tracking.
- If your kidneys are compromised, avoid using this medicine.

CHLORTHALIDONE (klor THAL i dohn)

Prescription Needed: Yes   **Controlled Drug:** No   **Generic:** Yes

Brand Names: Combipres [CD], Demi-Regroton [CD], Hygroton, Hylidone, Regroton [CD], Tenoretic [CD], Thalitone

Overview of BENEFITS versus RISKS	
Possible Benefits	*Possible Risks*
EFFECTIVE, WELL-TOLERATED DIURETIC	Loss of body potassium or magnesium
POSSIBLY EFFECTIVE IN MILD HYPERTENSION	Increased blood sugar
	Increased blood uric acid
ENHANCES EFFECTIVENESS OF OTHER ANTIHYPERTENSIVES	Increased blood calcium
	Blood cell disorders (rare)
Beneficial in treatment of diabetes insipidus	

See the thiazide diuretics profile for further information.

CHOLESTYRAMINE (koh LES tir a meen)

Prescription Needed: Yes   **Controlled Drug:** No   **Generic:** No

Brand Names: Cholybar, Questran, Questran Light

Overview of BENEFITS versus RISKS

Possible Benefits	*Possible Risks*
EFFECTIVE REDUCTION OF TOTAL CHOLESTEROL AND LOW-DENSITY CHOLESTEROL IN TYPE IIa CHOLESTEROL DISORDERS (15–25% reduction of total cholesterol, 25–35% reduction of LDL cholesterol)	Constipation (may be severe) Reduced absorption of fat, fat-soluble vitamins (A, D, E, and K), and folic acid Reduced formation of prothrombin with resultant bleeding
EFFECTIVE RELIEF OF ITCHING associated with biliary obstruction	
EFFECTIVE BINDING TO MEDICINES IN SOME DRUG OVERDOSES	

▷ **Illness This Medication Treats:**
  (1) Arteriohepatic dysplasia; (2) reduces abnormally high blood levels of total cholesterol and low-density (LDL) cholesterol in Type IIa cholesterol disorders; (3) relieves itching due to the deposit of bile acids in the skin associated with partial biliary obstruction; (4) reduces risk of heart disease in men with type II hyperlipoproteinemia.

▷ **Typical Dosage Range:** (Dosage or schedule must be determined by the doctor for each individual.)
  9 g powder (equivalent to 4 g cholestyramine) one to six times daily. Dose may be increased slowly, as needed and tolerated. The total daily dosage should not exceed 72 g powder (32 g cholestyramine).

▷ **How Best to Take This Medicine:** Always take this drug just before or with a meal; it is ineffective when taken without food. Mix the powder thoroughly in 4 to 6 oz of water, fruit juice, milk, thin soup, or a soft food such as applesauce; do not use carbonated beverages. **Do not take it in its dry form.**

▷ **How Long This Medicine Is Usually Taken:** Use on a regular schedule for up to 3 weeks is usually needed to see this drug's benefits in lowering high blood cholesterol. Duration of use should not exceed 3 months if no adequate response occurs. Long-term use (months to years) requires periodic physician evaluation.

▷ **Tell Your Doctor Before Taking This Medicine If You:**
- ever had an allergic reaction to it.
- have complete biliary obstruction.
- are prone to constipation.
- have peptic ulcer disease.
- have a bleeding disorder of any kind.
- have impaired kidney function.
- have phenylketonuria (PKU).

▷ **Possible Side Effects:**   Constipation; interference with normal fat digestion and absorption; reduced absorption of vitamins A, D, E, and K and folic acid. Acidosis.

▷ **Possible Adverse Effects:**
If any of the following develop, call your doctor promptly for guidance.
Some Mild Problems Drug Can Cause
Allergic reactions: skin rash, tongue irritation, anal itching.
Loss of appetite, abdominal discomfort, excessive gas, nausea, vomiting, diarrhea.
Some Serious Problems Drug Can Cause
Allergic reaction: asthmalike wheezing.
Vitamin K deficiency with resultant deficiency of prothrombin and increased tendency for bleeding.
Impaired absorption of calcium; predisposition to osteoporosis.
Gallbladder colic.

▷ **Possible Effects on Sex Life:**   Increased libido (questionable).

▷ *CAUTION*
1. The powder should never be taken in dry form; always mix thoroughly with a suitable liquid before swallowing.
2. Observe carefully for constipation; use stool softeners and laxatives as needed.
3. This drug may bind other drugs taken concurrently and impair their absorption. It is advisable to take *all other drugs* 1 to 2 hours before or 4 to 6 hours after taking this drug.
4. Safety and effectiveness of this drug for those under 6 years old are not established. Observe carefully for the possible development of acidosis and vitamin A or folic acid deficiency. Ask your doctor for guidance.
5. Those over 60 years old may face an increased risk of severe constipation. Impaired kidney function may predispose to acidosis.

Advisability of Use During Pregnancy or If Breast-Feeding:
Pregnancy Category: C. Use this drug only if clearly needed. Ensure adequate intake of vitamins and minerals, since this drug can re-

duce their availability to both mother and fetus. Ask your doctor for guidance. Not present in breast milk; will not effect breast-feeding.

▷ **Overdose Symptoms:** Progressive constipation.

▷ **Suggested Periodic Examinations While Taking This Drug:** (at doctor's discretion)

Measurements of blood levels of total cholesterol, LDL cholesterol, and HDL cholesterol.

Hemoglobin and red blood cell studies for possible anemia.

▷ **While Taking This Drug the Following Apply:**

Foods: Avoid foods that tend to constipate (cheeses, etc.).

Nutritional Support: Consult your doctor regarding the need for supplements of vitamins A, D, E, and K, folic acid, and calcium.

Beverages: Avoid carbonated beverages. Ensure adequate liquid intake (up to 2 qt daily). This medicine may be taken with milk.

Other Drugs:

Cholestyramine may *decrease* the effects of

- acetaminophen; take 2 hours before cholestyramine.
- digitoxin and digoxin; take 2 hours before cholestyramine.
- fluvastatin (Lescol).
- furosemide (Lasix).
- iron preparations; take 2 to 3 hours before cholestyramine.
- methotrexate: take 3 hours before cholestyramine.
- metronidazole (Flagyl).
- NSAIDs (some acidic ones such as piroxicam or sulindac).
- oral hypoglycemic agents (see Drug Classes).
- penicillin G.
- phenobarbital; take 2 hours before cholestyramine.
- thiazide diuretics (see Drug Classes); take 2 hours before cholestyramine.
- thyroxin; take 5 hours before cholestyramine.
- warfarin; take 6 hours after cholestyramine.

Cholestyramine *taken concurrently* with:

- amiodarone (Cordarone) can result in lowered amiodarone blood levels and decreased effectiveness.

Discontinuation: The dose of any potentially toxic drug taken at the same time as this medicine must be reduced appropriately if this drug is discontinued.

▷ **Saving Money When Using This Medicine:**

- Many medications are now available to treat cholesterol. Ask your doctor if this medicine offers the best combination of price and outcome for you.
- Ask your doctor if this medicine shows benefits similar to HMG CoA inhibitors.
- Discuss the benefits versus risks of alternate-day aspirin therapy.

CIMETIDINE (si MET i deen)

Prescription Needed: Yes   **Controlled Drug:** No   **Generic:** No

Brand Names: Tagamet, Tagamet HB (nonprescription)

Overview of BENEFITS versus RISKS

Possible Benefits	*Possible Risks*
EFFECTIVE TREATMENT OF PEPTIC ULCER DISEASE: relief of symptoms, acceleration of healing, prevention of recurrence	CONFUSIONAL STATES in the elderly and debilitated
CONTROL OF HYPERSECRETORY STOMACH DISORDERS	Blood cell and bone marrow disorders (rare)
EFFECTIVE TREATMENT OF EROSIVE REFLUX DISEASE OF ESOPHAGUS	Pancreatitis (rare)
	Liver damage (rare)
	Kidney damage (rare)

See the histamine (H2) blocking drugs profile for further information.

CIPROFLOXACIN (sip roh FLOX a sin)

Prescription Needed: Yes   **Controlled Drug:** No   **Generic:** No

Brand Names: Cipro

▷ **Warning:**   This drug may cause tendon rupture. If it is prescribed for you, ask if you should limit exercise or exertion during therapy. Call your doctor immediately if pain or inflammation appears while you are taking this medicine. A rare idiosyncratic reaction has been reported for medicines in this class, which starts as mental confusion and disorientation. Call your doctor if you notice a change in your thinking or the thinking of a loved one while they are taking this medicine.

```
┌─────────────────────────────────────────────────────────────┐
│              Overview of BENEFITS versus RISKS              │
│                                                             │
│     Possible Benefits            Possible Risks            │
│  HIGHLY EFFECTIVE           Very rare drug-induced colitis  │
│     TREATMENT FOR           Very rare hallucinations or     │
│     INFECTIONS OF THE          seizure                      │
│     LOWER RESPIRATORY       Very rare tendon rupture        │
│     TRACT, URINARY TRACT,                                   │
│     BONES, JOINTS, AND SKIN                                 │
│     TISSUES due to susceptible                              │
│     organisms                                               │
│  Effective treatment for some                               │
│     forms of bacterial                                      │
│     gastroenteritis (diarrhea)                              │
└─────────────────────────────────────────────────────────────┘
```

▷ **Illness This Medication Treats:**
Responsive infections (in adults) of: (1) the lower respiratory tract (lungs and bronchial tubes); (2) the urinary tract (kidneys, bladder, urethra, and prostate gland); (3) the digestive tract (small intestine and colon); (4) bones and joints; (5) skin and related tissues. (6) Ophthalmic preparation is used to treat a variety of eye infections including those caused by *Staphylococcus* and *Pseudomonas*.

▷ **Typical Dosage Range:** (Dosage or schedule must be determined by the doctor for each individual.)
250 to 750 mg every 12 hours, depending on the nature and severity of the infection. The total daily dosage should not exceed 1500 mg.
Ophthalmic: One or two drops instilled (placed) in the eye every 2 hours while you're awake for 2 days, then one or two drops every 4 hours while awake for 5 more days.

▷ **Conditions Requiring Dosing Adjustments:**
Liver function: Patients with severe liver failure should use this drug with caution.
Kidney function: The dose must be decreased or the time between doses increased for patients with compromised kidneys.
Cystic fibrosis: A loading dose of 750 mg as well as 750 mg every 8 hours is used.

▷ **How Best to Take This Medicine:**   May be taken with or without food; this drug should be taken 2 hours after eating. Drink fluids liberally during the entire course of treatment. Avoid antacids containing aluminum or magnesium for 2 hours before and after dosing. The tablet may be crushed for administration.

▷ **How Long This Medicine Is Usually Taken:**   Use on a regular schedule for 7 to 14 days is needed to see this drug's effectiveness. Continue for at least 2 days after all indications of infection have disappeared. Bone and joint infections may require treatment for 6 weeks or longer. Long-term use requires periodic physician evaluation of response.

> **Tell Your Doctor Before Taking This Medicine If You:**
- ever had an allergic reaction to it or to cinoxacin (Cinobac), nalidixic acid (NegGram), norfloxacin (Noroxin), or other quinolone drugs.
- are pregnant or breast-feeding.
- have an inadequately controlled seizure disorder, or a history of a seizure disorder or circulatory disorder of the brain.
- are given a prescription for a person under 18 years old.
- have a history of mental disorders (psychosis).
- have impaired liver or kidney function.
- are taking any form of probenecid or theophylline.

> **Possible Side Effects:**   Superinfections. Greenish tooth discoloration if used in infants. Problems in skeletal formation if used in those under 18 years old.

> **Possible Adverse Effects:**
> **If any of the following develop, call your doctor promptly for guidance.**
> *Some Mild Problems Drug Can Cause*
> Allergic reactions: rash, localized swelling.
> Dizziness, headache, migraine, anxiety, abnormal vision.
> Nausea, diarrhea, vomiting, indigestion.
> Burning sensation in the eye with the ophthalmic form.
> *Some Serious Problems Drug Can Cause*
> Idiosyncratic reactions: some drugs in this class have caused a change in mental status including confusion, inability to speak, and incapacitation.
> Central nervous system stimulation: restlessness, tremor, confusion, hallucinations, seizures (all very rare).
> Rare tendon rupture.
> Rare liver toxicity or kidney problems.
> Rare abnormal heartbeats or palpitations.

> *CAUTION*
1. With high doses or prolonged use, crystals may form in the kidney. This can be prevented by drinking copious amounts of water, up to 2 qt/24 hr.
2. Drugs of this class may decrease the formation of saliva and predispose to dental cavities or gum disease. Consult your dentist if dry mouth persists.
3. Those under 18 years old should avoid the use of this drug completely. It can impair normal bone growth and development.
4. For those over 60, impaired kidney function may require dosage

reduction. If you are taking theophylline concurrently, observe closely for possible theophylline accumulation and toxicity.

5. Dose MUST be decreased for the best effect for patients with kidney compromise.

6. Since tendon rupture has rarely been reported with this medicine, discuss with your doctor limits to exercise or heavy lifting while taking this medicine.

Advisability of Use During Pregnancy or If Breast-Feeding:

Pregnancy Category: C. The potential for adverse effects on fetal bone development contraindicates the use of this drug during entire pregnancy. Probably present in breast milk; avoid taking this drug or refrain from nursing.

▷ **Overdose Symptoms:** Headache, seizures, abdominal pain and nausea, liver toxicity.

▷ **Suggested Periodic Examinations While Taking This Drug:** (at doctor's discretion)

Liver function tests, urine analysis.

▷ **While Taking This Drug the Following Apply:**

Beverages: Caffeine-containing beverages will result in higher than expected blood levels and potential for exaggerated effects.

Other Drugs:

Ciprofloxacin may ***increase*** the effects of

• theophylline, causing theophylline toxicity.

Ciprofloxacin ***taken concurrently*** with

• azlocillin may result in toxicity.

• cyclosporine (Sandimmune) poses increased risk of kidney toxicity.

• foscarnet (Foscavir) may pose an increased seizure risk.

• phenytoin (Dilantin) can cause increased or decreased phenytoin levels.

• warfarin (Coumadin) can pose an increased risk of bleeding. More frequent INR (prothrombin time) testing is indicated.

The following drug may ***increase*** the effects of ciprofloxacin

• probenecid (Benemid).

The following drugs may ***decrease*** the effects of ciprofloxacin

• antacids containing aluminum or magnesium—can reduce the absorption of ciprofloxacin and lessen its effectiveness.

• calcium supplements.

• didanosine.

• iron salts.

• sucralfate (Carafate).

• zinc salts.

Driving, Hazardous Activities: May cause dizziness and impair vision. Restrict your activities as necessary.

Exposure to Sun: May rarely cause photosensitivity. Sunglasses are advised if your eyes are overly sensitive to bright light.

Discontinuation: If you experience no adverse effects, take the full course prescribed for maximal results. Consult your doctor regarding termination.

▷ **Saving Money When Using This Medicine:**
- Many antibiotics are available today. Ask your doctor if this medicine offers the best combination of price and outcomes for you—perhaps a penicillin could be used instead.

CISAPRIDE (SIS a pryde)

Prescription Needed: Yes   **Controlled Drug:** No   **Generic:** No

Brand Names: Propulsid

Overview of BENEFITS versus RISKS	
Possible Benefits	*Possible Risks*
EFFECTIVE TREATMENT OF NOCTURNAL HEARTBURN	Diarrhea
FEW CENTRAL NERVOUS SIDE EFFECTS	Joint pain
May have a role in helping diabetic gastroparesis	

▷ **Illness This Medication Treats:**
  (1) Reflux esophagitis symptoms; (2) decrease of nocturnal heartburn caused by gastroesophageal reflux disease.
  Other (unlabeled) generally accepted uses: (1) helps diabetic gastroparesis; (2) may help children with chronic constipation.

▷ **Typical Dosage Range:** (Dosage or schedule must be determined by the doctor for each individual.)
  Infants and Children: Safety and efficacy of this drug are not established for children or infants.
  12 to 60 Years of Age: For relief of nocturnal heartburn: 10 to 20 mg four times a day, taken 15 minutes before meals and at bedtime.
  For reflux esophagitis: 10 mg four times a day, combined with cimetidine 1 g/day.
  For diabetic gastroparesis: 10 mg four times a day, taken 15 minutes before meals and at bedtime.
  Over 60 Years of Age: Same as for 12 to 60 years.

▷ **Conditions Requiring Dosing Adjustments:**
  Liver function: Patients with liver failure should take 50% of the usual dose.

▷ **How Best to Take This Medicine:** This medicine should be taken 15 minutes before meals and at bedtime for the best effect.

▷ **How Long This Medicine Is Usually Taken:** Use on a regular schedule for 8 to 12 weeks may be needed to see the peak benefit of this drug in treating chronic functional constipation. Up to 12 weeks may be needed to realize the full therapeutic effect for reflux esophagitis. Long-term use (months to years) requires periodic physician evaluation of response and dosage adjustment.

▷ **Tell Your Doctor Before Taking This Medicine If You:**
- ever had an allergic reaction to it.
- have gastrointestinal obstruction, hemorrhage, or perforation.
- currently take a benzodiazepine drug.
- have an abnormally fast heartbeat.
- take prescription or nonprescription medicines that were not discussed when this drug was prescribed.

▷ **Possible Side Effects:** Sleepiness and fatigue.

▷ **Possible Adverse Effects:**
If any of the following develop, call your doctor promptly for guidance.
Some Mild Problems Drug Can Cause
Allergic reactions: skin rash and itching.
Somnolence and fatigue.
Occasional headache, dizziness, and sleep disturbances.
Rhinitis.
Diarrhea, rare urinary incontinence.
Some Serious Problems Drug Can Cause
Allergic reactions: anaphylactic reaction.
Rare increases in heart rate.

▷ *CAUTION*
1. Cisapride may cause increased heart rate. Notify your doctor if this occurs.
2. Report promptly any increased tendency to depression.
3. Safety and effectiveness of this drug for children are not established.
Advisability of Use During Pregnancy or If Breast-Feeding:
Pregnancy Category: C. Use of this drug is based on benefit-to-risk decision. Ask your doctor for guidance. Present in breast milk. Monitor nursing infant closely and discontinue this drug or nursing if adverse effects develop.

▷ **Overdose Symptoms:** Nausea, vomiting, flatulence, increased urination, and diarrhea.

▷ **Suggested Periodic Examinations While Taking This Drug:** (at doctor's discretion)

Periodic liver function tests.

▷ **While Taking This Drug the Following Apply:**

Alcohol: Sedative effects of alcohol are increased.

Marijuana Smoking: May cause additive drowsiness.

Other Drugs:

Cisapride may **decrease** the effects of

- warfarin (Coumadin), decreasing its benefits. More frequent INR (prothrombin times) testing are indicated.

Cisapride **taken concurrently** with

- cimetidine (Tagamet) results in increased cisapride levels and potential toxicity. Cisapride dose should be decreased by 40%.
- diazepam (Valium) can lead to a 17% increase in drug level.
- itraconazole (Sporanox), ketoconazole (Nizoral), fluconazole (Diflucan), or miconazole (Monistat) may lead to cisapride toxicity and abnormal heart effects.
- macrolide antibiotics such as clarithromycin (Biaxin), erythromycin (E-Mycin, others), or troleandomycin may lead to cisapride toxicity.

Driving, Hazardous Activities: This drug may cause some drowsiness. Restrict your activities as necessary.

Discontinuation: If this medication is stopped and you have been taking an anticoagulant, prothrombin time testing will be needed.

▷ **Saving Money When Using This Medicine:**

- Two medicines are currently in this class. Ask your doctor if this medicine offers the best combination of price and outcomes for you.

CLARITHROMYCIN (klar ith roh MY sin)

Prescription Needed: Yes   **Controlled Drug:** No   **Generic:** No

Brand Names: Biaxin

Overview of BENEFITS versus RISKS	
Possible Benefits	*Possible Risks*
EFFECTIVE TREATMENT OF RESPIRATORY TRACT INFECTIONS DUE TO SUSCEPTIBLE MICROORGANISMS	Mild gastrointestinal symptoms
	Drug-induced colitis (rare)
	Superinfections (rare)
EFFECTIVE TREATMENT OF SKIN INFECTIONS DUE TO SUSCEPTIBLE MICROORGANISMS	

▷ **Illness This Medication Treats:**
  (1) Certain upper respiratory tract infections—maxillary sinusitis, pharyngitis, tonsillitis; (2) certain lower respiratory tract infections—acute bronchitis and pneumonia; (3) certain skin (and skin structure) infections. Bacterial cultures and sensitivity testing should be performed as necessary. (4) Combination treatment of ulcers caused by *Helicobacter pylori*.

▷ **Typical Dosage Range:** (Dosage or schedule must be determined by the doctor for each individual.)
  Infants and Children: Otitis media: 7.5 mg per kilogram of body weight twice daily, up to a maximum of 500 mg twice a day for 10 days.
  12 to 60 Years of Age: For pharyngitis/tonsillitis: 250 mg/12 hr for 10 days.
  For maxillary sinusitis: 500 mg/12 hr for 14 days.
  For acute bronchitis: 250–500 mg/12 hr for 7 to 14 days.
  For pneumonia: 250 mg/12 hr for 7 to 14 days.
  For skin infections: 250 mg/12 hr for 7 to 14 days.
  Over 60 Years of Age: Same as for 12 to 60 years. If kidney function is impaired, reduce dose accordingly.

▷ **Conditions Requiring Dosing Adjustments:**
  Liver function: The liver plays a minor role (10–15%) in eliminating this medication. If the kidney function is normal, dosing adjustments are not needed for people with liver problems.
  Kidney function: The dose *must* be decreased or the dosing interval lengthened for patients with compromised kidneys.

▷ **How Best to Take This Medicine:**   May be taken with or without food. The tablet may be crushed.

▷ **How Long This Medicine Is Usually Taken:**   Use on a regular schedule for 4 to 6 days usually determines the effectiveness of this drug in controlling responsive infections. For streptococcal throat infections: No less than 10 consecutive days (without interruption), to reduce the possibility of developing rheumatic fever or glomerulonephritis. The duration of use should not exceed the time required to eliminate infection.

▷ **Tell Your Doctor Before Taking This Medicine If You:**
- ever had an allergic reaction to it or azithromycin, erythromycin, or troleandomycin.
- have impaired liver or kidney function.
- have a history of drug-induced colitis.
- have low blood platelets.
- are pregnant or planning pregnancy.

▷ **Possible Side Effects:**   Superinfections.

▷ **Possible Adverse Effects:**
If any of the following develop, call your doctor promptly for guidance.
Some Mild Problems Drug Can Cause
    Headache.
    Abnormal taste, nausea, stomach pain, diarrhea.
Some Serious Problems Drug Can Cause
    Drug-induced colitis (rare).
    Rare kidney toxicity or low blood platelets.
    Very rare acute psychosis (two case reports).

▷ *CAUTION*
1. If diarrhea develops and continues for more than 24 hours, call your doctor promptly. This could indicate the onset of drug-induced colitis.
2. Take the full dosage prescribed to prevent the possible emergence of resistant bacterial strains.
3. Safety and effectiveness of this drug for those under 12 years old are not established.
4. Dose must be adjusted if kidney function is severely impaired.

Advisability of Use During Pregnancy or If Breast-Feeding:
Pregnancy Category: C. This drug should not be used during pregnancy except when no alternative treatment is appropriate. Ask your doctor for guidance. Probably present in breast milk. Monitor nursing infant closely and discontinue taking this drug or nursing if adverse effects develop.

▷ **Overdose Symptoms:** Possible nausea, vomiting, abdominal discomfort, and diarrhea.

▷ **While Taking This Drug the Following Apply:**

Beverages: May be taken with milk.

Other Drugs:

Clarithromycin may ***increase*** the effects of

- carbamazepine (Tegretol); monitor blood levels of carbamazepine if appropriate.
- digoxin (Lanoxin).
- tacrolimus (Prograf).
- theophylline (Theo-Dur, Theolair, etc.); monitor blood levels of theophylline if appropriate.
- astemizole and terfenadine and may cause life-threatening heart rhythm abnormalities.
- warfarin and require dosing adjustments and more frequent INR (prothrombin time) testing.

Clarithromycin ***taken concurrently*** with

- cyclosporine (Sandimmune) may lead to toxicity.
- dihydroergotamine (and perhaps other ergots) can lead to dihydroergotamine toxicity.
- ergotamine can cause toxicity.
- zidovudine (AZT) may lead to decreased levels and lack of zidovudine effectiveness.

Driving, Hazardous Activities: This drug may cause nausea and/or diarrhea. Restrict your activities as necessary.

▷ **Saving Money When Using This Medicine:**

- Many antibiotics are available today. Ask your doctor if this medicine offers the best combination of price and outcomes for you— perhaps erythromycin could be used instead to treat the infection you face.
- If this medicine is being used to treat an ulcer (because we now know many ulcers are infections), it may offer better outcomes or be more cost-effective as combination therapy with omeprazole than traditional treatments in patients with *Helicobacter pylori*–associated ulcers.

CLINDAMYCIN (klin da MI sin)

Prescription Needed: Yes   **Controlled Drug:** No   **Generic:** Yes

Brand Names: Cleocin, Cleocin T

Overview of BENEFITS versus RISKS

Possible Benefits	*Possible Risks*
EFFECTIVE TREATMENT FOR SERIOUS INFECTIONS OF THE LOWER RESPIRATORY TRACT, ABDOMINAL CAVITY, GENITAL TRACT IN WOMEN, BLOODSTREAM (SEPTICEMIA), SKIN, AND RELATED TISSUES caused by susceptible organisms	SEVERE DRUG-INDUCED COLITIS (fatalities reported)
	Liver injury with jaundice (rare)
	Reduction in white blood cell and platelet counts (rare)
TREATMENT OF *PNEUMOCYSTIS CARINII* PNEUMONIA (PCP) ASSOCIATED WITH AIDS	
Effective for local treatment of acne	

▷ **Illness This Medication Treats:**
  (1) Serious and unusual infections of the lungs and bronchial tubes; abdominal cavity organs and tissues; the genital tract and pelvic organs in women; the skin and soft tissue structures; and generalized infections involving the bloodstream. (2) A more recent use is the prevention and treatment of *Pneumocystis carinii* pneumonia, frequently associated with AIDS. (3) Acne.

▷ **Typical Dosage Range:** (Dosage or schedule must be determined by the doctor for each individual.)
  For infections of average severity: 150 to 300 mg every 6 hours. For more severe infections: 300 to 450 mg every 6 hours. The total daily dosage should not exceed 1800 mg.
  For acne: The topical form is applied to the affected area twice daily.

CLOFAZIMINE (kloh FA zi meen)

Prescription Needed: Yes   **Controlled Drug:** No   **Generic:** No

Brand Names: Lamprene

Overview of BENEFITS versus RISKS	
Possible Benefits	*Possible Risks*
EFFECTIVE ADJUNCTIVE TREATMENT OF LEPROSY	RARE BOWEL OBSTRUCTION, GASTROINTESTINAL BLEEDING
Possibly effective adjunctive treatment of AIDS-related infection with *Mycobacterium avium-intracellulare* (MAI)	Rare liver damage
	Skin pigmentation (red to brownish-black) in large majority of users, lasting up to 5 years

▷ **Illness This Medication Treats:**

Leprosy, in combination with other antileprosy drugs,

Other (unlabeled) generally accepted uses: treatment of AIDS-related infections with *Mycobacterium avium-intracellulare*; used in combination with other antimycobacterials.

▷ **Typical Dosage Range:** (Dosage or schedule must be determined by the doctor for each individual.)

Infants and Children: Dosage not established.

12 to 60 Years of Age: For leprosy: 50 to 100 mg once daily.

For AIDS-related *Mycobacterium avium-intracellulare* (MAI) infections: 100 mg/8 hr in combination with a variety of other medicines. Total daily dosage should not exceed 300 mg.

Over 60 Years of Age: Same as for 12 to 60 years of age.

▷ **Conditions Requiring Dosing Adjustments:**

Liver function: The dose **must** be decreased for patients with liver compromise.

▷ **How Best to Take This Medicine:**   Take with food. Swallow capsule whole; do not alter or chew. Take with one or more other antileprosy drugs to prevent the emergence of drug-resistant strains of mycobacteria.

CLOMIPRAMINE (kloh MI pra meen)

Prescription Needed: Yes   **Controlled Drug:** No   **Generic:** No

Brand Names: Anafranil

Overview of BENEFITS versus RISKS

Possible Benefits	*Possible Risks*
EFFECTIVE TREATMENT OF SEVERE OBSESSIVE-COMPULSIVE NEUROSIS	DRUG-INDUCED SEIZURES ADVERSE BEHAVIORAL EFFECTS: confusion, delirium, disorientation, hallucinations, delusions, paranoia
Effective relief of symptoms of some types of endogenous depression	Conversion of depression to mania in manic-depressive disorders
	Aggravation of schizophrenia
	Rare liver toxicity
	Rare bone marrow depression and blood cell disorders

▷ **Illness This Medication Treats:**
Severe, disabling obsessive-compulsive disorder.

▷ **Typical Dosage Range:** (Dosage or schedule must be determined by the doctor for each individual.)
Initially 25 mg daily, taken in the evening. Dose may be increased cautiously, as needed and tolerated, by 25 mg daily at intervals of 3 to 4 days until a dose of 100 mg daily is reached in 2 weeks. This larger dose should be divided and taken after meals. The usual maintenance dose is 50 to 150 mg every 24 hours. The total daily dosage should not exceed 250 mg. (When determined, the optimal daily requirement may be taken at bedtime as a single dose.)

▷ **Conditions Requiring Dosing Adjustments:**
Liver function: The dose must decreased for patients with liver compromise.

▷ **How Best to Take This Medicine:** May be taken without regard to meals. If necessary, this drug may be taken with or following food to reduce stomach irritation. The capsule may be opened.

▷ **How Long This Medicine Is Usually Taken:** Use on a regular schedule for 3 to 4 weeks usually determines the effectiveness of this drug in controlling obsessive-compulsive behavior; optimal response may require 3 or more months of use. Long-term use (months to years) requires periodic evaluation of response and dosage adjustment. See your doctor regularly.

▷ **Tell Your Doctor Before Taking This Medicine If You:**
- ever had an allergic reaction to it.
- are taking, or have taken within the past 14 days, any MAO type A inhibitor.
- have active bone marrow depression or blood cell disorder, or a history of these conditions.
- have had a recent heart attack (myocardial infarction) or have any type of heart disease, especially coronary artery disease or a heart rhythm disorder.
- have narrow-angle glaucoma, or have increased internal eye pressure.
- have had an adverse reaction to any other antidepressant drug, especially one of the tricyclic class.
- have any type of seizure disorder.
- are subject to bronchial asthma.
- have impaired liver or kidney function.
- are taking thyroid medication or have any type of thyroid disorder.
- have an adrenaline-producing tumor.
- have prostatism.
- have a history of alcoholism or suicide attempts.
- plan to have surgery under general anesthesia soon.

▷ **Possible Side Effects:** Drowsiness, increased sweating, lightheadedness, blurred vision, dry mouth, constipation, impaired urination.

▷ **Possible Adverse Effects:**
If any of the following develop, call your doctor promptly for guidance.
Some Mild Problems Drug Can Cause
  Allergic reactions: skin rash, itching, drug fever.
  Headache, dizziness, nervousness, impaired memory, weakness, tremors, insomnia, muscle cramps, flushing.
  Increased appetite, weight gain.
  Altered taste, nausea, vomiting, diarrhea.
Some Serious Problems Drug Can Cause
  Allergic reactions: drug-induced hepatitis, with or without jaundice.
  Idiosyncratic reactions: neuroleptic malignant syndrome.
  Adverse behavioral effects: delirium, hallucinations, paranoia.
  Seizures; reduced control of epilepsy.
  Heart rhythm disturbances.
  Liver toxicity or serotonin syndrome.
  Bone marrow depression: fatigue, weakness, fever, sore throat, infections, abnormal bleeding or bruising.

▷ **Possible Effects on Sex Life:**   Altered libido, impaired ejaculation, impotence, inhibited male orgasm, inhibited female orgasm, female breast enlargement with milk production.

▷ *CAUTION*
1. Watch for early indications of toxicity or overdosage: confusion, agitation, rapid heart rate, heart irregularity. Measuring the drug's blood level clarifies the situation.
2. Use this drug with caution in the presence of schizophrenia. Watch closely for any deterioration of thinking or behavior.
3. Use this drug with caution in the presence of epilepsy. Watch for any change in the frequency or severity of seizures.
4. Safety and effectiveness of this drug for those under 10 years old are not established. Dosage and management should be supervised by a properly trained pediatrician. Total daily dosage should not exceed 200 mg.
5. For those over 60, small starting doses (10 mg at bedtime) are indicated. Dosage may be increased gradually as needed and tolerated to 75 mg daily in divided doses. During the first 2 weeks of treatment, observe for behavioral reactions: restlessness, agitation, forgetfulness, disorientation, delusions, or hallucinations. Also observe for unsteadiness and instability that may predispose to falling. This drug may aggravate prostatism.

Advisability of Use During Pregnancy or If Breast-Feeding:
Pregnancy Category: C. Use only if clearly needed. Avoid use of this drug during the last 3 months if possible, to prevent withdrawal symptoms in the newborn infant: irritability, tremors, seizures. Present in breast milk; avoid taking this drug or refrain from nursing.

▷ **Habit-Forming Potential:**   Psychological or physical dependence is rare and unexpected. This drug is not liable to abuse.

▷ **Overdose Symptoms:**   Confusion, delirium, hallucinations, drowsiness, tremors, unsteadiness, heart irregularity, seizures, stupor, sweating, fever.

▷ **Suggested Periodic Examinations While Taking This Drug:** (at doctor's discretion)
Monitoring of blood drug levels as appropriate. Complete blood cell counts; liver and kidney function tests. Serial blood pressure readings and electrocardiograms.
Measurement of internal eye pressure.

▷ **While Taking This Drug the Following Apply:**
Foods: You may need to limit your food intake to avoid excessive weight gain.
Beverages: May be taken with milk.

Alcohol: Avoid completely. This drug can markedly increase the intoxicating effects of alcohol; the combination can depress brain function significantly.

Tobacco Smoking: May delay the elimination of this drug and require dosage adjustment.

Marijuana Smoking: Increased drowsiness and mouth dryness; possible reduced effectiveness of this drug.

Other Drugs:

Clomipramine may *increase* the effects of
- all drugs with sedative effects; observe for excessive sedation.
- all drugs with atropinelike effects.

Clomipramine may *decrease* the effects of
- clonidine (Catapres).
- guanadrel (Hylorel).
- guanethidine (Ismelin, Esimil).

Clomipramine *taken concurrently* with
- anticonvulsants requires careful monitoring for changes in seizure patterns and adjustment of the anticonvulsant dosage.
- MAO type A inhibitors may cause high fever, seizures and excessive rise in blood pressure; avoid concurrent use of these drugs and provide periods of 14 days between administration of either.
- stimulants (amphetamine, cocaine, epinephrine, phenylpropanolamine, etc.) may cause severe high blood pressure and/or high fever.
- thyroid preparations may increase the risk of heart rhythm disorders.
- warfarin (Coumadin) requires more frequent INR (prothrombin time) testing in order to avoid bleeding.

The following drugs may *increase* the effects of clomipramine
- ACE inhibitors (see Drug Classes).
- cimetidine (Tagamet).
- estrogens.
- fluoxetine (Prozac).
- fluvoxamine (Luvox).
- haloperidol (Haldol).
- methylphenidate (Ritalin).
- oral contraceptives (birth control pills).
- phenothiazines (see Drug Classes).
- quinidine.
- ranitidine (Zantac).
- sertraline (Zoloft).
- verapamil (Calan, others).

The following drugs may *decrease* the effects of clomipramine
- barbiturates (see Drug Classes).
- carbamazepine (Tegretol).
- chloral hydrate (Noctec, Somnos, etc.).

- lithium (Lithobid, Lithotab, etc.).
- reserpine (Serpasil, Ser-Ap-Es, etc.).

Driving, Hazardous Activities: May cause seizures and impair mental alertness, judgment, physical coordination, and reaction time. Restrict your activities as necessary.

Exposure to Heat: Use caution. This drug may impair the body's adaptation to hot environments, increasing the risk of heatstroke. Avoid saunas.

Exposure to Environmental Chemicals: May mask the symptoms of poisoning due to handling certain insecticides (organophosphorous). Read their labels carefully.

Discontinuation: It is best to discontinue this drug gradually over a period of 3 to 4 weeks. Abrupt withdrawal after prolonged use may cause nausea, vomiting, diarrhea, headache, dizziness, malaise, disturbed sleep, and irritability. Obsessive-compulsive behavior may worsen when this drug is stopped. When this drug is discontinued, it may be necessary to adjust the dosages of other drugs taken concurrently.

▷ **Saving Money When Using This Medicine:**
- Many drugs are available today to treat conditions for which clomipramine is used. Ask your doctor if this medicine offers the best combination of price and outcome for you.

CLONAZEPAM (kloh NA ze pam)

Prescription Needed: Yes   **Controlled Drug:** C-IV*   **Generic:** No

Brand Names: Klonopin

▷ **Warning:**   The brand name Klonopin and the generic name clonidine are easily mistaken for each other, leading to serious medication errors. These names represent very different drugs. Klonopin (small round tablets colored yellow, blue, or white, according to strength) is the generic drug clonazepam; it is used to treat epilepsy. Clonidine (also available in small white tablets) is a generic drug used to treat high blood pressure. Verify that you are taking the correct drug.

*See Controlled Drug Schedules inside this book's cover.

Overview of BENEFITS versus RISKS

Possible Benefits	*Possible Risks*
EFFECTIVE CONTROL OF SOME TYPES OF PETIT MAL, AKINETIC, AND MYOCLONIC SEIZURES	Paradoxical reactions: excitement, agitation, hallucinations
Possibly effective in managing panic disorders	Minor impairment of mental functions
	Rare blood cell disorders: anemia, abnormally low white blood cell and platelet counts

---

▷ **Illness This Medication Treats:**

(1) Several types of epilepsy: petit mal, akinetic, myoclonic, simple and complex partial seizure patterns; (2) control of panic disorders.

▷ **Typical Dosage Range:** (Dosage or schedule must be determined by the doctor for each individual.)

Initially 0.5 mg three times daily. The dose may be increased by 0.5 to 1.0 mg every 3 days, as needed and tolerated, until seizures are controlled. Total daily dose should not exceed 20 mg.

▷ **Conditions Requiring Dosing Adjustments:**

Liver function: The dose must be decreased for patients with liver compromise.

Kidney function: Watch for signs and symptoms of accumulation.

▷ **How Best to Take This Medicine:** May be taken on empty stomach or with food or milk. The tablet may be crushed. Do not stop this drug abruptly if it is taken to control seizures, or if taken for more than 4 weeks to control panic attacks.

▷ **How Long This Medicine Is Usually Taken:** Use on a regular schedule for 2 to 3 weeks is usually needed to see this drug's benefit in reducing the frequency and severity of seizures. Optimal control requires careful dosage adjustments over a period of several months. Long-term use (months to years) requires ongoing physician supervision.

▷ **Tell Your Doctor Before Taking This Medicine If You:**
- ever had an allergic reaction to it.
- have acute narrow-angle glaucoma.
- have active liver disease, impaired liver or kidney function.
- are allergic to any benzodiazepine drug.
- have a history of alcoholism or drug abuse.
- are pregnant or planning pregnancy.
- have a history of serious depression or mental disorder.

- have any asthma, emphysema, chronic bronchitis, acute porphyria, or myasthenia gravis.

▷ **Possible Side Effects:** Drowsiness, lethargy, unsteadiness, increased salivation, weight gain.

▷ **Possible Adverse Effects:**
If any of the following develop, call your doctor promptly for guidance.
Some Mild Problems Drug Can Cause
   Allergic reactions: skin rash, hives, itching.
   Headache, dizziness, blurred vision, slurred speech, impaired memory, confusion, mental depression.
   Muscle weakness, trembling, uncontrolled body movements.
   Nausea, vomiting, constipation, diarrhea, impaired urination.
Some Serious Problems Drug Can Cause
   Idiosyncratic reactions: paradoxical responses of excitement, hyperactivity, agitation, anger, hostility.
   Rare blood cell disorders: abnormally low red blood cell, white blood cell, and platelet counts.
   Porphyria or abnormal eye movements.

▷ **Possible Effects on Sex Life:** Increased libido, enlargement of male breasts.

▷ *CAUTION*
   1. Clonazepam should not be stopped abruptly if it is being used to control seizures.
   2. The concurrent use of some over-the-counter drug products that contain antihistamines (allergy and cold preparations, sleep aids) can cause excessive sedation in sensitive individuals.
   3. Adverse behavioral reactions are more common in individuals with brain damage, mental retardation, or a history of psychiatric disorders.
   4. A decreased therapeutic response to this drug may occur in approximately 30% of users within 3 months after initiating treatment. Dosage adjustment may be necessary to restore seizure control.
   5. This drug is used to treat infants and children of all ages. Careful dosage adjustment based on weight and age is mandatory. Abnormal behavioral responses are more common in children.
   6. Small starting doses and longer amounts of time between doses are indicated in those over 60. Watch for possible development of lethargy, indifference, fatigue, weakness, unsteadiness, disturbing dreams, nightmares, and paradoxical reactions of excitement, agitation, anger, hostility, and rage.

Advisability of Use During Pregnancy or If Breast-Feeding:
Pregnancy Category: C. Avoid this drug during the first 3 months if

possible. Frequent use in late pregnancy may cause floppy infant syndrome in the newborn: weakness, lethargy, unresponsiveness, depressed breathing, low body temperature. Present in breast milk; avoid taking this drug or refrain from nursing.

▷ **Habit-Forming Potential:** This drug can produce psychological and/or physical dependence if used in large doses for an extended period of time. However, it is not prone to abuse.

▷ **Overdose Symptoms:** Marked drowsiness, weakness, confusion, slurred speech, staggering gait, tremor, stupor progressing to deep sleep or coma.

▷ **Suggested Periodic Examinations While Taking This Drug:** (at doctor's discretion)

During long-term use: complete blood cell counts; liver function tests.

▷ **While Taking This Drug the Following Apply:**

Beverages: May be taken with milk.

Alcohol: Alcohol may increase the depressant effects of this drug on the brain. Avoid alcohol completely—throughout the day and night—if you need to drive or engage in any hazardous activity.

Marijuana Smoking: Increased sedation and significant impairment of intellectual and physical performance.

Other Drugs:

Clonazepam *taken concurrently* with

- amiodarone (Cordarone) may blunt benefits of both drugs.
- desipramine and other tricyclic antidepressants (see Drug Classes) may blunt the tricyclic benefits.
- MAO inhibitors (see Drug Classes) may result in low blood pressure and worsening of breathing depression.
- valproic acid (Depakene, etc.) may cause continuous absence seizures.

The following drugs may *increase* the effects of clonazepam

- cimetidine (Tagamet).
- disulfiram (Antabuse).
- omeprazole (Prilosec).
- oral contraceptives.

The following drug may *decrease* the effects of clonazepam

- theophylline (aminophylline, Theo-Dur, etc.).

Driving, Hazardous Activities: This drug can impair mental alertness, judgment, physical coordination, and reaction time. Avoid hazardous activities accordingly.

Discontinuation: Avoid sudden discontinuation of this drug for seizure control, or if drug has been taken for more than 4 weeks for other conditions. Dosage should be tapered gradually to prevent a withdrawal syndrome that could include depression, confusion, hallucinations, tremor, seizures, muscle cramping, sweating, and vomiting.

▷ **Saving Money When Using This Medicine:**
- Many anticonvulsants are available today. Ask your doctor if this medicine offers the best combination of price and outcome for you.
- A new medicine called gabapentin has been approved for add-on therapy. Discuss this with your doctor if your seizures are not effectively controlled.

CLONIDINE (KLOH ni deen)

Prescription Needed: Yes   **Controlled Drug:** No   **Generic:** Yes

Brand Names: Catapres, Catapres-TTS, Combipres [CD]

Overview of BENEFITS versus RISKS	
Possible Benefits	*Possible Risks*
EFFECTIVE ANTIHYPERTENSIVE in mild to moderate high blood pressure	ACUTE WITHDRAWAL SYNDROME and hypertensive overshoot with abrupt discontinuation
Effective control of menopausal hot flashes (in selected cases)	Raynaud's phenomenon (cold fingers or toes)
Help in narcotic withdrawal	

▷ **Illness This Medication Treats:**
Mild to moderate high blood pressure. It is generally not used to start treatment. It may also be used as a step 3 or 4 drug in place of drugs that cause marked orthostatic hypotension.

Other (unlabeled) generally accepted uses: it is sometimes used to prevent migraine headache or hot flashes of menopause, and to treat menstrual cramps.

As Combination Drug Product [CD]: This step 2 antihypertensive is available in combination with the step 1 antihypertensive chlorthalidone, a diuretic. The differing methods of action complement each other to make the combination more effective.

▷ **Typical Dosage Range:** (Dosage or schedule must be determined by the doctor for each individual.)
Tablets: Initially 0.1 mg twice daily. Increase by 0.1 to 0.2 mg daily, as needed and tolerated. Usual range is 0.2 to 0.8 mg daily, taken in two doses. Total daily dosage should not exceed 2.4 mg. Medicated patches are applied once a week.

▷ **Conditions Requiring Dosing Adjustments:**
Liver function: The dose should be decreased for patients with liver compromise.

Kidney function: The dose MUST be decreased up to 50% of the usual dose at the usual dosing interval for patients with kidney compromise.

▷ **How Best to Take This Medicine:**   Tablets may be taken without regard to eating. The tablet may be crushed.

▷ **How Long This Medicine Is Usually Taken:**   Use on a regular schedule for 2 to 3 weeks is usually needed to see this drug's effectiveness in controlling high blood pressure. Long-term use (months to years) requires supervision and guidance by your doctor.

▷ **Tell Your Doctor Before Taking This Medicine If You:**
- ever had an allergic reaction to it.
- have a circulatory disorder of the brain.
- have angina or coronary artery disease.
- have or have had serious emotional depression.
- have Buerger's disease or Raynaud's phenomenon.
- are taking any sedative or hypnotic drugs or an antidepressant.
- plan to have surgery under general anesthesia soon.

▷ **Possible Side Effects:**   Drowsiness, dry nose and mouth, constipation (common), decreased heart rate, mild orthostatic hypotension.

▷ **Possible Adverse Effects:**
If any of the following develop, call your doctor promptly for guidance.
Some Mild Problems Drug Can Cause
  Allergic reactions: skin rash, localized swellings, itching.
  Headache, dizziness, fatigue, nervousness, dry and burning eyes.
  Painful parotid (salivary) gland, nausea, vomiting.
  Weight gain, urinary retention.
Some Serious Problems Drug Can Cause
  Idiosyncratic reaction: Raynaud's phenomenon.
  Aggravation of congestive heart failure, heart rhythm disorders, vivid dreaming, depression, hallucinations.
  Corneal ulcers (rare). Acute pancreatitis (rare).
  Very rare liver toxicity.

▷ **Possible Effects on Sex Life:**   At dosages of 0.2–0.8 mg/day: decreased libido and enlargement of the male breasts. At dosages of 0.5—3.6 mg/day: impotence. At any dosage: impaired ejaculation (rare).

▷ **CAUTION**
  1. **Do not stop taking this drug suddenly.** Sudden withdrawal can produce a severe and possibly fatal reaction.
  2. Hot weather and the fever associated with infection can reduce blood pressure significantly. Dosage adjustments may be necessary.
  3. Report the development of any tendency to emotional depression.

4. Safety and effectiveness of this drug for those under 12 years old are not established.
5. Those over 60 should **proceed cautiously** with the use of any antihypertensive drug. Unacceptably high blood pressure should be reduced without creating the risks associated with excessively low blood pressure. Small doses and frequent blood pressure checks are needed. Watch for development of light-headedness, dizziness, unsteadiness, fainting, and falling. Sedation and dry mouth occur in 50% of elderly users. Report promptly any changes in mood or behavior: depression, delusions, hallucinations.

Advisability of Use During Pregnancy or If Breast-Feeding:

Pregnancy Category: C. The manufacturer recommends avoidance of this drug by women who are or may become pregnant. Ask your doctor for guidance. Present in breast milk. This drug may impair milk production. Monitor nursing infant closely and discontinue drug or nursing if adverse effects develop.

▷ **Habit-Forming Potential:**   Rare reports of abuse of this drug have surfaced.

▷ **Overdose Symptoms:**   Marked drowsiness, weakness, dry mouth, slow pulse, low blood pressure, vomiting, stupor progressing to coma.

▷ **Suggested Periodic Examinations While Taking This Drug:** (at doctor's discretion)
Blood pressure measurements, monitoring of body weight.

▷ **While Taking This Drug the Following Apply:**

Foods: Avoid excessive salt. Ask your doctor for guidance regarding the degree of salt restriction.

Beverages: May be taken with milk.

Alcohol: Use with extreme caution. The combined effects can cause marked drowsiness and exaggerated reduction of blood pressure.

Other Drugs:

Clonidine may **decrease** the effects of
• levodopa (Larodopa, Sinemet, etc.), causing an increase in parkinsonism symptoms.

Clonidine **taken concurrently** with
• beta-adrenergic blockers (Inderal, Lopressor, etc.) may increase the risk of serious rebound hypertension if clonidine is discontinued first. It is best to stop the beta-blocker first and then gradually the clonidine.
• niacin may decrease the facial flushing effect of niacin.

The following drugs may **decrease** the effects of clonidine
• naloxone (Narcan)
• tricyclic antidepressants (Elavil, Sinequan, etc.); may reduce its effectiveness in lowering blood pressure.

Driving, Hazardous Activities: Use caution. This drug can cause drowsiness and impair mental alertness, judgment, and coordination.

Exposure to Heat: Use caution. Hot environments may reduce the blood pressure significantly; be alert to the possibility of orthostatic hypotension.

Exposure to Cold: Use caution. This drug may cause painful blanching and numbness of the hands and feet on exposure to cold air or water (Raynaud's phenomenon).

Heavy Exercise or Exertion: Use caution. Isometric exercises (the overload technique for strengthening individual · muscles) can significantly raise blood pressure. This drug may intensify the hypertensive response to isometric exercise. Ask your doctor for guidance.

Occurrence of Unrelated Illness: Fever may lower blood pressure significantly. Repeated vomiting may prevent the regular use of this drug, resulting in an acute withdrawal reaction. Consult your doctor.

Discontinuation: **Do not stop taking this drug suddenly.** A severe withdrawal reaction can occur within 12 to 48 hours after the last dose. The dose should be reduced gradually over 3 to 4 days, with periodic monitoring of the blood pressure.

▷ **Saving Money When Using This Medicine:**
- Many medicines are available today to treat high blood pressure. Ask your doctor if this medicine offers the best combination of price and outcome for you. Be certain to have your blood pressure periodically checked to make sure this medicine is still helping.
- A generic form is available.
- Talk with your doctor about stress management and exercise programs available in your community.

CLOTRIMAZOLE (kloh TRIM a zohl)

Prescription Needed: Yes   **Controlled Drug:** No   **Generic:** No

Brand Names: Clotrimaderm, Gyne-Lotrimin, Lotrimin, Mycelex

▷ **Warning:** The brand names Mycelex and Myoflex can be mistaken for each other, leading to serious medication errors. These names represent very different drugs. Mycelex (a large, white, round, flat lozenge) is the generic drug clotrimazole; it is used to treat yeast infections of the mouth and throat. Myoflex is a salicylate cream to relieve painful muscles and joints. Verify that you are using the correct drug.

Overview of BENEFITS versus RISKS

Possible Benefits	*Possible Risks*
EFFECTIVE TREATMENT AND PREVENTION OF *CANDIDA* (YEAST) INFECTIONS OF THE MOUTH AND THROAT (THRUSH)	Skin and mucous membrane irritation due to sensitization (drug-induced allergy)
EFFECTIVE TREATMENT OF *CANDIDA* INFECTIONS OF THE SKIN	Nausea, vomiting, stomach cramping, diarrhea (when swallowed)
EFFECTIVE TREATMENT OF *CANDIDA* INFECTIONS OF THE VULVA AND VAGINA	
EFFECTIVE TREATMENT OF TINEA (RINGWORM) INFECTIONS OF THE SKIN	

▷ **Illness This Medication Treats:**
(1) *Candida* (yeast) infections of the skin, mouth, throat, vulva, and vagina; (2) tinea and related infections: ringworm of the body, groin (jock itch), and feet (athlete's foot), due to susceptible fungal organisms.

▷ **Typical Dosage Ranges:** (Dosage or schedule must be determined by the doctor for each individual.)
Infants and Children: Use of lozenges is not recommended for children under 5 years old. For 5 years and older: Dissolve one lozenge slowly and completely in mouth five times a day for 14 days, longer if necessary.
12 to 60 Years of Age: For *Candida* infections of mouth and throat: Dissolve one lozenge slowly and completely in mouth five times a day for 14 days; extended treatment may be necessary for individuals with AIDS.
For *Candida* and tinea infections of skin: Apply cream, lotion, or solution to infected areas twice a day, morning and evening.
For *Candida* infections of vulva and vagina: One applicatorful (5 g) of cream intravaginally at bedtime for 7 to 14 consecutive days; or one 100 mg tablet intravaginally at bedtime for 7 days, or two 100 mg tablets intravaginally at bedtime for 3 days. One-dose treatment: One 500 mg tablet intravaginally at bedtime, once only.
Over 60 Years of Age: Same as for 12 to 60 years.

▷ **Conditions Requiring Dosing Adjustments:**
Liver function: The drug is mainly removed via the bile—the dose should be decreased if the bile duct is blocked.

▷ **How Best to Take This Medicine:** Dissolve lozenge in mouth slowly and completely, swallowing saliva as it accumulates. Do not chew the lozenge or swallow it whole. Take full course prescribed.

▷ **How Long This Medicine Is Usually Taken:** Use on a regular schedule for 1 to 2 weeks usually determines the effectiveness of this drug in controlling yeast or tinea infection. Long-term use (as in management of AIDS) requires periodic evaluation of response and dosage adjustment. See your doctor regularly.

▷ **Tell Your Doctor Before Taking This Medicine If You:**
- ever had an allergic reaction to it or fluconazole, itraconazole, ketoconazole, or miconazole.

▷ **Possible Adverse Effects:**

If any of the following develop, call your doctor promptly for guidance.

Some Mild Problems Drug Can Cause
Allergic reactions: skin rash, itching, burning, swelling, blistering.
Nausea, vomiting, stomach cramping, diarrhea (when swallowed).

Some Serious Problems Drug Can Cause
Allergic reactions: sensitization of tissues (where applied locally) that will allergically react with future drug application.
Rare liver toxicity with the oral form.

▷ **Possible Delayed Adverse Effects:** Local tissue sensitization to this drug.

▷ **CAUTION**
1. Avoid contact of cream, lotion, or solution with the eyes.
2. Do not cover local applications of cream or lotion with an occlusive dressing.
3. Use of lozenges by those under 5 years old is not recommended.

Advisability of Use During Pregnancy or If Breast-Feeding:
Pregnancy Category: B. Use this drug only if clearly needed. Ask your doctor for guidance. Presence in breast milk is unknown. Monitor the nursing infant closely and discontinue drug or nursing if adverse effects develop.

▷ **Overdose Symptoms:** Excessive use of lozenges may cause nausea, vomiting, or diarrhea.

▷ **While Taking This Drug the Following Apply:**
Other Drugs:
Clotrimazole *taken concurrently* with
- cyclosporine (Sandimmune) may result in cyclosporine toxicity.
- tacrolimus (Prograf) can result in kidney toxicity and increased potassium or glucose.

Discontinuation: As directed by your doctor.

▷ **Saving Money When Using This Medicine:**
- Many antifungals are available today. Ask your doctor if this medicine offers the best combination of price and outcome for you.

- Since some yeast medicines are now available without a prescription, talk with your doctor to make certain the symptoms you have are a yeast infection. If symptoms persist or worsen after starting therapy, call your doctor.

CLOXACILLIN (klox a SIL in)

Prescription Needed: Yes   **Controlled Drug:** No   **Generic:** Yes

Brand Names: Cloxapen, Tegopen

Overview of BENEFITS versus RISKS	
Possible Benefits	*Possible Risks*
EFFECTIVE TREATMENT OF INFECTIONS due to susceptible microorganisms	ALLERGIC REACTIONS, mild to severe
	Superinfections (yeast)
	Drug-induced colitis
	Blood cell disorders (rare)

▷ **Illness This Medication Treats:**
Infections caused by bacteria (often *Staphylococcus*) that have become resist to original penicillins; treatment of infections of skin and skin structures, the respiratory tract (including strep throat), and infections widely scattered throughout the body.

▷ **Typical Dosage Range:** (Dosage or schedule must be determined by the doctor for each individual.)
250 to 500 mg every 6 hours (4 doses/24 hr). The maximum dose is 6000 mg/24 hr. For children weighing less than 20 kg or 44 lb: 50–100 mg per kilogram of body weight divided into four doses. Children greater than 20 kg may receive the usual adult dose.

▷ **Conditions Requiring Dosing Adjustments:**
Liver function: The dose or dosing interval must be decreased for patients with liver disease.
Kidney function: This drug is eliminated through the bile and urine. Watch closely for adverse effects in cases of severe kidney compromise.

▷ **How Best to Take This Medicine:** Take on empty stomach, 1 hour before or 2 hours after eating, at the same times each day. Capsule may be opened for administration.

▷ **How Long This Medicine Is Usually Taken:** As long as necessary to eradicate the infection. For all streptococcal infections: not less than 10 consecutive days (without interruption), to reduce the possibility of rheumatic fever or glomerulonephritis.

▷ **Tell Your Doctor Before Taking This Medicine If You:**
- ever had an allergic reaction to it, are certain you are allergic to *any* form of penicillin, suspect you may be allergic to penicillin, or have a history of a previous reaction to it.
- are allergic to cephalosporin antibiotics (Ancef, Ceporan, Ceporex, Duricef, Kafocin, Keflex, Keflin, Kefzol, Loridine).
- are allergic by nature—hay fever, asthma, hives, eczema.
- have a history of kidney disease, regional enteritis, or ulcerative colitis.

▷ **Possible Side Effects:** Superinfections, often due to yeast organisms.

▷ **Possible Adverse Effects:**
If any of the following develop, call your doctor promptly for guidance.
Some Mild Problems Drug Can Cause
Allergic reactions: skin rashes, itching.
Irritations of mouth, unpleasant taste, nausea, vomiting, mild diarrhea.
Some Serious Problems Drug Can Cause
Allergic reactions: anaphylactic reaction, severe skin reactions, drug fever, swollen painful joints, sore throat.
Pseudomembranous colitis—severe diarrhea.
Rare blood clotting or liver problems.
Rare decreased white blood cell counts or kidney problems.

▷ *CAUTION*
1. Take the exact dose and the full course prescribed.
2. This drug should not be used concurrently with antibiotics such as erythromycin or tetracycline.
3. Dose for infants and children is based on age and weight. Consult your doctor for a precise dosage schedule.
4. For those over 60, evaluate kidney function before and during use to determine the need for dosage adjustment. Natural changes in the skin may predispose to prolonged itching reactions in the genital and anal regions. Report such reactions promptly.
5. Patient must be watched closely for adverse effects if there is severe kidney failure.

Advisability of Use During Pregnancy or If Breast-Feeding:
Pregnancy Category: B. Use this drug only if clearly needed. Ask your doctor for guidance. Probably present in breast milk. The nursing infant may be sensitized to penicillin and be at risk for diarrhea or yeast infections. Avoid taking this drug if possible or refrain from nursing.

▷ **Overdose Symptoms:** Possible nausea, vomiting, and/or diarrhea.

▷ **Suggested Periodic Examinations While Taking This Drug:** (at doctor's discretion)

Complete blood cell counts. Liver and kidney function tests with long-term use.

▷ **While Taking This Drug the Following Apply:**

Alcohol: No interactions expected, but excessive alcohol may blunt the immune response.

Other Drugs:

Cloxacillin may *decrease* the effects of

◆ oral contraceptives (birth control pills) in some women, impairing their effectiveness and possibly resulting in unwanted pregnancy.

Cloxacillin may *increase* the effects of

● warfarin (Coumadin) and increase risk of bleeding. More frequent INR (prothrombin time) testing is needed.

The following drugs may *decrease* the effects of cloxacillin

● antacids may reduce the absorption of cloxacillin.
● chloramphenicol (Chloromycetin).
● erythromycin (Erythrocin, E-Mycin, etc.).
● tetracyclines (Achromycin, Declomycin, Minocin, etc.).

Special Storage Instructions: Keep capsules in a tightly closed container at room temperature. Keep oral solution in the refrigerator.

Observe the Following Expiration Times: Oral solution kept refrigerated is good for 14 days; at room temperature, it is good for only 3 days.

▷ **Saving Money When Using This Medicine:**

● Several agents are available that work similarly. Ask your doctor if this drug offers the best combination of price and outcome for you.
● Make certain you understand how much and how often to take this medicine. Missing a dose or taking too little can let the infection return and promote resistant bacteria.

CLOZAPINE (KLOH za peen)

Prescription Needed: Yes   **Controlled Drug:** No   **Generic:** No

Brand Names: Clozaril

▷ **Note:** In the United States this drug is available only by special arrangement through the Clozaril Patient Management System (telephone: 1-800-648-1973). Ask your doctor for details.

Overview of BENEFITS versus RISKS

Possible Benefits	*Possible Risks*
EFFECTIVE CONTROL OF SEVERE SCHIZOPHRENIA that has failed to respond to other medicines	SERIOUS BLOOD CELL DISORDERS
Improvement in refractory cases	DRUG-INDUCED SEIZURES, depending on size of dose

---

▷ **Illness This Medication Treats:**
Severe schizophrenia that has failed to respond to adequate trials of at least two standard antipsychotic medications; because of its potential for causing serious blood cell disorders and seizures, it is used only for the severely ill schizophrenic patient.

▷ **Typical Dosage Range:** (Dosage or schedule must be determined by the doctor for each individual.)
Initially 25 mg one or two times a day; the dose is gradually increased by 25 to 50 mg daily as tolerated, to reach a dose of 300 to 450 mg daily by the end of 2 weeks. Subsequent increases should be limited to 100 mg one or two times a week. Average dosage requirements are 600 mg daily. Total daily dosage should not exceed 900 mg.

▷ **Conditions Requiring Dosing Adjustments:**
Liver function: Eliminated by liver; however, dose should be decreased for patients with liver compromise.
Kidney function: People with kidney compromise should be watched closely for adverse effects.

▷ **How Best to Take This Medicine:**   May be taken without regard to meals or with food if necessary to reduce stomach irritation. The tablet may be crushed.

▷ **How Long This Medicine Is Usually Taken:**   The benefits may be seen after 2 to 4 weeks of regular use. Peak effect usually requires 3 months. If no significant benefit is seen within 6 to 8 weeks, usage of this drug should be stopped. Long-term use (months to years) requires periodic physician evaluation of response.

▷ **Tell Your Doctor Before Taking This Medicine If You:**
- ever had an allergic reaction to it.
- have experienced severe bone marrow depression (impaired white blood cell production) with previous use of this drug.
- presently have any type of bone marrow or blood cell disorder, or you are currently taking any other drug that can cause bone marrow depression.
- have a history of any type of seizure disorder.
- have a history of narrow-angle glaucoma.

- have any type of heart or circulatory disorder, especially heart rhythm abnormalities or hypertension.
- have impaired liver or kidney function or prostatism.

▷ **Possible Side Effects:** Drowsiness, dizziness, light-headedness, orthostatic hypotension.

Blurred vision, salivation, dry mouth, impaired urination, constipation.

▷ **Possible Adverse Effects:**

If any of the following develop, call your doctor promptly for guidance.

Some Mild Problems Drug Can Cause

Allergic reactions: skin rash; drug fever—this usually happens within the first 3 weeks of therapy and goes away by itself.

Headache, tremor, fainting, nightmares, confusion, depression.

Rapid heartbeat, hypertension, chest pain.

Nausea, vomiting, diarrhea.

Some Serious Problems Drug Can Cause

Bone marrow depression.

Drug-induced seizures (dose-related).

Very rare neuroleptic malignant syndrome or anticholinergic syndrome.

▷ **Possible Effects on Sex Life:** Impotence (rare), abnormal ejaculation.

▷ *CAUTION*

1. White blood cell counts must be determined before clozapine treatment is started; follow-up counts must be made every week during the entire course of treatment and for 4 weeks after discontinuation.
2. Report promptly any indications of a possible infection: fever, sore throat, flu-like symptoms, skin infections, painful urination, etc.
3. Report promptly any tendency to light-headedness or dizziness on rising from a sitting or lying position; this could be an indication of orthostatic hypotension.
4. Call your doctor BEFORE taking any other medication while taking clozapine. This includes all prescription and over-the-counter drugs.
5. Safety and effectiveness of this drug for those under 16 years old are not established.
6. Those over 60 may be more susceptible to development of orthostatic hypotension, confusion, excitement, and prostatism. Report related symptoms promptly.

Advisability of Use During Pregnancy or If Breast-Feeding:

Pregnancy Category: B. Use this drug only if clearly needed. Presence in breast milk is unknown; avoid taking this drug or refrain from nursing.

▷ **Overdose Symptoms:** Marked drowsiness, delirium, hallucinations, rapid and irregular heartbeat, irregular breathing, fainting.

▷ **Suggested Periodic Examinations While Taking This Drug:** (at doctor's discretion)
White blood cell and differential counts before starting therapy, every week during therapy, and for 4 weeks after termination.
24-hour blood pressure measurements and electrocardiograms.

▷ **While Taking This Drug the Following Apply:**
Beverages: May be taken with milk.
Alcohol: Avoid completely. Alcohol can increase the sedative action of this drug and accentuate its depressant effects of brain function and blood pressure. This drug can increase the intoxicating effects of alcohol.
Tobacco Smoking: May accelerate the elimination and require increased dosage.
Marijuana Smoking: Moderate increase in drowsiness; accentuation of orthostatic hypotension; increased risk of aggravating psychosis.
Other Drugs:
Clozapine may **increase** the effects of
• drugs with sedative actions; observe for excessive sedation.
• drugs with atropinelike actions (see Drug Classes).
• antihypertensive drugs; observe for excessive reduction of blood pressure.
Clozapine **taken concurrently** with
• other bone marrow–depressant drugs may increase the risk of impaired white blood cell production
• erythromycin (E-Mycin, others) may result in increased clozapine concentrations and toxicity (only one case report, but caution is advised).
• fluvoxamine (Luvox) may result in clozapine toxicity.
• lithium (Lithobid, Lithotab, etc.) may increase the risk of confusional states, seizures, and neuroleptic malignant syndrome.
• cimetidine (Tagamet) can result in a toxic level of clozapine.
• phenytoin (Dilantin) can cause a decreased clozapine level and result in breakthrough schizophrenia.
• risperidone (Risperdal).
• warfarin (Coumadin) can cause increased bleeding risk. More frequent INR (prothrombin time) testing is indicated.
Driving, Hazardous Activities: May cause drowsiness, dizziness, blurred vision, confusion, and seizures. Restrict your activities as necessary.
Exposure to Heat: Use caution until your tolerance to environmental

heat is determined. This drug can cause fever and impair the body's adaptation to heat.

Occurrence of Unrelated Illness: Monitor all current infections very carefully and provide vigorous treatment. Observe white blood cell response to infection closely.

Discontinuation: If possible, discontinue this drug gradually over a period of 1 to 2 weeks. If abrupt withdrawal is necessary, observe carefully for recurrence of psychotic symptoms.

▷ **Saving Money When Using This Medicine:**

- Many agents are available to treat schizophrenia. This medicine should be tried only if you have failed to respond to two other medicines. Ask your doctor if this drug offers the best combination of price and outcome for you.

- A new agent called olanzapine has been approved, which appears to avoid some of the more common side effects of earlier agents. Talk to your doctor about this medicine.

- Stress management and an exercise program can help your outlook. Discuss available programs with your doctor.

CODEINE (KOH deen)

Prescription Needed: Yes   **Controlled Drug:** C-II*   **Generic:** Yes

Brand Names: Actifed w/Codeine [CD], Anacin w/Codeine [CD], Benylin Syrup w/Codeine [CD], Bufferin w/Codeine [CD], Dimetapp-C [CD], Empirin w/Codeine No. 2, 4 [CD], Fiorinal w/Codeine No. 1, 2, 3 [CD], Naldecon-CX [CD], Phenergan w/Codeine [CD], Robaxisal-C [CD], SK-Apap, Triaminic Expectorant w/Codeine [CD], Tylenol w/Codeine No. 1, 2, 3, 4 [CD]

Overview of BENEFITS versus RISKS	
Possible Benefits	*Possible Risks*
EFFECTIVE RELIEF OF MODERATE TO SEVERE PAIN	Low potential for habit formation (dependence)
EFFECTIVE CONTROL OF COUGH	Mild allergic reactions (infrequent)
	Nausea, constipation

▷ **Illness This Medication Treats:**

(1) Moderate to severe pain; (2) control of cough; (3) control of diarrhea. Its widest use is as an ingredient in analgesic preparations and cough remedies.

*See Controlled Drug Schedules inside this book's cover.

As Combination Drug Product [CD]: Codeine is commonly combined with milder analgesics to enhance effectiveness, notably aspirin and acetaminophen. It is frequently added to cough mixtures containing antihistamines, decongestants, and expectorants to make these "shotgun" preparations more effective in reducing the frequency and severity of cough.

▷ **Typical Dosage Range:** (Dosage or schedule must be determined by the doctor for each individual.)

As analgesic: 15 to 60 mg every 3 to 6 hours as needed. For cough: 10 to 20 mg every 4 to 6 hours as needed. For diarrhea: 30 mg/6 hr as needed. Total daily dosage should not exceed 200 mg for pain or 120 mg for cough or diarrhea.

▷ **Conditions Requiring Dosing Adjustments:**

Liver function: The dose must be decreased for patients with liver compromise.

Kidney function: For patients with moderate to severe kidney failure, the dose may have to be decreased by up to 75%.

▷ **How Best to Take This Medicine:** May be taken with or following food to reduce stomach irritation or nausea. Tablet may be crushed.

▷ **How Long This Medicine Is Usually Taken:** As required to control pain, cough, or diarrhea. Continual use should not exceed 5 to 7 days without interruption and reassessment of need.

▷ **Tell Your Doctor Before Taking This Medicine If You:**
- ever had an allergic reaction to it.
- are having an acute attack of asthma.
- have a history of drug abuse or alcoholism.
- have impaired liver or kidney function.
- have gallbladder disease, a seizure disorder, or an underactive thyroid gland.
- have chronic lung disease (COPD).
- have porphyria or a tendency to become constipated.
- are taking any other drugs that have a sedative effect.
- plan to have surgery under general anesthesia soon.

▷ **Possible Side Effects:** Drowsiness, light-headedness, dry mouth, urinary retention, constipation.

▷ **Possible Adverse Effects:**

If any of the following develop, call your doctor promptly for guidance.

Some Mild Problems Drug Can Cause

Allergic reactions: skin rash, itching.

Dizziness, sensation of drunkenness, confusion, depression, blurred or double vision.

Nausea, vomiting.

Some Serious Problems Drug Can Cause
Allergic reactions: anaphylaxis (rare), severe skin reactions.
Idiosyncratic reactions: delirium, hallucinations, increased pain sensitivity after the analgesic effect has worn off.
Seizures (rare), impaired breathing.
Rare porphyria.

▷ *CAUTION*
1. If you have asthma, chronic bronchitis, or emphysema, excessive use of this drug may cause significant respiratory difficulty, thickening of bronchial secretions, and suppression of coughing.
2. The concurrent use of this drug with atropinelike drugs can increase the risk of urinary retention and reduced intestinal function.
3. Do not take this drug following acute head injury.
4. Do not use this drug for children under 2 years old, because of their vulnerability to life-threatening respiratory depression.
5. For those over 60 years old, small starting doses are indicated initially, and increased as needed and tolerated. Use is limited to short-term treatment. There may be increased susceptibility to the development of drowsiness, dizziness, unsteadiness, falling, urinary retention, and constipation (often leading to fecal impaction).

Advisability of Use During Pregnancy or If Breast-Feeding:
Pregnancy Category: C. D if used in high doses or for prolonged periods near the time the baby is about to be born. Use this drug only if clearly needed and in small, infrequent doses. Present in breast milk in small amounts; avoid taking this drug or refrain from nursing.

▷ **Habit-Forming Potential:** Psychological and/or physical dependence can develop with use of large doses for an extended period of time. However, true dependence is infrequent and unlikely with prudent use.

▷ **Overdose Symptoms:** Drowsiness, restlessness, agitation, nausea, vomiting, dry mouth, vertigo, weakness, lethargy, stupor, coma, seizures.

▷ **Possible Effects of Long-Term Use:** Psychological and physical dependence, chronic constipation.

▷ **While Taking This Drug the Following Apply:**
Beverages: No restrictions. May be taken with milk.
Alcohol: Use extreme caution. Codeine can intensify the intoxicating effects of alcohol, and alcohol can intensify the depressant effects of codeine on brain function, breathing, and circulation.
Marijuana Smoking: Increase in drowsiness and pain relief; impairment of mental and physical performance.

Other Drugs:

Codeine may *increase* the effects of
- other drugs with sedative effects.
- atropinelike drugs, increasing the risk of constipation and urinary retention.
- monoamine oxidase inhibitors (MAOIs) and also increase central nervous system symptoms and depression.

Driving, Hazardous Activities: This drug can impair mental alertness, judgment, reaction time, and physical coordination. Avoid hazardous activities accordingly.

Discontinuation: Limit this drug to short-term use. If extended use is necessary, discontinuation should be gradual to minimize possible effects of withdrawal (usually mild with codeine).

▷ **Saving Money When Using This Medicine:**
- Effective pain management often involves the use of adjuvant drugs and the World Health Organization Pain Ladder. It is not unusual to combine medicines to more effectively reduce pain. Ask your doctor if this drug offers the best combination of price and outcomes for you, and if a second medicine in combination with the first might help treat the pain more effectively.
- Pain medicine benefits should be checked regularly (assessed) using a device called an algometer. Ask your doctor how your pain will be checked, and who will adjust medicine doses if needed.
- This medicine dose MUST be decreased for patients with liver compromise.
- If your pain is long-standing (chronic) in nature, talk with your doctor about the benefits of a visit to a pain management center.

COLCHICINE (KOL chi seen)

Prescription Needed: Yes   **Controlled Drug:** No   **Generic:** Yes

Brand Names: Colabid [CD], ColBenemid [CD], Cosalide, Proben-C [CD]

Overview of BENEFITS versus RISKS

Possible Benefits	*Possible Risks*
EFFECTIVE RELIEF OF ACUTE GOUT SYMPTOMS	Loss of hair
Prevention of recurrent gout attacks	Bone marrow depression (rare)
Prevention of attacks of Mediterranean fever	Peripheral neuritis (rare)
	Liver damage (rare)

▷ **Illness This Medication Treats:**

As Single Drug Product: Uses currently included in FDA-approved labeling: (1) reduces pain, swelling, and inflammation associated with acute attacks of gout; (2) used in smaller doses in prevention of recurrent gout attacks.

As Combination Drug Product [CD]: Colchicine is combined with probenecid to enhance its ability to prevent recurrent attacks of gout. Although colchicine is most effective in relieving the symptoms of acute gout, it has some effect in preventing recurrent and chronic discomfort. Probenecid increases the elimination of uric acid by the kidneys, thereby reducing its blood level to a point at which acute episodes of gout will not occur. This dual action is more effective than either drug used alone in the long-term management of gout.

▷ **Typical Dosage Range:** (Dosage or schedule must be determined by the doctor for each individual.)

For acute attack: 0.5 to 1.2 mg initially, followed by 0.5 to 0.65 mg every 1 to 2 hours until pain is relieved or nausea, vomiting, or diarrhea occurs. The total dose should not exceed 10 mg. For prevention of recurrent attacks: 0.5 to 0.65 mg one to three times every day.

▷ **Conditions Requiring Dosing Adjustments:**

Liver function: Caution must be used, and the dose decreased, for patients with obstruction or compromise of this route of elimination.

Kidney function: For patients with severe kidney failure (creatinine clearances of less than 10 ml/min), 50% of the usual dose should be taken at the typical dosing interval. Ongoing preventative use should be avoided if the creatinine clearance is less than 50 ml/min.

▷ **How Best to Take This Medicine:**   May be taken either on an empty stomach or with food to reduce nausea or stomach irritation. Start treatment at the earliest indication of an acute attack. Take the exact dose prescribed. The tablet may be crushed for administration.

▷ **How Long This Medicine Is Usually Taken:**   For acute attack— stop when pain is relieved or nausea, vomiting, or diarrhea occurs; do not resume for 3 days without consulting your doctor. For prevention—use the smallest effective dose for long-term management; consult your doctor regarding dosage schedule and duration.

▷ **Tell Your Doctor Before Taking This Medicine If You:**
  • ever had an allergic reaction to it.
  • have an active stomach or duodenal ulcer.
  • have active ulcerative colitis.
  • have a history of peptic ulcer disease or ulcerative colitis.
  • have any type of heart disease.
  • have impaired liver or kidney function.
  • plan to have surgery in the near future.

▷ **Possible Side Effects:**   Nausea, vomiting, abdominal cramping, diarrhea. Thrombophlebitis with intravenous use.

▷ **Possible Adverse Effects:**
If any of the following develop, call your doctor promptly for guidance.
Some Mild Problems Drug Can Cause
  Allergic reactions: skin rash, fever.
  Loss of hair.
Some Serious Problems Drug Can Cause
  Allergic reaction: anaphylactic reaction.
  Loss of hair.
  Drooping of the eyes (ptosis).
  Bone marrow depression.
  Peripheral neuritis.
  Inflammation of colon with bloody diarrhea.
  Liver damage.

▷ **Possible Effects on Sex Life:**   Reversible absence of sperm (azoospermia).

▷ **Natural Diseases or Disorders That May Be Activated by This Medicine:**   Peptic ulcer disease, ulcerative colitis.

▷ **Possible Effects on Laboratory Tests:**   Complete blood cell counts: decreased red cells, hemoglobin, white cells, and platelets; Increased white cells (follows initial decrease).
  INR (prothrombin time): Decreased (with concurrent use of warfarin).

Blood vitamin B12 level: Decreased.

Liver function tests: Increased liver enzymes (ALT/GPT, AST/GOT, and alkaline phosphatase), increased bilirubin.

Fecal occult blood test: Positive.

Sperm counts: Decreased (may be marked).

▷ **CAUTION**

1. If this drug causes vomiting and/or diarrhea before joint pain is relieved, discontinue it and call your doctor.

2. Try to limit each course of treatment for acute gout to 4 to 8 mg. Do not exceed 3 mg/24 hr or a total of 10 mg/course.

3. Omit taking this drug for 3 days between courses to avoid toxicity.

4. Carry this drug with you while traveling if you are subject to attacks of acute gout.

5. It is best to take colchicine preventively before and following surgery if you have recurrent gout. (Surgery often precipitates acute attacks of gout.) Ask your doctor for the proper dosage schedule.

6. Dosage of this drug has not been established for infants or children; ask your doctor for guidance.

7. This drug has a very narrow margin of safety for those over 60. Because the total dosage required to relieve the pain of acute gout often causes vomiting and/or diarrhea, extreme caution is advised when this drug is used by anyone with heart or circulatory disorders, reduced liver or kidney function, or general debility.

Advisability of Use During Pregnancy or If Breast-Feeding:

Pregnancy Category: C by one manufacturer, D by another. Avoid using this drug during entire pregnancy if possible. Ask your doctor for help. Present in breast milk; avoid taking this drug or refrain from nursing.

▷ **Overdose Symptoms:**   Nausea, vomiting, abdominal cramping, diarrhea (may be bloody), burning sensation in throat and skin, weak and rapid pulse, progressive paralysis, inability to breathe.

▷ **Possible Effects of Long-Term Use:**   Hair loss, aplastic anemia, peripheral neuritis.

▷ **Suggested Periodic Examinations While Taking This Drug:** (at doctor's discretion)

Complete blood cell counts, uric acid blood levels to monitor status of gout, sperm analysis for quantity and condition, liver function tests.

▷ **While Taking This Drug the Following Apply:**

Foods: Follow your doctor's advice regarding the need for a low-purine diet.

Beverages: It is best to drink no less than 3 qt of liquid every 24 hours. This drug may be taken with milk. Some herbal teas (promoted as being beneficial for arthritis) contain phenylbutazone and other potentially toxic ingredients. Avoid herbal teas if you are not certain of their source, content, and medicinal effects.

Alcohol: No interactions expected. However, alcohol may increase the risk of gastrointestinal irritation or bleeding. It also raises uric acid blood levels and could interfere with gout management.

Other Drugs:

Colchicine *taken concurrently* with

- allopurinol (Zyloprim), probenecid (Benemid), or sulfinpyrazone (Anturane) can prevent attacks of acute gout that often occur when treatment with these drugs is first started.
- cyanocobalamin will decrease B12 absorption.
- cyclosporine (Sandimmune) may increase cyclosporine levels and toxicity.
- erythromycins (E.E.S., and perhaps other macrolide antibiotics—see Drug Classes) may result in toxic colchicine blood levels.

Driving, Hazardous Activities: Usually no restrictions when this drug is taken continually in small (preventive) doses. Be alert to the possible occurrence of nausea, vomiting, and/or diarrhea with larger (treatment) doses.

Exposure to Cold: This drug can lower body temperature. Use caution to prevent hypothermia, especially if you are over 60 years old.

Occurrence of Unrelated Illness: Tell your doctor if you are injured or if you develop any new illness or disorder. During periods of such stress you may be subject to acute attacks of gout, and it may be necessary to adjust your medication schedule.

▷ **Saving Money When Using This Medicine:**

- Several agents are available that work similarly to this drug. Ask your doctor if this drug offers the best combination of price and outcomes for you.
- Colchicine should NOT be used to prevent gout by people with moderate kidney compromise (creatinine clearance [see Glossary] less than 50 ml/min).
- Talk with your doctor about the benefits of a low-purine diet.
- Your doctor may want to check lead levels and the health of your heart, as lead poisoning may be a culprit in gout, and gout is a risk factor for coronary heart disease.

COLESTIPOL   (koh LES ti pohl)

Prescription Needed: Yes   **Controlled Drug:** No   **Generic:** No

Brand Names: Colestid

Overview of BENEFITS versus RISKS

Possible Benefits	*Possible Risks*
EFFECTIVE REDUCTION OF TOTAL AND LOW-DENSITY (LDL) CHOLESTEROL IN TYPE IIa CHOLESTEROL DISORDERS	Constipation (may be severe)
	Reduced absorption of fat, fat-soluble vitamins (A, D, E, and K), and folic acid
EFFECTIVE RELIEF OF ITCHING associated with biliary obstruction	Reduced formation of prothrombin with resultant bleeding

---

▷ **Illness This Medication Treats:**
Uses currently included in FDA-approved labeling: (1) reduction of abnormally high blood levels of total and low-density (LDL) cholesterol in Type IIa cholesterol disorders; (2) relief of itching due to deposit of bile acids in the skin associated with partial biliary obstruction; (3) removal of interior blood vessel buildups (atherosclerosis).

▷ **Typical Dosage Range:** (Dosage or schedule must be determined by the doctor for each individual.)
Initially 5 g of powder three times daily. Dose may be increased slowly as needed and tolerated to 30 g daily in two to four divided doses.

▷ **Conditions Requiring Dosing Adjustments:**
Liver function: This medicine is eliminated in the feces; the liver is not involved. Caution must be used if this route is compromised, and dosing on an every-other-day basis should be considered.

▷ **How Best to Take This Medicine:** Always take just before or with a meal; this drug is ineffective when taken without food. Mix the powder thoroughly in 4 to 6 oz of water, fruit juice, tomato juice, milk, thin soup, or a soft food such as applesauce. **Do not take it in its dry form.**

▷ **How Long This Medicine Is Usually Taken:** Use on a regular schedule for 4 to 6 weeks is usually needed to see the effectiveness of this drug in lowering excessively high blood levels of cholesterol. If an acceptable response is not seen after 3 months, use of this drug should be stopped. Long-term use (months to years) requires periodic physician evaluation of response and dose adjustment.

▷ **Tell Your Doctor Before Taking This Medicine If You:**
- ever had an allergic reaction to it.
- have complete biliary obstruction.
- are prone to constipation.
- have peptic ulcer disease.
- have a bleeding disorder of any kind.
- have impaired kidney function.

▷ **Possible Side Effects:**   Constipation; interference with normal fat digestion and absorption; reduced absorption of vitamins A, D, E, and K and folic acid. Metabolic acidosis.

▷ **Possible Adverse Effects:**

If any of the following develop, call your doctor promptly for guidance.

Some Mild Problems Drug Can Cause

Allergic reactions: skin rash, hives, tongue irritation, anal itching.

Headache, dizziness, muscle and joint pains.

Loss of appetite, abdominal discomfort, excessive gas, nausea, vomiting, diarrhea.

Some Serious Adverse Effects

Vitamin K deficiency and increased bleeding tendency.

Impaired absorption of calcium; predisposition to osteoporosis.

Gallbladder colic (questionable).

Hypothyroidism.

▷ **Natural Diseases or Disorders That May Be Activated by This Medicine:**   Peptic ulcer disease; steatorrhea with large doses.

▷ **Possible Effects on Laboratory Tests:**   Blood cholesterol and triglyceride levels: decreased (therapeutic effect).

Blood thyroxine (T4) level: decreased when colestipol and niacin are taken concurrently (in presence of normal thyroid function).

▷ *CAUTION*

1. The powder should never be taken in dry form; always mix it thoroughly with a suitable liquid before swallowing.
2. Observe carefully for the development of constipation; use stool softeners and laxatives as needed.
3. This drug may bind other drugs taken concurrently and impair their absorption. It is advisable to take *all other drugs* 1 to 2 hours before or 4 to 6 hours after taking this drug.
4. Safety and effectiveness of this drug for those under 12 years old are not established. Observe carefully for possible development of acidosis and vitamin A or folic acid deficiency (ask your doctor for guidance).
5. People over 60 may be at increased risk of severe constipation. Impaired kidney function may predispose to the development of acidosis.

Advisability of Use During Pregnancy or If Breast-Feeding:

Pregnancy Category: C. Use this drug only if clearly needed. Ensure adequate intake of vitamins and minerals to satisfy the needs of the mother and fetus. Not present in breast milk. Breast-feeding is permitted.

▷ **Overdose Symptoms:**   Progressive constipation.

▷ **Possible Effects of Long-Term Use:**   Deficiencies of vitamins A, D, E, and K, and folic acid. Calcium deficiency, osteoporosis. Acidosis due to excessive retention of chloride.

▷ **Suggested Periodic Examinations While Taking This Drug:** (at doctor's discretion)
Measurements of blood levels of total, low-density (LDL), and high-density (HDL) cholesterol.
Hemoglobin and red blood cell studies for possible anemia.

▷ **While Taking This Drug the Following Apply:**
Foods: Avoid foods that tend to constipate (cheeses, etc.).
Nutritional Support: Consult your doctor regarding the need for supplements of vitamins A, D, E, and K, folic acid, and calcium.
Beverages: Ensure adequate liquid intake (up to 2 qt daily). This drug may be taken with milk.
Other Drugs:
Colestipol may *decrease* the effects of
• acetaminophen; take 2 hours before colestipol.
• aspirin; take 2 hours before colestipol.
• digitoxin and digoxin; take 2 hours before colestipol.
• furosemide; take 2 hours before colestipol.
• hydrocortisone; take 2 hours before colestipol.
• iron preparations; take 2 to 3 hours before colestipol.
• penicillin G; take 2 hours before colestipol.
• phenobarbital; take 2 hours before colestipol.
• tetracycline; take 2 hours before colestipol.
• thiazide diuretics (see Drug Classes); take 2 hours before colestipol.
• thyroxine; take 5 hours before colestipol.
• vitamin B12.
• warfarin; take 6 hours after colestipol.
Discontinuation: The dose of any potentially toxic drug taken concurrently must be appropriately reduced when this drug is discontinued. Following discontinuation of this drug, cholesterol blood levels usually return to pretreatment levels in approximately 1 month.

▷ **Saving Money When Using This Medicine:**
• Several agents are available to help lower cholesterol. Ask your doctor if this drug offers the best combination of price and outcomes for you. Newer data shows that HMG CoA inhibitors may actually reverse existing disease, and may lead to better outcomes.
• Make sure your doctor checks any sites where buildup (atherosclerosis) is present. Control of cholesterol may be able to halt the pro-

gression of this problem. If the situation worsens, an HMG CoA inhibitor drug may be needed.

- Talk with your doctor about the benefits versus risks of taking aspirin every other day.

CROMOLYN (KROH moh lin)

Other Names: Cromolyn sodium, sodium cromoglycate

Prescription Needed: Yes **Controlled Drug:** No **Generic:** No

Brand Names: Crolom, Gastrocrom, Intal, Nasalcrom, Opticrom

Overview of BENEFITS versus RISKS

Possible Benefits	*Possible Risks*
LONG-TERM PREVENTION OF RECURRENT ASTHMA ATTACKS	Anaphylactic reaction (rare)
Prevention of acute asthma due to allergens or exercise	Spasm of bronchial tubes, increased wheezing (rare)
Prevention and treatment of allergic rhinitis	Allergic pneumonitis (rare)
Relief of allergic conjunctivitis	
Treatment of giant papillary conjunctivitis	

▷ **Illness This Medication Treats:**

Uses currently included in FDA-approved labeling: (1) *prevention* of allergic reactions in the nose (allergic rhinitis, hay fever) and bronchial tubes (bronchial asthma; of no value in relieving asthma after the attack has begun); also in treating the symptoms of allergic rhinitis and conjunctivitis; (2) prevention of exercise-induced asthma, treatment of mastocytosis, and management of several allergy-related skin disorders.

Other (unlabeled) generally accepted use: may help modify reactions in food allergies.

▷ **Typical Dosage Range:** (Dosage or schedule must be determined by the doctor for each individual.)

Eyedrops: One drop four to six times daily at regular intervals.

Inhalation aerosol: 1.6 mg (two inhalations) four times daily at regular intervals for long-term prevention of asthma, or as a single dose 10 to 15 minutes before exposure to prevent acute allergen-induced or exercise-induced asthma.

Inhalation powder: 20 mg (one capsule) four times daily at regular intervals for long-term prevention of asthma; 20 mg (one capsule) as a single dose 10 to 15 minutes before exposure, to prevent acute allergen-induced or exercise-induced asthma. Total daily dosage should not exceed 160 mg (eight capsules).

Inhalation solution: Same as for inhalation powder.

Nasal insufflation: Initially 10 mg in each nostril every 4 to 6 hours as needed; reduce to every 8 to 12 hours for maintenance.

Nasal solution: 2.6 to 5.2 mg in each nostril three to six times daily, as needed.

▷ **Conditions Requiring Dosing Adjustments:**

Liver function: The dose must be decreased for patients with liver compromise.

Kidney function: The dose should be decreased for patients with kidney compromise; however, specific guidelines have not been developed.

▷ **How Best to Take This Medicine:** Follow carefully the dosing instructions provided with each dosage form, especially the inhalers. Do not swallow the capsules; the powder is intended for inhalation into the air passages of the lungs. (If swallowed inadvertently, the capsule will cause no beneficial or adverse effects.)

▷ **How Long This Medicine Is Usually Taken:** Use on a regular schedule for 4 to 6 weeks is usually needed to see the effectiveness of this drug in preventing recurrent attacks of asthma or allergic rhinitis. Long-term use (months to years) requires periodic physician evaluation.

▷ **Tell Your Doctor Before Taking This Medicine If You:**
- previously had an allergic reaction to any dosage form of it.
- are allergic to milk, milk products, or lactose (the inhalation powder contains lactose).
- have impaired liver or kidney function.
- have angina or a heart rhythm disorder (the inhalation aerosol contains propellants that could be hazardous).

▷ **Possible Side Effects:** Unpleasant taste with use of inhalation aerosol.

Mild throat irritation, hoarseness, cough (can be minimized by a few swallows of water after each inhalation of powder). Propellants in the metered dose inhaler may cause problems in patients with heart disease.

▷ **Possible Adverse Effects:**

If any of the following develop, call your doctor promptly for guidance.

Some Mild Problems Drug Can Cause
  Allergic reactions: skin rash, itching.
  Headache, dizziness.
  Nausea, vomiting, urinary urgency and pain, joint and muscle pain.
  Nosebleeds with nasal use.

Some Serious Problems Drug Can Cause
  Allergic reactions: rare anaphylactic reaction. Allergic pneumonitis
    (allergic reaction in lung tissue).
  Rare arteritis.

▷ **CAUTION**
  1. This drug only helps *prevent* bronchial asthma—use *before* the
     onset of acute bronchial constriction (asthmatic wheezing).
  2. *Do not* use this drug during an acute attack of asthma; it could
     worsen and prolong asthmatic wheezing.
  3. This drug does ***not*** interfere with the actions of those drugs used
     to relieve the acute asthma attack after it has begun. Cromolyn is
     used ***before and between*** acute attacks to prevent their develop-
     ment; bronchodilators are used ***during*** acute attacks to relieve
     them.
  4. If you are also using an inhalation bronchodilator drug, it is best
     to take it about 5 minutes before inhaling cromolyn.
  5. Safety and effectiveness of this drug for those under 5 years old
     are not established. Young children may find it easier to use the
     nebulized solution rather than the powder.
  6. This drug is not effective in management of chronic bronchitis or
     emphysema.

Advisability of Use During Pregnancy or If Breast-Feeding:
Pregnancy Category: B. Use this drug only if clearly needed. Presence in
  breast milk is unknown; avoid taking this drug or refrain from nursing.

▷ **Possible Effects of Long-Term Use:**   Allergic reaction of lung tissue
  (allergic pneumonitis, very rare).

▷ **While Taking This Drug the Following Apply:**
Foods: Follow the diet prescribed by your doctor. Avoid all foods to
  which you may be allergic.
Beverages: Avoid all beverages to which you may be allergic.
Other Drugs:
Cromolyn may make it possible to reduce the dosage of cortisonelike
  drugs for management of chronic asthma. Consult your doctor regarding dosage adjustment.
Driving, Hazardous Activities: May cause dizziness. Restrict your activities as necessary.
Heavy Exercise or Exertion: This drug may prevent exercise-induced
  asthma if taken 10 to 15 minutes before exertion. It is most effective
  in young people.

Discontinuation: If regular use has made it possible to reduce or discontinue maintenance doses of cortisonelike drugs and you find it necessary to discontinue cromolyn for any reason, watch closely for a sudden return of asthma. You may need to resume a cortisonelike drug and start other measures to keep your asthma under control.

Special Storage Instructions: Keep the powder cartridges in a dry, tightly closed container. Store in a cool place but not the refrigerator. Do not handle the cartridges or the inhaler when your hands are wet.

▷ **Saving Money When Using This Medicine:**

- Several agents are available that work similarly to this drug. Ask your doctor if this drug offers the best combination of price and outcome for you.
- Keep a diary outlining how many acute attacks you suffered in the past year, and continue it into your first year of cromolyn so an accurate comparison can be made.
- If ongoing cortisonelike (steroid) medicines are still needed, talk with your doctor about calcium supplements, exercise, and periodic bone mineral density testing to check your risk for osteoporosis.

CYCLOPHOSPHAMIDE (si kloh FOSS fa mide)

Prescription Needed: Yes   **Controlled Drug:** No   **Generic:** No

Brand Names: Cytoxan, Neosar

Overview of BENEFITS versus RISKS

Possible Benefits	*Possible Risks*
CURES OR CONTROLS CERTAIN TYPES OF CANCER	REDUCED WHITE BLOOD CELL COUNT
PREVENTION OF ORGAN TRANSPLANTATION REJECTION	SECONDARY INFECTION
	URINARY BLADDER BLEEDING
Possibly beneficial in the treatment of rheumatoid arthritis and lupus erythematosus	HEART, LUNG, LIVER, OR KIDNEY DAMAGE
Possibly beneficial in selected cases of nephrotic syndrome in children	Loss of hair

---

▷ **Illness This Medication Treats:**

(1) Various forms of cancer, notably malignant lymphomas, multiple myeloma, leukemias, and cancers of the breast and ovary (2) Because this drug suppresses the immune system, it also prevents organ transplantation rejection and treats certain autoimmune disorders. (3) Also approved for treating certain resistant forms of nephrotic syndrome (kidney dysfunction) in children.

▷ **Typical Dosage Range:** (Dosage or schedule must be determined by the doctor for each individual.)

1 to 5 mg per kilogram of body weight daily.

▷ **Conditions Requiring Dosing Adjustments:**

Liver function: If the bilirubin (a specific lab test of liver function) is from 3.1 to 5.0 and the SGOT is greater than 180, take 75% of the dose at the typical interval. If the bilirubin is greater than 5.0, the dose is omitted.

Kidney function: For patients with moderate to severe kidney failure the dose is decreased by 25 to 50% of the usual dose, taken at the usual interval.

▷ **How Best to Take This Medicine:** It is best to take the tablet on an empty stomach. However, if nausea or indigestion occurs, this drug may be taken with or following food. Total liquid intake should be NO LESS than 3 qt/24 hr to reduce the risk of bladder irritation. Tablets may be crushed.

▷ **How Long This Medicine Is Usually Taken:** Use on a regular schedule is required to achieve and maintain a significant remission of the cancer under treatment. Actual duration of use depends on the response of the cancer and the tolerance of the patient to the drug's effects. See your doctor regularly.

▷ **Tell Your Doctor Before Taking This Medicine If You:**
- ever had an allergic reaction to it.
- have an active infection of any kind.
- have bloody urine for any reason.
- have impaired liver or kidney function.
- have a blood cell or bone marrow disorder.
- have had chemotherapy or X-ray therapy for any type of cancer.
- are now taking, or have taken within the past year, any cortisonelike drug (see Drug Classes).
- have diabetes.
- are pregnant.
- plan to have surgery under general anesthesia soon.

▷ **Possible Side Effects:** Bone marrow depression—impaired production of primarily white blood cells and, to a lesser degree, red blood cells and blood platelets. Possible effects include fever, chills, sore throat, fatigue, weakness, abnormal bleeding or bruising.

Impairment of natural resistance (immunity) to infection. Ninefold increase in bladder cancer. Leukemia has been reported following treatment. Weakening of the heart muscle. Inflammation of the bladder.

▷ **Possible Adverse Effects:**
If any of the following develop, call your doctor promptly for guidance.
Some Mild Problems Drug Can Cause
   Allergic reaction: skin rash (rare).
   Headache, dizziness.
   Loss of scalp hair, darkening of skin and fingernails.
   Loss of appetite, nausea, vomiting, mouth ulcers, diarrhea.
   Excessive urination.
Some Serious Problems Drug Can Cause
   Idiosyncratic reaction: hemolytic anemia.
   Liver damage with jaundice—yellow eyes and skin.
   Kidney damage—reduced urine volume, bloody urine.
   Severe inflammation of bladder: painful urination, bloody urine.
   Drug-induced damage of heart and lung tissue.

▷ **Possible Effects on Sex Life:** Suppression of ovarian function—irregular menstrual pattern or cessation of menstruation.
Suppression of testicular function—reduction or cessation of sperm production.

▷ **Possible Delayed Adverse Effects:** Development of other types of cancer (secondary malignancies).

Development of severe cystitis with bleeding from the bladder wall (may occur many months after the last dose).

▷ *CAUTION*

1. This drug may interfere with the normal healing of wounds.
2. This drug can cause significant changes (mutations) in the chromosome structure of both sperm and eggs. Any adult taking this drug should understand its potential for causing serious defects in children conceived during or following the course of medication.
3. This drug can suppress natural resistance (immunity) to infection, resulting in life-threatening illness.
4. Avoid live-virus vaccines while taking this drug.
5. This drug should not be given if a child is dehydrated. Provide adequate fluid intake to ensure a copious urine volume for 4 hours following each dose. Prevent exposure of the child to anyone with active chickenpox or shingles. This drug may cause ovarian or testicular sterility.
6. For those over 60, there is a risk of developing serious chemical cystitis. It is necessary to maintain a copious volume of urine. This may increase the risk of urinary retention with prostatism.

Advisability of Use During Pregnancy or If Breast-Feeding:
Pregnancy Category: D. Avoid completely during the first 3 months. Use of this drug during the last 6 months must be carefully individualized. Present in breast milk; avoid taking this drug or refrain from nursing.

▷ **Overdose Symptoms:** Nausea, vomiting, diarrhea, bloody urine, water retention, weight gain, severe bone marrow depression, severe infections.

▷ **Suggested Periodic Examinations While Taking This Drug:** (at doctor's discretion)
Complete blood cell counts every 2 to 4 days during initial treatment, then every 3 to 4 weeks during maintenance treatment.
Liver and kidney function tests.
Thyroid function tests (if symptoms warrant).

▷ **While Taking This Drug the Following Apply:**
Beverages: May be taken with milk.
Other Drugs:
Cyclophosphamide *taken concurrently* with
- allopurinol (Zyloprim) may increase the degree of bone marrow depression.
- chloramphenicol can decrease cyclophosphamide's effectiveness.
- ciprofloxacin (Cipro) may blunt ciprofloxacin's benefits.

- digoxin (Lanoxin) may decrease absorption of digoxin and blunt digoxin's benefits.
- hydrochlorothiazide and other thiazide diuretics may worsen the lowering of white blood cells caused by cyclophosphamide.
- influenza vaccine may blunt this and probably other vaccine benefits.
- pentostatin may lead to fatal heart damage.
- succinylcholine can lead to toxicity.

Driving, Hazardous Activities: Use caution if dizziness occurs.

Occurrence of Unrelated Illness: Report promptly any indications of infection—fever, chills, sore throat, cough, flu-like symptoms. It may be necessary to discontinue this drug until the infection is controlled. See your doctor.

▷ **Saving Money When Using This Medicine:**
- Ask your doctor if this drug offers the best combination of price and outcome for you.
- Make sure you discuss new therapy options with your doctor, as there are several beneficial compounds under research.

CYCLOSPORINE (SI kloh spor een)

Other Names: Ciclosporin, cyclosporin A

Prescription Needed: Yes   **Controlled Drug:** No   **Generic:** No

Brand Names: Sandimmune, Neoral

Overview of BENEFITS versus RISKS	
Possible Benefits	*Possible Risks*
EFFECTIVE PREVENTION AND TREATMENT OF ORGAN TRANSPLANTATION REJECTION	MARKED KIDNEY TOXICITY DEVELOPMENT OF HYPERTENSION
Limited effectiveness in the treatment of Crohn's disease, myasthenia gravis, severe psoriasis, rheumatoid arthritis	Excessive hair growth
	Overgrowth of gums
	Liver toxicity
	Low white blood cell count
	Development of lymphoma

▷ **Illness This Medication Treats:**
(1) Organ rejection in kidney, liver, and heart transplantation in conjunction with cortisonelike drugs; (2) treatment for acute rejection of transplanted organs (rejection crisis).

Other (unlabeled) generally accepted uses: (1) used in transplantation of bone marrow. (2) Helps Sjögren's, Crohn's, and Grave's disease; psoriasis; myasthenia gravis; rheumatoid arthritis; aplastic anemia; and some cases of diabetes.

▷ **Typical Dosage Range:** (Dosage or schedule must be determined by the doctor for each individual.)

Initially 15 mg per kilogram of body weight per day, taken 4 to 12 hours before transplantation surgery. Continue this dose following surgery for 1 to 2 weeks, then gradually reduce the dose by 5% per week to a maintenance dose of 5 to 10 mg per kilogram of body weight per day. A new strategy that does NOT use weight, but instead uses the lowest blood level, has been developed. The micro-emulsion form offers more consistent blood level characteristics (pharmacokinetics). If Neoral is used, it should be taken at the same time each day in two equally divided doses. Cyclosporine blood levels are needed, particularly when changing from Sandimmune to Neoral.

▷ **Conditions Requiring Dosing Adjustments:**

Liver function: The dose must be adjusted (based on blood levels) for patients with liver compromise.

Kidney function: This drug is capable of causing marked kidney toxicity. A benefit-to-risk decision must be made if toxicity develops.

Hypercholesterolemia: If the blood cholesterol is 50% above normal, the dose must be decreased by 50% to avoid toxicity.

Obesity: Because of the way the drug is distributed in the body, the dosing of this medication **must** be based on ideal body weight (a calculation which helps eliminate fat).

Cystic fibrosis: It is very difficult to appropriately dose this medication for patients who have this disease. Some patients require as much as two times the usual dose. The dose should be adjusted to drug levels.

Diabetes: People with diabetes often need an increased dose of cyclosporine to achieve the desired effect. The dose should be determined based on blood levels.

Multiple organ transplants: People with multiple organ transplants, such as pancreas and kidney, should have their ongoing dose determined in response to blood levels.

▷ **How Best to Take This Medicine:** Preferably taken with or immediately following food to reduce stomach irritation. The capsule should be swallowed whole; do not open, crush, or chew. The oral solution should be mixed in orange juice (at room temperature) in a glass or ceramic cup; do not use a wax-lined or plastic container. Stir well and drink immediately. It is best to take this drug at the same time each day to maintain steady blood levels.

▷ **How Long This Medicine Is Usually Taken:** Use on a regular schedule for several weeks is usually needed to see this drug's effectiveness in preventing organ rejection or stopping rejection already underway. Long-term use (months to years) requires periodic physician evaluation of response, blood tests, and dosage adjustment.

▷ **Tell Your Doctor Before Taking This Medicine If You:**
- ever had an allergic reaction to it.
- are taking any immunosuppressant drug other than cortisonelike preparations.
- have an active lymphoma of any type.
- have an active, uncontrolled infection, especially chickenpox or shingles.
- are pregnant or breast-feeding.
- have a history of liver or kidney disease, or impaired liver or kidney function.
- have a history of hypertension or gout.
- have a chronic gastrointestinal disorder or a seizure disorder.
- are taking other medicines that may be toxic to the kidney.
- are taking a potassium supplement or drugs that can raise the blood level of potassium.

▷ **Possible Side Effects:** Predisposition to infections, low blood magnesium.

▷ **Possible Adverse Effects:**
If any of the following develop, call your doctor promptly for guidance.
Some Mild Problems Drug Can Cause
  Allergic reactions: skin rash, itching.
  Excessive hair growth, acne.
  Headache, confusion, tremors.
  Mouth sores, gum overgrowth, nausea/vomiting, diarrhea.
Some Serious Problems Drug Can Cause
  Allergic reactions: anaphylactic reaction.
  Severe kidney injury.
  Hypertension, mild to severe.
  Seizures.
  Low white blood cells or platelets.
  Liver injury.
  Lymphoma, possibly drug-induced.
  Elevation of blood potassium and uric acid levels.
  Rare pancreatitis or increased risk of skin cancers.

▷ **Possible Effects on Sex Life:** Enlargement and tenderness of male breast.

▷ *CAUTION*

1. Report promptly any indications of infection of any kind.
2. Report promptly any indication of swollen glands, sores or lumps in the skin, or abnormal bleeding or bruising.
3. Tell your doctor promptly if you become pregnant.
4. Comply fully with all instructions regarding periodic laboratory tests; these are mandatory to ensure safe and effective drug treatment.
5. It is advisable to avoid immunizations while taking this drug. Also, avoid contact with individuals who have recently taken oral poliovirus vaccine.
6. This drug has been used effectively and safely in children of all ages.
7. Reduced kidney function that accompanies normal aging may require adjustment of dosage. Kidney function tests and measurement of cyclosporine blood levels will provide guidance.
8. Since this medicine has a number of significant drug interactions, talk with your doctor or pharmacist BEFORE taking any prescription or nonprescription medicine.

Advisability of Use During Pregnancy or If Breast-Feeding:

Pregnancy Category: C. Avoid using this drug during entire pregnancy unless it is clearly needed. Present in breast milk; avoid taking this drug or refrain from nursing.

▷ **Overdose Symptoms:**   Headache, painful sensations in hands and feet, flushing of the face, gum soreness and bleeding, nausea, abdominal discomfort.

▷ **Suggested Periodic Examinations While Taking This Drug:** (at doctor's discretion)

Measurement of cyclosporine blood levels.
Complete blood cell counts.
Liver and kidney function tests.
Measurement of magnesium, potassium, and uric acid blood levels.
Serial blood pressure measurements.

▷ **While Taking This Drug the Following Apply:**

Foods: Avoid excessive intake of high-potassium foods (see Table 11, "High-Potassium Foods," Section Six).

Beverages: Grapefruit juice or milk may increase blood levels. If this medicine is to be taken with a liquid, orange juice may be used. Water may be used after the medicine/orange juice combination is taken.

Other Drugs:

Cyclosporine *taken concurrently* with

• ACE inhibitors (see Drug Classes) may increase risk of kidney problems.

- amphotericin B may lead to serious kidney toxicity.
- aspirin substitutes (nonsteroidal anti-inflammatory drugs) may increase kidney toxicity.
- aminoglycoside antibiotics (see Drug Classes) may increase kidney toxicity.
- azathioprine may increase immunosuppression.
- ciprofloxacin (Cipro) and possibly other fluoroquinolones may increase the risk of kidney toxicity.
- co-trimoxazole may decrease cyclosporine's effectiveness and increase risk of kidney toxicity.
- digoxin (Lanoxin) may result in serious digoxin toxicity.
- furosemide (Lasix) may increase the risk of gout.
- ganciclovir may result in increased risk of kidney toxicity.
- histamine (H2) blockers (see Drug Classes) or ketoconazole may result in decreased cyclosporine blood levels.
- imipenam-cilastatin may result in increased neurotoxicity.
- lovastatin, pravastatin, or simvastatin may increase the risk of muscle toxicity.
- lovastatin may result in sudden (acute) kidney failure.
- sulfamethoxazole and/or trimethoprim may increase kidney toxicity.
- methylprednisolone may cause seizures.
- azathioprine may increase immunosuppression.
- cyclophosphamide may increase immunosuppression.
- tacrolimus may result in kidney toxicity.
- vaccines may result in blunting of the vaccine response.
- verapamil (Calan, others) and possibly other calcium channel blockers may increase immunosuppression.

The following drugs may *increase* the effects of cyclosporine

- acetazolamide.
- allopurinol.
- amiodarone (Cordarone).
- azithromycin (Zithromax).
- ceftriaxone (Rocephin).
- clarithromycin (Biaxin).
- colchicine.
- danazol.
- diltiazem (Cardizem).
- econazole.
- erythromycin (E.E.S., others).
- fluconazole (Diflucan).
- itraconazole.
- ketoconazole.
- methyltestosterone.
- metoclopramide.

- miconazole.
- oral contraceptives (birth control pills).
- terconazole.

The following drugs may *decrease* the effects of cyclosporine

- carbamazepine (Tegretol).
- isoniazid.
- nafcillin.
- octreotide.
- phenobarbital.
- phenytoin.
- rifabutin.
- rifampin.
- sulfadimidine and/or trimethoprim.
- ticlopidine.

Driving, Hazardous Activities: May cause confusion or seizures. Restrict your activities as necessary.

Discontinuation: Do not stop taking this medicine without your doctor's guidance.

Special Storage Instructions: Keep the gelatin capsules in the blister packets until ready for use. Store below 77° F (25° C). Keep the oral solution in a tightly closed container. Store below 86° F (30° C). Do not refrigerate.

Observe the Following Expiration Times: The oral solution must be used within 2 months after opening.

▷ **Saving Money When Using This Medicine:**

- Ask your doctor if this drug offers the best combination of price and outcomes for you.

DAPSONE (DAP sohn)

Other Name: DDS

Prescription Needed: Yes   **Controlled Drug:** No   **Generic:** Yes

Brand Names: Generic only

Overview of BENEFITS versus RISKS

Possible Benefits	*Possible Risks*
EFFECTIVE ADJUNCTIVE TREATMENT OF ALL TYPES OF LEPROSY	HEMOLYTIC ANEMIA
	Aplastic anemia (rare)
	Rare skin reactions
EFFECTIVE TREATMENT OF DERMATITIS HERPETIFORMIS	Rare liver damage
	Rare peripheral neuritis
	Rare kidney damage
Effective adjunctive prevention and treatment of *Pneumocystis carinii* pneumonia (AIDS-related)	
Moderately effective adjunctive prevention of malaria (some types)	

▷ **Illness This Medication Treats:**

(1) All types of leprosy in combination with other antileprosy drugs; (2) dermatitis herpetiformis.

Other (unlabeled) generally accepted uses: (1) a third-line agent for prevention and treatment of *Pneumocystis carinii* pneumonia (PCP) in AIDS patients; (2) treatment of lupus erythematosus; (3) may have a role in rheumatoid arthritis as a step before gold or penicillamine therapy.

▷ **Typical Dosage Range:** (Dosage or schedule must be determined by the doctor for each individual.)

Infants and Children: For leprosy: 1.4 mg per kilogram of body weight, once daily.

To suppress dermatitis herpetiformis: Initially 2 mg per kilogram of body weight daily. Increase if needed and tolerated. As soon as possible, reduce to lowest effective maintenance dose.

To prevent *Pneumocystis carinii* pneumonia in children over 1 month old: 1 mg per kilogram of body weight, up to 100 mg daily.

12 to 60 Years of Age: For leprosy: 50 to 100 mg once daily, or 1.4 mg per kilogram of body weight once daily.

To suppress dermatitis herpetiformis: Initially 50 mg daily; as needed and tolerated, increase up to 300 mg daily. As soon as possible, reduce to lowest effective maintenance dose.

To prevent *Pneumocystis carinii* pneumonia: 50 to 100 mg once daily.

To treat *Pneumocystis carinii* pneumonia: 100 mg once daily, in combination with trimethoprim, 20 mg per kilogram of body weight daily, for 21 days.

To prevent malaria: 100 mg in combination with pyrimethamine (12.5 mg), once every 7 days.

Over 60 Years of Age: Same as for 12 to 60 years of age.

▷ **Conditions Requiring Dosing Adjustments:**

Liver function: Dapsone is capable of causing liver toxicity. Patients with liver compromise should use this drug with caution.

Kidney function: The dose must be decreased for patients with kidney compromise.

DESIPRAMINE (des IP ra meen)

Prescription Needed: Yes **Controlled Drug:** No **Generic:** No

Brand Names: Norpramin, Pertofrane

Overview of BENEFITS versus RISKS	
Possible Benefits	*Possible Risks*
EFFECTIVE RELIEF OF ENDOGENOUS DEPRESSION	ADVERSE BEHAVIORAL EFFECTS: confusion, disorientation, delusions, hallucinations
Possibly beneficial in other depressive disorders	CONVERSION OF DEPRESSION TO MANIA in manic-depressive affective disorders
	Aggravation of paranoia and schizophrenia
	Drug-induced heart rhythm disorders
	Abnormally low white blood cell and platelet counts

▷ **Illness This Medication Treats:**

Severe emotional depression; relief is more likely to be effective in primary (endogenous) depression than secondary reactive (exogenous) depression.

Other (unlabeled) generally accepted use: to treat chronic pain.

▷ **Typical Dosage Range:** (Dosage or schedule must be determined by the doctor for each individual.)

Initially 25 mg, two to four times daily. Dose may be increased cautiously as needed and tolerated by 25 mg daily at intervals of 1 week. The usual maintenance dose is 100 to 200 mg every 24 hours. The total daily dosage should not exceed 300 mg. (When determined, the optimal daily requirement may be taken at bedtime as a single dose.)

▷ **Conditions Requiring Dosing Adjustments:**

Liver function: Because of its potential to cause liver toxicity, this drug should be used with caution and the dose decreased for patients with compromised livers.

Kidney function: Patients with compromised kidneys should use this drug with caution, because it can cause urine retention.

▷ **How Best to Take This Medicine:** May be taken without regard to meals. The capsule may be opened and the tablet may be crushed for administration.

▷ **How Long This Medicine Is Usually Taken:** Use on a regular schedule for 3 to 4 weeks usually shows the effectiveness of this drug in relieving depression; optimal response may require 3 months of use. Long-term use (months to years) requires periodic evaluation of response and dosage adjustment. If used to help chronic pain, this drug may start to work very quickly.

▷ **Tell Your Doctor Before Taking This Medicine If You:**
- ever had an allergic reaction to it or have had an adverse reaction to any other antidepressant drug.
- are taking, or have taken within the past 14 days, any MAO type A inhibitor (see Drug Classes).
- have had a recent heart attack (myocardial infarction) or have any type of heart disease, especially a heart rhythm disorder.
- have narrow-angle glaucoma or increased internal eye pressure.
- have any type of seizure disorder.
- have any type of thyroid disorder or are taking thyroid medication.
- have diabetes or sugar intolerance.
- have prostatism.
- plan to have surgery under general anesthesia soon.

▷ **Possible Side Effects:** Mild drowsiness, light-headedness (low blood pressure), blurred vision, dry mouth, constipation, impaired urination.

▷ **Possible Adverse Effects:**
If any of the following develop, call your doctor promptly for guidance.

Some Mild Problems Drug Can Cause
Allergic reactions: skin rash, swelling of face or tongue, drug fever.
Headache, dizziness, weakness, tremors, fainting.
Irritation of tongue, altered taste, indigestion, nausea.
Fluctuations of blood sugar.

Some Serious Problems Drug Can Cause
Allergic reactions: drug-induced hepatitis, anaphylactic reaction.
Rare neuroleptic malignant syndrome.
Adverse behavioral effects: confusion, delusions, hallucinations.
Seizures; reduced control of epilepsy.
Aggravation of paranoid psychoses and schizophrenia.
Heart rhythm disturbances.
Parkinson-like disorders, peripheral neuritis.
Abnormally low white blood cell and platelet counts.

▷ **Possible Effects on Sex Life:**   Decreased libido, increased libido (antidepressant effect), impotence, painful male orgasm, male breast enlargement, female breast enlargement with milk production, swelling of testicles.

▷ *CAUTION*
  1. This drug should be used only when a true primary endogenous depression has been diagnosed, *not* to treat the symptoms of reactive depression associated with many life situations in the absence of affective illness.
  2. Observe for early indications of toxicity or overdosage: confusion, agitation, rapid heart rate, heart irregularity. Measurement of the blood level of this drug can clarify this situation.
  3. Withhold this drug if electroconvulsive therapy is to be used to treat the depression.
  4. Safety and effectiveness of this drug for use by those under 6 years old are not established.
  5. For those over 60, therapy is started with 25 mg one or two times daily to evaluate tolerance. During the first 2 weeks of treatment, observe for confusional reactions—restlessness, agitation, forgetfulness, disorientation, delusions, or hallucinations. Also observe for unsteadiness and instability that may predispose to falling. This drug may aggravate prostatism.

Advisability of Use During Pregnancy or If Breast-Feeding:
Pregnancy Category: C. Use only if clearly needed. Avoid using this drug during the first 3 months if possible. Present in breast milk in small amounts. Monitor nursing infant closely and discontinue drug or nursing if adverse effects develop.

▷ **Habit-Forming Potential:**   Psychological or physical dependence is rare and unexpected. This drug is not prone to abuse.

▷ **Overdose Symptoms:** Confusion, hallucinations, drowsiness, tremors, heart irregularity, seizures, stupor, hypothermia.

▷ **Suggested Periodic Examinations While Taking This Drug:** (at doctor's discretion)
Complete blood cell counts, liver function tests.
Serial blood pressure readings and electrocardiogram.

▷ **While Taking This Drug the Following Apply:**
Foods: You may need to limit your food intake to avoid excessive weight gain.
Beverages: May be taken with milk.
Alcohol: Avoid completely. This drug can markedly increase the intoxicating effects of alcohol; the combination can depress brain function significantly.
Tobacco Smoking: May accelerate the elimination of this drug and require increased dosage.
Marijuana Smoking:
Occasional (once or twice weekly): Transient increase in drowsiness and mouth dryness. Daily: Persistent drowsiness and mouth dryness; possible reduced effectiveness of this drug.
Other Drugs:
Desipramine may ***increase*** the effects of
- all drugs with sedative effects; watch for excessive sedation.
- all drugs with atropinelike effects (see Drug Classes).

Desipramine may ***decrease*** the effects of
- clonidine (Catapres).
- guanethidine (Ismelin, Esimil).
- guanfacine (Tenex).
- levodopa by decreasing the absorption of levodopa.

Desipramine ***taken concurrently*** with
- albuterol may increase the effect of albuterol on blood vessels.
- anticonvulsants requires careful monitoring for changes in seizure patterns and the need to adjust anticonvulsant dosage.
- ethchlorvynol (Placidyl) may cause delirium; avoid concurrent use.
- large doses of vitamin C (greater than 2 g) may lead to increased removal of desipramine from the body.
- MAO type A inhibitors (see Drug Classes) may cause high fever, seizures, and excessive rise in blood pressure; avoid concurrent use of these drugs and provide periods of 14 days between administration of either.
- quinidine may result in desipramine toxicity.
- stimulants (amphetamine, cocaine, epinephrine, phenylpropanolamine, etc.) may cause severe high blood pressure and/or high fever.
- thyroid preparations may increase the risk of heart rhythm disorders.

- warfarin (Coumadin) may lead to an increased risk of bleeding. More frequent INR (prothrombin time) testing is indicated.

The following drugs may **increase** the effects of desipramine

- cimetidine (Tagamet)
- fluoxetine (Prozac).
- fluvoxamine (Luvox).
- methylphenidate (Ritalin).
- phenothiazines (see Drug Classes).

The following drugs may **decrease** the effects of desipramine

- barbiturates (see Drug Classes).
- chloral hydrate (Noctec, Somnos, etc.).
- clonazepam.
- estrogen (see drug profile).
- lithium (Lithobid, Lithotab, etc.).
- oral contraceptives (see drug profile).
- reserpine (Serpasil, Ser-Ap-Es, etc.).

Driving, Hazardous Activities: May impair mental alertness, judgment, physical coordination, and reaction time. Restrict your activities as necessary.

Exposure to Sun: Use caution until your sensitivity has been determined. This drug may cause photosensitivity.

Exposure to Heat: Use caution. This drug can inhibit sweating and impair the body's adaptation to hot environments, increasing the risk of heatstroke. Avoid saunas.

Exposure to Cold: The elderly should use caution and avoid conditions conducive to hypothermia.

Exposure to Environmental Chemicals: This drug may mask the symptoms of poisoning from handling certain insecticides (organophosphorus types). Read their labels carefully.

Discontinuation: It is best to discontinue this drug gradually. Abrupt withdrawal after prolonged use may cause headache, malaise, and nausea. When this drug is stopped, it may be necessary to adjust the dosages of other drugs taken concurrently.

▷ **Saving Money When Using This Medicine:**

- Many medications are available to treat depression. Ask your doctor if this drug offers the best combination of price and outcome for you. Some newer antidepressants may have fewer side effects.
- If one medicine from a particular class does not work, a new medicine from a different class could be effective.
- Discuss the benefits of a well-balanced diet and regular exercise with your doctor.
- Depression has been recently found to have a link to osteoporosis. Talk with your doctor about calcium supplements and bone mineral density testing.

DEXAMETHASONE   (dex a METH a sohn)

Prescription Needed: Yes   **Controlled Drug:** No   **Generic:** Yes

Brand Names: Aeroseb-Dex, Ak-Trol, Decaderm, Decadron, Decadron-LA, Decadron Phosphate Ophthalmic, Decadron Phosphate Respihaler, Decadron w/Xylocaine [CD], Dexasone, Hexadrol, Maxidex

---

Overview of BENEFITS versus RISKS

Possible Benefits	*Possible Risks*
EFFECTIVE RELIEF OF SYMPTOMS IN A WIDE VARIETY OF INFLAMMATORY AND ALLERGIC DISORDERS	Short-term use (up to 10 days) is usually well tolerated
EFFECTIVE IMMUNOSUPPRESSION in selected benign and malignant disorders	Long-term use (exceeding 2 weeks) is associated with many possible adverse effects:
	ALTERED MOOD AND PERSONALITY
	CATARACTS, GLAUCOMA
	HYPERTENSION
	OSTEOPOROSIS
	PANCREATITIS
	ASEPTIC BONE NECROSIS
	INCREASED SUSCEPTIBILITY TO INFECTIONS

▷ **Illness This Medication Treats:**

(1) A wide variety of allergic and inflammatory conditions, most commonly in the management of serious skin disorders, asthma, regional enteritis, ulcerative colitis, and all types of major rheumatic disorders including bursitis, tendonitis, and most forms of arthritis. (2) Topical creams can help psoriasis, eczema, and other forms of dermatitis; (3) ophthalmic form can help a variety of steroid-responsive eye conditions.

▷ **Typical Dosage Range:** (Dosage or schedule must be determined by the doctor for each individual.)

Oral: 0.75 to 9 mg daily as a single dose or in divided doses. Other dosage forms vary with the condition being treated.

▷ **Conditions Requiring Dosing Adjustments:**

Liver function: The primary elimination of this medication is via the liver; however, specific guidelines for dosing adjustments are not available.

Kidney function: Use this drug with caution as it can cause alkalosis.

Obesity: Suggested dosing of the IV or oral form: 1 mg per kilogram of body weight per day, with measurement of free urinary cortisol.

▷ **How Best to Take This Medication:**   Take with or following food to prevent stomach irritation, preferably in the morning. The tablet may be crushed.

▷ **How Long This Medicine Is Usually Taken:**   For acute disorders: 4 to 10 days. For chronic disorders: According to individual requirements. The duration of use should not exceed the time necessary to obtain adequate symptomatic relief in acute self-limiting conditions or the time required to stabilize a chronic condition and permit gradual withdrawal. See your doctor regularly.

▷ **Tell Your Doctor Before Taking This Medicine If You:**
- ever had an allergic reaction to it.
- have active peptic ulcer disease.
- have an active infection of the eye caused by the herpes simplex virus.
- have active tuberculosis.
- have had an unfavorable reaction to any cortisonelike drug in the past.
- have psychoneurosis or psychosis.
- have osteoporosis.
- have a history of thrombophlebitis.
- have diabetes, glaucoma, high blood pressure, deficient thyroid function, or myasthenia gravis.
- plan to have surgery of any kind soon.

▷ **Possible Side Effects:**   Increased appetite, weight gain, retention of salt and water, excretion of potassium, increased susceptibility to infection.

▷ **Possible Adverse Effects:**
If any of the following develop, call your doctor promptly for guidance.
Some Mild Problems Drug Can Cause
  Allergic reaction: skin rash.
  Headache, dizziness, insomnia.
  Abdominal distention.
  Muscle cramping and weakness, easy bruising.
  Acne, excessive growth of facial hair.
Some Serious Problems Drug Can Cause
  Serious mental and emotional problems.
  Reactivation of latent tuberculosis.
  Development of peptic ulcer.
  Increased blood pressure.
  Low blood platelets.

Cataracts or glaucoma.
Cushing's syndrome.
High blood sugar.
Development of inflammation of the pancreas.
Bone death.
Thrombophlebitis—pain or tenderness in thigh or leg.
Pulmonary embolism.

▷ **Possible Effects on Sex Life:** Altered timing and pattern of menstruation.

▷ *CAUTION*
1. It is advisable to carry a personal identification card that states you are taking this drug, if your course of treatment exceeds 1 week.
2. Do not discontinue this drug abruptly if you are using it for long term treatment.
3. If vaccination against measles, rabies, smallpox, or yellow fever is required, discontinue this drug 72 hours before vaccination and do not resume it for at least 14 days after vaccination.
4. Avoid prolonged use of this drug in children if possible. During long-term use, observe for suppression of normal growth and the possibility of increased intracranial pressure. Following long-term use, the child may be at risk for adrenal gland deficiency during stress for as long as 18 months after this drug is stopped.
5. Cortisonelike drugs should be used very sparingly by people over 60 and only when the disorder under treatment is unresponsive to adequate trials of unrelated drugs. Avoid prolonged use of this drug. Continual use (even in small doses) can increase the severity of diabetes, enhance fluid retention, raise blood pressure, weaken resistance to infection, induce stomach ulcer, and accelerate the development of cataract and osteoporosis.
6. Wounds will heal less quickly and may be more likely to become infected. Talk with your doctor about this.

Advisability of Use During Pregnancy or If Breast-Feeding:
Pregnancy Category: C. Avoid using this drug completely during the first 3 months. Limit use during the last 6 months as much as possible. If this drug is used, examine the infant for possible deficiency of adrenal gland function. Present in breast milk; avoid taking this drug or refrain from nursing.

▷ **Habit-Forming Potential:** Use to suppress symptoms over an extended period may produce functional dependence. In the treatment of conditions such as asthma and rheumatoid arthritis, the dose should be kept as small as possible and the drug withdrawn after periods of reasonable improvement. Such procedures may reduce the degree of steroid rebound—the return of symptoms as the drug is withdrawn.

▷ **Overdose Symptoms:** Fatigue, muscle weakness, stomach irritation, acid indigestion, excessive sweating, facial flushing, fluid retention, swelling of extremities, increased blood pressure.

▷ **Suggested Periodic Examinations While Taking This Drug:** (at doctor's discretion)

Measurements of blood pressure, blood sugar, and potassium levels.

Complete eye examinations at regular intervals.

Chest X ray if you have a history of tuberculosis.

Determination of the growing child's rate of development, to detect retardation of normal growth.

Bone mineral density testing (BMD) to check risk of osteoporosis.

▷ **While Taking This Drug the Following Apply:**

Foods: Ask your doctor regarding the need to restrict salt intake or eat potassium-rich foods. During long-term use of this drug, a high-protein diet is advisable.

Nutritional Support: During long-term use, take a vitamin D supplement. During wound repair, take a zinc supplement.

Beverages: Drink all forms of milk liberally.

Alcohol: No interactions expected. Use caution if you are prone to peptic ulcer disease.

Tobacco Smoking: Nicotine increases the blood levels of naturally produced cortisone and related hormones. Heavy smoking may add to the expected actions of this drug and requires close observation for excessive effects.

Marijuana Smoking: May cause additional impairment of immunity.

Other Drugs:

Dexamethasone may *decrease* the effects of

• isoniazid (INH, Niconyl, etc.).

• salicylates (aspirin, sodium salicylate, etc.).

• vaccines, by blunting the immune response to them.

Dexamethasone *taken concurrently* with

• carbamazepine (Tegretol) reduces the effectiveness of dexamethasone.

• loop diuretics such as furosemide or bumetanide may result in additive potassium loss.

• oral anticoagulants may either increase or decrease their effectiveness; ask your doctor about the need for prothrombin time testing and dosage adjustment.

• oral hypoglycemic agents (see Drug Classes) or insulin may result in loss of glucose control.

The following drugs may *decrease* the effects of dexamethasone

• antacids may reduce its absorption.

• barbiturates (Amytal, Butisol, phenobarbital, etc.).

- phenobarbital.
- phenytoin (Dilantin, etc.).
- primidone.
- rifabutin.
- rifampin (Rifadin, Rimactane, etc.).

Driving, Hazardous Activities: Usually no restrictions. Be alert to the rare occurrence of dizziness.

Occurrence of Unrelated Illness: Dexamethasone may decrease your natural resistance to infection. Tell your doctor if you develop an infection of any kind. It may also reduce your body's ability to respond to the stress of acute illness, injury, or surgery. Keep your doctor fully informed of any significant changes in your state of health.

Discontinuation: If you have been taking this drug for an extended period, do not stop it abruptly. Ask your doctor for guidance regarding gradual withdrawal. For 2 years after discontinuing this drug, it is essential in the event of illness, injury, or surgery that you tell attending medical personnel that you have used this drug. The period of impaired response to stress following the use of cortisonelike drugs may last 1 to 2 years.

▷ **Saving Money When Using This Medicine:**
- Several agents are available that work similarly to this drug. Ask your doctor if this drug offers the best combination of price and outcome for you.

DIAZEPAM (di AZ e pam)

Prescription Needed: Yes   **Controlled Drug:** C-IV*   Generic: Yes

Brand Names: Diazepam Intensol, Valium, Valrelease, Vazepam, Zetran

---

Overview of BENEFITS versus RISKS

Possible Benefits	*Possible Risks*
RELIEF OF ANXIETY AND NERVOUS TENSION	Habit-forming potential with prolonged use
Wide margin of safety with therapeutic doses	Minor impairment of mental functions
	Very rare jaundice
	Very rare blood cell disorders

▷ **Illness This Medication Treats:**
(1) Mild to moderate anxiety; (2) relief of acute alcohol withdrawal symptoms: agitation, tremors, hallucinations, incipient delirium tremens; (3) relief of skeletal muscle spasm; (4) short-term control of certain types of seizures (epilepsy); (5) easing of severe muscle spasms.

▷ **Typical Dosage Range:** (Dosage or schedule must be determined by the doctor for each individual.)
2 to 10 mg two to four times daily. Dose may be increased cautiously as needed and tolerated. After 1 week of continual use, the total daily dose may be taken at bedtime. Total daily dose should not exceed 60 mg. The sustained-release form may enable some patients to take their medicine only once a day.

▷ **Conditions Requiring Dosing Adjustments:**
Liver function: The dose **must** be decreased by 50% for patients with liver compromise.
Kidney function: Caution must be used—when the total daily dose is greater than 15 mg, diazepam may accumulate.
Obesity: Obese patients may take longer than non-obese patients to accumulate this medicine, and then its removal from their bodies may take longer.

▷ **How Best to Take This Medicine:** May be taken on empty stomach or with food or milk. The prolonged-action capsule should not be opened, but the tablet may be crushed. Do not discontinue this drug abruptly if taken for more than 4 weeks.

*See Controlled Drug Schedules inside this book's cover.

▷ **How Long This Medicine Is Usually Taken:**   Continual use on a regular schedule for 3 to 5 days is usually necessary to determine this drug's effectiveness in relieving moderate anxiety. Limit continual use to 1 to 3 weeks. Avoid uninterrupted and prolonged use.

▷ **Tell Your Doctor Before Taking This Medicine If You:**
- ever had an allergic reaction to it.
- have acute narrow-angle glaucoma.
- are given a prescription for a child under 6 months old.
- are allergic to any benzodiazepine drug.
- have a history of alcoholism or drug abuse.
- are pregnant or planning pregnancy.
- have impaired liver or kidney function.
- have a history of serious depression or mental disorder.
- have asthma, emphysema, epilepsy, or myasthenia gravis.

▷ **Possible Side Effects:**   Drowsiness, lethargy, unsteadiness, hangover effects on the day following bedtime use.

▷ **Possible Adverse Effects:**
If any of the following develop, call your doctor promptly for guidance.
Some Mild Problems Drug Can Cause
Allergic reactions: rashes, hives.
Dizziness, fainting, blurred vision, slurred speech, sweating, nausea.
Some Serious Problems Drug Can Cause
Allergic reactions: liver damage with jaundice, abnormally low platelet count.
Amnesia.
Severe lowering of blood pressure following rapid intravenous doses.
Bone marrow depression.
Paradoxical responses of agitation, anger, rage.

▷ **Possible Effects on Sex Life:**   Altered timing and pattern of menstruation.
Small doses (2–5 mg/day) are used to allay the anxiety that accounts for many cases of impotence in men, and inhibited sexual responsiveness in women. Larger doses (10 mg/day or more) can decrease libido, impair potency in men, and inhibit orgasm in women.

▷ *CAUTION*
1. Diazepam should not be discontinued abruptly if it has been taken continually for more than 4 weeks.
2. The concurrent use of some over-the-counter drug products that contain antihistamines (allergy and cold preparations, sleep aids) can cause excessive sedation in sensitive individuals.

3. Safety and effectiveness of this drug for those under 6 months old are not established. This drug should not be used by the hyperactive or psychotic child of any age. Observe for excessive sedation and incoordination.

4. Diazepam is NOT advisable for use by those over 60, as there are many active metabolites and the drug tends to last much longer than expected. If it must be used, smaller doses at longer intervals are best to avoid overdosage. Watch for development of lethargy, indifference, fatigue, weakness, unsteadiness, disturbing dreams, nightmares, and paradoxical reactions of excitement, agitation, anger, hostility, and rage.

Advisability of Use During Pregnancy or If Breast-Feeding:

Pregnancy Category: D. Frequent use of this drug in late pregnancy can cause the floppy infant syndrome in the newborn: weakness, lethargy, unresponsiveness, depressed breathing, low body temperature. Avoid its use during entire pregnancy. Present in breast milk; avoid taking this drug or refrain from nursing.

▷ **Habit-Forming Potential:**   This drug can produce psychological and/or physical dependence if used in large doses for an extended period.

▷ **Overdose Symptoms:**   Marked drowsiness, weakness, feeling of drunkenness, staggering gait, tremor, stupor progressing to deep sleep or coma.

▷ **Suggested Periodic Examinations While Taking This Drug:** (at doctor's discretion)
Complete blood cell counts during long-term use.

▷ **While Taking This Drug the Following Apply:**

Beverages: Avoid excessive intake of caffeine-containing beverages: coffee, tea, cola, chocolate. This drug may be taken with milk.

Alcohol: Alcohol may increase the absorption of this drug and add to its depressant effects on the brain. It is advisable to avoid alcohol completely throughout the day and night, if driving or any hazardous activity is necessary.

Tobacco Smoking: Heavy smoking may reduce the calming action of this drug.

Marijuana Smoking: Increased sedation and significant impairment of intellectual and physical performance.

Other Drugs:

Diazepam may *increase* the effects of
• digoxin (Lanoxin), causing digoxin toxicity.
• phenytoin (Dilantin), causing phenytoin toxicity.

Diazepam may *decrease* the effects of
• levodopa (Sinemet, etc.), reducing its effectiveness in treating Parkinson's disease.

Diazepam *taken concurrently* with

- fluvoxamine (Luvox) may result in toxicity.
- narcotics or other centrally active medicines may result in additive depression of breathing.

The following drugs may *increase* the effects of diazepam

- cimetidine (Tagamet).
- disulfiram (Antabuse).
- isoniazid (INH, Rifamate, etc.).
- omeprazole (Prilosec).
- oral contraceptives (birth control pills).
- sertraline (Zoloft).
- valproic acid (Depakene).

The following drugs may *decrease* the effects of diazepam

- ranitidine (Zantac).
- rifabutin.
- rifampin (Rimactane, etc.).
- theophylline (aminophylline, Theo-Dur, etc.).

Driving, Hazardous Activities: This drug can impair mental alertness, judgment, physical coordination, and reaction time. Avoid hazardous activities accordingly.

Exposure to Heat: Use caution until the effect of excessive perspiration is determined. Because of reduced urine volume, this drug may accumulate in the body and produce overdosage effects.

Discontinuation: Avoid sudden discontinuation if this drug has been taken for more than 4 weeks without interruption. Dosage should be tapered gradually, to prevent a withdrawal syndrome that could include depression, confusion, hallucinations, tremor, seizures, muscle cramping, sweating, and vomiting.

▷ **Saving Money When Using This Medicine:**

- Several agents are available that work similarly to this drug. Ask your doctor if this drug offers the best combination of price and outcome for you.
- Talk with your doctor about stress management and exercise programs available in your community.

DICLOFENAC   (di KLOH fen ak)

Prescription Needed: Yes   **Controlled Drug:** No   **Generic:** No

Brand Names: Arthotec, Cataflam, Voltaren, Voltaren Ophthalmic

> ### Overview of BENEFITS versus RISKS
>
> | *Possible Benefits* | *Possible Risks* |
> |---|---|
> | EFFECTIVE RELIEF OF SYMPTOMS ASSOCIATED WITH MAJOR TYPES OF ARTHRITIS | PEPTIC ULCER DISEASE; associated bleeding and perforation |
> | Effective relief of symptoms associated with bursitis, tendonitis, and related conditions | Liver toxicity with jaundice
Aplastic anemia (rare)
Water retention
Kidney toxicity (rare) |
> | Effective relief of menstrual cramps | |

See the acetic acids (NSAIDs) profile for further information.

DIDANOSINE   (di DAN oh seen)

Other Names: Dideoxyinosine, DDI

Prescription Needed: Yes

Brand Names: Videx

> ### Overview of BENEFITS versus RISKS
>
> | *Possible Benefits* | *Possible Risks* |
> |---|---|
> | DELAYED PROGRESSION OF HIV to AIDS | DRUG-INDUCED PANCREATITIS
DRUG-INDUCED PERIPHERAL NEURITIS
Drug-induced seizures
Rare liver damage |

▷ **Illness This Medication Treats:**

Human immunodeficiency virus (HIV) infections in certain adults and children (6 months of age or older) with advanced disease who cannot tolerate zidovudine or who have shown significant deterioration during zidovudine therapy. This drug is not a cure for AIDS, and it does not reduce the risk of transmission of HIV infection to others through sexual contact or blood contamination.

Other (unlabeled) generally accepted use: part of combination therapy for AIDS.

▷ **Typical Dosage Range:** (Dosage or schedule must be determined by the doctor for each individual.)

Infants and Children: For those 6 months or older, dosage is based on the dosage form and body surface area:

Pediatric oral solution (reconstituted and mixed with buffers): 125 mg (12.5 ml) every 12 hours for body surface area of 1.1–1.4 square meters; 94 mg (9.5 ml) every 12 hours for body surface area of 0.8–1 square meters; 62 mg (6 ml) every 12 hours for body surface area of 0.5–0.7 square meters; 31 mg (3 ml) every 12 hours for body surface area of 0.4 square meters or less.

Chewable/dispersible tablets: 100 mg every 12 hours for body surface area of 1.1–1.4 square meters; 75 mg every 12 hours for body surface area of 0.8–1 square meters; 50 mg every 12 hours for body surface area of 0.5–0.7 square meters; 25 mg every 12 hours for body surface area of 0.4 square meters or less. For children 1 year of age or older, each dose should consist of two tablets to ensure that adequate buffering is provided to prevent degradation of the drug in stomach acid secretions; for children younger than 1 year old, one tablet provides adequate buffering.

12 to 60 Years of Age: Dosage is based on the dosage form and body weight:

Adult oral solution (buffered): 250 mg/12 hr for body weight of 60 kg or more; 167 mg/12 hr for body weight of less than 60 kg.

Chewable/dispersible tablets: 200 mg/12 hr for body weight of 60 kg or more; 125 mg/12 hr for body weight of less than 60 kg.

Over 60 Years of Age: Same as for 12 to 60 years. If liver or kidney function is impaired, reduce dosage accordingly.

▷ **Conditions Requiring Dosing Adjustments:**

Liver function: Up to 60% of a given dose is changed by the liver into chemical forms that are still not known. There is an increased risk of liver problems in people with compromised livers who take this drug. If this drug is used in this population, the dose must be decreased.

Kidney function: Dose **must** be decreased for patients with kidney compromise. Important: each tablet contains 15.7 mEq of magnesium—an element patients with renal compromise have difficulty removing. There is an increased risk of drug-induced pancreatitis if this drug is used by patients with kidney compromise.

▷ **How Best to Take This Medicine:**   This drug is most effective when taken on an empty stomach, 2 hours before or 2 hours after eating.

The pediatric oral solution is dispensed after unbuffered powder is first reconstituted with water and then buffered by equal quantities of antacid (such as Mylanta or Maalox). This mixture should be shaken very thoroughly before each dose is measured for administration.

The adult oral solution is prepared by stirring the contents of one packet into 120 ml (4 oz) of water until the powder is completely dissolved; this may require up to 3 minutes. The powder should not be mixed with fruit juice or other acidic liquid. The entire 4 oz of solution should be swallowed immediately.

The chewable/dispersible buffered tablets should be thoroughly chewed, crushed, or dispersed in water before swallowing. To disperse the tablet(s), stir the prescribed number in at least 30 ml (1 oz) of water until a uniform suspension is obtained. Swallow the entire preparation immediately.

▷ **How Long This Medicine Is Usually Taken:** Use on a regular schedule for several months is usually needed to determine this drug's effectiveness in slowing the progression of AIDS. Long-term use (months to years) requires periodic physician evaluation.

▷ **Tell Your Doctor Before Taking This Medicine If You:**
- ever had an allergic reaction to it or any drugs.
- have active liver disease.
- have had pancreatitis recently or have a history of pancreatitis or peripheral neuritis.
- are taking any other drugs currently.
- have a history of gout or high blood uric acid level.
- have a history of alcoholism.
- have a history of phenylketonuria.
- have a seizure disorder.
- have impaired liver or kidney function.

▷ **Possible Side Effects:** Mild decreases in red blood cell, white blood cell, and platelet counts. Mild increases in blood uric acid levels.

▷ **Possible Adverse Effects:**
If any of the following develop, call your doctor promptly for guidance.

Some Mild Problems Drug Can Cause

Allergic reactions: skin rash and itching.

Headache, dizziness, insomnia, nervousness.

Nausea, vomiting, and diarrhea, dry mouth and altered taste, yeast infection of mouth.

Loss of hair.

Muscle and joint pains.

Some Serious Problems Drug Can Cause

Pancreatitis, usually within the first 6 months of treatment.

Drug-induced peripheral neuritis, usually occurring after 2 to 6 months of treatment.

Seizures.

Serious skin rashes (Stevens-Johnson syndrome).

Rare liver or kidney damage.

Platelets may be lowered in 69% of pediatric patients.

▷ **Adverse Effects That May Mimic Natural Diseases or Disorders:**
Drug-induced liver reaction may suggest viral hepatitis.

▷ *CAUTION*

1. No drug can cure HIV infection. Taking didanosine does not reduce the risk of transmitting infection to others through sexual contact or contamination of blood.

2. Report promptly the development of stomach pain with nausea and vomiting; this could indicate the onset of pancreatitis. It may be necessary to discontinue this drug.

3. Report promptly the development of pain, numbness, tingling or burning in the hands or feet; this could indicate the onset of peripheral neuritis. It may be necessary to discontinue this drug.

4. Safety and effectiveness of this drug for those under 6 months old are not established. Children are also at risk for developing drug-induced pancreatitis and peripheral neuritis; monitor closely for significant symptoms. Because this drug has caused retinal damage in some children, detailed eye examinations are recommended every 6 months and any time visual disturbance occurs.

5. People over 60 with reduced kidney function may require dosage reduction.

Advisability of Use During Pregnancy or If Breast-Feeding:
Pregnancy Category: B. Ask your doctor for specific guidance. Presence in breast milk is unknown; avoid taking this drug or refrain from nursing.
Note: HIV has been found in human breast milk. Breast-feeding may result in transmission of HIV infection to the nursing infant.

▷ **Overdose Symptoms:**   Nausea, vomiting, stomach pain, diarrhea, pain in hands and feet, irritability, confusion.

▷ **Suggested Periodic Examinations While Taking This Drug:** (at doctor's discretion)
Complete blood cell counts before starting treatment and weekly thereafter until tolerance is established.
Blood amylase levels, fractionated for salivary gland and pancreatic origin. CD4 counts.
Liver and kidney function tests.
Viral load or burden to help check the success of treatment.

▷ **While Taking This Drug the Following Apply:**
Other Drugs:
Didanosine may *increase* the effects of
• zidovudine (Retrovir), and enhance its antiviral effect against HIV.
Didanosine may *decrease* the effects of
• dapsone, rendering it ineffective; avoid concurrent use.
• ketoconazole, if taken at the same time; take ketoconazole at least 2 hours before didanosine.

- ciprofloxacin (Cipro), if taken at the same time; take ciprofloxacin at least 2 hours before taking didanosine.
- itraconazole. Separate dosing by 2 hours.
- tetracylcines (see Drug Classes), if taken at the same time; take tetracyclines at least 2 hours before taking didanosine.

Didanosine *taken concurrently* with

- antacids will enhance the absorption of didanosine and increase its effectiveness.
- histamine (H2) blocking drugs (cimetidine, etc.), may increase didanosine toxicity.
- pentamidine or sulfamethoxazole may increase the risk of drug-induced pancreatitis; observe for significant symptoms.
- triazolam (Halcion) may cause confusion.
- zalcitabine (HIVID) may cause increased nerve toxicity.

The following drug may *increase* the effects of didanosine

- ribavirin—may enhance its antiviral effects.

Driving, Hazardous Activities: This drug may cause dizziness and impaired vision. Restrict your activities as necessary.

Discontinuation: Do not stop taking this drug without your doctor's knowledge and guidance.

▷ **Saving Money When Using This Medicine:**

- Ask your doctor if this drug offers the best combination of price and outcome for you. Current data favor combination therapy with three medicines from different classes.
- Current thinking in AIDS treatment finds many clinicians using combination therapy and measurements of viral burden or viral load to check the initial and ongoing success of treatment. This test can help make sure you are not continuing a medicine that has stopped working.
- Talk with your doctor about new agents coming to market or in clinical trials. Many new medicines are being researched.
- Discuss any needed vaccinations with your doctor.

DIFLUNISAL (di FLU ni sal)

Prescription Needed: Yes   **Controlled Drug:** No   **Generic:** No

Brand Names: Dolobid

Overview of BENEFITS versus RISKS	
Possible Benefits	*Possible Risks*
EFFECTIVE RELIEF OF MILD TO MODERATE PAIN AND INFLAMMATION	Gastrointestinal pain, ulceration, bleeding (rare) Liver or kidney damage (rare) Fluid retention (rare)

See the propionic acid (NSAIDs) profile for further information.

DIGITOXIN (di ji TOX in)

Prescription Needed: Yes   **Controlled Drug:** No   **Generic:** Yes

Brand Names: Crystodigin

Overview of BENEFITS versus RISKS	
Possible Benefits	*Possible Risks*
EFFECTIVE HEART STIMULANT IN CONGESTIVE HEART FAILURE EFFECTIVE PREVENTION AND TREATMENT OF CERTAIN HEART RHYTHM DISORDERS	NARROW TREATMENT RANGE (treatment dose is 60% of toxic dose) Frequent and sometimes serious disturbances of heart rhythm Abnormally low blood platelet counts (rare)

See the digoxin profile for further information.

DIGOXIN (di JOX in)

Prescription Needed: Yes   **Controlled Drug:** No   **Generic:** Yes

Brand Names: Lanoxicaps, Lanoxin, SK-Digoxin

Overview of BENEFITS versus RISKS

Possible Benefits	*Possible Risks*
EFFECTIVE HEART STIMULANT IN CONGESTIVE HEART FAILURE	NARROW TREATMENT RANGE (treatment dose is 60% of toxic dose)
EFFECTIVE PREVENTION AND TREATMENT OF CERTAIN HEART RHYTHM DISORDERS	Frequent and sometimes serious disturbances of heart rhythm

---

▷ **Illness This Medication Treats:**

(1) Congestive heart failure; (2) restoration and maintenance of normal heart rate and rhythm in such disorders as atrial fibrillation, atrial flutter, and atrial/supraventricular tachycardia.

▷ **Typical Dosage Range:** (Dosage or schedule must be determined by the doctor for each individual.)

Loading dose: 10 mcg per kilogram of lean body weight. 10–15 mcg per kilogram of body weight may be used if digoxin is being used to control abnormal heart rhythms (such as atrial fibrillation). This loading dose can be taken by mouth or intravenously. Once the dose is calculated, it is often taken with 50% in the first dose and the rest divided into smaller doses taken at 6- to 8-hour intervals until the desired response is achieved. The usual ongoing dose is 0.125–0.25 mg/day.

▷ **Conditions Requiring Dosing Adjustments:**

Liver function: Use this drug with caution; blood levels should be obtained more frequently.

Kidney function: Dose MUST be adjusted for patients with kidney compromise. Smaller doses and dosing every other day may be needed.

▷ **How Best to Take This Medicine:**   Take at the same time each day, preferably on an empty stomach to ensure uniform absorption. May be taken with or following food if desired; milk and dairy products may delay absorption but do not reduce the amount of drug absorbed. The tablet may be crushed; the capsule should be swallowed whole.

▷ **How Long This Medicine Is Usually Taken:** Use on a regular schedule for 7 to 10 days is usually necessary to determine this drug's effectiveness in relieving heart failure or controlling heart rhythm disorders. Long-term use requires doctor's supervision and periodic assessment of continued need.

▷ **Tell Your Doctor Before Taking This Medicine If You:**
- ever had an allergic reaction to it.
- have experienced any unfavorable reaction to a digitalis preparation in the past.
- have taken any digitalis preparation within the past 2 weeks.
- have a history of severe lung disease or some kinds of abnormal heart rhythms.
- are now taking (or have recently taken) any diuretic (urine-producing) drug.
- have impaired liver or kidney function.
- have a history of thyroid function disorder.

▷ **Possible Side Effects:** Slow heart rate, rare enlargement and/or sensitivity of the male breast tissue.

▷ **Possible Adverse Effects:**
If any of the following develop, call your doctor promptly for guidance.
Some Mild Problems Drug Can Cause
Allergic reactions: skin rash, hives.
Headache, lethargy, confusion, changes in vision: halo effect, blurring.
Nightmares.
Loss of appetite, nausea, vomiting, diarrhea—early toxicity signs in adults.
Some Serious Problems Drug Can Cause
Idiosyncratic reactions: hallucinations, facial neuralgias, peripheral neuralgias, blindness (very rare).
Disorientation, most common in the elderly.
Rare serious skin rashes.
Heart rhythm disturbances.

▷ **Possible Effects on Sex Life:** Decreased libido and impotence in 35% of male users. Enlargement and tenderness of male breasts. Both effects are attributed to digoxin's estrogenlike action.

▷ **Adverse Effects That May Mimic Natural Diseases or Disorders:** Drug-induced mental disturbances in the elderly may be mistaken for senile dementia or psychosis.

▷ *CAUTION*
1. This drug has a narrow margin of safe use. Adhere strictly to prescribed dosage schedules. Do not raise or lower the dose without first consulting your doctor.

2. If you are taking calcium supplements, ask your doctor for guidance. Avoid large doses.
3. It is advisable to carry a personal identification card that states you are taking this drug.
4. Avoid taking over-the-counter antacids and cold, cough, and allergy remedies without asking your doctor.
5. Infants and children should be closely watched for signs of toxicity: slow heart rate (below 60 beats/min), irregular heart rhythms.
6. Those over 60 may have a reduced tolerance for this drug; smaller doses are advisable. Watch for headache, dizziness, fatigue, weakness, lethargy, depression, confusion, nervousness, agitation, delusions, difficulty with reading. Report the development of any of these effects promptly to your doctor.

Advisability of Use During Pregnancy or If Breast-Feeding:
Pregnancy Category: C. Use this drug only if clearly needed. Overdosage can be harmful to the fetus. Present in breast milk. Monitor nursing infant closely and discontinue drug or nursing if adverse effects develop.

▷ **Overdose Symptoms:** Loss of appetite, excessive saliva, nausea, vomiting, diarrhea, serious disturbances of heart rate and rhythm, intestinal bleeding, drowsiness, headache, confusion, delirium, hallucinations, convulsions.

▷ **Suggested Periodic Examinations While Taking This Drug:** (at doctor's discretion)
Measurements of blood levels of digoxin, calcium, magnesium, and potassium; electrocardiograms.
Time to sample blood for digoxin level: 6 to 8 hours after last dose, or just before next dose.
Recommended therapeutic range: 0.5–2.0 ng/ml.

▷ **While Taking This Drug the Following Apply:**
Foods: Ask your doctor regarding the advisability of eating high-potassium foods.
Beverages: Avoid excessive amounts of caffeine-containing beverages: coffee, tea, cola. May be taken with milk.
Tobacco Smoking: Nicotine can cause irritability of the heart muscle and predispose to serious rhythm disturbances. It is advisable to abstain from all forms of tobacco.
Marijuana Smoking: Possible accentuation of heart failure; reduced digoxin effect; changes in electrocardiogram, confusing interpretation.
Other Drugs:
Digoxin **taken concurrently** with
• intravenous calcium may cause a fatal interaction.
• digoxin immune FAB (Digibind) will result in decreased blood levels; this is a therapy for digoxin toxicity.

- diuretics (other than spironolactone and triamterene) may result in serious heart rhythm disturbances due to excessive loss of potassium and magnesium.
- propranolol (Inderal) or other beta-blockers (see Drug Classes) may result in very slow heart rates.
- quinidine may result in decreased digoxin effectiveness and increased digoxin toxicity; careful dosage adjustments are necessary.

The following drugs may *increase* the effects of digoxin

- alprazolam (Xanax).
- amiloride (Midamor).
- amiodarone (Cordarone).
- amphotericin B (Fungizone or Abelcet).
- benzodiazepines (Librium, Valium, etc.).
- captopril (Capoten, Capozide).
- cyclosporine (Sandimmune).
- diltiazem (Cardizem) and perhaps other calcium channel blockers.
- erythromycin (E.E.S., Erythrocin, etc.).
- ethacrynic acid.
- flecainide (Tambocor).
- hydroxychloroquine.
- ibuprofen (Advil, Medipren, Motrin, Nuprin, etc.).
- indomethacin (Indocin).
- itraconazole.
- methimazole (Tapazole).
- nifedipine (Adalat, Procardia).
- propafenone (Rythmol).
- propylthiouracil (Propacil).
- quinine.
- tetracyclines.
- tolbutamide (Orinase).
- trazodone (Desyrel).
- verapamil (Isoptin).

The following drugs may *decrease* the effects of digoxin

- aluminum-containing antacids (Amphojel, Maalox, etc.).
- bleomycin (Blenoxane).
- carmustine (BiCNU).
- cholestyramine (Questran).
- colestipol (Colestid).
- cyclophosphamide (Cytoxan).
- cytarabine (Cytosar).
- doxorubicin (Adriamycin).
- fluvoxamine (Luvox).
- kaolin (Kaolin-Pectin, Donagel, others).
- methotrexate (Mexate).
- metoclopramide (Reglan).
- neomycin.

- penicillamine (Cuprimine, Depen).
- procarbazine (Matulane).
- rifampin or rifabutin.
- sucralfate (Carafate).
- sulfa antibiotics or sulfasalazine.
- thyroid hormones.
- vincristine (Oncovin).

Driving, Hazardous Activities: Usually no restrictions. However, this drug may cause drowsiness, vision changes, and nausea. Restrict your activities as necessary.

Occurrence of Unrelated Illness: Any illness that causes vomiting or diarrhea can seriously alter this drug's effectiveness. Notify your doctor promptly.

Discontinuation: This drug may be continued indefinitely. Do not stop taking it without asking your doctor.

▷ **Saving Money When Using This Medicine:**
- Drug levels are very expensive. Ask your doctor about the needed frequency of levels.
- Just because you are older does NOT mean you automatically need digoxin. Ask your doctor if this drug offers the best combination of price and outcome for you.
- If you are taking a water pill (diuretic) in addition to digoxin, make sure you have your potassium and magnesium levels checked. Low blood potassium can lead to digoxin toxicity with "normal blood levels." Low magnesium may increase risk of heart problems.

DILTIAZEM (dil TI a zem)

Prescription Needed: Yes **Controlled Drug:** No **Generic:** Yes

Brand Names: Cardizem, Cardizem CD, Cardizem SR, Dilacor SR, Dilacor XR, Diltiazem, Teczem [CD], Tiamate (extended release), Tiazac

Controversies in Medicine: Results of several studies have indicated that medicines in this chemical family should NOT be used in some patients with extremely compromised hearts. Amlodipine (Norvasc) is the only calcium channel blocker that presently has data to show that it is SAFE, even in the most severely ill congestive heart failure patients. Amlodipine is the only calcium channel blocker to be FDA-approved as safe for use in treating hypertension or angina in patients who also have congestive heart failure. There have been several FDA hearings on calcium channel blockers in general.

One retrospective chart review yielded data showing that there was increased risk if nifedipine immediate-release forms were used for treating conditions other than angina in those over 71. There was a caution advised, but the form of nifedipine in question was not approved for uses other than angina. A recent FDA panel found medicines in this class to be safe and effective. A study of nearly 6,000 patients at Tel Aviv Medical Center found that there was no statistically significant risk of death in patients who took calcium channel blockers versus those who did not take these medicines.

Overview of BENEFITS versus RISKS	
Possible Benefits	*Possible Risks*
EFFECTIVE PREVENTION OF BOTH MAJOR TYPES OF ANGINA	Depression, confusion
	Low blood pressure
	Heart rhythm disturbance
EFFECTIVE CONTROL OF MILD TO MODERATE HYPERTENSION	Fluid retention
	Very rare liver damage
	Rare muscle damage

▷ **Illness This Medication Treats:**
(1) Angina pectoris due to coronary artery spasm (Prinzmetal's variant angina) that occurs spontaneously and is not associated with exertion; (2) classical angina-of-effort in individuals who have not responded to or cannot tolerate the nitrates and beta-blockers customarily used to treat this disorder; (3) mild to moderate hypertension.

▷ **Typical Dosage Range:** (Dosage or schedule must be determined by the doctor for each individual.)
Initially 30 mg three or four times daily. Dose may be increased gradually at 1- to 2-day intervals as needed and tolerated. Total daily dosage should not exceed 360 mg. Prolonged-release forms may allow less frequent dosing.
Author's note: A new combination form called Teczem has been approved, which contains diltiazem in combination with enalapril.

▷ **Conditions Requiring Dosing Adjustments:**
Liver function: The maximum daily dose for patients with liver compromise should be 90 mg. This medication is also a rare cause of liver toxicity, requiring a benefit-to-risk decision for patients with compromised livers.
Kidney function: Diltiazem may be one of the best calcium channel blockers for patients with renal compromise to use, as a large percentage of it is metabolized by the liver and excreted in feces. Cau-

tion must still be used, however, because the drug itself is a rare cause of compromised kidneys.

▷ **How Best to Take This Medicine:**   Preferably taken before meals and at bedtime. Tablet may be crushed.

▷ **How Long This Medicine Is Usually Taken:**   Use on a regular schedule for 2 to 4 weeks is usually necessary to determine this drug's effectiveness in reducing the frequency and severity of angina and lowering blood pressure. The smallest effective dose should be used in long-term therapy (months to years).

▷ **Tell Your Doctor Before Taking This Medicine If You:**
- ever had an allergic reaction to it.
- have a sick sinus syndrome (and are not wearing an artificial pacemaker).
- have been told you have a second-degree or third-degree heart block.
- have low blood pressure (systolic pressure below 90).
- have had an unfavorable response to any calcium blockers in the past.
- have stenosis of the aorta.
- are currently taking any form of digitalis or a beta-blocker.
- have a history of congestive heart failure.
- have impaired liver or kidney function.
- have a history of drug-induced liver damage.

▷ **Possible Side Effects:**   Fatigue, light-headedness, heart rate and rhythm changes in predisposed individuals.

▷ **Possible Adverse Effects:**
If any of the following develop, call your doctor promptly for guidance.
Some Mild Problems Drug Can Cause
Allergic reactions: skin rash, itching.
Headache, drowsiness, dizziness, nervousness, insomnia, depression, hallucinations.
Flushing, palpitations, fainting, slow heart rate, low blood pressure.
Very rare desire to be in constant motion (akathisia).
Nausea, vomiting, diarrhea, constipation.
Some Serious Problems Drug Can Cause
Serious disturbances of heart rate and/or rhythm, fluid retention, congestive heart failure.
Very rare lowering of blood platelets or white blood cells (granulocytes).
Very rare muscle damage (myopathy).
Drug-induced liver damage (very rare).

▷ **Possible Effects on Sex Life:**   Impotence is reported in less than 1% of users. Rare cases of swelling or tenderness of male breast tissue (gynecomastia). One reported case of heavy vaginal bleeding.

▷ *CAUTION*
1. Be sure to tell all health care providers who treat you that you are taking this drug. Note its use on your personal identification card.
2. You may use nitroglycerin and other nitrate drugs as needed to relieve acute episodes of angina pain. However, if you detect that your angina attacks are becoming more frequent or intense, tell your doctor promptly.
3. Safety and effectiveness of this drug for those under 12 years old are not established.
4. Those over 60 may be more susceptible to the development of weakness, dizziness, fainting, and falling. Take necessary precautions to prevent injury. Report promptly any changes in your pattern of thirst and urination.

Advisability of Use During Pregnancy or If Breast-Feeding:
Pregnancy Category: C. Avoid taking this drug during the first 3 months. Use during the last 6 months only if clearly needed. Ask your doctor for guidance. Present in breast milk; avoid taking this drug or refrain from nursing.

▷ **Overdose Symptoms:**   Weakness, light-headedness, fainting, slow pulse, low blood pressure, shortness of breath, congestive heart failure.

▷ **Suggested Periodic Examinations While Taking This Drug:** (at doctor's discretion)
Evaluations of heart function, including electrocardiogram; liver and kidney function tests with long-term use.

▷ **While Taking This Drug the Following Apply:**
Foods: Avoid excessive salt intake.
Beverages: May be taken with milk.
Alcohol: Use with caution until combined effects have been determined. Alcohol may exaggerate the drop in blood pressure some individuals experience.
Tobacco Smoking: Nicotine may reduce the effectiveness of this drug.
Marijuana Smoking: Possible reduced effectiveness of this drug; mild to moderate increase in angina; possible changes in electrocardiogram, confusing interpretation.
Other Drugs:
Diltiazem *taken concurrently* with
• aspirin can result in prolonged bleeding time or hemorrhage.
• beta-blockers or digitalis preparations (see Drug Classes) may affect heart rate and rhythm adversely. Careful monitoring by your doctor is necessary if these drugs are taken concurrently.

- carbamazepine (Tegretol) may result in toxicity and seizures.
- digoxin (Lanoxin) can lead to digoxin toxicity.
- lithium (Lithobid, others) may result in nerve toxicity or psychosis.
- oral hypoglycemic agents (see Drug Classes) may result in exaggerated lowering of blood sugar.
- phenytoin (Dilantin) may lead to phenytoin toxicity.
- rifampin or rifabutin may lead to decreased diltiazem effectiveness.
- tacrolimus (Prograf) may lead to tacrolimus toxicity.

The following drugs may *increase* the effects of diltiazem
- cimetidine (Tagamet).
- fluvoxamine (Luvox).
- ranitidine (Zantac).

Driving, Hazardous Activities: Usually no restrictions. This drug may cause drowsiness or dizziness. Restrict your activities as necessary.

Exposure to Sun: Use caution until your sensitivity has been determined. This drug may cause photosensitivity.

Exposure to Heat: Caution is advised. Hot environments can exaggerate the blood pressure–lowering effects of this drug. Watch for lightheadedness or weakness.

Heavy Exercise or Exertion: This drug may improve your ability to be more active without resulting angina pain. Use caution and avoid excessive exercise that could impair heart function in the absence of warning pain.

Discontinuation: Do not stop taking this drug abruptly. Consult your doctor regarding gradual withdrawal.

▷ **Saving Money When Using This Medicine:**
- Several agents are available that work similarly to this drug. Ask your doctor if this drug offers the best combination of price and outcome for you.
- Talk with your doctor about the benefits of stress management for you.
- If your high blood pressure is accompanied with buildup of material inside your veins (atherosclerosis) and increased cholesterol, talk with your doctor about an HMG CoA inhibitor.
- Discuss the benefits versus risks of taking aspirin every other day in order to help prevent a heart attack.

DIPHENHYDRAMINE (di fen HI dra meen)

Prescription Needed: Varies   **Controlled Drug:** No*
Generic: Yes

Brand Names: Acetaminophen-PM, Ambenyl Syrup [CD], Benadryl, Benadryl 25, Benylin, Compoz, Excedrin P.M. [CD], Nytol, Sleep-Eze 3, Sominex 2

Overview of BENEFITS versus RISKS

Possible Benefits	*Possible Risks*
EFFECTIVE RELIEF OF ALLERGIC RHINITIS AND ALLERGIC SKIN DISORDERS	Marked sedation
	Atropinelike effects
	Accentuation of prostatism
EFFECTIVE, NONADDICTIVE SEDATIVE AND HYPNOTIC	
Prevention and relief of motion sickness	
Partial relief of symptoms of Parkinson's disease	
Treatment of anaphylaxis	

▷ **Illness This Medication Treats:**

(1) Motion sickness (control of dizziness, nausea, and vomiting); (2) symptoms associated with Parkinson's disease; (3) drug-induced parkinsonian reactions, especially in children and the elderly; (4) conditions caused by histamine release, such as allergic reactions; (5) cough.

As Combination Drug Product [CD]: This drug may have a mild suppressant effect on coughing. It is combined with expectorants and either codeine or dextromethorphan in some cough preparations.

▷ **Typical Dosage Range:** (Dosage or schedule must be determined by the doctor for each individual.)

25 to 50 mg every 4 to 6 hours. Total daily dosage should not exceed 300 mg.

▷ **Conditions Requiring Dosing Adjustments:**

Liver function: Single doses are not expected to be a problem; however, the use of multiple doses by patients with liver compromise has not been studied.

Kidney function: If the creatinine clearance is 50 to 80 ml/min, the usual dose can be used and taken every 6 hours. If the creatinine

---

*Ambenyl Syrup is C-V. See Controlled Drug Schedules inside this book's cover.

clearance is 10 to 50 ml/min, the usual dose can be taken every 6 to 12 hours. If the creatinine clearance is less than 10 ml/min, diphenhydramine can be taken every 12 to 18 hours.

▷ **How Best to Take This Medicine:** Preferably taken with or following food to reduce stomach irritation. Tablet may be crushed and capsule opened for administration.

▷ **How Long This Medicine Is Usually Taken:** Use on a regular schedule for 2 to 3 days usually determines the effectiveness of this drug in relieving the symptoms of allergic rhinitis and dermatosis. If not effective after 5 days, this drug should be stopped. As a bedtime sedative (hypnotic), use only as needed. Avoid long-term use without interruption.

▷ **Tell Your Doctor Before Taking This Medicine If You:**
- ever had an allergic reaction to it.
- are taking, or have taken during the past 2 weeks, any MAO type A inhibitors.
- had an unfavorable response to any antihistamine drug in the past.
- have narrow-angle glaucoma.
- have peptic ulcer disease, with any degree of pyloric obstruction.
- think you have chickenpox.
- have a G6PD deficiency.
- have prostatism.
- are subject to bronchial asthma or seizures (epilepsy).

▷ **Possible Side Effects:** Drowsiness; sense of weakness; dryness of nose, mouth, and throat; constipation.

▷ **Possible Adverse Effects:**
If any of the following develop, call your doctor promptly for guidance.
Some Mild Problems Drug Can Cause
Allergic reactions: skin rash, hives.
Headache, dizziness, nervousness, blurred vision, difficult urination.
Reduced tolerance for contact lenses.
Nausea, vomiting, diarrhea.
Some Serious Problems Drug Can Cause
Allergic reaction: anaphylactic reaction.
Idiosyncratic reactions: insomnia, confusion.
Hemolytic anemia.
Rare movement disorders or porphyria.
Rare reduced white blood cell count—fever, infections.
Rare blood platelet destruction—abnormal bleeding or bruising.

▷ **Possible Effects on Sex Life:** Shortened menstrual cycle (early arrival of expected menstrual onset).

▷ *CAUTION*

1. Stop this drug 5 days before diagnostic skin testing procedures, to prevent false-negative test results.
2. Do not use this drug if you have active bronchial asthma, bronchitis, or pneumonia. It can thicken bronchial mucus and make it more difficult to remove (by absorption or coughing).
3. This drug should not be used in newborns. Doses for children should be small. The young child is especially sensitive to the effects of antihistamines on the brain and nervous system. Avoid using this drug in the child with chickenpox or a flu-like infection; although unproven, this drug may adversely affect the course of Reye's syndrome developed during the illness.
4. Those over 60 may be more susceptible to drowsiness, dizziness, and unsteadiness, and to impaired thinking, judgment, and memory. This drug can worsen problems in urinating that are associated with prostate gland enlargement. The sedative effects of antihistamines in the elderly can cause a syndrome of underactivity that may be misinterpreted as senility or emotional depression.

Advisability of Use During Pregnancy or If Breast-Feeding:
Pregnancy Category: B. Avoid using this drug during the last 3 months. Use sparingly during the first 6 months only if clearly needed. Present in breast milk; avoid taking this drug or refrain from nursing.

▷ **Overdose Symptoms:**   Marked drowsiness, confusion, incoordination, unsteadiness, muscle tremors, stupor, coma, seizures, fever, flushed face, dilated pupils, weak pulse, shallow breathing.

▷ **Suggested Periodic Examinations While Taking This Drug:** (at doctor's discretion)
Complete blood cell counts.

▷ **While Taking This Drug the Following Apply:**
Beverages: May be taken with milk.
Alcohol: Use with extreme caution until the combined effect has been determined. The combination of alcohol and antihistamines can cause rapid and marked sedation.
Marijuana Smoking: Increased drowsiness and mouth dryness; possible accentuation of impaired thinking.
Other Drugs:
Diphenhydramine may *increase* the effects of
• amitriptyline and cause urinary retention.
• all drugs with a sedative effect, causing oversedation.
• atropine and atropinelike drugs.
Diphenhydramine *taken concurrently* with
• phenothiazines (see Drug Classes) may result in difficult urination or intestinal obstruction.

- temazepam in pregnancy may lead to increased risk of fetal death.
- tricyclic antidepressants (see Drug Classes) may cause increased risk of urinary retention.

The following drugs may *increase* the effects of diphenhydramine

- MAO type A inhibitors—may delay its elimination, thus exaggerating and prolonging its action.

Driving, Hazardous Activities: May impair mental alertness, judgment, physical coordination, and reaction time. Restrict your activities as necessary.

Exposure to Sun: Use caution until your sensitivity has been determined. This drug may cause photosensitivity.

Exposure to Environmental Chemicals: The insecticides Aldrin, Dieldrin, and Chlordane may decrease the effectiveness of this drug. The insecticide Sevin may increase its sedative effects.

▷ **Saving Money When Using This Medicine:**
- Several agents are available that work similarly to this drug. Ask your doctor if this drug offers the best combination of price and outcome for you.
- Talk with your doctor about the use of a nonsedating antihistamine if your symptoms continue.

DIPYRIDAMOLE (di peer ID a mohl)

Prescription Needed: Yes   **Controlled Drug:** No   **Generic:** Yes

Brand Names: Persantine, Pyridamole, SK-Dipyridamole

Overview of BENEFITS versus RISKS	
Possible Benefits	*Possible Risks*
EFFECTIVE PREVENTION OF THROMBOEMBOLISM (BLOOD CLOTS) FOLLOWING HEART VALVE SURGERY	Mild low blood pressure with dizziness and fainting (infrequent) Mild indigestion

▷ **Illness This Medication Treats:**
   (1) Prevention of thromboembolism (blood clot formation and migration) following heart valve surgery; (2) intravenously as an alternative to exercise in heart testing.

▷ **Typical Dosage Range:** (Dosage or schedule must be determined by the doctor for each individual.)
   50 to 100 mg three or four times daily. Total daily dosage should not exceed 400 mg. Intravenous dosing varies with the protocol.

DISOPYRAMIDE (di so PEER a mide)

Prescription Needed: Yes   **Controlled Drug:** No   **Generic:** Yes

Brand Names: Napamide, Norpace, Norpace CR, Pisopyramide

Overview of BENEFITS versus RISKS	
Possible Benefits	*Possible Risks*
EFFECTIVE TREATMENT OF SELECTED HEART RHYTHM DISORDERS	NARROW TREATMENT RANGE
	FREQUENT ADVERSE EFFECTS
	LOW BLOOD PRESSURE
	CONGESTIVE HEART FAILURE
	Rare agranulocytosis
	Rare peripheral neuropathy or liver toxicity
	Heart conduction and rhythm abnormalities
	Frequent atropinelike side effects

▷ **Illness This Medication Treats:**
Abnormal rhythms in the ventricles (lower chambers) of the heart.

▷ **Typical Dosage Range:** (Dosage or schedule must be determined by the doctor for each individual.)
100 to 200 mg every 6 hours. Dosage should not exceed 200 mg/6 hr or 800 mg/24 hr (1600 mg/24 hr has been used occasionally). A loading dose of 300 mg of the immediate-release form may be used by patients weighing more than 50 kg if a more rapid response is needed.

▷ **Conditions Requiring Dosing Adjustments:**
Liver function: The dose should be decreased for patients with liver compromise.
Kidney function: The dose MUST be decreased for patients with kidney compromise. For patients with moderate to severe kidney failure, the typical immediate-release form dose is taken only every 12 to 24 hours. This drug may cause urinary retention and should be used with caution by patients with urinary outflow problems.

▷ **How Best to Take This Medicine:** Best taken on an empty stomach, 1 hour before or 2 hours after eating. However, it may be taken with or following food to reduce stomach irritation. The regular capsules may be opened for administration; however, the prolonged-action capsules should not be opened, chewed, or crushed.

▷ **How Long This Medicine Is Usually Taken:** Use for 2 to 4 days is needed to determine this drug's effectiveness in correcting or preventing responsive rhythm disorders. Long-term use requires physician supervision and periodic evaluation.

▷ **Tell Your Doctor Before Taking This Medicine If You:**
- ever had an allergic reaction to it.
- have second- or third-degree heart block (determined by electrocardiogram).
- have had any unfavorable reactions to other antiarrhythmic drugs in the past.
- have a history of heart disease of any kind, especially heart block.
- have a history of low blood pressure.
- have impaired liver or kidney function.
- have glaucoma or a family history of glaucoma.
- have an enlarged prostate gland.
- have low blood potassium or low white blood cells.
- have myasthenia gravis.
- are taking any form of digitalis or diuretic drug that can cause excessive loss of body potassium (ask your doctor).

▷ **Possible Side Effects:** Drop in blood pressure in susceptible individuals.
Dry mouth, constipation, blurred vision, impaired urination.

▷ **Possible Adverse Effects:**
If any of the following develop, call your doctor promptly for guidance.
Some Mild Problems Drug Can Cause
  Allergic reactions: skin rash, itching.
  Headache, nervousness, fatigue, muscular weakness, mild aches.
  Loss of appetite, indigestion, nausea, vomiting, diarrhea.
  Lowered blood sugar level (hypoglycemia).
Some Serious Problems Drug Can Cause
  Idiosyncratic reaction: acute psychotic behavior (rare).
  Severe drop in blood pressure, fainting.
  Progressive heart weakness, predisposing to congestive heart failure.
  Inability to empty urinary bladder, prostatism.
  Jaundice.
  Peripheral neuropathy.
  Rare porphyria.
  Rare abnormally low white blood cell count.

▷ **Possible Effects on Sex Life:** Rare reports of impotence (300 mg/day); enlargement and tenderness of male breasts (gynecomastia).

▷ *CAUTION*
1. Thorough evaluation of your heart function (including an electrocardiogram) is necessary before using this drug.
2. Periodic evaluation of your heart function is necessary to determine your response to this drug. Some people may experience worsening of their heart rhythm disorder and/or deterioration of heart function. Close monitoring of heart rate, rhythm, and overall performance is essential.
3. The dosage of this drug must be adjusted carefully for each individual. Do not change your dosage without the knowledge and supervision of your doctor.
4. Do not take any other antiarrhythmic drug while taking this drug unless directed to do so by your doctor.
5. Dosing is accomplished on a milligram-per-kilogram-of-weight basis in children. Initial use of this drug requires hospitalization and supervision by a qualified pediatrician.
6. Reduced kidney function may require reduced dosage. This drug can aggravate existing prostatism and promote constipation. Observe carefully for light-headedness, dizziness, unsteadiness, and tendency to fall, especially in older people.

Advisability of Use During Pregnancy or If Breast-Feeding:
Pregnancy Category: C. Use this drug only if clearly needed. Ask your doctor for guidance. Present in breast milk; avoid taking this drug or refrain from nursing.

▷ **Overdose Symptoms:** Dryness of eyes, nose, mouth, and throat; impaired urination; constipation; marked drop in blood pressure; abnormal heart rhythms; congestive heart failure.

▷ **Suggested Periodic Examinations While Taking This Drug:** (at doctor's discretion)
Electrocardiogram, complete blood cell count, measurement of potassium blood levels.

▷ **While Taking This Drug the Following Apply:**
Foods: Ask your doctor regarding the need for salt restriction and advisability of eating potassium-rich foods.
Beverages: May be taken with milk.
Alcohol: Alcohol can increase the drug's blood pressure–lowering effects and the blood sugar–lowering effects; its use is not advised.
Tobacco Smoking: Nicotine can cause irritability of the heart and reduce the effectiveness of this drug.
Other Drugs:
Disopyramide may *increase* the effects of
• antihypertensive drugs, causing excessive lowering of blood pressure.

- atropinelike drugs (see Drug Classes).
- warfarin (Coumadin, etc.); monitor INR (prothrombin times) and adjust dosage accordingly.

Disopyramide may *decrease* the effects of

- ambenonium (Mytelase).
- neostigmine (Prostigmin).
- pyridostigmine (Mestinon).

The beneficial effects of these three drugs in treating myasthenia gravis may be reduced.

Disopyramide *taken concurrently* with

- amiodarone (Cordarone) may result in an abnormal heart effect.
- beta-blockers (see Drug Classes) may result in abnormally low heart rates.
- digoxin (Lanoxin, others) may result in digoxin toxicity.
- erythromycin (E.E.S., others) and perhaps other macrolide antibiotics (see Drug Classes) may lead to disopyramide toxicity.
- insulin or oral hypoglycemic agents (see Drug Classes) may lead to abnormally low blood sugar.
- phenobarbital may decrease disopyramide's effectiveness.
- phenytoin (Dilantin) may decrease disopyramide's benefits and increase risk of anticholinergic effects.
- potassium supplements may lead to disopyramide toxicity.
- quinidine may increase disopyramide levels and decrease therapeutic benefit of quinidine.
- verapamil (Calan, others) may precipitate or worsen congestive heart failure.
- warfarin may pose an increased risk of bleeding. INR (prothrombin time) should be checked more frequently, and dosing adjusted to lab results.

The following drugs may *decrease* the effects of disopyramide

- all diuretics that promote potassium loss.
- rifabutin.
- rifampin (Rimactane, Rifadin).

Driving, Hazardous Activities: May cause dizziness or blurred vision. Restrict your activities as necessary.

Exposure to Sun: Use caution. This drug is reported to cause photosensitization in susceptible individuals.

Exposure to Heat: Use caution. The use of this drug in hot environments may increase the risk of heatstroke.

Occurrence of Unrelated Illness: Disorders that cause vomiting, diarrhea, or dehydration can adversely affect this drug's action. Report such developments promptly.

Discontinuation: This drug should not be discontinued abruptly following long-term use. Ask your doctor for guidance regarding gradual dose reduction.

▷ **Saving Money When Using This Medicine:**
- Several agents are available that work similarly to this drug. Ask your doctor if this drug offers the best combination of price and outcome for you.
- Periodic checks of the ongoing success of this medicine in suppressing abnormal heartbeats are prudent.
- Talk with your doctor about taking aspirin every other day in order to help prevent a heart attack.

DISULFIRAM (di SULF i ram)

Prescription Needed: Yes   **Controlled Drug:** No   **Generic:** Yes

Brand Names: Antabuse

Overview of BENEFITS versus RISKS

Possible Benefits	*Possible Risks*
EFFECTIVE ADJUNCT IN THE TREATMENT OF CHRONIC ALCOHOLISM	DANGEROUS REACTIONS WITH ALCOHOL INGESTION
	Acute psychotic reactions (uncommon)
	Drug-induced liver damage (rare)
	Drug-induced optic and/or peripheral neuritis (rare)
	Low blood platelets

▷ **Illness This Medication Treats:**
Abusive drinking of alcoholic beverages. It does not abolish the craving or impulse to drink. It is of value in treating alcoholism because of the psychological reinforcement it provides, reminding the patient of the dire consequences of ingesting alcohol.

▷ **Typical Dosage Range:** (Dosage or schedule must be determined by the doctor for each individual.)
In the absence of all signs of alcoholic intoxication and no less than 12 hours after the last ingestion of alcohol, treatment is started with a single dose of 500 mg/day for 1 to 2 weeks. This is followed by a maintenance dose of 250 mg/day. The maintenance range of 125–500 mg/day is determined by experience with each individual. The total daily dosage should not exceed 1000 mg.

▷ **Conditions Requiring Dosing Adjustments:**

Liver function: The literature is contradictory as to the use of this drug by patients with liver dysfunction. Use of this drug by patients with mild liver compromise is a benefit-to-risk decision. Disulfiram should NOT be taken by people with portal hypertension or active hepatitis.

Kidney function: Dosing adjustments are not indicated.

Lung disease: The dose may need to be decreased for patients with severe lung dysfunction.

Diabetes: Diabetics may have an increased risk for blood vessel (micro- and macrovascular) problems if they take this medicine.

▷ **How Best to Take This Medicine:** May be taken with or following food to reduce stomach irritation. Tablet may be crushed for administration.

▷ **How Long This Medicine Is Usually Taken:** Use on a regular schedule for several months is usually necessary to determine this drug's effectiveness in deterring alcohol consumption. If well tolerated, disulfiram use should continue until a basis for permanent self-control and sobriety is established. See your doctor regularly.

▷ **Tell Your Doctor Before Taking This Medicine If You:**

- have used disulfiram or have experienced a severe allergic reaction to it. Note: Interaction of disulfiram and alcohol is *not an allergic* reaction.
- have ingested any form of alcohol in any amount within the past 12 hours.
- are taking (or have taken recently) metronidazole (Flagyl).
- have coronary heart disease or a serious heart rhythm disorder.
- do not intend to avoid alcohol completely while taking this drug.
- have not been given a full explanation of the reaction you will experience if you drink alcohol while taking this drug.
- are pregnant or planning pregnancy in the near future.
- have a history of diabetes, epilepsy, or kidney or liver disease.
- are currently taking oral anticoagulants, digitalis, isoniazid, paraldehyde, or phenytoin (Dilantin).
- plan to have surgery under general anesthesia while taking this drug.

▷ **Possible Side Effects:** Drowsiness, lethargy during early use. Offensive breath and body odor.

▷ **Possible Adverse Effects:**
If any of the following develop, call your doctor promptly for guidance.

Some Mild Problems Drug Can Cause
Allergic reactions: skin rash, hives.
Headache, dizziness, restlessness, tremor.

Metallic or garliclike taste, indigestion. (These usually subside after 2 weeks of use.)

Some Serious Problems Drug Can Cause

Allergic reactions: severe skin rashes, drug-induced hepatitis (rare).

Idiosyncratic reaction: acute toxic effect on brain, psychotic behavior.

Seizures, decreased thyroid function.

Very rare lowered blood platelets.

Carpal tunnel syndrome.

Optic or peripheral neuritis.

▷ **Possible Effects on Sex Life:** Decreased libido and/or impaired erection in 30% of users taking recommended doses of 125 to 500 mg per day.

▷ *CAUTION*

1. This drug should never be taken by anyone in a state of alcoholic intoxication.
2. The patient should be fully informed regarding the purpose and actions of this drug *before* treatment is started.
3. During long-term use, your doctor should examine you for any indication of reduced thyroid function.
4. Carry a personal identification card noting that you are taking this drug.
5. Safety and effectiveness of this drug for those under 12 years old are not established.
6. Those over 60 should watch for excessive sedation during the early use of this drug. *Do not* perform an alcohol trial to determine this drug's effects.

Advisability of Use During Pregnancy or If Breast-Feeding:

Pregnancy Category: X. Avoid using this drug completely if possible. Presence in breast milk is unknown; avoid taking this drug or refrain from nursing.

▷ **Overdose Symptoms:** Marked lethargy, impaired memory, altered behavior, confusion, unsteadiness, weakness, stomach pain, nausea, vomiting, diarrhea.

▷ **Suggested Periodic Examinations While Taking This Drug:** (at doctor's discretion)

Visual acuity, liver function tests.

▷ **While Taking This Drug the Following Apply:**

Foods: Avoid all foods prepared with alcohol, including sauces, marinades, vinegars, desserts. When dining out, inquire about the use of alcohol in food preparation.

Beverages: Avoid all punches or fruit drinks that may contain alcohol. This drug may be taken with milk.

Alcohol: **Avoid completely in all forms** while taking this drug and for 14 days following the last dose. The combination of disulfiram and alcohol, even in small amounts, produces the disulfiram (Antabuse) reaction within 5 to 10 minutes after ingesting alcohol—intense flushing and warming of the face, a severe throbbing headache, shortness of breath, chest pains, nausea, repeated vomiting, sweating, and weakness. If the amount of alcohol ingested is large enough, the reaction may progress to blurred vision, vertigo, confusion, marked drop in blood pressure, and loss of consciousness. Severe reactions may lead to convulsions and death. The reaction may last from 30 minutes to several hours, depending on the amount of alcohol and disulfiram in the body. As the symptoms subside, the individual is exhausted and usually sleeps for several hours.

Marijuana Smoking: Possible increase in drowsiness and lethargy.

Other Drugs:

Disulfiram may **increase** the effects of

- oral anticoagulants (warfarin, etc.), and increase the risk of bleeding; increased INRs (prothrombin time tests) and dosage adjustments may be necessary.
- barbiturates, causing oversedation.
- chlordiazepoxide (Librium) and diazepam (Valium), causing oversedation.
- paraldehyde, causing excessive depression of brain function.
- phenytoin (Dilantin), causing toxic effects on the brain; dosage adjustments may be necessary.

Disulfiram may **decrease** the effects of

- perphenazine (Trilafon, etc.).

Disulfiram **taken concurrently** with

- cisplatin (Platinol) can increase cisplatin toxicity.
- cyclosporine (Sandimmune) may result in a disulfiram reaction if intravenous cyclosporine is used.
- isoniazid (INH, etc.) may cause acute mental disturbance and incoordination, making it necessary to discontinue treatment.
- metronidazole (Flagyl) may cause acute mental and behavioral disturbances, making it necessary to discontinue treatment.
- over-the-counter cough syrups, tonics, etc. containing alcohol may cause a disulfiram reaction; avoid concurrent use.
- paraldehyde may lead to a disulfiram reaction.
- theophylline (Theo-Dur, others) may lead to theophylline toxicity.

The following drug may **increase** the effects of disulfiram

- amitriptyline (Elavil) may enhance the disulfiram + alcohol interaction; avoid concurrent use of these drugs.

Driving, Hazardous Activities: This drug may cause drowsiness or dizziness. Restrict your activities as necessary.

Exposure to Environmental Chemicals: Thiram, a pesticide, and carbon disulfide, a pesticide and industrial solvent, can have additive toxic effects during use of this drug. Observe for toxic effects on the brain and nervous system.

Discontinuation: Treatment with this drug is only part of your total treatment program. Do not stop taking it without the knowledge and guidance of your doctor. Abrupt withdrawal does not cause any symptoms; however, no alcohol should be ingested for 14 days following discontinuation.

▷ **Saving Money When Using This Medicine:**
- This drug has the best outcome when combined with ongoing support groups or similar guidance. Ask your doctor whether this drug offers the best combination of price and outcome for you.
- Naltrexone (ReVia) works in a different way than this medicine and may help stop alcohol craving. Discuss this medicine with your doctor if craving a drink is a particular problem for you.
- Talk with your doctor about stress management and exercise programs that are available in your community.

DORNASE ALFA (DOOR nase AL fa)

Prescription Needed: Yes   **Controlled Drug:** No   **Generic:** No

Brand Names: Pulmozyme

Overview of BENEFITS versus RISKS	
Possible Benefits	*Possible Risks*
DECREASED MUCUS VISCOSITY	Hoarseness
IMPROVED LUNG FUNCTION	Antibodies to DNA
DECREASED OCCURRENCE OF RESPIRATORY INFECTIONS	Facial swelling
DECREASED frequency of HOSPITALIZATION	

▷ **Illness This Medication Treats:**
Cystic fibrosis in conjunction with standard therapies.

▷ **Typical Dosage Range:** (Dosage or schedule must be determined by the doctor for each individual.)
Infants and Children: Safety and efficacy of this drug for those under 5 years old are not established.
5 to 60 Years of Age: One 2.5 mg dose administered by one of the tested nebulizers each day. Some selected patients (older patients) may benefit from twice-daily dosing.

▷ **How Best to Take This Medicine:** The solution must be kept in the refrigerator and protected from strong light. This drug should not be used if it is cloudy or discolored. Do NOT mix dornase with other medications. Clinical trials have been conducted only with the Hudson T Up-draft ll, Marquest Acorn ll, and Pulmo-Aide compressor. The reusable PARI LC Jet nebulizer and PARI PRONEB compressor were also tested. Do NOT use this drug with other equipment.

▷ **How Long This Medicine Is Usually Taken:** Use on a regular schedule for 8 days usually determines the effectiveness of this drug in treating cystic fibrosis. Long-term use (up to 12 months has been studied) requires periodic doctor's evaluation of response and dosage adjustment.

▷ **Tell Your Doctor Before Taking This Medicine If You:**
- ever had an allergic reaction to it.
- had a rash after the last dose was taken.
- are uncertain how to use the nebulizer or compressor.
- have an allergy to Chinese hamster ovary cells.

▷ **Possible Side Effects:** Hoarseness.

▷ **Possible Adverse Effects:**
If any of the following develop, call your doctor promptly for guidance.
Some Mild Problems Drug Can Cause
Allergic reactions: rash.
Pharyngitis.
Laryngitis.
Rare facial swelling.
Some Serious Problems Drug Can Cause
Antibodies to DNA.

▷ *CAUTION*
1. Use dornase only with one of the studied nebulizers and compressors.
2. Do not use this drug if it is cloudy or discolored.
3. Safety and effectiveness of this drug for those under 5 years old are not established.
Advisability of Use During Pregnancy or If Breast-Feeding:
Pregnancy Category: B. Ask your doctor for guidance. Presence in breast milk is unknown; avoid taking this drug or refrain from nursing.

▷ **Overdose Symptoms:** Single doses of up to 180 times the usual human dose have been well tolerated in rats and monkeys.

▷ **Suggested Periodic Examinations While Taking This Drug:** (at doctor's discretion)
Periodic pulmonary function tests.

▷ **While Taking This Drug the Following Apply:**

Nutritional Support: Continued enzyme and nutritional augmentation is still needed.

Alcohol: Follow your doctor's advice regarding alcohol use.

Other Drugs:

Clinical studies have revealed that dornase is compatible with medications typically used in managing cystic fibrosis. Specific adverse drug interactions are not documented at present.

Driving, Hazardous Activities: Specific limitations because of drug effects are not defined at present.

Discontinuation: Use of this drug must be continued indefinitely to derive any benefit.

Special Storage Instructions: This medicine should be stored in the refrigerator in its protective pouch.

▷ **Saving Money When Using This Medicine:**

- No other agents presently available work similarly to this drug. Ask your doctor if this drug offers the best combination of price and outcome for you.
- If your insurance takes issue with the use of this medicine, discuss the cost of hospitalizations versus the cost of the medicine.
- If this medicine is started, keep a diary of the number of infections and hospitalizations that occur after it is started.

DOXAZOSIN (dox AY zoh sin)

Prescription Needed: Yes   **Controlled Drug:** No   **Generic:** No

Brand Names: Cardura

Overview of BENEFITS versus RISKS	
Possible Benefits	*Possible Risks*
EFFECTIVE TREATMENT OF MILD TO MODERATE HYPERTENSION when used alone or in combination with other antihypertensive drugs	First-dose drop in blood pressure
	Dizziness
	Fluid retention
	Rapid heart rate

▷ **Illness This Medication Treats:**

(1) Mild to moderate hypertension with once-daily treatment; (2) prostate problems (benign prostatic hyperplasia).

▷ **Typical Dosage Range:** (Dosage or schedule must be determined by the doctor for each individual.)

Initiate treatment with a test dose of 1 mg to determine the response within the first 6 hours. If it is tolerated satisfactorily, increase dose cautiously (as needed and tolerated) by doubling it every 2 weeks and taking it as a single dose at bedtime. Doses in excess of 4 mg may increase the occurrence of light-headedness or dizziness, indicating low blood pressure. Total daily dosage should not exceed 16 mg.

▷ **Conditions Requiring Dosing Adjustments:**
Liver function: Extreme caution **must** be taken and lower doses taken if this drug is used by patients with liver compromise.
Kidney function: Doses of 1 to 8 mg have been used. In one study on renal compromise, 1 mg decreased the blood pressure for 3 days.

▷ **How Best to Take This Medicine:**   Preferably taken at bedtime to avoid orthostatic hypotension. May be taken without regard to food. The tablet may be crushed.

▷ **How Long This Medicine Is Usually Taken:**   Use on a regular schedule for 6 to 8 weeks is needed to see this drug's effectiveness in controlling hypertension. Long-term use (months to years) requires periodic physician evaluation.

▷ **Tell Your Doctor Before Taking This Medicine If You:**
- ever had an allergic reaction to this drug, prazosin (Minipres), or terazosin (Hytrin).
- are experiencing or have a history of mental depression.
- have active liver disease.
- have angina (active coronary artery disease) and are not taking a beta-blocker (see your doctor).
- have experienced orthostatic hypotension when using other antihypertensive drugs.
- have impaired circulation to the brain or a history of stroke.
- have coronary artery disease.
- have active liver disease or impaired liver function.
- have impaired kidney function.
- plan to have surgery under general anesthesia soon.

▷ **Possible Side Effects:**   Orthostatic hypotension, drowsiness, salt and water retention, dry mouth, nasal congestion, constipation.

▷ **Possible Adverse Effects:**
If any of the following develop, call your doctor promptly for guidance.
Some Mild Problems Drug Can Cause
Allergic reaction: skin rash, itching.
Headache, dizziness, fatigue, nervousness, numbness and tingling, blurred vision.
Palpitation, rapid heart rate, shortness of breath.
Nausea, diarrhea.

Some Serious Problems Drug Can Cause
  Mental depression.
  Arrhythmias.

▷ **Possible Effects on Sex Life:**   Impotence.

▷ *CAUTION*
  1. Observe for the possible first-dose response of a precipitous drop in blood pressure, with or without fainting; this usually occurs within the first 6 hours. Limit initial doses to 1 mg taken at bedtime for the first week; remain supine after taking these trial doses.
  2. Impaired liver function may increase your sensitivity to this drug and require smaller than usual doses.
  3. Call your doctor if you plan to use over-the-counter remedies for allergic rhinitis or head colds; these preparations contain drugs that may interact with doxazosin.
  4. Safety and effectiveness of this drug for those under 12 years old are not established.
  5. For those over 60, therapy is started with no more than 1 mg/day for the first week. Subsequent increases in dose must be very gradual and carefully supervised by your doctor. The occurrence of orthostatic hypotension can cause unexpected falls and injury; sit or lie down promptly if you feel light-headed or dizzy. Report any indications of dizziness or chest pain promptly.
  6. The dose of this drug MUST be decreased when used by the elderly.
  7. Lower doses of this drug must be used by patients with liver or kidney compromise.

  Advisability of Use During Pregnancy or If Breast-Feeding:
  Pregnancy Category: B. Use this drug only if clearly needed. Ask your doctor for guidance. Presence in breast milk is unknown. Monitor nursing infant closely and discontinue drug or nursing if adverse effects develop.

▷ **Overdose Symptoms:**   Orthostatic hypotension, headache, generalized flushing, rapid heart rate, extreme weakness, irregular heart rhythm, circulatory collapse.

▷ **Suggested Periodic Examinations While Taking This Drug:** (at doctor's discretion)
  Measurements of blood pressure in lying, sitting, and standing positions.
  Measurements of body weight to detect fluid retention.

▷ **While Taking This Drug the Following Apply:**
  Foods: Avoid excessive salt intake.
  Beverages: May be taken with milk.

Alcohol: CAUTION—alcohol can exaggerate the blood pressure–lowering actions of this drug, causing excessive reduction.

Tobacco Smoking: Nicotine can contribute significantly to this drug's ability to intensify coronary insufficiency in susceptible individuals. All forms of tobacco should be avoided.

Other Drugs:

The following drugs may *increase* the effects of doxazosin

- beta-adrenergic blockers; may increase the severity and duration of the first-dose hypotensive response.

The following drugs may *decrease* the effects of doxazosin

- estrogens.
- indomethacin (Indocin) and other NSAIDs (see Drug Classes).

Driving, Hazardous Activities: This drug may cause dizziness or drowsiness. Restrict your activities as necessary.

Exposure to Cold: Use caution until combined effect has been determined. Cold environments may increase this drug's ability to cause coronary insufficiency (angina) and hypothermia in susceptible individuals.

Heavy Exercise or Exertion: Excessive exertion can augment this drug's ability to induce angina.

Discontinuation: If you are taking this drug as part of your treatment program for congestive heart failure, do not discontinue it abruptly. Ask your doctor for guidance.

▷ **Saving Money When Using This Medicine:**

- Several agents are available that work similarly to this drug. Ask your doctor if this drug offers the best combination of price and outcome for you.
- If this medicine is being used to treat high blood pressure, ask your doctor if taking aspirin every other day makes sense for you.
- If this drug is used to treat hypertension, have your blood pressure checked periodically to ensure continuation of this drug's benefits

DOXEPIN (DOX e pin)

Prescription Needed: Yes   **Controlled Drug:** No   **Generic:** Yes

Brand Names: Adapin, Sinequan, Zonalon

Overview of BENEFITS versus RISKS

Possible Benefits	*Possible Risks*
EFFECTIVE RELIEF OF ENDOGENOUS DEPRESSION	ADVERSE BEHAVIORAL EFFECTS: confusion, disorientation, hallucinations, delusions
EFFECTIVE RELIEF OF ANXIETY AND NERVOUS TENSION	CONVERSION OF DEPRESSION TO MANIA in manic-depressive disorder
Possibly beneficial in other depressive disorders	Aggravation of schizophrenia and paranoia
	Rare blood cell disorders
	Rare liver toxicity
	Lowered blood pressure on standing

▷ **Illness This Medication Treats:**
  (1) Symptoms associated with spontaneous (endogenous) depression, refractory depression, neurotic depression, mixed depression anxiety, and depression and anxiety in alcoholism; (2) treatment of sleep disturbances.

▷ **Typical Dosage Range:** (Dosage or schedule must be determined by the doctor for each individual.)
  Initially 25 mg two to four times daily. Dose may be increased cautiously as needed and tolerated, by 10 to 25 mg daily at intervals of 1 week. Usual maintenance dose is 75 to 150 mg every 24 hours. Total dose should not exceed 300 mg/24 hr. When the optimal requirement is determined, it may be taken at bedtime as one dose.

▷ **Conditions Requiring Dosing Adjustments:**
  Liver function: This drug rarely causes hepatitis. This drug should be used with caution by patients with liver compromise. No specific guidelines for dosing adjustment have been developed.
  Kidney function: This drug should be used with caution by patients with compromised kidneys and urine outflow problems.

▷ **How Best to Take This Medicine:**   May be taken without regard to meals. Capsule may be opened for administration.

▷ **How Long This Medicine Is Usually Taken:**   Some benefit may be apparent within to 2 weeks, but adequate response may require continual use for 10 to 12 weeks or longer. Long-term use should not exceed 6 months without evaluation of the need for continuation. See your doctor regularly.

▷ **Tell Your Doctor Before Taking This Medicine If You:**
- ever had an allergic reaction to it.
- are taking or have taken within the past 14 days any MAO type A inhibitors.
- are recovering from a recent heart attack.
- have narrow-angle glaucoma.
- are allergic or sensitive to any other tricyclic antidepressant.
- have a history of diabetes, epilepsy, glaucoma, heart disease, prostate gland enlargement, or overactive thyroid function.
- are pregnant or planning pregnancy.
- plan to have surgery under general anesthesia soon.

▷ **Possible Side Effects:** Drowsiness, blurred vision, dry mouth, constipation, impaired urination. Decreased blood pressure on standing.

▷ **Possible Adverse Effects:**
If any of the following develop, call your doctor promptly for guidance.

Some Mild Problems Drug Can Cause
Allergic reactions: skin rash, swelling of face or tongue, drug fever.
Headache, dizziness, fainting, unsteady gait, tremors.
Peculiar taste, irritation of mouth, nausea.
Fluctuation of blood sugar levels.

Some Serious Problems Drug Can Cause
Allergic reactions: hepatitis with or without jaundice.
Hallucinations, agitation, delusions.
Bone marrow depression (reported for other drugs of this class).
Peripheral neuritis—numbness, tingling.
Rare seizures, kidney damage, or abnormal heart rhythm.
Parkinson-like disorders—usually mild and infrequent; most likely in the elderly.

▷ **Possible Effects on Sex Life:** Female breast enlargement with milk production; swelling of testicles. Ejaculation disorders, painful and persistent erection (priapism). Enlargement and tenderness of male breast tissue (gynecomastia).

▷ *CAUTION*
1. Dosage of this drug must be adjusted for each person individually. Report for follow-up evaluation and laboratory tests as directed by your doctor.
2. It is advisable to withhold this drug if electroconvulsive therapy is used to treat your depression.
3. Safety and effectiveness of this drug for those under 12 years old are not established.
4. Those over 60 should watch during the first 2 weeks of treatment for development of confusion, agitation, forgetfulness, disorienta-

tion, delusions, and hallucinations. Reduction of dosage or discontinuation may be necessary. Unsteadiness may predispose to falling and injury. This drug may increase the degree of impaired urination associated with prostate gland enlargement.

Advisability of Use During Pregnancy or If Breast-Feeding:

Pregnancy Category: C. Use only if clearly needed. If possible, avoid use of this drug during the first 3 months and the last month. Ask your doctor for guidance. Present in breast milk. Monitor the nursing infant closely and discontinue drug or nursing if adverse effects develop.

▷ **Overdose Symptoms:** Confusion, hallucinations, marked drowsiness, heart palpitations, dilated pupils, tremors, stupor, deep sleep, coma, convulsions.

▷ **Suggested Periodic Examinations While Taking This Drug:** (at doctor's discretion)

Complete blood cell counts, liver function tests, serial blood pressure readings, and electrocardiogram.

▷ **While Taking This Drug the Following Apply:**

Foods: This drug may increase your appetite and cause excessive weight gain.

Beverages: May be taken with milk.

Alcohol: Avoid completely. This drug can markedly increase the intoxicating effects of alcohol and accentuate its depressant action on brain function.

Tobacco Smoking: May hasten the elimination of this drug. Higher doses may be necessary.

Other Drugs:

Doxepin may *increase* the effects of

- albuterol—may increase the effect of albuterol on blood vessels.
- atropinelike drugs.
- dicumarol, increasing the risk of bleeding; dosage adjustments may be necessary.
- other medicines with central nervous system effects (narcotics, benzodiazepines, etc.).
- phenytoin (Dilantin).
- thyroid hormones.

Doxepin may *decrease* the effects of

- clonidine (Catapres).
- guanethidine (Ismelin).

Doxepin *taken concurrently* with

- MAO type A inhibitors may cause high fever, delirium, and convulsions.
- carbamazepine (Tegretol) may decrease the effectiveness of doxepin.

- cimetidine (Tagamet) may result in doxepin toxicity (urine retention, dry mouth).
- diphenhydramine (Benadryl) or other medicines with anticholinergic actions may lead to increased urine retention or bowel obstruction.
- epinephrine will cause an exaggerated increase in blood pressure.
- fluoxetine (Prozac), propoxyphene (Darvon), or quinidine (Quinaglute) may result in doxepin toxicity.
- meperidene (Demerol) may result in an increased risk of respiratory depression.
- methylphenidate (Ritalin) may lead to doxepin toxicity.
- paroxetine (Paxil) can cause an increased doxepin level and toxicity.
- pseudoephedrine (caution—this may be found in nonprescription products) may lead to abnormal increases in blood pressure.
- propoxyphene (Darvon) can lead to doxepin toxicity.
- quinidine (Quinaglute) can lead to doxepin toxicity.
- sertraline (Zoloft) may lead to doxepin toxicity.
- verapamil (Calan, Verelan) may lead to increased doxepin levels.
- warfarin (Coumadin) may prolong the anticoagulant action of warfarin. More frequent INR (prothrombin time) testing is needed.

Driving, Hazardous Activities: This drug may impair mental alertness, judgment, physical coordination, and reaction time. Avoid hazardous activities.

Exposure to Sun: Use caution until your sensitivity to the sun has been determined. This drug may cause photosensitivity.

Exposure to Heat: Doxepin can inhibit sweating and impair the body's adaptation to hot environments, increasing the risk of heatstroke. Avoid saunas.

Exposure to Cold: The elderly should use caution and avoid conditions conducive to hypothermia.

Discontinuation: It is advisable to discontinue this drug gradually. Abrupt withdrawal after long-term use can cause headache, malaise, and nausea.

▷ **Saving Money When Using This Medicine:**

- Several agents are available that work similarly to this drug. Ask your doctor if this drug offers the best combination of price and outcome for you.
- Some of the newer agents may have fewer side effects than older ones. Talk with your doctor about newer medicines if side effects become a problem for you.
- Recently depression has been found to be a potential risk factor for osteoporosis. Ask your doctor about calcium supplements, exercise, risk factors, and bone mineral density testing.

DOXYCYCLINE (dox ee SI kleen)

Prescription Needed: Yes   **Controlled Drug:** No   **Generic:** Yes

Brand Names: Doryx, Doxychel, Vibramycin, Vibra-Tabs, Vivox

Overview of BENEFITS versus RISKS

Possible Benefits	*Possible Risks*
EFFECTIVE TREATMENT OF INFECTIONS due to susceptible microorganisms	ALLERGIC REACTIONS, mild to severe
	Liver reaction with jaundice (rare)
	Fungal superinfections
	Drug-induced colitis
	Blood cell disorders

▷ **Illness This Medication Treats:**
  (1) A broad range of infections caused by susceptible bacteria and protozoa; (2) prevents traveler's diarrhea; (3) syphilis in penicillin-allergic patients.
  Other (unlabeled) generally accepted uses: (1) used to treat early Lyme disease; (2) may help some cases of infertility of unexplained origin.

▷ **Typical Dosage Range:** (Dosage or schedule must be determined by the doctor for each individual.)
  100 mg every 12 hours the first day, then 100 to 200 mg once daily or 50 to 100 mg every 12 hours. Total daily dosage should not exceed 300 mg.

▷ **Conditions Requiring Dosing Adjustments:**
  Liver function: People with both liver and kidney compromise should decrease the dose; however, no dosage decrease is needed for patients with mild to moderate liver compromise. This drug can cause liver dysfunction; its use by patients with liver compromise requires a benefit-to-risk decision.
  Kidney function: Patients with creatinine clearances of 50 to 80 ml/min should take the usual dose every 12 hours. Those with creatinine clearances of 10 to 50 ml/min should take the usual dose every 12 to 18 hours. Patients with creatinine clearances of less than 10 ml/min should take the usual dose every 18 to 24 hours.
  Malnutrition: The half-life of this drug may decrease in patients with malnutrition. If clinical progress is not what is expected, the dose may need to be increased.

▷ **How Best to Take This Medicine:** Best taken on an empty stomach, 1 hour before or 2 hours after eating. However, if stomach irritation occurs, it may be taken with food or milk. (Unlike other tetracyclines, doxycycline absorption is not significantly affected by ingestion of food or milk.) Take this drug at the same time each day, with a full glass of water or milk. Take the full course prescribed. The tablet may be crushed and the capsule may be opened for administration.

▷ **How Long This Medicine Is Usually Taken:** The time required to control the infection and be free of fever and symptoms for 48 hours; this varies with the nature of the infection.

▷ **Tell Your Doctor Before Taking This Medicine If You:**
- are allergic to any tetracycline drug.
- are pregnant or breast-feeding.
- are given a prescription for a child under 8 years old.
- have a history of liver or kidney disease.
- have systemic lupus erythematosus.
- are taking any penicillin drug.
- are taking any anticoagulant drug.
- plan to have surgery under general anesthesia soon.

▷ **Possible Side Effects:** Superinfections, often due to yeast organisms. These can occur in the mouth, intestinal tract, or rectum and/or vagina, resulting in rectal and vaginal itching.

▷ **Possible Adverse Effects:**
If any of the following develop, call your doctor promptly for guidance.
Some Mild Problems Drug Can Cause
Allergic reactions: skin rash, itching of hands and feet, swelling of face or extremities.
Loss of appetite, nausea, vomiting, diarrhea.
Irritation of mouth, sore throat, abdominal cramping.
Some Serious Problems Drug Can Cause
Allergic reactions: anaphylactic reaction, asthma, fever, swollen joints, abnormal bleeding or bruising, jaundice.
Permanent discoloration and/or malformation of teeth when taken by children under 8 years old, including infants and the fetuses of pregnant mothers.
Rare liver toxicity or systemic lupus erythematosus.
Rare serious skin reactions (Stevens-Johnson syndrome) or kidney toxicity.

▷ *CAUTION*
1. Antacids and preparations containing aluminum, bismuth, iron, magnesium, or zinc can prevent adequate absorption of this drug and reduce its effectiveness significantly.
2. Troublesome and persistent diarrhea can develop in sensitive individuals. If diarrhea persists for more than 24 hours, discontinue taking this drug and call your doctor.

3. Tetracyclines should not be given to children under 8 years old because of the risk of permanent discoloration and deformity of the teeth. Rarely young infants may develop increased intracranial pressure within the first 4 days of receiving this drug. Tetracyclines may inhibit normal bone growth and development.

4. For those over 60, natural skin changes may predispose to severe and prolonged itching reactions in the genital and anal regions.

Advisability of Use During Pregnancy or If Breast-Feeding:

Pregnancy Category: D. Avoid completely during entire pregnancy. Present in breast milk; avoid taking this drug or refrain from nursing.

▷ **Overdose Symptoms:**   Nausea, vomiting, diarrhea, acute liver damage (rare).

▷ **Suggested Periodic Examinations While Taking This Drug:** (at doctor's discretion)

Complete blood cell counts, liver and kidney function tests.

During extended use, sputum and stool examinations may detect early superinfection due to yeast organisms.

▷ **While Taking This Drug the Following Apply:**

Foods: Avoid meats and iron-fortified cereals and supplements for 2 hours before and after taking this drug.

Beverages: May be taken with milk or carbonated beverages.

Alcohol: No interactions expected. However, it is best avoided if you have active liver disease.

Other Drugs:

Doxycycline may *increase* the effects of

- oral anticoagulants, making it necessary to reduce their dosage.
- digoxin (Lanoxin), causing digitalis toxicity.
- lithium (Eskalith, Lithane, etc.), increasing the risk of lithium toxicity.

Doxycycline may *decrease* the effects of

- oral contraceptives (birth control pills), impairing their effectiveness in pregnancy prevention.
- penicillins, impairing their effectiveness in treating infections.

The following drugs may *decrease* the effects of doxycycline

- antacids (aluminum and magnesium preparations, sodium bicarbonate, etc.); may reduce drug absorption.
- barbiturates (see Drug Classes).
- bismuth preparations (Pepto-Bismol, etc.).
- calcium supplements.
- carbamazepine (Tegretol).
- cimetidine (Tagamet).
- phenobarbital.
- phenytoin (Dilantin).
- iron and mineral preparations—may reduce drug absorption.

Driving, Hazardous Activities: Usually no restrictions. Be alert to the possible occurrence of nausea or diarrhea.

Exposure to Sun: Use caution until your sensitivity has been determined. Tetracyclines can cause photosensitivity.

▷ **Saving Money When Using This Medicine:**
- Several agents are available that work similarly to this drug. Ask your doctor if this drug offers the best combination of price and outcome for you.
- Ask your doctor if the infection-fighting potential of this medicine matches the severity of your infection.

ENALAPRIL (e NAL a pril)

Prescription Needed: Yes   **Controlled Drug:** No   **Generic:** No

Brand Names: Vaseretic [CD], Vasotec

Overview of BENEFITS versus RISKS	
Possible Benefits	*Possible Risks*
EFFECTIVE CONTROL OF MILD TO SEVERE HIGH BLOOD PRESSURE	Low blood pressure
	Bone marrow depression (rare)
Possibly beneficial as adjunctive treatment in selected cases of congestive heart failure	Allergic swelling of face, tongue, or vocal cords

▷ **Illness This Medication Treats:**
(1) High blood pressure. Mild to moderate high blood pressure usually responds to low doses; severe high blood pressure may require higher doses, with greater risk of serious adverse effects. (2) Used adjunctively to treat heart failure that does not respond to digitalis and diuretics.

▷ **Typical Dosage Range:** (Dosage or schedule must be determined by the doctor for each individual.)
Initially 5 mg once daily for weeks. Usual maintenance dose is 10 to 40 mg per day in a single dose or two divided doses. Total daily dose should not exceed 40 mg if kidney function is impaired.
Heart failure: 2.5 to 10 mg once or twice daily.

▷ **Conditions Requiring Dosing Adjustments:**
Liver function: For patients with liver compromise the dose may need to be increased, because less of the drug is changed to the active form.
Kidney function: Patients with moderate to severe kidney compromise

may need only 2.5 mg/day. Enalapril should NOT be used by patients with progressive kidney failure.

Diabetes: Diabetics with decreased creatinine clearance and proteinuria (protein in the urine) should take decreased doses.

▷ **How Best to Take This Medicine:**   Take on an empty stomach or with food at same time each day. Tablet may be crushed for administration.

▷ **How Long This Medicine Is Usually Taken:**   Use on a regular schedule for several weeks usually determines the effectiveness of this drug in controlling high blood pressure. The proper treatment of high blood pressure usually requires the long-term use of effective medications. See your doctor regularly.

▷ **Tell Your Doctor Before Taking This Medicine If You:**
- ever had an allergic reaction to it.
- are in the last 6 months of pregnancy or are planning pregnancy.
- currently have a blood cell or bone marrow disorder.
- have active liver disease.
- have an abnormally high level of blood potassium.
- had an allergic reaction (or other adverse effect) to any other ACE inhibitor.
- have a history of kidney disease or impaired kidney function.
- have scleroderma or systemic lupus erythematosus.
- have any form of heart disease.
- have diabetes.
- are taking any other antihypertensives, diuretics, immunosuppressants, nitrates, or potassium supplements.
- plan to have surgery under general anesthesia soon.

▷ **Possible Side Effects:**   Dizziness, light-headedness, fainting (excessive drop in blood pressure).

▷ **Possible Adverse Effects:**
If any of the following develop, call your doctor promptly for guidance.
Some Mild Problems Drug Can Cause
   Allergic reactions: skin rash, itching.
   Headache, drowsiness, nervousness, numbness and tingling, insomnia.
   Rare baldness.
   Rapid heart rate, palpitations.
   Nausea, vomiting, diarrhea.
   Excessive sweating, muscle cramps.
Some Serious Problems Drug Can Cause
   Allergic reactions: swelling (angioedema) of face, tongue, and/or vocal cords; can be life-threatening.

Bone marrow depression—fatigue, weakness, fever, sore throat, abnormal bleeding or bruising (very rare).

Rare pancreatitis, depression. hallucinations, or liver or kidney toxicity.

Rare peripheral neuropathy.

▷ **Possible Effects on Sex Life:** Rare report of impotence, swelling or tenderness of male breast tissue; rare itching of the vulva or vagina.

▷ *CAUTION*

1. Ask your doctor about the advisability of discontinuing other antihypertensives (especially diuretics) for 1 week before starting this drug.
2. **Tell your doctor immediately if you become pregnant.** This drug should not be taken beyond the first 3 months of pregnancy.
3. Call your doctor immediately if your face or tongue starts to swell after taking this medicine.
4. **Report promptly** any indications of infection (fever, sore throat) and any indications of water retention (weight gain, puffiness, swollen feet or ankles).
5. Do not use a salt substitute without your doctor's knowledge and approval. (Many salt substitutes contain potassium.)
6. It is advisable to obtain blood cell counts and urine analyses **before** starting this drug.
7. Safety and effectiveness of this drug for infants and children are not established.
8. For those over 60, small doses are advisable until tolerance has been determined. Sudden and excessive lowering of blood pressure can predispose to stroke or heart attack in those with impaired brain circulation or coronary artery heart disease.

Advisability of Use During Pregnancy or If Breast-Feeding:
Pregnancy Category: D. Avoid using this drug completely during the last 6 months. C during the first 3 months of pregnancy; use this drug only if clearly needed. Ask your doctor for guidance. Present in breast milk. Monitor the nursing infant closely and discontinue drug or nursing if adverse effects develop.

▷ **Overdose Symptoms:** Excessive drop in blood pressure: light-headedness, dizziness, fainting.

▷ **Suggested Periodic Examinations While Taking This Drug:** (at doctor's discretion)
Before starting drug: complete blood cell counts; urine analysis with measurement of protein content; blood potassium level.
During use of drug: blood cell counts; measurements of blood potassium.

▷ **While Taking This Drug the Following Apply:**
Foods: Ask your doctor about salt intake.

Nutritional Support: **Do not take** potassium supplements unless directed by your doctor.

Beverages: May be taken with milk.

Alcohol: Use caution until combined effect has been determined. Alcohol may enhance this drug's blood pressure–lowering effect.

Other Drugs:

Enalapril **taken concurrently** with

- allopurinol may lead to serious skin reactions.
- aspirin or other NSAIDs (see Drug Classes) may blunt therapeutic effects of enalapril.
- azathioprine can lead to severe impairment of blood formation.
- cyclosporine (Sandimmune) can lead to acute kidney failure.
- ethacrynic acid can cause excessive lowering of blood pressure.
- lithium (Lithobid, others) can lead to lithium toxicity.
- loop diuretics can lead to severe lowering of blood pressure on standing.
- oral hypoglycemic agents (see Drug Classes) may lead to decreased insulin resistance and require a decrease in the oral hypoglycemic agent dose to avoid excessive lowering of the blood sugar.
- phenothiazines (see Drug Classes) can cause additive lowering of blood pressure.
- potassium preparations (K-Lyte, Slow-K, etc.) may cause increased blood levels of potassium, with risk of serious heart rhythm disturbances.
- potassium-sparing diuretics, such as amiloride (Moduretic), spironolactone (Aldactazide), or triamterene (Dyazide), may cause increased blood levels of potassium with risk of serious heart rhythm disturbances.
- rifampin or rifabutin may blunt the therapeutic benefit of enalapril.
- thiazide diuretics may result in increased levels of the active medicine and exaggerated lowering of the blood pressure.

Driving, Hazardous Activities: Usually no restrictions. Be aware of possible drops in blood pressure with resultant dizziness or faintness.

Exposure to Sun: Caution is advised. A similar drug of this class can cause photosensitivity.

Exposure to Heat: Caution is advised. Avoid excessive perspiring with resultant loss of body water and drop in blood pressure.

Occurrence of Unrelated Illness: Report promptly any disorder that causes nausea, vomiting, or diarrhea. Fluid and chemical imbalances must be corrected as soon as possible.

▷ **Saving Money When Using This Medicine:**
- Many ACE inhibitors are available (agents that work similarly to

this drug). Ask your doctor if this drug offers the best combination of price and outcome for you.

- Talk with your doctor to see if taking aspirin every other day makes sense for you.
- Ask your doctor about stress management and exercise programs available in your area.

EPINEPHRINE (ep i NEF rin)

Other Name: Adrenaline

Prescription Needed: Varies   **Controlled Drug:** No   **Generic:** Yes

Brand Names: Adrenalin, Bronkaid Mist, Epifrin, E-Pilo Preparations [CD], EpiPen, Epitrate, Glaucon, Medihaler-Epi Preparations, Primatene Mist, Sus-Phrine, Vaponefrin

---

Overview of BENEFITS versus RISKS

Possible Benefits	*Possible Risks*
EFFECTIVE RELIEF OF SEVERE ALLERGIC (ANAPHYLACTIC) REACTIONS	Significant increase in blood pressure (in sensitive people)
TEMPORARY RELIEF OF ACUTE BRONCHIAL ASTHMA	Idiosyncratic reaction: pulmonary edema (fluid formation in lungs)
Reduction of internal eye pressure (treatment of glaucoma)	Heart rhythm disorders
Relief of allergic congestion of the nose and sinuses	

▷ **Illness This Medication Treats:**
  (1) Acute bronchial asthma attacks; (2) less frequently as a decongestant for symptomatic relief of allergic nasal congestion and as eyedrops in the management of glaucoma.

▷ **Typical Dosage Range:** (Dosage or schedule must be determined by the doctor for each individual.)
  Aerosols: One inhalation, repeated in 1 to 2 minutes if needed; wait 4 hours before next inhalation. Eyedrops: One drop every 12 hours. Dosage may vary with product; follow printed instructions and label directions.

▷ **Conditions Requiring Dosing Adjustments:**
Kidney function: Dosage adjustment of this drug is not defined for patients with kidney compromise.

▷ **How Best to Take This Medicine:** Aerosols and inhalation solutions: After the first inhalation, wait 1 to 2 minutes to determine if a second inhalation is necessary. If relief does not occur within 20 minutes and difficult breathing persists, seek medical attention promptly. Avoid prolonged and excessive use. Eyedrops: During instillation of drops and for the following 2 minutes, press a finger against the tear sac (inner corner of eye) to prevent rapid absorption of drug into body circulation.

▷ **How Long This Medicine Is Usually Taken:** According to individual needs. Long-term use requires supervision and periodic evaluation by your doctor.

▷ **Tell Your Doctor Before Taking This Medicine If You:**
- ever had an allergic reaction to it.
- have narrow-angle glaucoma.
- have experienced a recent stroke or heart attack.
- have any degree of high blood pressure.
- have any form of heart disease, especially coronary heart disease (with or without angina), or a heart rhythm disorder.
- have diabetes or overactive thyroid function.
- have a history of stroke.
- are taking any MAO type A inhibitors, phenothiazines, digitalis preparations, or quinidine.

▷ **Possible Side Effects:** In sensitive people: restlessness, anxiety, headache, tremor, palpitation, coldness of hands and feet, dryness of mouth and throat (with use of aerosol).

▷ **Possible Adverse Effects:**
If any of the following develop, call your doctor promptly for guidance.
Some Mild Problems Drug Can Cause
Allergic reactions: skin rash; eyedrops may cause redness, swelling, and itching of the eyelids.
Weakness, dizziness, pallor.
Some Serious Problems Drug Can Cause
Idiosyncratic reaction: excessive fluid in the lungs (pulmonary edema).
In predisposed individuals: excessive rise in blood pressure with risk of stroke (cerebral hemorrhage).
Rapid heart rate and potential arrhythmias.
Rare seizures, porphyria, or kidney toxicity.

▷ **CAUTION**

1. If this drug is used frequently in a short period of time, it may no longer work. If this happens, avoid its use completely for 12 hours, at which time a normal response should return.

2. Excessive use of aerosol preparations in treating asthma has been associated with sudden death.

3. This drug can cause significant irritability of the nerve pathways (conduction system) and muscles of the heart, predisposing to serious heart rhythm disorders. If you have any form of heart disorder, call your doctor.

4. This drug can increase the blood sugar level. If you have diabetes, test for urine sugar frequently to detect significant changes.

5. If you become unresponsive to this drug and intend to substitute isoproterenol (Isuprel), allow an interval of 4 hours between the usage of these two drugs.

6. Promptly discard all preparations of this drug at the first appearance of discoloration (pink to red to brown) or cloudiness (precipitation). Such changes indicate drug deterioration.

7. Use this drug cautiously in infants and children, in small doses until tolerance is determined. Watch for any indications of weakness, light-headedness, or inclination to faint.

8. For those over 60, caution and small doses are recommended until tolerance is determined. Watch for excessive stimulation: nervousness, headache, tremor, rapid heart rate. This drug may aggravate arteriosclerosis, heart disease, high blood pressure, Parkinson's disease, or prostatism. Ask your doctor for guidance.

Advisability of Use During Pregnancy or If Breast-Feeding:
Pregnancy Category. C. This drug can cause significant reduction of oxygen supply to the fetus. Use it only if clearly needed and in small, infrequent doses. Avoid usage during the first 3 months and during labor and delivery. Present in breast milk; avoid taking this drug or refrain from nursing.

▷ **Habit-Forming Potential:** Tolerance to this drug can develop with frequent use, but dependence does not occur.

▷ **Overdose Symptoms:** Nervousness, throbbing headache, dizziness, tremor, palpitations, disturbance of heart rhythm, difficult breathing, abdominal pain, vomiting of blood.

▷ **Suggested Periodic Examinations While Taking This Drug:** (at doctor's discretion)
Blood pressure measurements; blood or urine sugar measurements in presence of diabetes; vision testing and measurement of internal eye pressure in presence of glaucoma.

▷ **While Taking This Drug the Following Apply:**

Foods: No restrictions, except those that cause asthma.

Alcohol: Alcoholic beverages can increase the urinary excretion of this drug.

Other Drugs:

Epinephrine *taken concurrently* with

- certain beta-blockers (nadolol, propranolol) may increase blood pressure and decrease heart rate.
- chlorpromazine (Thorazine) may decrease blood pressure and increase heart rate.
- furazolidone (Furoxone) may cause increased blood pressure and high fever.
- guanethidine (Esimil, Ismelin) may increase blood pressure.
- halothane may lead to abnormal heartbeats.
- pilocarpine (Ocusert) may cause increased myopia.
- tricyclic antidepressants (amitriptyline, etc.) may cause increased blood pressure and heart rhythm disturbances.

Driving, Hazardous Activities: This drug may cause dizziness or excessive nervousness. Restrict your activities as necessary.

Heavy Exercise or Exertion: No interactions expected. However, exercise can induce asthma in sensitive individuals.

Occurrence of Unrelated Illness: Use caution in the presence of severe burns. This drug can increase drainage from burned tissue and cause significant loss of tissue fluids and blood proteins.

Discontinuation: If this drug fails to provide relief after an adequate trial, discontinue it and consult your doctor. It is dangerous to increase the dosage or frequency of use.

Special Storage Instructions: Protect this drug from exposure to air, light, and heat. Keep it in a cool place, preferably the refrigerator.

▷ **Saving Money When Using This Medicine:**

- Several agents are available that work similarly to this drug. Ask your doctor if this drug offers the best combination of price and outcome for you.
- Lidocaine made available by nebulization has some recent data showing benefits in treating asthma. Discuss this with your doctor.
- Ask your doctor if nedocromil or cromolyn should be considered for preventing acute asthma attacks.

ERGOTAMINE (er GOT a meen)

Prescription Needed: Yes   **Controlled Drug:** No   **Generic:** No

Brand Names: Bellergal-S [CD], Cafergot [CD], Cafergot P-B [CD], Ercaf [CD], Ergomar, Ergostat, Medihaler Ergotamine, Wigraine [CD], Wigrettes

---

Overview of BENEFITS versus RISKS

Possible Benefits	*Possible Risks*
PREVENTION AND RELIEF OF VASCULAR HEADACHES: MIGRAINE, MIGRAINE-LIKE, AND HISTAMINE HEADACHES	GANGRENE OF THE FINGERS, TOES, OR INTESTINE AGGRAVATION OF CORONARY ARTERY DISEASE (ANGINA) ABORTION

▷ **Illness This Medication Treats:**

Vascular headaches, especially migraine and cluster headaches. It should not be used continually to prevent migraine attacks, but it is often effective in terminating the headache if taken within the first hour following the onset of pain. It may be used on a short-term basis to prevent or abort cluster headaches during the period of their occurrence. The inhalation form provides rapid onset of action.

As Combination Drug Product [CD]: Combined with caffeine this drug takes advantage of caffeine's ability to enhance its absorption. This permits a smaller dose to be effective and reduces the risk of adverse effects with repeated use. This drug is also combined with belladonna (atropine) and a barbiturate to provide preparations that are useful in relieving the symptoms of premenstrual tension and menopausal syndrome: nervousness, nausea, hot flushes, and sweating.

▷ **Typical Dosage Range:** (Dosage or schedule must be determined by the doctor for each individual.)

Inhalation: One spray (0.36 mg) at the onset of headache; repeat one spray every 5 to 10 minutes as needed for relief, up to a maximum of 6 sprays/24 hr. Do not exceed 15 sprays/week. Sublingual tablets: Dissolve 1 mg under the tongue at the onset of headache; repeat 1 mg every 30 to 60 minutes as needed, up to a maximum of 5 mg per attack. Do not exceed 5 mg/24 hr or 10 mg/week. Determine the optimal dose required (up to 5 mg) to abort the headache in a single dose at the onset of pain.

▷ **Conditions Requiring Dosing Adjustments:**

Liver function: This drug should be used with caution by patients with liver compromise.

Kidney function: This drug is a rare cause of acute renal failure; however, it should be used with caution by patients with compromised kidneys.

▷ **How Best to Take This Medicine:**   Follow written instructions carefully. Do not exceed prescribed doses. The regular tablets (combination drug) may be crushed; sustained-release tablets should be taken whole (not crushed). Sublingual tablets should be dissolved under the tongue, not swallowed.

▷ **How Long This Medicine Is Usually Taken:**   Continual use on a regular schedule for several episodes of headache is usually necessary to determine this drug's effectiveness in aborting or relieving the pain of vascular headache. Do not exceed recommended dosage schedules. If headaches are not controlled after several trials of maximal doses, consult your doctor for alternative treatment.

▷ **Tell Your Doctor Before Taking This Medicine If You:**
- ever had an allergic reaction to it or are allergic or overly sensitive to *any* ergot preparation.
- are pregnant.
- have a severe infection.
- have angina pectoris (coronary artery disease), Buerger's disease, hardening of the arteries (arteriosclerosis), high blood pressure (severe hypertension), kidney disease or impaired kidney function, liver disease or impaired liver function, Raynaud's phenomenon, thrombophlebitis, severe itching.
- are planning to have a face-lift (rhytidectomy), as this medicine may cause skin flap problems.

▷ **Possible Side Effects:**   Usually infrequent and mild with recommended doses.
Susceptible individuals may notice a sensation of cold hands and feet, with mild numbness and tingling.

▷ **Possible Adverse Effects:**
If any of the following develop, call your doctor promptly for guidance.
Some Mild Problems Drug Can Cause
Allergic reactions: localized swellings (angioedema), itching.
Headache, drowsiness, dizziness, confusion.
Chest pain, numbness and tingling, muscle pains in arms or legs.
Nausea, vomiting, diarrhea.
Some Serious Problems Drug Can Cause
Gangrene of the extremities—coldness; numbness; pain; dark discoloration; eventual loss of fingers, toes, or feet.
Gangrene of the intestine—severe abdominal pain and swelling; emergency surgery required.

Retroperitoneal fibrosis, pain syndromes (reflex sympathetic dystrophy), or rare porphyrias.

Fibrous changes in the lung or kidney failure.

▷ **CAUTION**

1. Excessive use of this drug can actually provoke migraine headache and increase its occurrence.
2. Do not exceed a total dose of 5 mg/24 hr or 10 mg/week.
3. Individual sensitivity to the effects of this drug vary greatly. Some may experience early toxic effects even while taking recommended doses. Report promptly any indications of impaired circulation: numbness in fingers or toes, muscle cramping, chest pain.
4. Safety and effectiveness of this drug for those under 12 years old are not established.
5. Those over 60 may have natural changes in blood vessels and circulation that make them more susceptible to this drug's serious adverse effects. See the preceding list of disorders that contraindicate the use of this drug.
6. This drug should NOT be used by patients with progressive kidney failure.

Advisability of Use During Pregnancy or If Breast-Feeding:

Pregnancy Category: X. This drug should be avoided during the entire pregnancy. Present in breast milk; avoid taking this drug or refrain from nursing.

▷ **Overdose Symptoms:** Manifestations of ergotism: coldness of skin; severe muscle pains; tingling and burning pain in hands and feet; loss of blood supply to extremities, resulting in gangrene in fingers and toes. Acute ergot poisoning: nausea, vomiting, diarrhea, cold skin, numbness of extremities, confusion, seizures, coma.

▷ **Possible Effects of Long-Term Use:** A form of functional dependence may develop, resulting in withdrawal headaches when the drug is discontinued.

▷ **Suggested Periodic Examinations While Taking This Drug:** (at doctor's discretion)

Evaluation of circulation to the extremities.

▷ **While Taking This Drug the Following Apply:**

Foods: Avoid all foods to which you are allergic; some migraine headaches are due to food allergies.

Alcohol: Best avoided; alcohol can intensify vascular headache.

Tobacco Smoking: Best avoided; nicotine can further reduce the restricted blood flow produced by this drug.

Marijuana Smoking: Best avoided; additive effects can increase the coldness of hands and feet.

Other Drugs:

Ergotamine may ***decrease*** the effects of

- nitroglycerin, reducing its effectiveness in preventing or relieving angina pain.

The following drugs may ***increase*** the effects of ergotamine

- beta-blockers (see Drug Classes).
- dopamine.
- erythromycin (E-Mycin, ERYC, etc.).
- sumatriptan (Imitrex); may extend spasms of the blood vessels.
- troleandomycin (Tao).

Driving, Hazardous Activities: This drug may cause drowsiness or dizziness. Restrict your activities as necessary.

Exposure to Cold: Avoid as much as possible. Cold environments and handling of cold objects further reduces the restricted blood flow to the extremities.

Discontinuation: Following long-term use, it may be necessary to withdraw this drug gradually to prevent withdrawal headache. Ask your doctor for guidance.

▷ **Saving Money When Using This Medicine:**

- Several agents are available to treat migraines. Ask your doctor if this drug offers the best combination of price and outcomes for you.
- Talk with your doctor about any one of the many agents used to PREVENT migraines.

ERYTHROMYCIN (er ith roh MY sin)

Prescription Needed: Yes **Controlled Drug:** No **Generic:** Yes

Brand Names: This is a representative list only. E.E.S., E-Mycin, ERYC, Eryderm, EryPed, Erythrocin, Ilosone, Pediazole [CD], Robimycin, T-Stat, Wyamycin S

Overview of BENEFITS versus RISKS

Possible Benefits	*Possible Risks*
EFFECTIVE TREATMENT OF INFECTIONS DUE TO SUSCEPTIBLE MICROORGANISMS	Allergic reactions, mild and infrequent
	Liver reaction (most common with erythromycin estolate)
	Drug-induced colitis (rare)
	Superinfections (rare)

▷ **Illness This Medication Treats:**

(1) Skin and skin structure infections, such as acne and *Streptococcus*; (2) respiratory tract infections, including strep throat, diphtheria, and several types of pneumonia; (3) gonorrhea and syphilis; (4) amebic dysentery; (5) Legionnaire's disease; (6) long-term prevention of recurrences of rheumatic fever.

▷ **Typical Dosage Range:** (Dosage or schedule must be determined by the doctor for each individual.)

Oral form: 250 to 1000 mg every 6 hours, according to nature and severity of infection. Total daily dosage should not exceed 8 g. For endocarditis prophylaxis: 1 g 2 hours before procedure and 500 mg 6 hours later.

▷ **Conditions Requiring Dosing Adjustments:**

Liver function: This drug must be used with caution by patients with liver compromise. It should also be used with caution by patients with biliary tract disease.

Kidney function: Patients with severe kidney compromise can take 50 to 75% of the usual dose at the usual time. It is a rare cause of interstitial nephritis (inflammation of a specific part of the kidney).

▷ **How Best to Take This Medicine:** Nonenteric-coated preparations should be taken 1 hour before or 2 hours after eating. Enteric-coated preparations may be taken without regard to food. Regular uncoated capsules may be opened and tablets crushed for administration; coated and prolonged-action preparations should be swallowed whole. Ask your pharmacist for guidance.

▷ **How Long This Medicine Is Usually Taken:** Use on a regular schedule for 3 to 5 days usually determines this drug's effectiveness in controlling responsive infections. For streptococcal infections:

not less than 10 consecutive days (without interruption) to reduce the possibility of rheumatic fever or glomerulonephritis. The duration of use should not exceed the time required to eliminate the infection.

▷ **Tell Your Doctor Before Taking This Medicine If You:**
- ever had an allergic reaction to it.
- have active liver disease.
- are allergic by nature: hay fever, asthma, hives, eczema.
- previously have taken the estolate form of erythromycin.

▷ **Possible Side Effects:**   Superinfections.

▷ **Possible Adverse Effects:**
If any of the following develop, call your doctor promptly for guidance.

Some Mild Problems Drug Can Cause
Allergic reactions: skin rash, itching.
Nausea, vomiting, diarrhea, abdominal cramping.

Some Serious Problems Drug Can Cause
Allergic reaction: rare anaphylactic reaction.
Idiosyncratic reactions: liver reaction—nausea, vomiting, fever, jaundice (usually but not exclusively associated with erythromycin estolate).
Rare pancreatitis, decreased white blood cells, abnormal heart rhythm, low body temperature, or worsening of myasthenia gravis.
Drug-induced colitis, transient loss of hearing.

▷ *CAUTION*
1. Take the full dosage prescribed to prevent the possible emergence of resistant bacterial strains.
2. If you have a history of liver disease or impaired liver function, avoid any form of erythromycin estolate.
3. If diarrhea develops and continues for more than 24 hours, call your doctor promptly.
4. Watch allergic children closely for signs of allergy. Watch for evidence of gastrointestinal irritation.
5. People over 60 may be at increased risk for itching reactions in the genital and anal regions, often due to yeast superinfections. Watch for evidence of hearing loss. Report such developments promptly.

Advisability of Use During Pregnancy or If Breast-Feeding:
Pregnancy Category: B. Use of this drug is generally thought to be safe during entire pregnancy, *except for erythromycin estolate*; this form of erythromycin can cause toxic liver reactions during pregnancy and should be avoided. Present in breast milk. Monitor the nursing infant closely and discontinue this drug or nursing if adverse effects develop.

▷ **Overdose Symptoms:** Possible nausea, vomiting, diarrhea, and abdominal discomfort.

▷ **Suggested Periodic Examinations While Taking This Drug:** (at doctor's discretion)
Liver function tests if the estolate form is used.

▷ **While Taking This Drug the Following Apply:**
Beverages: Avoid fruit juices and carbonated beverages for 1 hour after taking any nonenteric-coated preparation. May be taken with milk.
Alcohol: Avoid if you have impaired liver function or are taking the estolate form of this drug.
Other Drugs:
Erythromycin may ***increase*** the effects of
- carbamazepine (Tegretol), causing toxicity.
- digoxin (Lanoxin), causing toxicity.
- ergotamine (Cafergot, Ergostat, etc.), causing impaired circulation to extremities.
- methylprednisolone (Medrol), causing excess steroid effects.
- theophylline (aminophylline, Theo-Dur, etc.), causing toxicity.
- warfarin (Coumadin), increasing the risk of bleeding.

Erythromycin may ***decrease*** the effects of
- clindamycin.
- penicillins.

Erythromycin ***taken concurrently*** with
- astemizole may lead to serious heart arrhythmias.
- oral contraceptives (birth control pills) can cause loss of effectiveness and result in pregnancy if another method is not substituted.
- cyclosporine (Sandimmune) may lead to cyclosporine toxicity.
- disopyramide (Norpace) can lead to arrhythmias.
- loratadine (Claritin) may result in increased blood levels, but does not appear to result in heart problems like some other nonsedating antihistamines.
- lovastatin may lead to serious muscle damage.
- midazolam may lead to excessive central nervous system depression.
- terfenadine (Seldane) may lead to serious heart arrhythmias.
- triazolam may lead to toxicity.
- trimetrexate may lead to toxic trimetrexate levels.
- valproic acid can lead to toxic valproic acid levels.

Driving, Hazardous Activities: This drug may cause nausea and/or diarrhea. Restrict your activities as necessary.
Special Storage Instructions: Keep liquid forms refrigerated.
Observe the Following Expiration Times: Freshly mixed oral suspension: 14 days. Premixed oral suspension: 18 months. Ask your pharmacist for guidance.

▷ **Saving Money When Using This Medicine:**

- Many antibiotics work similarly to this drug. Ask your doctor if this drug offers the best combination of price and outcome for you.
- Talk with your doctor about how soon you should experience a response to this medicine. Ask what to do if the expected beneficial response does not occur.

ESTROGENS (ES troh jenz)

Other Names: Chlorotrianisene, conjugated estrogens, esterified estrogens, estradiol, estriol, estrone, estropipate, quinestrol

Prescription Needed: Yes

Brand Names: DV, Estinyl, Estrace, Estraderm, Menrium [CD], Milprem [CD], Ogen, PMB [CD], Premarin, Premphase, Prempro, TACE, Vivelle

Overview of BENEFITS versus RISKS	
Possible Benefits	*Possible Risks*
EFFECTIVE RELIEF OF MENOPAUSAL HOT FLUSHES AND NIGHT SWEATS	INCREASED RISK OF CANCER OF THE UTERUS with 3+ years of continual use
PREVENTION OR RELIEF OF ATROPHIC VAGINITIS, ATROPHY OF THE VULVA AND URETHRA	INCREASED RISK OF BREAST CANCER (even if combined with a progesterone)
PREVENTION OF OSTEOPOROSIS	Increased frequency of gallstones
Prevention of thinning of the skin	Accelerated growth of preexisting fibroid tumors of the uterus
Mental tonic effect	Fluid retention
Prevention of postmenopausal cardiovascular disease	Postmenopausal bleeding
	Deep vein thrombophlebitis and thromboembolism (less likely with conjugated estrogens; more likely with synthetic unconjugated hormones)
	Increased blood pressure (rare)
	Decreased sugar tolerance (rare)

▷ **Illness This Medication Treats:**

(1) Ovarian failure or removal in young women; (2) menopausal syndrome; (3) postmenopausal atrophy of genital tissues; and (4) post-

menopausal osteoporosis. Also used in selected cases of breast cancer and prostate cancer.

As Combination Drug Product [CD]: Estrogen is available in combination with chlordiazepoxide (Librium) and meprobamate (Equanil, Miltown). These mild tranquilizers provide a calming effect that makes the combination more effective in selected cases of menopausal syndrome. See the oral contraceptives drug profile for a discussion of the combination of estrogens and progestins.

▷ **Typical Dosage Range:** (Dosage or schedule must be determined by the doctor for each individual.)

For conjugated and esterified estrogens: 0.3 to 1.25 mg daily for 21 days. Omit for 7 days. Repeat cyclically as needed. For other forms of estrogen: Consult your doctor. Patch forms may offer significant convenience.

▷ **Conditions Requiring Dosing Adjustments:**

Liver function: This drug should not be used by patients with acute or severe liver compromise. This drug can be lithogenic (capable of causing stones) to the bile.

Kidney function: Reduction in dosage is not defined for patients with kidney compromise.

▷ **How Best to Take This Medicine:** May be taken without regard to food. The tablets may be crushed for administration. The capsules should be taken whole.

▷ **How Long This Medicine Is Usually Taken:** Continual use on a regular schedule for 10 to 20 days is needed to see the effect of this drug in relieving menopausal symptoms. Long-term use requires supervision and periodic evaluation by your doctor every 6 months.

▷ **Tell Your Doctor Before Taking This Medicine If You:**
- ever have had an allergic reaction to it.
- have a history of thrombophlebitis, embolism, heart attack, or stroke.
- have seriously impaired liver function.
- have abnormal and unexplained vaginal bleeding.
- have sickle cell disease.
- are pregnant.
- had an unfavorable reaction to estrogen therapy.
- have a history of cancer of the breast or reproductive organs.
- have fibrocystic breast changes, fibroid tumors of the uterus, endometriosis, migrainelike headaches, blood clotting disorder, epilepsy, asthma, heart disease, high blood pressure, gallbladder disease, diabetes, or porphyria.
- smoke tobacco on a regular basis.
- plan to have surgery soon.

▷ **Possible Side Effects:** Fluid retention, weight gain, breakthrough
bleeding (spotting in middle of menstrual cycle), altered menstrual
pattern, resumption of menstrual flow after a period of natural cessation (postmenopausal bleeding), increased susceptibility to yeast
infection of the genital tissues.

▷ **Possible Adverse Effects:**
**If any of the following develop, call your doctor promptly for
guidance.**
Some Mild Problems Drug Can Cause
Allergic reactions: skin rash, hives, itching.
Headache, nervous tension, accentuation of migraine headaches.
Nausea, vomiting, bloating, diarrhea.
Tannish pigmentation of the face.
Some Serious Problems Drug Can Cause
Idiosyncratic reaction: cutaneous porphyria—fragile scarring of the
skin.
Emotional depression, rise in blood pressure.
Gallbladder disease, benign liver tumors, jaundice, rise in blood
sugar.
Erosion of uterine cervix, enlargement of uterine fibroid tumors.
Thrombophlebitis (vein inflammation and formation of blood clot).
Pulmonary embolism.
Stroke—headaches, blackouts, altered vision, slurred speech, in-
ability to speak.
Benign liver tumors.
Retinal thrombosis—sudden change or loss of vision.
Heart attack (blood clot in coronary artery)—sudden pain in chest,
neck, jaw, or arm; weakness; sweating; nausea.
Conjugated estrogens were not associated with increased relative
risk of breast cancer in one study.

▷ **Possible Effects on Sex Life:** Swelling and tenderness of breasts,
milk production.
Increased vaginal secretions.

▷ **Possible Delayed Adverse Effects:** Estrogens taken during pregnancy can predispose the female child to development of cancer of
the vagina or cervix following puberty.

▷ *CAUTION*
1. Estrogens should be taken in cycles of 3 weeks on, and 1 week off,
medication.
2. Estrogen vaginal creams can be absorbed systemically by the
woman, or through the penis during intercourse.
3. This drug is of very limited usefulness for people over 60; its use is
restricted to those women who are at increased risk for developing osteoporosis. Hot flushes should be treated with nonestro-

genic medications. If estrogen is used, report promptly any signs of impaired circulation: speech disturbances, altered vision, sudden hearing loss, vertigo, sudden weakness or paralysis, angina, leg pains.

4. Estrogens should NOT be used by patients with severe liver compromise.

Advisability of Use During Pregnancy or If Breast-Feeding:

Pregnancy Category: X. Estrogens taken during pregnancy can predispose the female child to cancer of the vagina or cervix following puberty. ***Avoid estrogens completely during entire pregnancy.*** Present in breast milk in very small amounts. High-dose estrogens suppress milk formation, although breast-feeding is considered to be safe while using estrogens.

▷ **Overdose Symptoms:** Headache, drowsiness, nausea, vomiting, fluid retention, abnormal vaginal bleeding, breast enlargement and discomfort.

▷ **Suggested Periodic Examinations While Taking This Drug:** (at doctor's discretion)

Regular (every 6 months) evaluation of the breasts and pelvic organs, including Pap smears. Liver function tests as indicated.

▷ **While Taking This Drug the Following Apply:**

Foods: Avoid excessive use of salt if fluid retention occurs.

Beverages: May be taken with milk.

Tobacco Smoking: Heavy smoking (15 or more cigarettes daily) with the use of estrogen-containing oral contraceptives significantly increases the risk of heart attack (coronary thrombosis). Avoid heavy smoking.

Other Drugs:

Estrogens *taken concurrently* with

- antidiabetic drugs may cause unpredictable fluctuations of blood sugar.
- oral hypoglycemic agents (see Drug Classes) may result in loss of sugar control.
- thyroid hormones may result in the need for increased thyroid dose.
- tricyclic antidepressants (Elavil, Sinequan, etc.) may enhance adverse effects and reduce their antidepressant effectiveness.
- vitamin C (ascorbic acid) may result in increased estrogen effects.
- warfarin (Coumadin) can alter prothrombin activity.

The following drugs may ***decrease*** the effects of estrogens

- carbamazepine (Tegretol).
- phenobarbital.
- phenytoin (Dilantin).
- primidone (Mysoline).
- rifampin (Rifadin, Rimactane).

Driving, Hazardous Activities: Usually no restrictions. See your doctor for assessment of individual risk and guidance.

Exposure to Sun: Use caution; estrogens can cause photosensitivity.

Discontinuation: It is advisable to discontinue usage of estrogens periodically to determine if they are still needed. Reduce the dose gradually to prevent acute withdrawal hot flushes. Stop usage altogether when a definite need for therapy no longer exists. Ask your doctor for guidance.

▷ **Saving Money When Using This Medicine:**
- Ask your doctor if this drug offers the best combination of price and outcome for you.
- Talk with your doctor about calcium supplements, exercise, periodic measures of height, and bone mineral density testing and osteoporosis.
- If this medicine is being used after menopause, talk with your doctor about adding progesterone.
- If you decide to start this medicine, ask your doctor if periodic checks of bone mineral density are a good idea.

ETHAMBUTOL (eth AM byu tohl)

Prescription Needed: Yes   **Controlled Drug:** No   **Generic:** No

Brand Names: Myambutol

Overview of BENEFITS versus RISKS	
Possible Benefits	*Possible Risks*
EFFECTIVE ADJUNCTIVE TREATMENT OF PULMONARY TUBERCULOSIS	RARE OPTIC NEURITIS WITH IMPAIRMENT OR LOSS OF VISION
EFFECTIVE ADJUNCTIVE TREATMENT OF AIDS-RELATED *MYCOBACTERIUM AVIUM-INTRACELLULARE* INFECTIONS	Rare peripheral neuritis Activation of gout
Possibly effective treatment of tuberculous meningitis	

▷ **Illness This Medication Treats:**
Pulmonary tuberculosis, in combination with other antitubercular drugs.

Other (unlabeled) generally accepted use: treatment of *Mycobacterium avium-intracellulare* complex in combination with other medicines.

▷ **Typical Dosage Range:** (Dosage or schedule must be determined by the doctor for each individual.)

Infants and Children: Dosage not established. Some authorities recommend that children under 6 years old not be given this drug.

13 to 60 Years of Age: For initial treatment of tuberculosis: 15 mg per kilogram of body weight, once daily. The total daily dose should not exceed 500 to 1500 mg.

For retreatment of tuberculosis: 25 mg per kilogram of body weight, once daily for 60 days; then 15 mg per kilogram of body weight. The total daily dose should not exceed 900 to 2500 mg.

For tuberculous meningitis or AIDS-related *Mycobacterium avium-intracellulare* (MAI) infections: 15 to 25 mg per kilogram of body weight, once daily.

Over 60 Years of Age: Same as for 13 to 60 years of age.

▷ **Conditions Requiring Dosing Adjustments:**

Liver function: No dosage decreases are anticipated for patients with mild to moderate hepatic (liver) compromise.

Kidney function: For patients with mild to moderate kidney failure, the usual dose can be taken every 24 to 36 hours. Patients with severe kidney failure may need only the usual dose every 48 hours.

▷ **How Best to Take This Medicine:** May be taken with food to reduce stomach irritation. The tablet may be crushed. Take the full course prescribed.

▷ **How Long This Medicine Is Usually Taken:** Use on a regular schedule for 4 to 6 weeks is needed to determine this drug's effectiveness in controlling infections. Long-term use (6 months to 2 or more years) requires periodic physician evaluation.

▷ **Tell Your Doctor Before Taking This Medicine If You:**
- ever had an allergic reaction to it.
- currently have optic or peripheral neuritis, or have a history of either.
- currently have active gout or a history of low blood platelets.
- have diabetes or a history of alcoholism.
- have impaired kidney function.

▷ **Possible Side Effects:** Increased blood level of uric acid and gouty arthritis.

▷ **Possible Adverse Effects:**
If any of the following develop, call your doctor promptly for guidance.

Some Mild Problems Drug Can Cause
   Allergic reactions: skin rash, itching, fever.
   Headache, confusion, disorientation.
   Loss of appetite, nausea, vomiting, stomach pain.
Some Serious Problems Drug Can Cause
   Allergic reactions: severe skin reactions, painful joints.
   Optic neuritis: eye pain, blurred vision, red–green color blindness.
   Peripheral neuritis: numbness, tingling.
   Rare hallucinations, low blood platelets or white blood cells.

▷ **Possible Delayed Adverse Effects:**   Optic neuritis may not occur until after many months of treatment. Visual loss may persist for up to a year after this drug is discontinued; rarely is visual loss permanent.

▷ **Natural Diseases or Disorders That May Be Activated by This Medicine:**   Latent gout.

▷ *CAUTION*
   1. Report promptly any changes in vision; these could indicate the onset of optic neuritis. Immediate evaluation is mandatory.
   2. Report promptly any unusual sensations in the hands or feet; these could indicate the onset of peripheral neuritis. Careful evaluation is advisable.
   3. Safety and effectiveness of this drug for those under 13 years old are not established.
   4. Those over 60 may be more likely to experience confusion or disorientation. Age-related decrease in kidney function may require adjustment of dosage.
   5. The dose must be decreased for patients with mild to moderate kidney failure.

   Advisability of Use During Pregnancy or If Breast-Feeding:
   Pregnancy Category: B. Use this drug only if clearly needed. Ask your doctor for guidance. Present in breast milk; avoid taking this drug or refrain from nursing.

▷ **Overdose Symptoms:**   Nausea, vomiting, stomach discomfort, confusion, possible blurred vision.

▷ **Suggested Periodic Examinations While Taking This Drug:** (at doctor's discretion)
   Complete eye examinations (including visual fields and color vision) should be performed before treatment is started, and then monthly during treatment.
   Blood uric acid levels.
   Liver and kidney function tests.

▷ **While Taking This Drug the Following Apply:**
   Foods: Follow your doctor's advice regarding high-purine foods.
   Beverages: Avoid excessively caffeinated coffee.

Other Drugs:
The following drugs may **decrease** the effects of ethambutol
- antacids containing aluminum salts—can slow and reduce the absorption of ethambutol.

Ethambutol **taken concurrently** with
- BCG vaccine may blunt the immune response from the vaccine.

Driving, Hazardous Activities: This drug may cause confusion, disorientation, and impaired vision. Restrict your activities as necessary.

Discontinuation: This drug is generally used for long-term treatment—months to years. Talk with your doctor regarding the appropriate time to consider discontinuation.

▷ **Saving Money When Using This Medicine:**
- There is an epidemic of resistant tuberculosis in this country. Therapy for resistant tuberculosis MUST combine several agents. Ask your doctor which combination of drugs offers the best balance of price and outcome for you.

ETHANOL (ETH an all)

Other Names: Nonprescription: Moonshine, alcohol, jack, white lightning, wine, beer, whiskey, vodka, etc.

Prescription Needed: Yes (for intravenous) **Controlled Drug:** No **Generic:** Yes (only generic IV available)

Brand Names:
Prescription: Tuss-Ornade (5%), Vicks 44D, Temaril (5.7%), Nyquil Nightime Cold Medicine, Novahistine DMX Liquid, Eskaphen B
Nonprescription: Robert Alison Chardonnay (12% by volume), Budweiser, Smirnoff (40% by volume), others

▷ **Warning:** The clinical use of this medication is limited to intravenous treatment of methanol and antifreeze (ethylene glycol) poisoning, and as a preservative. Past use has included treatment of premature labor (tocolytic).
This drug is widely used in its nonprescription form as an antianxiety agent, and may offer prevention of certain cardiovascular problems when used in moderation.

```
┌─────────────────────────────────────────────────────────────┐
│              Overview of BENEFITS versus RISKS              │
│      Possible Benefits              Possible Risks          │
│  EFFECTIVE TREATMENT OF         WITHDRAWAL SYMPTOMS         │
│    POISONING                    SEIZURES                    │
│  MODERATE USE MAY               LIVER DAMAGE (with          │
│    PREVENT SOME HEART             prolonged use)            │
│    PROBLEMS                     Pancreatitis                │
│                                 Encephalopathy              │
│                                 Low white blood cell counts │
│                                   and anemia                │
│                                 Myopathy                    │
└─────────────────────────────────────────────────────────────┘
```

▷ **Illness This Medication Treats:**
Supplementation of caloric intake (intravenously) in very specific cases.
Other (unlabeled) generally accepted uses: (1) treatment of methanol or antifreeze (ethylene glycol) poisoning; (2) adjunctive treatment of cancer pain; (3) intravenous treatment of DTs (delirium tremens) (4) sclerosing esophageal varices and stopping bleeding; (5) treatment of hepatocellular cancer where severe liver problems preclude surgery; (6) sclerosing thyroid cysts; (7) destruction of nerve tissue (neurolytic block) in chronic pain therapy; (8) in nonprescription form for antianxiety; (9) recent data appears to show that use ranging up to moderate (no greater than 0.7 mg per kilogram of body weight for 3 days in a row) may actually help PREVENT coronary heart disease and heart attacks.

As Combination Drug Product [CD]: Ethanol is widely present in elixirs and other liquid vehicles for drugs as a preservative, and partial drug action enhancer.

Warning: Some people may experience no mental or physical changes even though a breath or blood alcohol level shows they are "legally drunk."

Nonprescription form: Each ounce of 100 proof whiskey has 15 ml of ethanol; 6 oz (12%) wine has 22 ml of ethanol; 12 oz of beer (4.9%) has 18 ml of ethanol.

▷ **Typical Dosage Range:** (Dosage or schedule must be determined by the doctor for each individual.)
Infants and Children: Methanol or ethylene glycol poisoning: 40 ml per kilogram of body weight per day.
18 to 60 Years of Age: Methanol or ethylene glycol poisoning: A loading dose of 0.6 mg per kilogram of body weight is given, followed by 109 to 125 mg per kilogram of body weight per hour to maintain a blood level of 100 mg/dl.
Over 60 Years of Age: Same as for 12 to 60 years of age for poisonings.

The amount consumed versus the collective mental and physical effects may decrease in older people for the nonprescription products—that is, it takes less to get drunk. It generally takes a milder dose to cause an equal or greater change in coordination or mental ability. There is also an increased risk of hypothermia.

▷ **Conditions Requiring Dosing Adjustments:**
Liver function: Ethanol is extensively changed in the liver to acetaldehyde and acetyl CoA. The drug is also a clear cause of liver toxicity. The dose must be decreased for patients with liver compromise.
Kidney function: The kidney is minimally involved in the elimination of this drug, and no dosing changes are needed.

▷ **How Best to Take This Medicine:**   If methanol or ethylene glycol poisoning is suspected: The nearest poison control center should be contacted, and oral dosing (use of a strong vodka mixed in orange juice) may be of benefit, depending on your distance from a hospital or freestanding emergency center.

For nonprescription antianxiety use: The specific dose of this drug and the resulting blood level of alcohol depends on many factors; however, the most important ones are the person's weight, the metabolic activity of the liver, food content in the stomach, the strength of the alcohol in the consumed beverage, the number of drinks consumed over a given period of time, and how well-hydrated (whether there has been extreme exercise and fluid loss) the person is. Again, although a blood or breath alcohol level may be a marker for mental or physical changes, some people may have no physical or mental changes and still have a blood or breath alcohol level in the state-defined range of "legally drunk."

Each 10 ml of ethanol increases the blood ethanol level of an average 150 lb (70-kg) man by 16.6 mg % (3.6 mm/l). The legal definition of intoxication is a blood alcohol level of 0.10, or 100 mg/dl. "Under the influence" in Maryland is 0.07, or 70 mg/dl. Driving impairment may occur at blood levels of 0.05 (50 mg/dl) or lower.

▷ **How Long This Medicine Is Usually Taken:**   Use on a regular schedule for 48 hours determines the effectiveness of this drug for methanol overdose. Long-term use of ethanol as an antianxiety agent is NOT recommended.

▷ **Tell Your Doctor Before Taking This Medicine If You:**
- ever had an allergic reaction to it.
- have epilepsy.
- have a history of alcohol addiction.
- have liver or kidney compromise.
- have gout.
- are prone to low blood sugars or have a urinary tract infection.

- have diabetes or have suffered a diabetic coma.
- have congestive heart failure.

▷ **Possible Side Effects:**   Intoxication; perception, coordination, and mood changes.

▷ **Possible Adverse Effects:**
If any of the following develop, call your doctor promptly for guidance.
Some Mild Problems Drug Can Cause
  Allergic reactions: itching, rash, hives, and flushing.
  Headache.
  Hangover: nausea, headache, malaise.
  Sedation (dose-dependent).
  Disorientation.
  Color blindness (with chronic use).
  Neuropathy (tingling, burning, or numbness).
  Memory loss.
  Vitamin deficiency.
  Stomach irritation.
Some Serious Problems This Drug Can Cause
  Allergic reactions: anaphylaxis—rash, swelling of tongue, breathing problems, flushing.
  Bronchospasm (asthmatics at increased risk).
  Respiratory depression.
  Elevated or decreased white blood cell count.
  Increased or decreased platelets.
  Anemia (megaloblastic with chronic use).
  Heart dysfunction (myopathy with chronic use).
  High blood pressure.
  Abnormal heart rhythms (atrial and ventricular).
  Chest pain (angina).
  Liver toxicity (cirrhosis with chronic use).
  Osteoporosis (with chronic use).
  Pancreatitis.
  Encephalopathy (with chronic use).
  Cerebrovascular bleeding (dose-dependent).
  Low blood sugar (especially if meals are missed).
  Ketoacidosis (with chronic use).
  Vitamin deficiency with chronic use (folic acid, vitamin B1 and B6).
  Low magnesium (with chronic use).
  Low potassium (especially with acute intoxication in children).
  Gout (precipitated by alcohol use in those with gout).
  Tolerance (with chronic use).
  Withdrawal: nausea, fever, rapid heart rate, hallucinations.

May progress to DTs (delirium tremens): profound confusion, hallucinations, etc.

▷ **Possible Effects on Sex Life:** Decreased libido, impotence (with excessive chronic use). Difficulty achieving an erection in males and decreased vaginal dilation in females. Chronic alcohol use may lead to tenderness and swelling of male and female breast tissue, testicular atrophy, low sperm counts, decreased menstrual blood flow, and diminished capability for orgasm in females.

▷ **Possible Delayed Adverse Effects:** Liver toxicity, anemia, low or high platelets, vitamin deficiency.

▷ *CAUTION*

1. This drug in its nonprescription form may cause fatal increases in blood pressure if combined with cocaine.
2. With high doses (nearly pure grain alcohol) or many drinks (frequent dosing) over a short period of time, fatal blood alcohol levels may be reached with the nonprescription form.
3. Safety and effectiveness of this drug for those under 12 years old are not established. Accidental and unsupervised drinking of the nonprescription form or liquids—such as mouthwash with high alcohol content—may have severe consequences in children. Alcohol found in mouthwash or perfume may poison small children. Seriously low blood sugar may occur up to 6 hours after drinking. Low potassium may also occur with high ethanol levels. Therapy is guided by blood sugar, potassium, and blood alcohol (ethanol) levels. Fatality caused by low blood sugar was reported in a 4-year-old child who drank 12 oz of a mouthwash containing 10% ethanol.
4. For those over 60, poisoning from methanol or ethylene glycol is an emergency situation, and although their sensitivity to effects may increase, dosing is adjusted to blood levels. The nonprescription form dosage (number of drinks) tolerated would be expected to decrease with increasing age. Again, some people may have blood or breath alcohol levels in the "legally drunk" range and still have no symptoms.

Advisability of Use During Pregnancy or If Breast-Feeding:
Pregnancy Category: D, X if used for long periods. Avoid use of ethanol during your ENTIRE pregnancy. Present in breast milk; avoid using this drug or refrain from nursing.

▷ **Habit-Forming Potential:** Clearly defined alcoholism exists and occurs.

▷ **Overdose Symptoms:** Toxic levels result in ataxia, loss of consciousness progressing to coma, anesthesia, respiratory failure, and death. Levels of 150–300 mg/dl may result in exaggerated emotional states, confusion, and incoordination. Fatalities most often result with blood concentrations greater than 400 mg/dl. Fatal blood levels vary greatly, however, and death has been reported following levels as low as 260 mg/dl. Again, some people have no mental or physical changes with an alcohol level in the "legally drunk" range.

▷ **Suggested Periodic Examinations While Taking This Drug:** (at doctor's discretion)

Blood alcohol levels and methanol or ethylene glycol levels guide therapy in poisonings.

Chronic alcohol abuse: complete blood counts, liver function tests, amylase and lipase, electrocardiograms.

▷ **While Taking This Drug the Following Apply:**

Nutritional Support: Vitamin support, particularly thiamine (B1), folic acid, and B6, is needed with chronic use. Magnesium replacement is also needed.

Marijuana Smoking: Additive central nervous system depression.

Other Drugs:

Ethanol may *increase* the effects of

- central nervous system depressants such as benzodiazepines, barbiturates, opioids, and anesthetic agents.
- chlorpromazine (Thorazine), resulting in increased sedation.
- cocaine, resulting in dangerous increases in blood pressure.
- cyclosporine (Sandimmune) if taken with ethanol in large doses.
- diphenhydramine (Benadryl, others), increasing sedation.
- warfarin (Coumadin) and requires more frequent INR (prothrombin time) testing.

Ethanol may *decrease* the effects of

- phenytoin (Dilantin) by reducing blood phenytoin levels.
- propranolol (Inderal) by increasing propranolol elimination.

Ethanol *taken concurrently* with

- acetaminophen (Tylenol) poses an increased risk of liver damage.
- some antihistamines can pose an increased risk of sedation.
- aspirin and potentially other NSAIDs (see Drug Classes) may result in increased blood loss from the stomach.
- cefamandole (Mandol), cefotetan (Cefotan), metronidazole (Flagyl), and cefoperazone (Cefobid) may result in disulfiramlike reaction.
- cimetidine (Tagamet) may decrease the amount of alcohol it takes to get drunk.
- disulfiram (Antabuse) will result in severe vomiting and intolerance.
- griseofulvin can increase the effects of alcohol.
- insulin may result in potential severe hypoglycemia.
- isoniazid may result in elevated isoniazid levels.
- ketoconazole may result in disulfiramlike reactions.

- lithium (Lithobid) may result in worsened incoordination and intoxication.
- methotrexate may increase risk of liver damage.
- nitroglycerin (Nitrostat, others) may result in excessive decreases in blood pressure.
- oral hypoglycemic agents (see Drug Classes) poses an increased risk of seriously low glucose levels.
- tricyclic antidepressants may result in increased antidepressant levels and toxicity.
- verapamil (Calan, others) may increase the amount of time ethanol stays in the body.

Driving, Hazardous Activities: Ethanol may cause drowsiness, mental impairment, and coordination problems. Driving skill may be impaired at very low blood levels, with the perception that capabilities are NOT reduced. Drinking and driving are NOT recommended. Restrict your activities as necessary.

Exposure to Sun: May result in additive dehydration.

Heavy Exercise or Exertion: May worsen the adverse effects of this drug.

Discontinuation: Abrupt discontinuation after chronic use of this drug may result in a serious withdrawal syndrome known as delirium tremens (DTs).

▷ **Saving Money When Using This Medicine:**

- As an antidote for antifreeze or methanol poisoning, there is no other option to ethanol.
- Many medications are available to treat anxiety and help with life-crisis situations. Ask your doctor for an alternative that provides the best combination of cost and outcome for you.
- If you recognize a developing dependence on alcohol, ask your doctor for help immediately. The serious side effects occur particularly with long-term use.

ETHOSUXIMIDE (eth oh SUX i mide)

Prescription Needed: Yes   **Controlled Drug:** No   **Generic:** No

Brand Names: Zarontin

Overview of BENEFITS versus RISKS

Possible Benefits	*Possible Risks*
EFFECTIVE CONTROL OF ABSENCE SEIZURES (PETIT MAL EPILEPSY) EFFECTIVE CONTROL OF MYOCLONIC AND AKINETIC EPILEPSY	RARE APLASTIC ANEMIA Rare decrease in white blood cells and blood platelets

---

▷ **Illness This Medication Treats:**
Petit mal epilepsy; a drug of choice in absence seizures.

▷ **Typical Dosage Range:** (Dosage or schedule must be determined by the doctor for each individual.)
20 to 40 mg per kilogram of body weight every 24 hours. Initially 500 mg/24 hr. Dosage may be increased cautiously by 250 mg every 4 to 7 days until satisfactory control is achieved. The total daily dosage should not exceed 1500 mg. Blood levels increase more quickly in females (using the same dose) than males.

▷ **Conditions Requiring Dosing Adjustments:**
Liver function: Blood levels are recommended if this medication is used by patients with liver compromise.
Kidney function: Dose must be adjusted for patients with severe kidney failure, and only 75% of the usual dose taken.

▷ **How Best to Take This Medicine:** May be taken with food to reduce stomach irritation. Capsule may be opened for administration.

▷ **How Long This Medicine Is Usually Taken:** Use on a regular schedule for 1 to 2 weeks usually determines the effectiveness of this drug in reducing the frequency of absence seizures. Long-term use requires supervision and periodic evaluation by your doctor.

▷ **Tell Your Doctor Before Taking This Medicine If You:**
• are allergic to this or any other succinimide drug.
• have active liver disease.
• currently have a blood cell or bone marrow disorder.
• have a history of liver or kidney disease.
• have any blood disorder, especially one caused by drugs.
• have a history of serious depression or other mental illness.

▷ **Possible Side Effects:**   Drowsiness, lethargy, fatigue.

▷ **Possible Adverse Effects:**
If any of the following develop, call your doctor promptly for guidance.
Some Mild Problems Drug Can Cause
Allergic reactions: skin rash, hives.
Headache, dizziness, euphoria, impaired vision, numbness and tingling in extremities.
Loss of appetite, nausea, vomiting, hiccups, diarrhea.
Excessive growth of hair.
Some Serious Problems Drug Can Cause
Allergic reaction: swelling of tongue.
Thickening and overgrowth of gums.
Nervousness, hyperactivity, disturbed sleep, night terrors.
Aggravation of emotional depression and paranoid mental disorders.
Severe bone marrow depression.

▷ **Possible Effects on Sex Life:**   Increased libido (questionable); non-menstrual vaginal bleeding.

▷ *CAUTION*
1. This drug may increase the frequency of grand mal seizures in individuals with mixed seizure disorders.
2. Compliance with your doctor's request for periodic blood counts and other tests deemed necessary is mandatory.
3. If a single daily dose causes nausea or vomiting in infants or children, give in two or three divided doses 8 to 12 hours apart. Marked individual variation in response occurs; the use of blood levels for monitoring is advised. Observe for a possible lupuslike reaction: fever, rash, arthritis.
4. This drug is rarely prescribed for those over 60 years old.

Advisability of Use During Pregnancy or If Breast-Feeding:
Pregnancy Category: C. Avoid using this drug during the first 3 months. Use only if clearly needed during the last 6 months. Present in breast milk. Monitor the nursing infant closely and discontinue drug or nursing if adverse effects develop. If the mother requires high doses, she should refrain from nursing. Ask your doctor for guidance.

▷ **Overdose Symptoms:**   Increased drowsiness, lethargy, weakness, dizziness, unsteadiness, nausea, vomiting, stupor progressing to coma.

▷ **Suggested Periodic Examinations While Taking This Drug:** (at doctor's discretion)
Complete blood cell counts every 2 weeks during the first month of use, then monthly thereafter; liver and kidney function tests.

▷ **While Taking This Drug the Following Apply:**

Beverages: May be taken with milk.

Alcohol: Caution—this drug may increase the sedative effects of alcohol. Excessive alcohol may precipitate seizures.

Other Drugs:

Ethosuximide may ***increase*** the effects of
- phenytoin (Dilantin) by slowing its elimination.

Ethosuximide ***taken concurrently*** with
- carbamazepine (Tegretol) may change ethosuximide levels.
- phenobarbital may decrease seizure control.
- valproic acid (Depakene) may alter the effects of ethosuximide unpredictably.

The following drug may ***increase*** the effects of ethosuximide
- isoniazid (INH, Niconyl, etc.).

Driving, Hazardous Activities: This drug may cause drowsiness, dizziness, unsteadiness, and impaired vision. Restrict your activities as necessary.

Discontinuation: Do not stop taking this drug abruptly. Ask your doctor for guidance regarding gradual reduction of dosage.

▷ **Saving Money When Using This Medicine:**
- Many medications are available to treat seizures. Ask your doctor for an alternative that provides the best combination of cost and outcome for you.
- It may be possible (after a significant seizure-free period) to discontinue this medicine. Ask your doctor for help.
- Blood levels are expensive. Talk with your doctor to ensure they are obtained at prudent, not excessive, intervals.
- A new medicine called gabapentin is available as add-on therapy. Ask your doctor if this medicine could be of help if your seizures are not well controlled.

ETIDRONATE (e ti DROH nate)

Prescription Needed: Yes   **Controlled Drug:** No   **Generic:** No

Brand Names: Didronel

Overview of BENEFITS versus RISKS

Possible Benefits	*Possible Risks*
PARTIAL RELIEF OF SYMPTOMS OF PAGET'S DISEASE OF BONE	Increased bone pain
	Bone fractures
EFFECTIVE PREVENTION AND TREATMENT OF ABNORMAL CALCIFICATION	Kidney failure
	Focal osteomalacia
Effective adjunctive treatment of abnormally high blood calcium levels (associated with malignant disease)	
Treatment of postmenopausal osteoporosis	

▷ **Illness This Medication Treats:**

(1) Symptomatic Paget's disease of bone (excessive bone growth of skull, spine, and long bones); (2) prevention and treatment of abnormal bone formation following total hip replacement or spinal cord injury; (3) adjunctive treatment of excessively high blood calcium levels due to malignant bone disease.

Other (unlabeled) generally accepted uses: treatment of postmenopausal osteoporosis (newer agents may have supplanted this use).

▷ **Typical Dosage Range:** (Dosage or schedule must be determined by the doctor for each individual.)

Infants and Children: Dosage not established.

12 to 60 Years of Age: For Paget's disease: Initially 5 mg per kilogram of body weight daily, as a single dose, for 6 months. Discontinue for a drug-free period of 6 months. As needed, repeat the alternating 6-month courses of drug treatment and drug abstention.

For ossification associated with hip replacement: 20 mg per kilogram of body weight daily for 1 month before and 3 months after surgery.

For ossification associated with spinal cord injury: Initially 20 mg per kilogram of body weight daily for 2 weeks after injury; then decrease dose to 10 mg per kilogram of body weight daily for an additional 10 weeks.

For high blood calcium associated with malignant bone disease: 20 mg per kilogram of body weight daily for 30 days; if needed and tolerated, continue for a maximum of 90 days.

The total daily dose should not exceed 20 mg per kilogram of body weight.

Over 60 Years of Age: Same as for 12 to 60 years of age.

▷ **Conditions Requiring Dosing Adjustments:**

Liver function: This drug is not known to be metabolized in the liver.

Kidney function: Patients with steady-state creatinines greater than 2.5 mg/min should use this drug with caution, if at all.

▷ **How Best to Take This Medicine:**   Take with water on an empty stomach 2 hours before or after food. Suggested times: on arising, midmorning, or at bedtime. Do not take with milk. If nausea or diarrhea occurs, the daily dose may be divided into two or three portions. The tablet may be crushed.

▷ **How Long This Medicine Is Usually Taken:**   Use on a regular schedule for 1 to 3 months usually determines the effectiveness of this drug for relieving the symptoms of Paget's disease. If it is effective, the standard course of treatment is 6 months. Long-term use (months to years) requires periodic physician evaluation.

▷ **Tell Your Doctor Before Taking This Medicine If You:**
- ever had an allergic reaction to it.
- recently fractured a bone that has not healed completely.
- have a history of heart disease, especially congestive heart failure.
- have impaired kidney function.
- are subject to enterocolitis or recurrent diarrhea.

▷ **Possible Side Effects:**   Increased bone pain or tenderness (usually beginning within 4 to 6 weeks after starting treatment).

▷ **Possible Adverse Effects:**

If any of the following develop, call your doctor promptly for guidance.

Some Mild Problems Drug Can Cause

Allergic reactions: skin rash, hives, itching.

Nausea, diarrhea.

Some Serious Problems Drug Can Cause

Allergic reactions: angioedema (swelling of face, lips, tongue, throat, and/or vocal cords); may be life-threatening.

Osteomalacia (thinning and weakening of bone) with fractures.

Rare ulcers or kidney failure.

▷ *CAUTION*

1. Maintain a well-balanced diet with adequate calcium and vitamin D content.

2. Mineral supplements and drugs containing aluminum, calcium, iron, or magnesium can prevent absorption; separate their intake and etidronate dosage by at least 2 hours.

3. Tell your doctor if nausea or diarrhea persists; dosage adjustment (multiple small doses) can correct this.

4. Tell your doctor if bone pain persists or increases while taking this drug.

5. Large doses or prolonged use in infants and children should be avoided to reduce the possibility of rickets.

6. Those over 60 should watch their fluid balance carefully if this drug is taken intravenously to lower blood calcium levels.

Advisability of Use During Pregnancy or If Breast-Feeding:

Pregnancy Category: C. Use this drug only if clearly needed. Ask your doctor for guidance. Presence in breast milk is unknown; avoid taking this drug or refrain from nursing.

▷ **Overdose Symptoms:** Nausea, vomiting, diarrhea.

▷ **Suggested Periodic Examinations While Taking This Drug:** (at doctor's discretion)

Measurements of blood calcium, phosphate, and alkaline phosphatase levels.

Measurement of urine hydroxyproline content.

Kidney function tests.

Bone mineral density tests.

▷ **While Taking This Drug the Following Apply:**

Foods: Avoid all foods, especially dairy products, for 2 hours before and after taking this drug.

Nutritional Support: Ensure adequate intake of calcium and vitamin D.

Beverages: Take this drug with water. Avoid all forms of milk for 2 hours before and after taking this drug.

Other Drugs:

The following drugs may *decrease* the effects of etidronate
• all antacids containing aluminum, calcium, or magnesium.
• all iron preparations.

Etidronate *taken concurrently* with
• foscarnet (Foscavir) may lead to additive decreases in calcium.
• plicamycin may lead to additive calcium decreases.

Discontinuation: Adhere strictly to the time schedules given under "Typical Dosage Range," above. Your doctor should determine when to discontinue this drug.

▷ **Saving Money When Using This Medicine:**

• Ask your doctor if this drug provides the best combination of cost and outcome for you.

• If this medicine is used for postmenopausal osteoporosis, ask your doctor if the newer agents may lead to better outcomes.

ETODOLAC (e TOE do lak)

Prescription Needed: Yes   **Controlled Drug:** No   **Generic:** No

Brand Names: Lodine

Overview of BENEFITS versus RISKS	
Possible Benefits	*Possible Risks*
EFFECTIVE TREATMENT OF MILD TO MODERATE INFLAMMATION AND PAIN DECREASED GASTROINTESTINAL BLEEDING RISK	Gastrointestinal pain, ulceration, or bleeding (rare) Blood cell disorders: low platelet counts, anemia (rare) Fluid retention Rare kidney damage Rare liver damage Hearing toxicity

See the acetic acids (NSAIDs) drug profile for further information.

ETRETINATE (e TRET i nayt)

Prescription Needed: Yes   **Controlled Drug:** No   **Generic:** No

Brand Names: Tegison

Overview of BENEFITS versus RISKS	
Possible Benefits	*Possible Risks*
EFFECTIVE TREATMENT FOR SEVERE, RESISTANT PSORIASIS in most treated cases	MAJOR DRUG-INDUCED BIRTH DEFECTS DRUG-INDUCED HEPATITIS (rare) Adverse effects on eyes and vision; musculoskeletal structures; blood cholesterol and triglycerides Increased intracranial pressure (very rare) Delayed blood clotting (partial thromboplastin time [PTT] extended)

▷ **Illness This Medication Treats:**
   Severe, generalized forms of psoriasis (and related skin disorders) that
   have failed to respond to conventional, less hazardous treatments.

▷ **Typical Dosage Range:** (Dosage or schedule must be determined by the doctor for each individual.)

Initially 1 mg per kilogram of body weight per day, in divided doses, until satisfactory response is obtained (usually 8 to 16 weeks). Maintenance: 0.5 to 0.75 mg per kilogram of body weight per day, beginning after initial response. Total daily dosage should not exceed 1.5 mg per kilogram of body weight per day.

▷ **Conditions Requiring Dosing Adjustments:**

Liver function: This drug is a rare cause of hepatitis. It should be used with caution by patients with liver compromise, and the dose decreased.

Kidney function: This drug is a rare cause of nephrotoxicity. It should be used with caution by patients with compromised kidneys.

▷ **How Best to Take This Medicine:** Take with or immediately following meals, preferably with whole milk. Do not suck or chew the capsule; swallow it whole.

▷ **How Long This Medicine Is Usually Taken:** Use on a regular schedule for 2 to 4 weeks is usually necessary to determine this drug's effectiveness in reversing the skin changes of psoriasis. The full effect of treatment may not be apparent until after 2 to 3 months of continual use. Long-term use (months to years) requires periodic physician evaluation. Due to the potential for drug accumulation and toxicity with long-term use, this drug should be temporarily discontinued after 18 months; it may be resumed as needed.

▷ **Tell Your Doctor Before Taking This Medicine If You:**
- ever had an allergic reaction to it.
- are pregnant or breast-feeding.
- plan to donate blood in the near future.
- are allergic to vitamin A or other vitamin A derivatives: isotretinoin (Accutane), tretinoin (Retin-A).
- are allergic to parabens (preservatives).
- have cerebral or coronary artery disease.
- have high cholesterol or triglyceride blood levels.
- have diabetes.
- have impaired liver or kidney function.
- are an alcoholic.
- find your night vision is critical to you.
- have a history of Crohn's disease or ulcerative colitis.

▷ **Possible Side Effects:** Dry nose, nosebleeds, dry lips, sore mouth and tongue, bleeding gums.

Loss of hair, skin peeling of hands and feet, dry skin, itching, bruising, nail deformities.

Thickening of bone (hyperostosis), calcification of tendons and ligaments, bone and joint pain.

▷ **Possible Adverse Effects:**
If any of the following develop, call your doctor promptly for guidance.
Some Mild Problems Drug Can Cause
Allergic reactions: skin rash, itching.
Headache, dizziness, fatigue, fever, irritability.
Eye irritation, blurred vision, sensitivity to bright light, decreased tolerance for contact lenses, earache, impaired hearing.
Altered taste, loss of appetite, nausea, constipation, diarrhea.
Painful urination.
Some Serious Problems Drug Can Cause
Increased intracranial pressure; headache, nausea, vomiting, visual disturbances.
Hepatitis; some reported deaths worldwide.
Nephrotoxicity (kidney) (very rare).
Eye reactions: corneal erosion, abrasion, staining; cataract; retinal hemorrhage; visual field defects; reduced night vision.
Inflammatory bowel disease (Crohn's disease), rare.
Altered blood fat levels: increased triglycerides and total cholesterol; decreased HDL cholesterol. Any of these changes may increase the risk for the development of atherosclerotic heart disease.
Rare lowering of blood platelets.
Ear toxicity (ototoxicity).

▷ **Possible Effects on Sex Life:**   Altered timing and pattern of menstruation, loss of libido, erectile problems.

▷ **Possible Delayed Adverse Effects:**   This drug has been found in the blood 2.9 years following termination of its use and potentially induces birth defects during this time. It has not been determined how long pregnancy should be avoided after discontinuation of treatment.

▷ **CAUTION**
1. *This drug should not be taken during pregnancy.* A pregnancy test should be performed within 2 weeks prior to taking this drug. In the absence of pregnancy, the drug should be started on the second or third day of the next normal menstrual period. An effective form of contraception should be used for 1 month before the drug is started, during the entire period of treatment, and for an indefinite period (minimum of 3 years) after the drug is discontinued. If pregnancy does occur, stop taking this drug immediately and call your doctor.
2. *Do not donate blood to a blood bank if you are taking this drug.* Blood containing this drug could pose a serious risk to the devel-

oping fetus of a pregnant patient. Avoid blood donation for a minimum of 3 years if use of the blood is beyond your control.

3. ***Comply fully with your doctor's recommendations for periodic examinations before, during, and following treatment with this drug.*** These are mandatory for safe and effective use.

4. Avoid the concurrent use of vitamin A supplements.

5. If you experience significant eye reactions or altered vision, call your doctor promptly.

6. It is common for psoriasis to appear to worsen during the early period of treatment. Call your doctor if symptoms become severe or prolonged.

7. If dry mouth or sore and bleeding gums persist, consult your dentist.

8. This drug should be used by children only after all less hazardous treatments have failed. It is advisable to obtain pretreatment X rays to determine bone age and monitor bone growth and development by yearly X-ray studies. This drug can impair normal bone maturation.

9. Those over 60 should watch for anemia, impaired kidney function, and fluctuating blood potassium levels.

Advisability of Use During Pregnancy or If Breast-Feeding:
Pregnancy Category: X. Avoid using this drug completely during entire pregnancy. See *"CAUTION"* above. Presence in breast milk is unknown; avoid taking this drug or refrain from nursing.

▷ **Overdose Symptoms:** Severe headache, irritability, drowsiness, itching, nausea, vomiting.

▷ **Suggested Periodic Examinations While Taking This Drug:** (at doctor's discretion)
Complete blood cell counts; measurements of blood sugar, potassium, sodium, and chloride.
Blood cholesterol profiles, before and during treatment.
Liver and kidney function tests.
Complete eye examinations.
Bone X rays, especially for children.

▷ **While Taking This Drug the Following Apply:**
Foods: High-fat foods increase absorption of this drug.
Beverages: No restrictions. Whole milk increases absorption of this drug.
Alcohol: Use moderately; excessive intake can increase blood triglyceride levels.
Other Drugs:
Etretinate may ***increase*** the effects of
• vitamin A and its derivatives (isotretinoin and tretinoin) and increase the risk of vitamin A toxicity.

Etretinate *taken concurrently* with

- carbamazepine (Tegretol) may result in decreased etretinate effectiveness.
- methotrexate may increase the risk of liver toxicity.
- tetracyclines may increase the risk of elevated intracranial pressure.
- warfarin (Coumadin) may decrease the effectiveness of warfarin.

Driving, Hazardous Activities: This drug may cause dizziness and blurred vision. Restrict your activities as necessary.

Exposure to Sun: Use caution; this drug can cause photosensitivity.

Discontinuation: If this drug is not significantly beneficial after 4 months of continual use, its use should be stopped. If the response is adequate to justify its long-term use, it should be discontinued temporarily ("drug holiday") after 18 months of continual treatment. Once the skin has cleared satisfactorily, this drug should be discontinued. Most people experience some recurrence after 2 months. Subsequent treatment courses of 4 to 9 months can be instituted as required.

▷ **Saving Money When Using This Medicine:**

- Ask your doctor if this drug offers the best combination of cost and outcome for you.
- Discuss the use of less toxic agents before this medicine is considered.

FAMCICLOVIR (fam SEYE klo veer)

Prescription Needed: Yes   **Controlled Drug:** No   **Generic:** No

Brand Names: Famvir

Overview of BENEFITS versus RISKS

Possible Benefits	*Possible Risks*
EFFECTIVE TREATMENT OF HERPES ZOSTER (SHINGLES)	Diarrhea
	Purpura
	Paresthesias
TREATS AN INFECTION THAT MAY BE LIFE-THREATENING IN AIDS AND MARROW TRANSPLANT PATIENTS	
TREATS RECURRENT GENITAL HERPES	

▷ **Illness This Medication Treats:**

(1) Acute herpes zoster (shingles); (2) recurrent genital herpes.

▷ **Typical Dosage Range:** (Dosage or schedule must be determined by the doctor for each individual.)

Infants and Children: Safety and efficacy of this drug for those under 18 years old are not established.

18 to 60 Years of Age: 500 mg is taken every 8 hours for 7 days. It is important to start this medicine promptly after the diagnosis is made.

For recurrent genital herpes: 125 mg twice daily for 5 days.

Over 60 Years of Age: Same as for 12 to 60 years of age.

▷ **Conditions Requiring Dosing Adjustments:**

Liver function: No dose changes are needed for patients with well-compensated liver impairment.

Kidney function: People with moderate compromise should take 500 mg/12 hr. Patients with severe compromise only need 500 mg once a day.

▷ **How Best to Take This Medicine:** Use on a regular schedule for 2 days usually determines this drug's effectiveness in treating herpes zoster, and the medicine is usually taken for 7 days. Physician evaluation is needed to determine when this medicine should be stopped.

▷ **Tell Your Doctor Before Taking This Medicine If You:**

- ever had an allergic reaction to it.
- have a history of liver or kidney problems.
- know your immune system is compromised.

▷ **Possible Adverse Effects:**
If any of the following develop, call your doctor promptly for guidance.
Some Mild Problems Drug Can Cause
  Allergic reactions: itching
  Diarrhea.
  Headache.
  Nausea.
  Paresthesias.
Some Serious Problems Drug Can Cause
  Allergic reactions: unknown.
  Purpura.
  Rigors.

▷ *CAUTION*
  1. The best effect is achieved if this drug is started very soon after the condition is diagnosed.
  2. Safety and effectiveness of this drug for those under 18 years old are not established.
  3. This drug MUST be adjusted for patients with moderate to severe kidney compromise. Ask your doctor if your dose has been appropriately adjusted.

Advisability of Use During Pregnancy or If Breast-Feeding:
Pregnancy Category: B. Adequate studies of pregnant women are not available. Presence in breast milk is unknown; avoid using this drug or refrain from nursing.

▷ **While Taking This Drug the Following Apply:**   *Driving, Hazardous Activities:* This drug may cause dizziness or fatigue. Restrict your activities as necessary.

▷ **Saving Money When Using This Medicine:**
  • Pain after a shingles infection is often very intense. By decreasing the length of time and severity of pain, this drug saves money.
  • Ask your doctor if this drug provides the best combination of cost and outcome for you.
  • The best approach is to prevent this illness. Since shingles actually results from an earlier case of chickenpox, talk with your doctor about getting the newly available chickenpox vaccine (varicella virus vaccine or Varivax) if you have never had chickenpox.
  • A new medicine called valacyclovir may achieve with oral dosing the intravenous levels of acyclovir. Discuss this medicine with your doctor.

FAMOTIDINE (fa MOH te deen)

Prescription Needed: Yes   **Controlled Drug:** No   **Generic:** No

Brand Names: Pepcid, Pepcid AC (nonprescription form)

Overview of BENEFITS versus RISKS	
Possible Benefits	*Possible Risks*
EFFECTIVE TREATMENT OF PEPTIC ULCER DISEASE: relief of symptoms, acceleration of healing, prevention of recurrence	Headache, dizziness
CONTROL OF HYPERSECRETORY STOMACH DISORDERS	
Beneficial in treatment of reflux esophagitis	

See the histamine (H2) blocking drug profile for further information.

FELBAMATE (FELL ba mate)

Prescription Needed: Yes   **Controlled Drug:** No   **Generic:** No

Brand Names: Felbatol

▷ **Warning:** THIS DRUG HAS BEEN FOUND TO CAUSE APLASTIC ANEMIA, WHICH MAY BE FATAL. It also may cause FATAL LIVER DISEASE. This drug presently remains on the market, reserved only for those for whom the benefit of seizure control outweighs the risk. This drug should NOT be stopped abruptly because the risk of seizures will be increased, unless a suitable antiseizure drug that appropriately covers the specific seizure type being treated has been started.

Combined with phenytoin (Dilantin), this medicine may lead to serious increases in phenytoin levels unless the phenytoin dose is adjusted.

Overview of BENEFITS versus RISKS	
Possible Benefits	*Possible Risks*
CONTROLS VARIOUS SEIZURE FORMS OF LENNOX-GASTAUT SYNDROME	FATAL APLASTIC ANEMIA LOW WHITE BLOOD CELL COUNTS AND PLATELETS (RARE)
CONTROLS SEIZURES REFRACTORY TO CARBAMAZEPINE OR PHENYTOIN	ACUTE AND POTENTIALLY FATAL LIVER DISEASE Stevens-Johnson syndrome (serious rash—rare) Agitation

▷ **Illness This Medication Treats**
   (1) Combination therapy for controlling seizures of Lennox-Gastaut syndrome; (2) effective in controlling refractory partial seizures; (3) combination treatment of partial seizures not controlled by appropriate levels of carbamazepine or phenytoin. USE OF FELBAMATE IS RESTRICTED TO THOSE PATIENTS FOR WHOM THE BENEFIT OUTWEIGHS THE RISK.

▷ **Typical Dosage Range:** (Dosage or schedule must be determined by the doctor for each individual.)
   Infants and Children: In children with Lennox-Gastaut syndrome: Start at 15 mg per kilogram of body weight daily, taken in three or four divided doses. Concurrent anticonvulsants are decreased by 20%. Felbamate is subsequently increased as needed and tolerated by 15 mg per kilogram of body weight per day at weekly intervals to a maximum dose of 45 mg per kilogram of body weight per day. Other anticonvulsant drugs used concomitantly are adjusted based on drug levels or side effects. Safety and efficacy of this drug in infants or in children who do not have Lennox-Gastaut syndrome are not established.
   12 to 60 Years of Age: Dosing is started with 400 mg three times daily (1200 mg/day). Can be increased by 600 mg/day at 2-week intervals to a maximum dose of 3600 mg daily for people who were not previously treated.
   Monotherapy: Starting dose of 1200 mg daily and reduction of other anticonvulsant doses by one-third; then increased weekly as needed and tolerated by 1200 mg/day to the 3600 mg/day maximum. Other anticonvulsants are decreased by one-third with each increase in felbamate dose, until they are stopped.
   Adjunctive therapy: Start at 400 mg three times a day (1200 mg/day) with a concomitant 20% reduction of other anticonvulsant drugs. Felbamate is subsequently increased as needed and tolerated to the

maximum 3600 mg daily dose. Other anticonvulsant doses are adjusted according to drug levels or side effects.

Over 60 Years of Age: This drug should be used with caution, particularly by people with compromised livers or kidneys.

▷ **Conditions Requiring Dosing Adjustments:**

Liver function: Dosing should be adjusted based on blood levels of patients with compromised livers. THIS DRUG MAY CAUSE FATAL LIVER FAILURE.

Kidney function: Most of this drug is eliminated unchanged in the kidney; dosing should be adjusted based on blood levels of people with kidney compromise.

FELODIPINE (fe LOH di peen)

Prescription Needed: Yes   **Controlled Drug:** No   **Generic:** No

Brand Names: Plendil

Controversies in Medicine: Results of several studies have indicated that medicines in this chemical family should NOT be used in some patients with extremely compromised hearts. Amlodipine (Norvasc) is the only calcium channel blocker that presently has data to show that it is SAFE, even in the most severely ill congestive heart failure patients. Amlodipine is the only calcium channel blocker to be FDA-approved as safe for use in treating hypertension or angina in patients who also have congestive heart failure. There have been several FDA hearings on calcium channel blockers in general.

One retrospective chart review yielded data showing that there was increased risk if nifedipine immediate-release forms were used for treating conditions other than angina in those over 71. There was a caution advised, but the form of nifedipine in question was not approved for uses other than angina. A recent FDA panel found medicines in this class to be safe and effective. A study of nearly 6,000 patients at Tel Aviv Medical Center found that there was no statistically significant risk of death in patients who took calcium channel blockers versus those who did not take these medicines.

Overview of BENEFITS versus RISKS

Possible Benefits

EFFECTIVE TREATMENT OF
MILD TO MODERATE
HYPERTENSION

Possible Risks

Peripheral edema (in feet and
ankles)

▷ **Illness This Medication Treats:**
Mild to moderate hypertension.

▷ **Typical Dosage Range:** (Dosage or schedule must be determined by
the doctor for each individual.)
Infants and Children: Dosage not established.
12 to 60 Years of Age: Initially 5 mg once daily. Increase dose as needed
and tolerated at intervals of 2 weeks. The usual dosage range is 5 to
10 mg once daily. The total daily dose should not exceed 20 mg once
daily.
Over 60 Years of Age: Starting dose is 2.5 mg/day. Total daily dose
should not exceed 10 mg once daily.

▷ **Conditions Requiring Dosing Adjustments:**
Liver function: For patients with liver compromise the starting dose
should be 2.5 mg/day.

▷ **How Best to Take This Medicine:**   May be taken with or following
food to reduce stomach irritation. The tablet should be swallowed
whole; do not crush or chew.

▷ **How Long This Medicine Is Usually Taken:**   Use on a regular
schedule for 2 to 4 weeks is needed to determine this drug's effectiveness in controlling hypertension. The smallest effective dose
should be used in long-term (months to years) therapy. Supervision
and periodic evaluation by your doctor are essential. See your doctor regularly.

▷ **Tell Your Doctor Before Taking This Medicine If You:**
- ever had an allergic reaction to it.
- have active liver disease.
- have uncorrected congestive heart failure.
- have had an unfavorable response to any calcium blocker in the
past.
- are currently taking any form of digitalis or a beta-blocker.
- are taking any other drugs that lower blood pressure.
- have a history of congestive heart failure, heart attack, or stroke.
- have a history of muscular dystrophy, myasthenia gravis, or atrial
fibrillation.
- are subject to heart rhythm disturbances.
- have a history of impaired liver or kidney function.

▷ **Possible Side Effects:**   Swelling of feet and ankles (dose- and age-dependent), flushing and sensation of warmth. Abnormal growth of the gums.

▷ **Possible Adverse Effects:**

If any of the following develop, call your doctor promptly for guidance.

Some Mild Problems Drug Can Cause
  Allergic reactions: skin rash.
  Headache, sleep disorders, dizziness, fatigue.
  Nausea, stomach pain, constipation, or diarrhea.

Some Serious Problems This Drug Can Cause
  Aggravation of angina.
  Extremely rare decreases in hemoglobin, hematocrit, or red blood cell count.

▷ **Possible Effects on Sex Life:**   Impotence.

▷ *CAUTION*

  1. Be sure to inform all doctors and dentists who provide care for you that you are taking this drug. Note the use of this drug on your personal identification card.
  2. You may use nitroglycerin and other nitrate drugs as needed to relieve acute episodes of angina pain. However, if your angina attacks are becoming more frequent or intense, notify your doctor promptly.
  3. Safety and effectiveness of this drug for those under 12 years old are not established.
  4. Those under 60 may be more susceptible to the development of weakness, dizziness, fainting, and falling. Take necessary precautions to prevent injury.

Advisability of Use During Pregnancy or If Breast-Feeding:

Pregnancy Category: C. Avoid this drug during the first 3 months. Use it during the last 6 months only if clearly needed. Ask your doctor for guidance. Presence in breast milk is unknown; avoid taking this drug or refrain from nursing.

▷ **Overdose Symptoms:**   Weakness, light-headedness, fainting, fast pulse, low blood pressure, shortness of breath, flushed and warm skin, tremors.

▷ **Suggested Periodic Examinations While Taking This Drug:** (at doctor's discretion)

Evaluations of heart function, including electrocardiograms; measurements of blood pressure in supine, sitting, and standing positions.

▷ **While Taking This Drug the Following Apply:**

Foods: Avoid excessive salt intake.

Beverages: Grapefruit juice may cause a serious increase in the absorption of this drug and lead to toxicity. DO NOT take this medicine with grapefruit juice; it may be taken with milk or water.

Alcohol: Use with caution until combined effects have been determined. Alcohol may exaggerate the drop in blood pressure in some people.

Tobacco Smoking: Nicotine may reduce the effectiveness of this drug.

Other Drugs:

Felodipine *taken concurrently* with

- adenosine may result in slowing of the heart.
- beta-blockers or digitalis preparations may adversely affect heart rate and rhythm. Careful monitoring by your doctor is necessary.
- carbamazepine (Tegretol) may blunt felodipine's effectiveness.
- digoxin (Lanoxin) may result in digoxin toxicity.
- magnesium may cause low blood pressure.
- phenobarbital may blunt felodipine's benefits.
- phenytoin (Dilantin) may decrease phenytoin levels and blunt the benefit it offers.
- rifampin may decrease felodipine's benefits (this has NOT been reported specifically for felodipine, but for other medicines in its class).

The following drugs may *increase* the effects of felodipine

- cimetidine (Tagamet).
- erythromycin and other macrolide (see Drug Classes) antibiotics.

Driving, Hazardous Activities: Usually no restrictions. This drug may cause dizziness. Restrict your activities as necessary.

Exposure to Heat: Caution is advised. Hot environments can exaggerate the blood pressure–lowering effects of this drug. Observe for light-headedness or weakness.

Discontinuation: Do not stop taking this drug abruptly. Ask your doctor about gradual withdrawal. Watch for possible rebound hypertension.

▷ **Saving Money When Using This Medicine:**

- Dosage of this drug MUST be adjusted for patients with liver compromise, and the starting dose decreased to 5 mg/day. Ask your doctor if your dose has been appropriately adjusted.
- Many calcium channel blockers are available in this country. Ask your doctor if this drug provides the best combination of cost and outcome for you.
- Have your blood pressure checked periodically to ensure that this medicine is continuing to keep your blood pressure under control. Call your doctor if it is not.
- Talk with your doctor about the advisability of the use of aspirin every other day in order to help prevent a heart attack.

FENAMATES

(Nonsteroidal Anti-Inflammatory Drug Combination)
Meclofenamate (MEK low fen a mate)
Mefenamic acid (MEF en amik a sid)

Prescription Needed: Yes   **Controlled Drug:**   No **Generic:** Yes

Brand Names: Meclofenamate: Meclodium, Meclomen, Mefenamic acid: Ponstel, Ponstan

---

Overview of BENEFITS versus RISKS

Possible Benefits	*Possible Risks*
EFFECTIVE RELIEF OF MILD TO MODERATE PAIN AND INFLAMMATION	Gastrointestinal pain, ulceration, bleeding (rare) Rare: kidney damage; fluid retention; bone marrow depression; hemolytic anemia (mefenamic acid); systemic lupus erythematosus (mefenamic acid); pancreatitis (mefenamic acid)

▷ **Illness This Medication Treats:**
(1) Meclofenamate for pain relief of osteoarthritis and rheumatoid arthritis; (2) mefenamic acid for chronic pain relief, painful menstruation (dysmenorrhea), and postoperative pain.
Other (unlabeled) generally accepted uses: (1) meclofenamate for treatment of temporal arteritis and nephrotic syndrome; (2) mefenamic acid for treatment of PMS and temporal arteritis.

▷ **Typical Dosage Range:** (Dosage or schedule must be determined by the doctor for each individual.)
Meclofenamate: 200 to 400 mg daily, in three or four divided doses. Total daily dosage should not exceed 400 mg.
Mefenamic acid: 500 mg initially, then 250 mg/6 hr, taken with food.

▷ **Conditions Requiring Dosing Adjustments:**
Liver function: Changes in dosing are not presently recommended for patients with liver compromise.
Kidney function: Meclofenamate is eliminated by the kidneys; however, specific dosing guidelines have not been elaborated. Mefenamic acid is contraindicated for patients with kidney failure.

▷ **How Best to Take This Medicine:**   Take with food or milk to prevent stomach irritation. Take with a full glass of water and remain upright (do not lie down) for 30 minutes. The capsule may be opened for administration.

▷ **How Long This Medicine Is Usually Taken:**   Meclofenamate: Use on a regular schedule for 2 to 3 weeks usually determines the effectiveness of this drug in arthritis therapy. Long-term use (months to years) requires physician supervision and periodic evaluation.

Mefenamic acid: Peak levels occur in up to 4 hours. Use beyond 7 days is not recommended.

▷ **Tell Your Doctor Before Taking This Medicine If You:**
- ever had an allergic reaction to it.
- are subject to asthma or nasal polyps caused by aspirin.
- have active peptic ulcer disease, regional enteritis, ulcerative colitis, or any form of gastrointestinal bleeding.
- have a bleeding disorder or a blood cell disorder, or a history of any type of bleeding disorder.
- have severe impairment of kidney function.
- have systemic lupus erythematosus (mefenamic acid)
- have recently had pancreatitis (mefenamic acid).
- are allergic to aspirin or aspirin substitutes.
- have a history of peptic ulcer disease, regional enteritis, or ulcerative colitis.
- have impaired liver or kidney function.
- have high blood pressure or a history of heart failure.
- take acetaminophen, aspirin or aspirin substitutes, anticoagulants, oral antidiabetics, or cortisonelike drugs.

▷ **Possible Side Effects:**   Ringing in ears, fluid retention.

▷ **Possible Adverse Effects:**
If any of the following develop, call your doctor promptly for guidance.

Some Mild Problems Drug Can Cause
　　Allergic reactions: skin rash, itching.
　　Headache, dizziness, altered vision, depression.
　　Mouth sores, nausea, vomiting, diarrhea.

Some Serious Problems Drug Can Cause
　　Allergic reactions: severe skin reactions, drug fever.
　　Active peptic ulcer, with or without bleeding.
　　Kidney damage: painful urination, bloody urine, reduced urine.
　　Rare bone marrow depression.
　　Mefenamic acid: May also cause rare hemolytic anemia, liver damage, pancreatitis, and systemic lupus erythematosus.

▷ *CAUTION*
　　1. Dosage should always be limited to the smallest amount that produces reasonable improvement.
　　2. These drugs may mask early indications of infection. Inform your doctor if you think you are developing an infection.

3. Mefenamic acid should be used for a maximum of 7 days.
4. Safety and effectiveness have not been established for those under 14 years old for meclofenamate or 18 years old for mefenamic acid.
5. Small doses are advisable for people over 60 until tolerance is determined. Watch for any indications of liver or kidney toxicity, fluid retention, dizziness, confusion, impaired memory, stomach bleeding, or diarrhea.

Advisability of Use During Pregnancy or If Breast-Feeding:
Pregnancy Category: Meclofenamate: B normally and D in the last 3 months of pregnancy. Mefenamic acid: C. The manufacturer does not recommend the use of meclofenamate during pregnancy. Use of mefenamic acid in late pregnancy should be avoided. Ask your doctor for help regarding mefenamic acid use during pregnancy. Present in breast milk; avoid using these drugs or refrain from nursing.

▷ **Overdose Symptoms:** Drowsiness, nausea, vomiting, diarrhea, marked agitation, irrational behavior, metabolic acidosis, and seizures.

▷ **Suggested Periodic Examinations While Taking This Drug:** (at doctor's discretion)
Complete blood cell counts, kidney function tests, complete eye examinations if vision is altered in any way.

▷ **While Taking This Drug the Following Apply:**
Beverages: These drugs may be taken with milk.
Alcohol: Use with caution. Alcohol irritates the stomach lining; added to the irritant action of these drugs, it may increase the risk of stomach ulceration and/or bleeding.
Other Drugs.
Meclofenamate may *increase* the effects of
• acetaminophen (Tylenol, etc.), increasing the risk of kidney damage; avoid prolonged use of this combination.
• anticoagulants (Coumadin, etc.), increasing the risk of bleeding; monitor prothrombin time and adjust dose accordingly.
Meclofenamate *taken concurrently* with the following drugs may increase the risk of bleeding; avoid these combinations:
• aspirin and perhaps other NSAIDs (see Drug Classes).
• dipyridamole (Persantine).
• sulfinpyrazone (Anturane).
• valproic acid (Depakene).
Mefenamic acid *taken concurrently with*
• cyclosporine (Sandimmune) may result in cyclosporine toxicity.
• antacids containing magnesium may result in rapid mefenamic acid toxicity.

- anticoagulants (Coumadin, etc.) will displace the drugs from binding sites and increase bleeding risk.
- aspirin, dipyridamole, or sulfinpyrazone may result in increased bleeding risk.

Meclofenamate or mefenamic acid *taken concurrently with*

- diuretics (see Drug Classes) may result in decreased effectiveness of the diuretic.
- enoxaparin may result in increased surgical blood loss.
- lithium (Lithobid, others) will increase blood lithium levels over time and may result in toxicity.
- methotrexate can result in serious methotrexate toxicity.

Driving, Hazardous Activities: These drugs may cause dizziness or altered vision. Restrict your activities as necessary.

▷ **Saving Money When Using These Medicines:**

- Meclofenamate dosing should be decreased for patients with kidney compromise and should NOT be used by patients with kidney failure. Nonsteroidal anti-inflammatory drugs (NSAIDs) must be considered as a benefit-to-risk decision for patients with kidney compromise.
- Many NSAIDs are available in this country. Ask your doctor if either of these drugs provides the best combination of cost and outcome for you.
- Talk with your doctor about visiting a chronic pain center if use of these medications is to continue.
- Call the Arthritis Foundation to check for the latest facts on arthritis: 1-800-283-7800.

FENOPROFEN (fen oh PROH fen)

Prescription Needed: Yes   **Controlled Drug:** No   **Generic:** Yes

Brand Names: Nalfon

Overview of BENEFITS versus RISKS	
Possible Benefits	*Possible Risks*
EFFECTIVE RELIEF OF MILD TO MODERATE PAIN AND INFLAMMATION	Gastrointestinal pain, ulceration, bleeding (rare)
	Rare liver or kidney damage; fluid retention; bone marrow depression

See the propionic acids (NSAIDs) drug profile for further information.

FENTANYL TRANSDERMAL (FEN ta nil)

Prescription Needed: Yes   **Controlled Drug:** C-ll*   **Generic:** No

Brand Names: Duragesic, Fentanyl Oralet

Overview of BENEFITS versus RISKS	
Possible Benefits	*Possible Risks*
EFFECTIVE PAIN RELIEF WITH A PATCH APPLIED TO THE SKIN	Habit-forming potential with prolonged use
PATCH APPLICATION NEEDED ONLY ONCE EVERY 3 DAYS	Impairment of mental function
	Methemoglobinemia (rare)
EFFECTIVE PAIN RELIEF WITH A CONVENIENT SUCKER FORM	Respiratory depression

▷ **Illness This Medication Treats:**
Use currently included in FDA-approved labeling: treatment of pain.

▷ **Typical Dosage Range:** (Dosage or schedule must be determined by the doctor for each individual.)

Infants and Children: Safety and efficacy of this drug for those under 12 years old are not established.

18 to 60 Years of Age: Patch: Not indicated for patients 18 years old who weigh less than 50 kg (110 lb).

For patients who have not been using opioids such as morphine, the 25 mcg/hr (2.5 mg) patch should be used.

For people who previously used opioids, the amount needed to control pain on a 24-hour basis is calculated, converted to an equal amount of morphine (morphine equianalgesic dose), and then converted to fentanyl

Sucker: Used to treat pain and control anxiety prior to surgery. 400 mcg is usually suggested for those weighing 50 kg or more.

Over 60 Years of Age: These people should receive the 25 mcg/hr (2.5 mg) patch, unless they were already receiving the equivalent of 135 mg of oral morphine daily. Intravenous fentanyl clears more slowly in this population than in younger patients, and careful observation should be made for overdose.

▷ **Conditions Requiring Dosing Adjustments:**
Liver function: The dose must be decreased for patients with liver compromise.

*See Controlled Drug Schedules inside this book's cover.

Kidney function: For patients with moderate to severe kidney failure, 75% of the usual dose should be taken. For patients with severe kidney failure, the dose should be reduced by 50%.

▷ **How Best to Take This Medicine:** The patch should be removed from its protective pouch and the stiff protective liner removed from the sticky side. Do not cut or damage the system. The sticky side of the patch should be applied to a nonhairy, dry area such as the back, chest, flank, or upper arm. Avoid any skin that is burned, irritated, or excessively oily. Wash your hands once you have successfully applied the patch. After 3 days a new patch should be applied to a different area. The exhausted patch should be folded onto itself and flushed down the toilet. Avoid exposing the patch to external heat sources such as electric blankets or heating pads.

The sucker form should be allowed to slowly dissolve in the mouth and not bitten.

▷ **How Long This Medicine Is Usually Taken:** Use on a regular schedule for 1 to 3 days usually determines the effectiveness of this drug in controlling pain. An immediate-release form of morphine or similar opioid should be available for pain control while this drug reaches its peak effect. Long-term use (months) requires periodic physician evaluation of response and dosage adjustment of both the patch and an immediate-release form of morphine or similar drug.

▷ **Tell Your Doctor Before Taking This Medicine If You:**
- ever had an allergic reaction to it.
- have mild or intermittent pain.
- have acute or postoperative pain without opportunity for proper dose adjustment.
- have liver or kidney compromise.
- have chronic lung disease.
- have an abnormally slow heartbeat or other heart disease.
- are taking an MAO inhibitor (see Drug Classes).
- weigh less than 50 kg or are less than 18 years old.
- develop a high fever.
- have a history of alcoholism or drug abuse.
- take other prescription or nonprescription medicines that were not discussed when transdermal fentanyl was prescribed.

▷ **Possible Side Effects:**   Constipation, dry mouth, and sleepiness.

▷ **Possible Adverse Effects:**
If any of the following develop, call your doctor promptly for guidance.
Some Mild Problems Drug Can Cause
   Allergic reactions: skin rash and itching.
   Nausea and vomiting.

Sleepiness and confusion.

Sweatiness and constipation.

Blurred vision.

Some Serious Problems Drug Can Cause

Allergic reactions: exfoliative dermatitis and/or anaphylactic reactions.

Arrhythmias (rare).

Paranoid reaction (rare).

Seizures (rare).

Rare porphyrias.

Respiratory depression.

▷ **Possible Effects on Sex Life:** Impotence and blunted orgasm sensation in men. Irregular menstrual periods and blunted orgasm sensation in women.

▷ **Possible Delayed Adverse Effects:** Dependence and tolerance.

▷ *CAUTION*

1. Extreme caution should be used if this drug is combined with other opioids, narcotic drugs, benzodiazepines, or alcohol.
2. This drug may cause serious constipation in older patients.
3. Do not expose the patch site to external sources of heat such as heating pads or electric blankets, as an increased rate of drug release may occur.
4. Safety and effectiveness of this drug for those under 12 years old are not established.
5. For people over 60, the 25 mcg patch should be used as a starting dose unless a daily dose of over 135 mg of morphine is already being taken. Those with cardiac, respiratory, kidney, or liver compromise should take low doses and be carefully monitored.

Advisability of Use During Pregnancy or If Breast-Feeding:
Pregnancy Category: C. D if taken in high doses or for a long time. Ask your doctor for guidance. Present in breast milk; avoid taking this drug or refrain from nursing.

▷ **Habit-Forming Potential:** A Schedule II narcotic, fentanyl can cause physical and psychological dependence resembling morphine dependence, and tolerance with repeated use.

▷ **Overdose Symptoms:** Dizziness, amnesia, and stupor. Respiratory depression and apnea may occur.

▷ **Possible Effects of Long-Term Use:** Tolerance and physical or psychological dependence.

▷ **Suggested Periodic Examinations While Taking This Drug:** (at doctor's discretion)

Liver function tests.

▷ **While Taking This Drug the Following Apply:**

Alcohol: DO NOT DRINK ALCOHOL. Additive effects in loss of mental status, respiratory depression, and confusion.

Marijuana Smoking: Additive adverse effects; however, marijuana may block the vomiting effect of fentanyl.

Other Drugs:

Fentanyl may ***increase*** the effects of

- benzodiazepines such as diazepam (Valium) and alprazolam (Xanax).
- central nervous system depressants such as opiates, barbiturates, tranquilizers, and tricyclic antidepressants.

Fentanyl ***taken concurrently*** with

- amiodarone (Cordarone) may result in heart toxicity.
- clonidine (Catapres) may result in greater than expected fentanyl effects.
- MAO inhibitors (see Drug Classes) may worsen lowering of blood pressure and breathing depression sometimes seen with fentanyl.

Driving, Hazardous Activities: This drug may cause drowsiness, sedation, and respiratory depression. Restrict your activities as necessary.

Discontinuation: The patch may be removed if the drug is not tolerated or is to be stopped. Once the patch is removed, fentanyl continues to be released from the patch site for 17 hours or more. Ideally, if pain medicine is still needed, the chosen alternative should be substituted and fentanyl transdermal slowly tapered.

▷ **Saving Money When Using This Medicine:**

- Pain therapy currently combines medications from several drug classes. This drug may be combined with a tricyclic antidepressant such as amitriptyline (Elavil) or an NSAID such as ibuprofen (Motrin). Such combinations attack the cause of the pain by several mechanisms, often allowing the opioid dose (such as fentanyl) to be decreased.
- This drug MUST be adjusted in dosage for patients with moderate to severe kidney compromise or liver compromise. Ask your doctor if your dose has been appropriately adjusted.
- Many medications are available to treat pain. Ask your doctor if this drug provides the best combination of cost and outcome for you. Ask your doctor who will assess your pain and who will adjust your medicine dose if needed.
- Ask your doctor how long this drug is usually taken to treat your condition.

FINASTERIDE (fin ASS tur ide)

Prescription Needed: Yes   **Controlled Drug:** No   **Generic:** No

Brand Names: Proscar

Overview of BENEFITS versus RISKS

Possible Benefits	*Possible Risks*
NONSURGICAL TREATMENT OF SYMPTOMATIC BENIGN PROSTATIC HYPERPLASIA: shrinkage of prostatic tissue, and increase in urine flow Hair growth	IMPOTENCE, decreased libido, hypersensitivity reactions

---

Author's note: A recent study has questioned the effectiveness of this medicine in prostatic hyperplasia, but more data are needed.

▷ **Illness This Medication Treats:**

Use currently included in FDA-approved labeling: treatment of symptomatic benign prostatic hyperplasia (BPH). Maximum shrinkage of the prostate has occurred after 6 months of therapy.

Other (unlabeled) generally accepted use: may have a role in restoring hair loss.

▷ **Typical Dosage Range:** (Dosage or schedule must be determined by the doctor for each individual.)

Infants and Children: Not indicated.

12 to 60 Years of Age: Symptomatic benign prostatic hyperplasia (BPH) often does not occur in the younger end of this adult dosing range; however, the dose for this age range is 5 mg/day taken by mouth.

Over 60 Years of Age: Same as for 12 to 60 years of age, unless liver function has decreased.

▷ **Conditions Requiring Dosing Adjustments:**

Liver function: People with abnormal liver function tests were not included in the original study data. Your doctor must decide if this drug is the best one for you.

Kidney function: At present there appears to be no need to adjust the dose for patients with mild to moderate kidney failure.

▷ **How Best to Take This Medicine:** This medicine is best taken on an empty stomach. Food changes the peak blood concentration, and may decrease the total amount absorbed.

▷ **How Long This Medicine Is Usually Taken:** Use on a regular schedule for at least 6 months usually determines the effectiveness of this drug in shrinking the prostate and decreasing symptoms of benign prostatic hyperplasia. See your doctor regularly.

▷ **Tell Your Doctor Before Taking This Medicine If You:**
- ever had an allergic reaction to it.
- have a history of impaired liver function or liver disease.
- have kidney problems of any nature.
- are planning to have a child or your sexual partner is pregnant.

▷ **Possible Side Effects:** Usually increases testosterone levels; however, the significance of this effect is not known.

▷ **Possible Adverse Effects:**
If any of the following develop, call your doctor promptly for guidance.
Some Mild Problems Drug Can Cause
Allergic reactions: rare skin rash, hives.
Some Serious Problems Drug Can Cause
Allergic reactions: rare hypersensitivity reactions.

▷ **Possible Effects on Sex Life:** Impotence.
Decreased libido.
Decreased volume of ejaculate.
Swelling and tenderness of male breast tissue (gynecomastia).

▷ **Possible Effects on Laboratory Tests:** Decreased PSA (prostate specific antigen).

▷ *CAUTION*
1. You should have a digital rectal examination and other examinations for prostate cancer before starting this medication.
2. If your liver function changes, tell your doctor.
3. If your sexual partner is pregnant, avoid exposing your partner to your semen. Exposure to finasteride-containing semen may cause genital abnormalities in male offspring.
4. Safety and effectiveness of this drug for use in infants and children have not been established.

Advisability of Use During Pregnancy or If Breast-Feeding:
Pregnancy Category: X. Women who are pregnant should avoid exposure to crushed finasteride tablets and semen of a sexual partner who is on finasteride. Ask your doctor for guidance. Refrain from nursing if you have been exposed to finasteride or finasteride-containing semen.

▷ **Overdose Symptoms:** Multiple doses of up to 80 mg/day have been taken without adverse effect.

▷ **While Taking This Drug the Following Apply:**
 Foods: This medicine is best taken on an empty stomach.
 Other Drugs:
 Finasteride may *decrease* the effects of
 • theophylline (Theo-Dur, others).

▷ **Saving Money When Using This Medicine:**
 • Two medications are now approved to treat prostate hyperplasia, and a third for unlabeled use.
 • Ask your doctor if this drug provides the best combination of cost and outcome for you.

FLUCONAZOLE   (flu KOHN a zohl)

Prescription Needed: Yes   **Controlled Drug:** No   **Generic:** No

Brand Names: Diflucan

Overview of BENEFITS versus RISKS	
Possible Benefits	*Possible Risks*
EFFECTIVE TREATMENT AND SUPPRESSION OF CRYPTOCOCCAL MENINGITIS	Severe skin reactions (rare)
	Possible liver damage (rare)
EFFECTIVE TREATMENT OF *CANDIDA* INFECTIONS OF THE MOUTH, THROAT, AND ESOPHAGUS	
EFFECTIVE TREATMENT OF SYSTEMIC *CANDIDA* INFECTIONS	

▷ **Illness This Medication Treats:**
 (1) Cryptococcal (yeast) meningitis (may be AIDS-related); (2) *Candida* (yeast) infections of the mouth, throat, and esophagus (may be AIDS-related); (3) systemic *Candida* infections—pneumonia, peritonitis, urinary tract infections (may be AIDS-related); (4) vaginal yeast infections through one-dose treatment.

▷ **Typical Dosage Range:** (Dosage or schedule must be determined by the doctor for each individual.)
 Infants and Children: From 3 to 13 years old: 3–6 mg per kilogram of body weight daily.
 13 to 60 Years of Age: For treatment of cryptococcal meningitis: 400 mg once daily until significant improvement occurs; then 200 to 400

mg once daily for 10 to 12 weeks after the cerebrospinal fluid (CSF) culture becomes negative.

For suppression of cryptococcal meningitis: 200 mg once daily.

For treatment of *Candida* infections of mouth and throat: 200 mg on the first day; then 100 mg once daily for 2 weeks.

For treatment of *Candida* infection of the esophagus: 200 mg on the first day, then 100 mg once daily for at least 3 weeks; continue treatment for 2 weeks after clearance of all symptoms of infection. If necessary, doses up to 400 mg once daily may be used.

For treatment of systemic *Candida* infections: 400 mg on the first day, then 200 mg once daily for at least 4 weeks; continue treatment for 2 weeks after clearance of all symptoms of infection.

Over 60 Years of Age: Same as for 13 to 60 years of age. Dosage must be adjusted for patients with impaired kidney function.

▷ **Conditions Requiring Dosing Adjustments:**

Liver function: This drug is a rare cause of hepatitis and should be used with caution by patients with liver compromise.

Kidney function: For patients with mild to moderate kidney failure, 50% of the usual dose should be taken every 48 hours. For patients with severe kidney failure, 25% of the usual dose should be taken every 48 hours.

▷ **How Best to Take This Medicine:** Preferably taken on an empty stomach; may be taken with or after food to reduce stomach irritation. The tablet may be crushed for administration.

▷ **How Long This Medicine Is Usually Taken:** Use on a regular schedule for 2 to 4 weeks usually determines the effectiveness of this drug in controlling infections due to *Candida* or *Cryptococcus* yeasts. Actual cures or long-term suppression often require continual treatment for many months. This drug may be continuous therapy for AIDS patients.

▷ **Tell Your Doctor Before Taking This Medicine If You:**
- ever had an allergic reaction to it or are allergic to related antifungal drugs: clotrimazole, itraconazole, ketoconazole, miconazole.
- have active liver disease.
- have impaired liver or kidney function.
- currently are taking any other drugs.

▷ **Possible Adverse Effects:**

If any of the following develop, call your doctor promptly for guidance.

Some Mild Problems Drug Can Cause

Allergic reactions: skin rash.

Headache.

Nausea, vomiting, diarrhea.

Some Serious Problems This Drug Can Cause
Allergic reactions: severe dermatitis (very rare).
Liver toxicity (very rare and questionable).
Abnormally low blood platelet counts: abnormal bruising or bleeding.
Rare seizures, adrenal suppression, or low white blood cell counts.

▷ **Possible Effects on Sex Life:**   Very rare amenorrhea (questionable cause).

▷ **Adverse Effects That May Mimic Natural Diseases or Disorders:**
Liver reaction may suggest viral hepatitis.

▷ *CAUTION*
1. Safety and effectiveness of this drug for those under 13 years old are not established.
2. Age-related decrease in kidney function may require adjustment of dosage.

Advisability of Use During Pregnancy or If Breast-Feeding:
Pregnancy Category: C. Use this drug only if clearly needed. Ask your doctor for guidance. Presence in breast milk is unknown; avoid taking this drug or refrain from nursing.

▷ **Overdose Symptoms:**   Possible nausea, vomiting, diarrhea.

▷ **Suggested Periodic Examinations While Taking This Drug:** (at doctor's discretion)
Liver and kidney function tests.

▷ **While Taking This Drug the Following Apply:**
Beverages: May be taken with milk.
Other Drugs:
Fluconazole may *increase* the effects of
• oral antidiabetics (chlorpropamide, glipizide, glyburide, tolbutamide), causing hypoglycemia; monitor blood glucose levels carefully.
• cyclosporine (Sandimmune).
• phenytoin (Dilantin, etc.), causing phenytoin toxicity; monitor phenytoin blood levels.
• trimetrexate (Neutrexin).
• warfarin (Coumadin), causing unwanted bleeding; monitor prothrombin times as necessary.
• zidovudine (AZT) and result in toxicity.
Fluconazole *taken concurrently* with
• astemizole (Hismanal) may result in serious heart toxicity.
• hydrochlorothiazide (Esidrix, others) may interact.
• loratadine (Claritin) may result in increased loratadine blood levels, but this has not been associated with heart toxicity. However, since

blood levels will be increased by this combination, it is prudent to decrease the loratadine dose if these medicines are combined.

- oral hypoglycemic agents (see Drug Classes) may increase lowering of blood sugar.
- terfenadine (Seldane) may result in serious heart toxicity.
- trimetrexate may increase trimetrexate toxicity.

The following drugs may *decrease* the effects of fluconazole

- cimetidine (Tagamet).
- rifampin (Rifadin, Rimactane, etc.).

Discontinuation: Take the full course prescribed. Continual treatment for several months may be necessary. Ask your doctor about the appropriate time to consider discontinuation.

▷ **Saving Money When Using This Medicine:**
- Many medications are available to treat fungal infections. Ask your doctor if this drug provides the best combination of cost and outcome for you.
- It may be possible (after a significant infection-free period) to stop this medicine. Ask your doctor for help.

FLUCYTOSINE   (flu SI toh seen)

Other Names: 5-fluorocytosine, 5-FC

Prescription Needed: Yes

Brand Names: Ancobon

Overview of BENEFITS versus RISKS	
Possible Benefits	*Possible Risks*
EFFECTIVE ADJUNCTIVE TREATMENT OF CERTAIN INFECTIONS CAUSED BY *CANDIDA* AND *CRYPTOCOCCUS* FUNGI OR *ASPERGILLUS*	BONE MARROW DEPRESSION DRUG-INDUCED LIVER DAMAGE
Effective adjunctive treatment of chromomycosis infection.	Peripheral neuritis Ulcerative colitis (rare)

▷ **Illness This Medication Treats:**
(1) Endocarditis, pneumonia, septicemia, and urinary tract infections caused by *Candida*; (2) meningitis, pneumonia, septicemia, and urinary tract infections caused by *Cryptococcus*. These infections are often AIDS-related.

Note: Flucytosine is usually combined with amphotericin B to treat disseminated fungal infections.

▷ **Typical Dosage Range:** (Dosage or schedule must be determined by the doctor for each individual.)

Infants and Children: 50 to 150 mg per kilogram of body weight, divided into four doses given every 6 hours.

12 to 60 Years of Age: 50 to 150 mg per kilogram of body weight every 6 hours.

Over 60 Years of Age: Same as for 12 to 60 years of age. If kidney function is impaired, reduced dosage is mandatory.

▷ **Conditions Requiring Dosing Adjustments:**

Liver function: For patients with mild to moderate liver compromise, changes in dosage do not appear to be needed at the present. Flucytosine can cause liver toxicity (especially with blood levels greater than 100 mcg/ml), and should be used with caution by patients with liver compromise.

Kidney function: For patients with mild to moderate kidney failure the usual dose can be taken every 12 to 24 hours. For patients with severe kidney failure the usual dose can be taken every 24 to 48 hours.

▷ **How Best to Take This Medicine:** If a single dosage requires more than one capsule, space administration over a period of 15 minutes to reduce stomach irritation and nausea. May be taken with or after food. The capsule may be opened for administration.

▷ **How Long This Medicine Is Usually Taken:** Use on a regular schedule for 4 to 6 weeks usually determines the effectiveness of this drug in controlling candidal or cryptococcal infection. Long-term use (months to years) requires periodic physician evaluation.

▷ **Tell Your Doctor Before Taking This Medicine If You:**
- ever had an allergic reaction to it.
- have an active blood cell or bone marrow disorder or impaired liver or kidney function.
- have active liver or kidney disease.
- have active Crohn's disease, ulcerative colitis, or a history of either.
- have a history of drug-induced bone marrow depression.
- have a history of peripheral neuritis.

▷ **Possible Adverse Effects:**
If any of the following develop, call your doctor promptly for guidance.

Some Mild Problems Drug Can Cause

Allergic reactions: skin rash, itching.

Headache, dizziness, drowsiness, hallucinations.

Loss of appetite, nausea, vomiting, diarrhea.

Some Serious Problems Drug Can Cause
Bone marrow depression.
Liver damage, with or without jaundice.
Peripheral neuritis.
Rare bowel perforation or kidney damage.

▷ *CAUTION*
1. When this drug is used alone, infecting fungi may rapidly develop resistance to its effect; it is usually used concurrently with amphotericin B (taken intravenously).
2. If kidney function is significantly impaired, reduced dosage is mandatory to prevent toxic reactions.
3. No specific information is available on special precautions for use of this drug by infants or children.
4. Those over 60 may need a dosage adjustment to compensate for age-related decrease in kidney function.

Advisability of Use During Pregnancy or If Breast-Feeding:
Pregnancy Category: C. Use this drug only if clearly needed. Ask your doctor for guidance. Present in breast milk; avoid taking this drug or refrain from nursing.

▷ **Overdose Symptoms:** Nausea, vomiting, stomach pain, diarrhea, confusion.

▷ **Suggested Periodic Examinations While Taking This Drug:** (at doctor's discretion)
Measurement of blood levels of flucytosine.
Complete blood cell counts.
Liver and kidney function tests.

▷ **While Taking This Drug the Following Apply:**
Beverages: May be taken with milk.
Other Drugs:
The following drugs may *decrease* the effects of flucytosine
• antacids.
• cytarabine (Cytosar); may reduce its antifungal effect.
Flucytosine *taken concurrently* with
• amphotericin B may result in increased risk of kidney toxicity.
• zidovudine (AZT) may result in additive and serious blood toxicity.
Driving, Hazardous Activities: This drug may cause dizziness, drowsiness, or confusion. Restrict your activities as necessary.
Exposure to Sun: Use caution until your sensitivity is determined. This drug may cause photosensitivity.
Discontinuation: It may be necessary to use this drug for an extended period of time. Your doctor should determine the appropriate time for discontinuation.

▷ **Saving Money When Using This Medicine:**
- Many medications are available to treat fungal infections. Ask your doctor if this drug provides the best combination of cost and outcome for you.
- A new medicine that is lipid-associated may have greater activity against *Cryptococcus*. Talk to your doctor.

FLUNISOLIDE (flu NIS oh lide)

Prescription Needed: Yes   **Controlled Drug:** No   **Generic:** No

Brand Names: AeroBid, Nasalide, Nasarel

Overview of BENEFITS versus RISKS	
Possible Benefits	*Possible Risks*
EFFECTIVE CONTROL OF SEVERE CHRONIC BRONCHIAL ASTHMA	Yeast infections of mouth and throat
	Increased susceptibility to respiratory tract infections
	Localized areas of allergic pneumonia

▷ **Illness This Medication Treats:**
(1) Chronic bronchial asthma in people who require cortisonelike drugs for asthma control. Inhalation dosing is better than cortisone taken by mouth or injection; it helps the respiratory tract without going through the entire body. This prevents the more serious adverse effects that usually result from the long term use of cortisone taken for systemic effects. (2) Various kinds of hay fever (allergic rhinitis).

▷ **Typical Dosage Range:** (Dosage or schedule must be determined by the doctor for each individual.)

Infants and Children: Up to 6 years old: Dosage not established.

6 years and older: 0.5 mg (two metered sprays) two times a day, morning and evening. Limit total daily dosage to 1 mg.

15 to 60 Years of Age: Oral inhalation: 0.5 to 1 mg (two to four metered sprays) two times a day, morning and evening. Limit total daily dose to 2 mg.

Nasal inhalation: Two sprays per nostril per day. Maximum dose is eight sprays (400 mcg) per day. Once the peak effect is seen, the dose should be reduced to the smallest dose and frequency that works.

Aqueous nasal form: Two sprays in each nostril twice daily to start. Ongoing dose should be the smallest dose and frequency that works.

Over 60 Years of Age: Same as for 15 to 60 years of age.

▷ **Conditions Requiring Dosing Adjustments:**
Liver function: Specific guidelines are not available for dosage adjustment for patients with liver compromise.
Kidney function: No specific changes are recommended for patients with compromised kidneys.

▷ **How Best to Take This Medicine:**   May be used as needed without regard to eating. Shake the container well before using. Carefully follow the printed patient instructions provided. Rinse the mouth and throat (gargle) with water thoroughly after each inhalation.

▷ **How Long This Medicine Is Usually Taken:**   Use on a regular schedule for 1 to 4 weeks is usually necessary to determine this drug's effectiveness in controlling severe chronic asthma. Long-term use requires physician supervision and guidance.

▷ **Tell Your Doctor Before Taking This Medicine If You:**
- ever had an allergic reaction to it.
- are experiencing severe acute asthma or status asthmaticus that requires more intense treatment for prompt relief.
- have a form of nonallergic bronchitis with asthmatic features.
- have a herpes infection of the eye or chickenpox.
- are now taking or have recently taken any cortisone-related drug (including ACTH by injection) for any reason.
- have a history of tuberculosis of the lungs.
- have chronic bronchitis or bronchiectasis.
- think you may have an active infection of any kind, especially a respiratory infection.

▷ **Possible Side Effects:**   Yeast infections (thrush) of the mouth and throat.
Unpleasant taste.

▷ **Possible Adverse Effects:**
If any of the following develop, call your doctor promptly for guidance.
Some Mild Problems Drug Can Cause
Allergic reactions: skin rash, itching.
Headache, dizziness, nervousness, loss of smell or taste.
Upper respiratory infections, cough.
Heart palpitation, increased blood pressure, swelling of feet and ankles.
Loss of appetite, nausea, vomiting, diarrhea.
Some Serious Problems This Drug Can Cause
Allergic reaction: localized "allergic" pneumonitis (lung inflammation).
Bronchospasm, asthmatic wheezing (rare).
Tachycardia or hypertension with the inhalation form.

▷ *CAUTION*

1. This drug should NOT be relied on for the immediate relief of acute asthma.

2. If you were using any cortisone-related drugs for treatment of your asthma *before* transferring to this inhaler drug, it may be necessary to resume them if you are injured or get an infection of any kind, or if you require surgery. Be sure to tell your doctor of your prior use of cortisone-related drugs.

3. If severe asthma returns while you use this drug, notify your doctor immediately so that additional supportive treatment with cortisone-related drugs can be provided as needed.

4. Carry a personal identification card with a notation (if applicable) that you have used cortisone-related drugs within the past year. During periods of stress it may be necessary to resume cortisone treatment in adequate dosage.

5. An interval of approximately 5 to 10 minutes should separate the inhalation of bronchodilators such as albuterol, bitolterol, epinephrine, and pirbuterol (which should be used first) and the inhalation of this drug. This sequence permits greater penetration of flunisolide into the bronchial tubes. The delay between inhalations also reduces the possibility of adverse effects from the propellants used in the two inhalers.

6. Safety and effectiveness of the oral inhaler for those under 4 years old have not been established. To ensure adequate penetration of the drug and obtain maximal benefit, the use of a spacer device is recommended for inhalation therapy.

7. People over 60 with chronic bronchitis or bronchiectasis should be watched closely for lung infections.

Advisability of Use During Pregnancy or If Breast-Feeding:
Pregnancy Category: C. Avoid during the first 3 months. Use infrequently and only as clearly needed during the last 6 months. Presence in breast milk is unknown; avoid taking this drug or refrain from nursing.

▷ **Habit-Forming Potential:**   With the recommended dosage a state of functional dependence is not likely to develop.

▷ **Overdose Symptoms:**   Indications of cortisone excess (due to systemic absorption)—fluid retention, flushing of the face, stomach irritation, nervousness.

▷ **Suggested Periodic Examinations While Taking This Drug:** (at doctor's discretion)
Inspection of mouth and throat for evidence of yeast infection.
Assessment of the status of adrenal function in individuals who have used cortisone-related drugs over an extended period before using this drug.

X-ray examination of the lungs of individuals with a history of tuber-culosis.

▷ **While Taking This Drug the Following Apply:**

Foods: No specific restrictions beyond those advised by your doctor.

Tobacco Smoking: No interactions expected. However, smoking can affect the condition under treatment and reduce the effectiveness of this drug.

Other Drugs:

The following drugs may *increase* the effects of flunisolide

- inhalant bronchodilators (albuterol, bitolterol, epinephrine, pir-buterol, etc.).
- oral bronchodilators (aminophylline, ephedrine, terbutaline, theo-phylline, etc.).

Flunisolide *taken concurrently* with

- stanozolol may result in increased risk of acne or edema.

Occurrence of Unrelated Illness: Acute infections, serious injuries, and surgical procedures can create an urgent need for additional sup-portive cortisone-related drugs, by mouth and/or injection. Tell your doctor immediately about a new illness or injury of any kind.

Discontinuation: If regular use has made it possible to reduce or dis-continue maintenance doses of cortisonelike drugs by mouth, *do not* discontinue this drug abruptly. If you find it necessary to dis-continue this drug for any reason, consult your doctor promptly. It may be necessary to resume cortisone preparations and institute other measures for satisfactory management.

Special Storage Instructions: Store at room temperature. Avoid expo-sure to temperatures above 120° F (49° C). Do not store or use this inhaler near heat or open flame.

▷ **Saving Money When Using This Medicine:**

- Ask your doctor if this drug provides the best combination of cost and outcome for you.
- It may be possible (after a significant asthma-free period) to discon-tinue this medicine. Ask your doctor for help.
- If you have had to continue cortisonelike drugs (steroids), talk with your doctor about exercise, calcium supplements, and bone mineral density testing.

FLUOXETINE (flu OX e teen)

Prescription Needed: Yes   **Controlled Drug:** No   **Generic:** No

Brand Names: Prozac

Overview of BENEFITS versus RISKS

Possible Benefits	*Possible Risks*
EFFECTIVE TREATMENT OF MAJOR DEPRESSIVE DISORDERS	Serious allergic reactions
	Conversion of depression to mania in manic-depressive disorders
Possibly effective in relieving the symptoms of obsessive-compulsive disorder	Seizures

---

▷ **Illness This Medication Treats:**
 (1) Major forms of depression that have not responded well to other therapies; (2) obsessive-compulsive disorder.
 Author's note: The FDA advisory board has recommended that fluoxetine be approved for treatment of bulimia. As this book went to press approval was pending.

▷ **Typical Dosage Range:** (Dosage or schedule must be determined by the doctor for each individual.)
 Initially 20 mg every 1 to 3 days as a single morning dose; if no improvement occurs after 4 weeks of treatment, the dose may be increased by 20 mg/day as needed and tolerated. Doses over 20 mg/day should be taken in two divided doses—early morning and noon. Total daily dosage should not exceed 80 mg.

▷ **Conditions Requiring Dosing Adjustments:**
 Liver function: The dose should be decreased or the dosing interval lengthened for patients with liver compromise. Fluoxetine is also a rare cause of hepatotoxicity, and should be used with caution in this patient population.
 Kidney function: The dose should be decreased or the dosing interval lengthened for patients with severe renal compromise.

▷ **How Best to Take This Medicine:** May be taken without regard to food. The capsule may be opened for administration and the contents mixed with any convenient food. To facilitate smaller doses, the contents may be mixed with orange juice or apple juice and refrigerated; doses of 5 to 10 mg may prove effective and be better tolerated.

▷ **How Long This Medicine Is Usually Taken:** Use on a regular schedule for 4 to 8 weeks is usually necessary to determine: (1) this drug's effectiveness in relieving depression; and (2) the pattern of both favorable and unfavorable drug effects. Long-term use (months to years) requires periodic physician evaluation.

▷ **Tell Your Doctor Before Taking This Medicine If You:**
 • ever had an allergic reaction to it.
 • are currently taking or have taken within the past 14 days any MAO type A inhibitor.

- have experienced any adverse effects from antidepressants used in the past.
- have impaired liver or kidney function.
- have Parkinson's disease.
- have a seizure disorder.
- are pregnant or plan pregnancy while taking this drug.

▷ **Possible Side Effects:**   Decreased appetite, weight loss, abnormal and excessive urination (SIADH).

▷ **Possible Adverse Effects:**
If any of the following develop, call your doctor promptly for guidance.
Some Mild Problems Drug Can Cause
   Allergic reactions: skin rash, itching.
   Headache, nervousness, insomnia, drowsiness, dizziness, impaired concentration.
   Altered taste, nausea, diarrhea.
Some Serious Problems This Drug Can Cause
   Allergic reactions: serum sickness–like syndrome: fever, weakness, joint swelling, swollen lymph glands, fluid retention, skin rash.
   Rare psychosis, hallucinations, or liver toxicity.
   Drug-induced seizures.
   Worsening of Parkinson's disease.
   Intense suicidal preoccupation in severe depression that does not respond to this drug (see "Current Controversies in Drug Management," below).

▷ **Possible Effects on Sex Life:**   Impaired erection, inhibition of ejaculation, and inhibited orgasm in men and women.

▷ *CAUTION*
   1. If any type of skin reaction develops (rash, hives, etc.), discontinue this drug and tell your doctor promptly.
   2. If dryness of the mouth develops and persists for more than 2 weeks, consult your dentist for guidance.
   3. Consult your doctor before taking any other prescription or over-the-counter drug with this drug.
   4. If you are advised to take any MAO type A inhibitor, allow an interval of 5 weeks after discontinuing this drug before starting it.
   5. It is advisable to withhold this drug if electroconvulsive therapy is to be used to treat your depression.
   6. Safety and effectiveness of this drug for those under 12 years old are not established.
   7. Those over 60 should have a maximum daily dose of 60 mg.
Advisability of Use During Pregnancy or If Breast-Feeding:
Pregnancy Category: B. Use only if clearly needed. Present in breast milk; avoid taking this drug or refrain from nursing.

▷ **Habit-Forming Potential:** Some rare reports of patients abusing Prozac with higher than prescribed doses or combinations with alcohol have surfaced. A euphoric effect and some abuse potential may exist.

▷ **Overdose Symptoms:** Agitation, restlessness, excitement, nausea, vomiting, seizures.

▷ **While Taking This Drug the Following Apply:**
Beverages: May be taken with milk.
Alcohol: Avoid completely.
Other Drugs:
Fluoxetine may *increase* the effects of
- diazepam (Valium).
- digitalis preparations (digitoxin, digoxin).
- warfarin (Coumadin) and related oral anticoagulants.
- phenytoin (Dilantin) by increasing the drug level.

Fluoxetine *taken concurrently* with
- antidiabetic drugs (insulin, oral hypoglycemics) may increase the risk of hypoglycemic reactions; monitor blood and urine sugar levels carefully.
- astemizole (Hismanal) or terfenadine (Seldane) or similar drugs may result in increased risk of heart arrhythmias. Avoid combining.
- MAO type A inhibitors may cause confusion, agitation, high fever, seizures, and dangerous elevations of blood pressure. Avoid the concurrent use of these drugs.
- carbamazepine (Tegretol) may increase the carbamazepine level. Drug levels are critical if these medications are combined.
- dextromethorphan (a cough suppressant found in many nonprescription products labeled "DM") may lead to visual hallucinations if combined. DO NOT combine.
- ketorolac (Toradol) may result in hallucinations. DO NOT combine these medicines.
- lithium (Lithobid, etc.) may result in increased lithium levels and an increased risk of neurotoxicity.
- loratadine (Claritin) may result in increased loratadine levels, but does not presently appear to result in abnormal heart rhythms. Since the blood level will be increased, it appears prudent to decrease the loratadine dose if these medicines are to be combined.
- tryptophan may result in central nervous system toxicity. Avoid this combination.
- any tricyclic antidepressant (amitriptyline, nortriptyline, etc.—see Drug Classes) may result in increased antidepressant levels that will persist for weeks.
- haloperidol (Haldol) may increase haloperidol levels. Decreased dose and blood levels are needed.

- buspirone (BuSpar) may increase underlying anxiety. Avoid this combination.
- terfenadine (Seldane) or similar drugs may result in increased terfenadine levels and risk of abnormal heartbeats. AVOID combining.
- selegiline (Eldepryl) can result in serotonin toxicity syndrome. DO NOT COMBINE these drugs.

Driving, Hazardous Activities: This drug may cause drowsiness, dizziness, impaired judgment, and delayed reaction time. Restrict your activities as necessary.

Discontinuation: The slow elimination of this drug from the body makes any withdrawal effects from abrupt discontinuation unlikely. However, ask your doctor if you plan to discontinue this drug for any reason.

▷ **Current Controversies in Drug Management:** In 1990 it was reported that six patients being treated with fluoxetine experienced the onset of intense suicidal preoccupation. All six had severe depression that had not responded to fluoxetine for 2 to 7 weeks. For most of them, suicidal mentality persisted for 2 to 3 months after the drug was discontinued. The resultant adverse publicity suggested that this experience may be somewhat characteristic of fluoxetine in contrast to other antidepressant drugs.

A review of relevant literature on this subject reveals that the development or intensification of suicidal thoughts during treatment (regardless of the severity of depression) has been documented repeatedly for many antidepressant drugs in wide use. It is apparent that suicidal thinking may emerge during treatment with any antidepressant. Recent reports establish that for some patients, switching to fluoxetine stops suicidal thinking and satisfactorily relieves depression.

This experience is an example of the marked variability of individual response to drug therapy. Successful management requires clinical judgment (based on experience), close monitoring, and appropriate dosage adjustments.

▷ **Saving Money When Using This Medicine:**
- Many medications are available to treat depression. Ask your doctor if this drug provides the best combination of cost and outcome for you.
- It may be possible (after a significant depression-free period) to stop taking this medicine. Ask your doctor for help.
- The dose or dosing interval MUST be adjusted for patients with kidney and liver compromise. Ask your doctor if this has occurred.
- A recent study associated osteoporosis with depression. Talk with your doctor about your exercise, diet, and other risk factors for osteoporosis. Bone mineral density testing may also be needed.

FLUPHENAZINE (flu FEN a zeen)

Prescription Needed: Yes   **Controlled Drug:** No   **Generic:** No

Brand Names: Permitil, Prolixin

```
+-------------------------------------------------------------+
|               Overview of BENEFITS versus RISKS             |
|        Possible Benefits              Possible Risks         |
|    EFFECTIVE CONTROL OF          SERIOUS TOXIC EFFECTS ON    |
|      ACUTE MENTAL                  BRAIN with long-term use  |
|      DISORDERS in most patients  Liver damage with jaundice  |
|    Beneficial effects on thinking,  Rare blood cell disorders:|
|      mood, and behavior             abnormally low white blood|
|                                     cell counts              |
+-------------------------------------------------------------+
```

▷ **Illness This Medication Treats:**
Schizophrenia.

▷ **Typical Dosage Range:** (Dosage or schedule must be determined by the doctor for each individual.)
2.5 to 10 mg three to four times per day; adjust dosage as needed and tolerated. Total daily dosage should not exceed 40 mg.

▷ **Conditions Requiring Dosing Adjustments:**
Liver function: This drug should be used with caution by patients with both liver and kidney compromise.
Kidney function: Fluphenazine should be used with caution by patients with compromised kidneys.

▷ **How Best to Take This Medicine:** May be taken with or following meals to reduce stomach irritation. Regular tablets may be crushed for administration. Prolonged-action tablets should be swallowed whole (not crushed). The concentrate must be diluted in 4 to 6 oz of water, milk, fruit juice, or carbonated beverage.

▷ **How Long This Medicine Is Usually Taken:** Use on a regular schedule for several weeks usually determines the effectiveness of this drug in controlling psychotic disorders. If not significantly beneficial within 6 weeks, use of this drug should be discontinued. Long-term use (months to years) requires periodic physician evaluation.

▷ **Tell Your Doctor Before Taking This Medicine If You:**
• ever had an allergic reaction to it.
• have a history of brain damage.
• have active liver disease.
• have cancer of the breast.
• have a current blood cell or bone marrow disorder.

- are allergic or abnormally sensitive to any phenothiazine.
- have impaired liver or kidney function.
- have any type of seizure disorder.
- have diabetes, glaucoma, heart disease, or chronic lung disease.
- have a history of lupus erythematosus.
- are taking any drug with sedative effects.
- plan to have surgery under general or spinal anesthesia soon.

▷ **Possible Side Effects:**   Drowsiness (usually during the first 2 weeks), orthostatic hypotension, blurred vision, dry mouth, nasal congestion, constipation, impaired urination (all mild).

▷ **Possible Adverse Effects:**
If any of the following develop, call your doctor promptly for guidance.
Some Mild Problems Drug Can Cause
   Allergic reactions: skin rash, itching.
   Lowering of body temperature, especially in the elderly.
   Headache, dizziness, weakness, excitement, unusual dreaming.
   Increased appetite and weight gain.
Some Serious Problems Drug Can Cause
   Allergic reactions: hepatitis with jaundice, usually between second and fourth week; anaphylactic reaction.
   Idiosyncratic reaction: neuroleptic malignant syndrome.
   Impaired production of white blood cells.
   Parkinson-like disorders; muscle spasms of face, jaw, neck, back, extremities.
   Depression.
   Rare porphyria, seizures, or pituitary tumors.
   Prolonged drop in blood pressure with weakness, perspiration, and fainting.

▷ **Possible Effects on Sex Life:**   Decreased male libido; increased female libido. Impaired erection; complete impotence. Inhibited male orgasm; inhibited female orgasm. Inhibited ejaculation. Altered timing and pattern of menstruation. Female breast enlargement and milk production. Male breast enlargement and tenderness. May help treat sexual hyperactivity.

▷ **Adverse Effects That May Mimic Natural Diseases or Disorders:**
   Nervous system reactions may suggest Parkinson's disease.
   Liver reactions may suggest viral hepatitis.
   Reactions resembling systemic lupus erythematosus may occur.

▷ *CAUTION*
   1. Many over-the-counter medications for allergies, colds, and coughs contain drugs that can interact unfavorably with this drug. Ask your doctor or pharmacist for help before using any such medications.

2. Antacids that contain aluminum and/or magnesium can prevent the absorption of this drug and reduce its effectiveness.
3. Obtain prompt evaluation of any change or disturbance of vision.
4. This drug is not for use by infants under 6 months old, or children of any age with symptoms suggestive of Reye's syndrome. Monitor carefully for blood cell changes.
5. Those over 60 should take small doses until individual response has been determined. You may be more susceptible to the development of drowsiness, lethargy, constipation, lowering of body temperature, and orthostatic hypotension. This drug can enhance existing prostatism. You may also be more susceptible to the development of Parkinson-like reactions and/or tardive dyskinesia. These reactions must be recognized early since they may become unresponsive to treatment and irreversible.

Advisability of Use During Pregnancy or If Breast-Feeding:
Pregnancy Category: C. Avoid using this drug during the first 3 months and during the last month because of possible effects on the newborn infant. Present in breast milk; avoid taking this drug or refrain from nursing.

▷ **Overdose Symptoms:** Marked drowsiness, weakness, tremor, agitation, unsteadiness, deep sleep, coma, convulsions.

▷ **Suggested Periodic Examinations While Taking This Drug:** (at doctor's discretion)
Complete blood cell counts, especially between the fourth and tenth weeks of treatment.
Liver function tests, electrocardiograms.
Complete eye examinations—eye structures and vision.
Careful inspection of the tongue for early evidence of fine, involuntary, wavelike movements that could indicate tardive dyskinesia.

▷ **While Taking This Drug the Following Apply:**
Beverages: May be taken with milk.
Alcohol: Avoid completely. Alcohol can increase the sedative action of phenothiazines and accentuate their depressant effects on brain function and blood pressure. Phenothiazines can increase the intoxicating effects of alcohol
Tobacco Smoking: Possible reduction of drowsiness from drug.
Marijuana Smoking: Moderate increase in drowsiness; accentuation of orthostatic hypotension; increased risk of precipitating latent psychoses, confusing the interpretation of mental status and drug responses.
Other Drugs:
Fluphenazine may *increase* the effects of
• all sedative drugs, causing excessive sedation.
• all atropinelike drugs, causing nervous system toxicity.

Fluphenazine may *decrease* the effects of
- guanethidine (Ismelin, Esimil), reducing its effectiveness in lowering blood pressure.

Fluphenazine *taken concurrently* with
- beta-blockers may cause increased effects of both drugs; monitor drug effects closely, and adjust dosages as necessary.
- clonidine (Catapres, others) may result in acute organic brain syndrome (disorientation, delirium). DO NOT COMBINE.
- lithium (Lithobid, others) may result in increased nerve toxicity.
- MAO inhibitors (see Drug Classes) may cause very low blood pressure or worsening of respiratory depression.
- oral hypoglycemic agents (see Drug Classes) may result in lower blood sugar levels than expected.
- vitamin C (ascorbic acid) may decrease the therapeutic benefits of fluphenazine.

The following drugs may *decrease* the effects of fluphenazine
- antacids containing aluminum and/or magnesium.
- benztropine (Cogentin).
- trihexyphenidyl (Artane).

Driving, Hazardous Activities: This drug can impair mental alertness, judgment, and physical coordination. Avoid hazardous activities.

Exposure to Sun: Use caution until your sensitivity has been determined. Some phenothiazines can cause photosensitivity.

Exposure to Heat: Use caution and avoid excessive heat as much as possible. This drug may impair the regulation of body temperature and increase the risk of heatstroke.

Exposure to Cold: Use caution and dress warmly. This drug can increase the risk of hypothermia in the elderly.

Discontinuation: After a period of long-term use, do not discontinue this drug suddenly. Gradual withdrawal over 2 to 3 weeks under the supervision of your doctor is recommended. Do not discontinue this drug without your doctor's knowledge and approval. The relapse rate of schizophrenia after discontinuation is 50 to 60%.

▷ **Saving Money When Using This Medicine:**
- A large number of drugs are available to provide similar effectiveness. Ask your doctor to prescribe the one that offers the best combination of cost and outcome.
- It may be possible (after a significant symptom-free period) to stop taking this medicine. Ask your doctor for help.
- If you have liver and kidney compromise, the dose must be adjusted. Ask your doctor if this has been done.
- A new medicine called olanzapine may offer fewer side effects while producing favorable outcomes.

FLURAZEPAM (floor AZ e pam)

Prescription Needed: Yes   **Controlled Drug:** C-IV*   **Generic:** Yes

Brand Names: Dalmane, Durapam

Overview of BENEFITS versus RISKS	
Possible Benefits	*Possible Risks*
EFFECTIVE HYPNOTIC	Habit-forming potential with
NO SUPPRESSION OF RAPID	long-term use
EYE MOVEMENT (REM)	Minor impairment of mental
SLEEP	functions (hangover effect)
NO REM SLEEP REBOUND	Very rare jaundice
after discontinuation	Very rare blood cell disorder
Wide margin of safety with	Suppression of stage-4 sleep
therapeutic doses	with reduced quality of sleep

▷ **Illness This Medication Treats:**

Short-term treatment of insomnia consisting of difficulty in falling asleep, frequent nighttime awakenings, and/or early morning awakenings.

▷ **Typical Dosage Range:** (Dosage or schedule must be determined by the doctor for each individual.)

Infants and Children: Up to 15 years old: Use of this drug not recommended.

15 to 60 Years of Age: Initially 15 mg at bedtime; increase to 30 mg only if needed and tolerated.

Over 60 Years of Age: Same as for 15 to 60 years of age. Usually 15 mg is adequate; use higher doses with caution.

▷ **Conditions Requiring Dosing Adjustments:**

Liver function: The dose **must** be decreased for patients with liver compromise. Flurazepam is also a rare cause of liver toxicity, and its use by patients with compromised livers is a benefit-to-risk decision.

▷ **How Best to Take This Medicine:** May be taken on an empty stomach or with food or milk. The capsule may be opened for administration. Do not discontinue this drug abruptly if taken for more than 4 weeks.

▷ **How Long This Medicine Is Usually Taken:** Use for 3 nights is usually necessary to evaluate this drug's effectiveness in relieving insomnia. If possible, this drug should be used for periods of 3 to 5 nights intermittently, repeated as needed with appropriate dosage

*See Controlled Drug Schedules inside this book's cover.

adjustment. Avoid uninterrupted and prolonged use. The duration of use should not exceed 2 weeks without reappraisal of continued need.

▷ **Tell Your Doctor Before Taking This Medicine If You:**
- ever had an allergic reaction to it.
- are pregnant or planning pregnancy.
- have acute narrow-angle glaucoma.
- are allergic to any benzodiazepine drug.
- have a history of alcoholism or drug abuse.
- have impaired liver or kidney function.
- have a history of serious depression or mental disorder.
- are taking other drugs with sedative effects.
- have asthma, emphysema, epilepsy, or myasthenia gravis.

▷ **Possible Side Effects:** "Hangover" effects on arising: drowsiness, lethargy, and unsteadiness.

▷ **Possible Adverse Effects:**
If any of the following develop, call your doctor promptly for guidance.
Some Mild Problems Drug Can Cause
   Allergic reactions: skin rash, burning eyes, swelling of tongue.
   Dizziness, fainting, blurred vision, slurred speech, nausea.
   Ringing in the ears.
Some Serious Problems Drug Can Cause
   Allergic reactions: rare liver damage with jaundice.
   Idiosyncratic reactions: nervousness, irritability, euphoria, hallucinations.
   Rare liver toxicity.
   Rare bone marrow depression.
   Risk of falls if used in those over 60.

▷ **Adverse Effects That May Mimic Natural Diseases or Disorders:**
   Liver reaction with jaundice may suggest viral hepatitis.

▷ *CAUTION*
   1. This drug should not be discontinued abruptly if it has been taken continually for more than 4 weeks.
   2. The concurrent use of some over-the-counter drugs that contain antihistamines (allergy and cold preparations, sleep aids) can cause excessive sedation in sensitive individuals.
   3. Regular nightly use of any hypnotic drug should be avoided.
   4. This drug is transformed by the liver into long-acting forms that can persist in the body for 24 hours or more. With continual daily use of this drug, these active drug forms accumulate and produce increasing sedation. If you experience a "hangover" effect, avoid hazardous activities (driving, etc.) and the use of alcohol.

5. Safety and effectiveness of this drug for those under 15 years old have not been established.

6. Those over 60 should take smaller starting doses and take them less often then usual. It may be prudent to use a drug with fewer active metabolites. Watch for development of lethargy, indifference, fatigue, weakness, unsteadiness, disturbing dreams, nightmares, and paradoxical reactions of excitement, agitation, anger, hostility, and rage. Long-acting benzodiazepines may cause residual sluggishness and unsteadiness, with increased risk of falling during the day following bedtime use. May also increase the number of sleep apnea episodes in this age group.

Advisability of Use During Pregnancy or If Breast-Feeding:

Pregnancy Category: X. Avoid use of this drug during entire pregnancy. Probably present in breast milk. Avoid taking this drug or refrain from nursing.

▷ **Habit-Forming Potential:** This drug can produce psychological and/or physical dependence if used in large doses for an extended period. Avoid continual use.

▷ **Overdose Symptoms:** Marked drowsiness, weakness, feeling of drunkenness, staggering gait, tremor, stupor progressing to deep sleep or coma.

▷ **Suggested Periodic Examinations While Taking This Drug:** (at doctor's discretion)

Complete blood cell counts and liver function tests during long-term use.

▷ **While Taking This Drug the Following Apply:**

Beverages: Avoid excessive intake of caffeine-containing beverages (coffee, tea, cola, chocolate) within 4 hours of taking this drug. May be taken with milk.

Alcohol: Use with extreme caution—alcohol may increase the absorption of this drug and add to its depressant effects on the brain. It is best to avoid alcohol completely—throughout the day and night—if you must drive or engage in any hazardous activity.

Tobacco Smoking: Heavy smoking may reduce the hypnotic action of this drug.

Marijuana Smoking: Increased sedation and significant impairment of intellectual and physical performance.

Other Drugs:

Flurazepam may *increase* the effects of

• digoxin (Lanoxin), causing digoxin toxicity.
• lithium (Lithobid, others) and cause additive drowsiness.
• phenytoin (Dilantin), causing phenytoin toxicity.

Flurazepam may *decrease* the effects of

• levodopa (Sinemet, etc.), reducing its effectiveness in treating Parkinson's disease.

Flurazepam *taken concurrently* with
- narcotics, other benzodiazepines, phenothiazines, or antihistamines (see Drug Classes) may result in additive sedation.

The following drugs may *increase* the effects of flurazepam
- cimetidine (Tagamet).
- disulfiram (Antabuse).
- isoniazid (INH, Rifamate, etc.).
- omeprazole (Prilosec).
- oral contraceptives (birth control pills).
- valproic acid (Depakene).

The following drugs may *decrease* the effects of flurazepam
- rifampin (Rimactane, etc.).
- theophylline (aminophylline, Theo-Dur, etc.).

Driving, Hazardous Activities: This drug can impair mental alertness, judgment, physical coordination, and reaction time. Avoid hazardous activities accordingly.

Exposure to Heat: Use caution until the effect of excessive perspiration is determined. Because of reduced urine volume, this drug may accumulate in the body and produce overdosage effects.

Discontinuation: Avoid sudden discontinuation if this drug has been taken for more than 4 weeks without interruption. Dosage should be tapered gradually to prevent a withdrawal syndrome that could include depression, confusion, hallucinations, tremor, seizures, muscle cramping, sweating, and vomiting.

▷ **Saving Money When Using This Medicine:**
- A large number of drugs are available that provide similar effectiveness. Ask your doctor to prescribe the drug that offers the best combination of cost and outcome.
- This drug is for SHORT-TERM use. Ask your doctor for help.
- Make sure you talk with your doctor about caffeine use (coffee, tea, sodas, and chocolate) as well as prescription, nonprescription, or herbal medicines you take. These can have an impact on sleeplessness.
- Talk with your doctor about stress management and exercise programs available in your community.

FLURBIPROFEN   (flur BI pro fen)

Prescription Needed: Yes   **Controlled Drug:** No   **Generic:** No

Brand Names: Ansaid

Overview of BENEFITS versus RISKS	
Possible Benefits	*Possible Risks*
EFFECTIVE RELIEF OF SYMPTOMS ASSOCIATED WITH MAJOR TYPES OF ARTHRITIS	PEPTIC ULCER DISEASE with associated bleeding and perforation
Effective relief of symptoms associated with bursitis, tendonitis, and related conditions	Liver toxicity with jaundice
	Water retention
	Rare kidney toxicity
	Rare aplastic anemia
Effective relief of menstrual cramps	

See the propionic acids (NSAID) drug profile for further information.

FLUTAMIDE (FLU ta mide)

Prescription Needed: Yes   **Controlled Drug:** No   **Generic:** No

Brand Names: Eulexin

Overview of BENEFITS versus RISKS	
Possible Benefits	*Possible Risks*
EFFECTIVE ADJUNCTIVE TREATMENT OF PROSTATE CANCER	Rare drug-induced hepatitis
	Breast enlargement and tenderness
	Hot flashes

▷ **Illness This Medication Treats:**
Metastatic prostate cancer; used concurrently with leuprolide (taken by injection).

▷ **Typical Dosage Range:** (Dosage or schedule must be determined by the doctor for each individual.)
Infants and Children: Not used in this age group.
12 to 60 Years of Age: 250 mg every 8 hours. Taken concurrently with leuprolide; the usual dose of leuprolide is 7.5 mg taken by injection once a month.
Over 60 Years of Age: Same as for 12 to 60 years of age.

▷ **Conditions Requiring Dosing Adjustments:**
Liver function: This drug should be used with caution by patients with liver compromise. It is also a rare cause of cholestatic jaundice.
Kidney function: This drug should be used with caution by patients with renal compromise.

▷ **How Best to Take This Medicine:**   May be taken without regard to food. The capsule may be opened and the tablet may be crushed for administration.

▷ **How Long This Medicine Is Usually Taken:**   Use on a regular schedule for 2 to 3 months usually determines the effectiveness of this drug in controlling prostate cancer. Long-term use (months to years) requires periodic physician evaluation.

▷ **Tell Your Doctor Before Taking This Medicine If You:**
- ever had an allergic reaction to it.
- have a history of liver disease or impaired liver function.
- have hypertension.

▷ **Possible Side Effects:**   Hot flashes, loss of libido, impotence, breast enlargement and tenderness.

▷ **Possible Adverse Effects:**
If any of the following develop, call your doctor promptly for guidance.
Some Mild Problems Drug Can Cause
    Allergic reactions: skin rash.
    Drowsiness, nervousness.
    Nausea/vomiting, diarrhea.
    Fluid retention (edema) of legs.
    Rare blurred vision.
Some Serious Problems Drug Can Cause
    Drug-induced hepatitis with jaundice.
    Rare lupus erythematosus or heart attack.
    Low blood platelets or white blood cells, or anemia.

▷ **Possible Effects on Sex Life:**   See "Possible Side Effects," above. Sexual changes are probably a result of the combination therapy approach.

▷ *CAUTION*
1. For best results, flutamide and leuprolide should be started and continued together for the duration of treatment.
2. During combined treatment with flutamide and leuprolide, symptoms of prostate cancer (difficult urination, bone pain, etc.) may worsen temporarily; these are transient and not significant.
3. This drug is excreted more slowly by the elderly. If digestive symptoms or edema are troublesome, ask your doctor about your dosage schedule.

Advisability of Use During Pregnancy or If Breast-Feeding:
Pregnancy Category: D.

▷ **Overdose Symptoms:**   Possible drowsiness, unsteadiness, nausea, vomiting.

▷ **Suggested Periodic Examinations While Taking This Drug:** (at doctor's discretion)

Prostatic specific antigen (PSA) assays.

Complete blood cell counts.

Liver function tests.

▷ **While Taking This Drug the Following Apply:**

Beverages: May be taken with milk.

Other Drugs:

Flutamide *taken concurrently* with

- flu (influenza), pneumococcal, or yellow fever vaccine may result in blunting of the immune response and hence the benefit from these vaccines.

Driving, Hazardous Activities: This drug may cause drowsiness. Restrict your activities as necessary.

Exposure to Sun: Use caution until full effect is known. This drug may cause photosensitivity.

Discontinuation: To be determined by your doctor.

▷ **Saving Money When Using This Medicine:**

- Ask your doctor if this drug offers the best combination of cost and outcome for you.
- Since a considerable amount of research occurs in oncology, talk with your doctor about medicines currently under research or those that are newly approved.

FLUVOXAMINE (FLEW vox a meen)

Prescription Needed: Yes **Controlled Drug:** No **Generic:** No

Brand Names: Luvox

Overview of BENEFITS versus RISKS	
Possible Benefits	*Possible Risks*
TREATMENT OF OBSESSIVE-COMPULSIVE DISORDER	Nausea or vomiting (often resolves with time)

▷ **Illness This Medication Treats:**

Obsessive-compulsive disorder.

Other (unlabeled) generally accepted uses: (1) may have a role in treating resistant depression; (2) can help control binge eating; (3) may help panic attacks; (4) may help chronic tension headaches.

▷ **Typical Dosage Range:** (Dosage or schedule must be determined by the doctor for each individual.)

Infants and Children: Safety and efficacy of this drug are not established for those under 18 years old.

18 to 60 Years of Age: Dosing is started with 50 mg taken at bedtime. Further increases are made as needed or tolerated in 50-mg steps every 4 to 7 days. Maximum dose is 300 mg daily. If the patient needs more than 100 mg daily, the dose should be divided into two equal doses taken twice daily.

Over 65 Years of Age: Careful adjustment with lower starting doses and slow increases are recommended. This medicine is removed 50% more slowly by this population than by younger patients.

▷ **Conditions Requiring Dosing Adjustments:**

Liver function: Since fluvoxamine is extensively changed in the liver, lower starting doses and slow increases are prudent.

Kidney function: Lower starting doses and careful patient monitoring is needed.

▷ **How Best to Take This Medicine:**   Take this medicine exactly as prescribed and at the same time daily. This medicine may be taken with or without food. Call your doctor if vomiting (a possible side effect) continues for more than 2 days after you start therapy.

▷ **How Long This Medicine Is Usually Taken:**   Regular use for 4 to 14 days usually determines effectiveness. Long-term use requires periodic checks of response and possible dosing adjustments. Keep follow-up appointments with your doctor.

▷ **Tell Your Doctor Before Taking This Medicine If You:**
- ever had an allergic reaction to it.
- have a severely damaged liver or kidneys.
- have taken terfenadine or astemizole, or have taken a monoamine oxidase inhibitor (MAOI) (see Drug Classes).
- have a history of seizures.
- have a history of heart problems.

▷ **Possible Side Effects:**   Nausea or vomiting (usually subsides).

▷ **Possible Adverse Effects:**
If any of the following develop, call your doctor promptly for guidance.

Some Mild Problems This Drug Can Cause
    Allergic reactions: skin rash.
    Headache, sleep disorders.
    Constipation or anorexia.

Some Serious Problems This Drug Can Cause
    Allergic reactions: anaphylactic reaction.
    Rare liver toxicity, seizures, mania, serious skin rash (toxic epidermal necrolysis or TEN) or lowering of blood sodium (SIADH).

▷ **Possible Effects on Sex Life:** Delayed or absent orgasm, failure to ejaculate.

▷ *CAUTION*

1. This medicine has several important drug-drug interactions. Be certain to tell those who prescribe medicines for you that you are taking fluvoxamine.
2. Safety and effectiveness of this drug for those less than 18 years old are not established.
3. Those over 60 should use this drug with caution and lower starting doses.
4. Tell your doctor if you started vomiting after taking this medicine, and it continues for more than 2 days.

Advisability of Use During Pregnancy or If Breast-Feeding:

Pregnancy Category: C. Adequate studies of pregnant women are not available. Ask your doctor for guidance. Present in breast milk. Watch the nursing infant closely, and stop breast-feeding or discuss stopping this medicine with your doctor if adverse effects develop.

▷ **Overdose Symptoms:** Nausea, vomiting, or seizures.

▷ **Suggested Periodic Examinations While Taking This Drug:** (at doctor's discretion)

Periodic checks of liver enzymes.

▷ **While Taking This Drug the Following Apply:**

Alcohol: Alcohol may intensify the drowsiness this medicine can cause.

Tobacco Smoking: Smoking shortens the length of time this medicine stays in your body.

Other Drugs:

Fluvoxamine *taken concurrently* with

- amitriptyline (Elavil, others) can lead to amitriptyline toxicity
- astemizole (Hismanal) may cause serious heart arrhythmias. DO NOT combine.
- benzodiazepines (see Drug Classes) may cause toxicity.
- beta-blockers (see Drug Classes) may cause toxicity.
- carbamazepine (Tegretol) can cause toxicity.
- clomipramine (Anafranil) may cause toxicity.
- imipramine (Tofranil, others) can cause toxicity.
- lithium (Lithobid, others) can cause serotonin syndrome.
- monoamine oxidase inhibitors (MAOIs—see Drug Classes) may lead to toxicity. DO NOT combine.
- maprotiline can cause maprotiline toxicity.
- methadone can cause increased methadone effects.
- oral hypoglycemics (see Drug Classes) may stay in the body longer than expected, and cause excessive blood sugar lowering. This has been reported with sertraline, a similar medicine.
- phenytoin (Dilantin) may lead to phenytoin toxicity.

- terfenadine (Seldane) can cause **serious heart arrhythmias**. DO NOT combine.
- theophylline (Theo-Dur, others) can lead to toxicity.
- warfarin (Coumadin) can lead to bleeding. Increased INR (pro-thrombin time) testing is needed, with doses adjusted to laboratory test results.

Driving, Hazardous Activities: Caution: This medicine may cause drowsiness. Use caution until you know the degree of this effect on you.

Discontinuation; A withdrawal syndrome has been reported if this medicine is suddenly stopped. Talk with your doctor about tapering this medicine if it must be stopped.

▷ **Saving Money When Using This Medicine:**

- Effective control of symptoms of obsessive-compulsive disorder (OCD) or depression can allow patients to return to work and productive lives.
- Talk with your doctor to make sure that this medicine offers you the best balance of price and outcomes.

FOSCARNET (fos KAR net)

Prescription Needed: Yes   **Controlled Drug:** No   **Generic:** No

Brand Names: Foscavir

Overview of BENEFITS versus RISKS	
Possible Benefits	*Possible Risks*
TREATMENT OF CYTOMEGALOVIRUS (CMV) RETINITIS IN AIDS PATIENTS	SEIZURES
	ENCEPHALOPATHY (RARE)
	CARDIAC ARREST (RARE)
SIGNIFICANT DELAY IN PROGRESSION OF EYE DISEASE	SIGNIFICANT KIDNEY IMPAIRMENT
	ELECTROLYTE ABNORMALITIES
	Low blood platelets
	Anemia
	Bronchospasm

▷ **Illness This Medication Treats:**

(1) Cytomegalovirus (CMV) retinitis in patients with AIDS; (2) combination therapy with ganciclovir of CMV retinitis; (3) acyclovir-resistant herpes simplex infections in people with compromised immune systems.

FOSINOPRIL (FOH sin oh pril)

Prescription Needed: Yes **Controlled Drug:** No **Generic:** No

Brand Names: Monopril

Overview of BENEFITS versus RISKS

Possible Benefits	*Possible Risks*
EFFECTIVE CONTROL OF MILD TO MODERATE HIGH BLOOD PRESSURE	Low blood pressure Allergic swelling: face, tongue, throat, vocal cords

---

▷ **Illness This Medication Treats:**
(1) Mild to moderate high blood pressure, alone or concurrently with a thiazide diuretic; (2) help in decreasing enlarged left side of the heart.

▷ **Typical Dosage Range:** (Dosage or schedule must be determined by the doctor for each individual.)
Infants and Children: Dosage not established.
18 to 60 Years of Age: Initially 10 mg once daily for those not taking a diuretic; 5 mg once daily for those taking a diuretic. Usual maintenance dose is 20 to 40 mg per day, taken in a single dose. Total daily dosage should not exceed 80 mg.
Over 60 Years of Age: Same as for 18 to 60 years of age.

▷ **Conditions Requiring Dosing Adjustments:**
Liver function: As a prodrug, fosinopril is changed into fosinoprilat (the active form) by the liver. Patients with liver compromise should use this drug with caution and in lower doses
Kidney function: This drug is removed by both the liver and bile and via the kidneys. Patients with renal compromise (especially renal artery stenosis) should start with a decreased dose, increasing it as needed and tolerated.

▷ **How Best to Take This Medicine:** Take on an empty stomach or with food at same time each day. The tablet may be crushed for administration.

▷ **How Long This Medicine Is Usually Taken:** Use on a regular schedule for 2 to 3 weeks determines the effectiveness of this drug in controlling high blood pressure. The proper treatment of high blood pressure usually requires the long-term use of effective medications. Consult your doctor regularly.

▷ **Tell Your Doctor Before Taking This Medicine If You:**
• ever had an allergic reaction to it or to another ACE inhibitor.
• are in the last 6 months of pregnancy or are planning pregnancy.

- currently have a blood cell or bone marrow disorder.
- have an abnormally high level of blood potassium.
- have a history of kidney disease or impaired kidney function.
- have scleroderma or systemic lupus erythematosus.
- have cerebral artery disease.
- have any form of heart disease.
- are taking any other antihypertensives, diuretics, nitrates, or potassium supplements.
- plan to have surgery under general anesthesia soon.

▷ **Possible Side Effects:** Dizziness, orthostatic hypotension, increased blood potassium level.

▷ **Possible Adverse Effects:**
If any of the following develop, call your doctor promptly for guidance.
Some Mild Problems Drug Can Cause
    Allergic reactions: skin rash, itching.
    Headache, fatigue, drowsiness, numbness, and tingling.
    Chest pain, palpitation, cough.
    Indigestion, nausea and vomiting, diarrhea.
Some Serious Problems Drug Can Cause
    Allergic reactions: swelling (angioedema) of face, tongue, and/or vocal cords, which can be life-threatening.
    Impairment of kidney function.
    Pancreatitis has been reported with members of the same pharmacologic family.
    Rare decreased white blood cells.

▷ **Possible Effects on Sex Life:** Decreased libido. Rare abnormal swelling of male breast tissue (gynecomastia). Impotence has been reported with members of the same pharmacologic family.

▷ *CAUTION*
1. Ask your doctor about the advisability of discontinuing other antihypertensive drugs (especially diuretics) for 1 week before starting this drug.
2. **Tell your doctor immediately if you become pregnant.** This drug should not be taken beyond the first 3 months of pregnancy.
3. **Report promptly** any indications of infection (fever, sore throat) or water retention (weight gain, puffiness, swollen feet or ankles).
4. Do not use a salt substitute without your doctor's knowledge and approval (many contain potassium).
5. It is advisable to obtain blood cell counts and urine analyses **before** starting this drug.
6. Safety and effectiveness of this drug for those under 18 years old are not established.
7. Those over 60 should take small doses until tolerance has been

determined. Sudden and excessive lowering of blood pressure can predispose to stroke or heart attack in those with impaired brain circulation or coronary artery disease.

Advisability of Use During Pregnancy or If Breast-Feeding:

Pregnancy Category: D. Avoid using this drug completely during the last 6 months. C during the first 3 months of pregnancy; use only if clearly needed. Ask your doctor for guidance. Present in breast milk; avoid taking this drug or refrain from nursing.

▷ **Overdose Symptoms:** Excessive drop in blood pressure, light-headedness, dizziness, fainting.

▷ **Suggested Periodic Examinations While Taking This Drug:** (at doctor's discretion)

Before starting drug: complete blood cell counts; urine analysis with measurement of protein content; blood potassium level.

During use: blood cell counts; blood potassium measurements.

▷ **While Taking This Drug the Following Apply:**

Foods: Consult your doctor regarding salt intake.

Nutritional Support: Do not take potassium supplements unless directed by your doctor.

Beverages: May be taken with milk.

Alcohol: Use caution until combined effect has been determined. Alcohol may enhance the blood pressure–lowering effect of this drug.

Other Drugs:

Fosinopril *taken concurrently* with

- lithium (Lithobid, others) may cause increased lithium blood levels and toxicity; monitor blood levels and adjust dosage as necessary.
- NSAIDs (see Drug Classes), such as aspirin or ketorolac (Toradol), may result in blunting of the benefits of fosinopril.
- potassium preparations (K-Lyte, Slow-K, etc.) may cause increased blood levels of potassium with risk of serious heart rhythm disturbances.
- potassium-sparing diuretics such as amiloride (Moduretic), spironolactone (Aldactazide), or triamterene (Dyazide) may increase blood levels of potassium with risk of serious heart rhythm disturbances.
- chlorpromazine (Thorazine) can cause large increases in blood pressure. AVOID this combination.
- cyclosporine (Sandimmune) can cause a large decrease in kidney function.
- loop diuretics—furosemide (Lasix) or bumetanide (Bumex)—can markedly lower blood pressure on standing (postural hypotension).

Driving, Hazardous Activities: Usually no restrictions. Be aware of possible drops in blood pressure, with resultant dizziness or faintness.

Exposure to Sun: Caution is advised. A similar drug of this class can cause photosensitivity.

Exposure to Heat: Caution is advised. Avoid excessive perspiring with resultant loss of body water and drop in blood pressure.

Occurrence of Unrelated Illness: Report promptly any disorder that causes nausea, vomiting, or diarrhea. Fluid and chemical imbalances must be corrected as soon as possible.

Discontinuation: This drug may be stopped abruptly without a sudden increase in blood pressure. However, you should consult your doctor regarding withdrawal for any reason.

▷ **Saving Money When Using This Medicine:**
- A large number of ACE inhibitors are available to provide similar effectiveness. Ask your doctor to prescribe the drug that offers the best combination of cost and outcome for you.
- Talk with your doctor about stress management and exercise programs available in your area.
- Discuss with your doctor the benefits and risks of taking aspirin every other day.

FUROSEMIDE   (fur OH se mide)

Prescription Needed: Yes   **Controlled Drug:** No   **Generic:** Yes

Brand Names: Lasix, Furocot, Lasaject, Luramide, SK-Furosemide

Overview of BENEFITS versus RISKS	
Possible Benefits	*Possible Risks*
PROMPT, EFFECTIVE, RELIABLE DIURETIC	WATER AND ELECTROLYTE DEPLETION with excessive use
MODEST ANTIHYPERTENSIVE IN MILD TO MODERATE HYPERTENSION	Excessive potassium loss
	Increased blood sugar level
	Increased blood uric acid level
ENHANCES EFFECTIVENESS OF OTHER ANTIHYPERTENSIVES	Decreased blood calcium level
	Liver damage (rare)
	Blood cell disorder (rare)

▷ **Illness This Medication Treats:**
(1) Congestive heart failure and some liver, lung, or kidney diseases; removal of excessive water (edema); (2) high blood pressure, usually in conjunction with other antihypertensives.

▷ **Typical Dosage Range:**   As antihypertensive: 40 mg/12 hr initially; increase dose as needed and tolerated. As diuretic: 20 to 80 mg in a single dose initially; if necessary, increase the dose by 20 to 40 mg every 6 to 8 hours. The smallest effective dose should be determined. The total daily dose should not exceed 640 mg. In general other medicines should be added before the dose is increased above 80 mg per day.

▷ **Conditions Requiring Dosing Adjustments:**

Liver function: Larger doses may be needed for patients with liver compromise; however, extreme care must be taken to maintain critical electrolytes.

Kidney function: Larger initial doses may be needed for people with compromised kidneys before an effect is seen. Patients with renal compromise should use this drug with caution.

Cystic fibrosis: People with this disease may be more sensitive to this drug, and smaller starting doses are prudent.

▷ **How Best to Take This Medicine:** May be taken with or following meals to reduce stomach irritation. Best taken in the morning to avoid nighttime urination. The tablet may be crushed for administration.

▷ **How Long This Medicine Is Usually Taken:** Use on a regular schedule for 2 to 3 weeks determines the effectiveness of this drug in lowering high blood pressure. Long-term use (months to years) requires periodic physician evaluation of response.

▷ **Tell Your Doctor Before Taking This Medicine If You:**
- ever had an allergic reaction to it.
- are allergic to any form of sulfa drug.
- are pregnant or planning pregnancy.
- have a history of kidney or liver disease.
- have diabetes, gout, or lupus erythematosus.
- are taking any form of cortisone, digitalis, oral antidiabetic, or insulin.
- plan to have surgery under general anesthesia soon.

▷ **Possible Side Effects:** Light-headedness on arising from sitting or lying position.

Increased blood sugar level, affecting control of diabetes.

Increased blood uric acid level, affecting control of gout.

Decreased blood potassium level, causing muscle weakness and cramping.

Decreased thiamine level.

Decreased magnesium level.

▷ **Possible Adverse Effects:**
If any of the following develop, call your doctor promptly for guidance.
Some Mild Problems Drug Can Cause
Allergic reactions: skin rashes, hives, drug fever.

Headache, dizziness, blurred or yellow vision, ringing in ears, numbness and tingling.

Reduced appetite, indigestion, nausea, vomiting, diarrhea.

Some Serious Problems Drug Can Cause

Allergic reactions: hepatitis with jaundice, anaphylactic reaction, severe skin reactions.

Idiosyncratic reaction: fluid accumulation in lungs.

Temporary hearing loss.

Inflammation of the pancreas—severe abdominal pain.

Bone marrow depression.

Rare porphyria, kidney stones, liver toxicity, or skin lesions (erythema multiforme).

Stevens-Johnson syndrome.

May increase risk of hip fracture.

▷ **Possible Effects on Sex Life:**   Impotence using recommended dosage of 20 to 80 mg per day.

▷ *CAUTION*

1. Do not exceed recommended doses. Increased dosage can cause excessive loss of sodium and potassium, with resultant loss of appetite, nausea, fatigue, weakness, confusion, and tingling in the extremities.

2. If you are also taking a digitalis preparation (digitoxin, digoxin), ensure an adequate intake of high-potassium foods to prevent potassium deficiency, a potential cause of digitalis toxicity.

3. In infants and children overdosage can cause serious dehydration. Significant potassium loss can occur within the first 2 weeks of drug use.

4. Those over 60 should take small doses until individual response has been determined. You may be more susceptible to the development of impaired thinking, orthostatic hypotension, potassium loss, and blood sugar increase. Overdosage and extended use can cause excessive loss of body water, blood thickening, and increased tendency for clotting—predisposing to stroke, heart attack, or thrombophlebitis.

Advisability of Use During Pregnancy or If Breast-Feeding:

Pregnancy Category: C. Avoid during pregnancy unless a very serious complication occurs for which this drug is significantly beneficial. Avoid completely during the first 3 months. Ask your doctor for guidance. Present in breast milk; avoid taking this drug or refrain from nursing.

▷ **Overdose Symptoms:**   Dry mouth, thirst, lethargy, weakness, muscle cramping, nausea, vomiting, drowsiness progressing to stupor or coma.

▷ **Suggested Periodic Examinations While Taking This Drug:** (at doctor's discretion)

Complete blood cell counts; measurements of sodium, potassium, chloride, magnesium, sugar, and uric acid blood levels.

Kidney and liver function tests.

▷ **While Taking This Drug the Following Apply:**

Foods: Ask your doctor about the advisability of eating foods rich in potassium (see Table 11, "High-Potassium Foods," Section Six). Follow your doctor's advice regarding the use of salt.

Beverages: This drug may be taken with milk.

Alcohol: Use with caution until the combined effects have been determined. Alcohol may exaggerate this drug's blood pressure–lowering effects and cause orthostatic hypotension.

Other Drugs:

Furosemide may *increase* the effects of

- other antihypertensive drugs; dosage adjustments may be necessary to prevent excessive blood pressure lowering.
- digoxin (Lanoxin), resulting in digoxin toxicity even with "normal" digoxin levels.
- lithium (Lithobid, others), causing lithium toxicity.

Furosemide may *decrease* the effects of

- oral antidiabetics (sulfonylureas); dosage adjustments may be necessary for proper control of blood sugar.

Furosemide *taken concurrently* with

- aminoglycoside antibiotics (see Drug Classes) may lead to hearing toxicity.
- cephalosporin antibiotics may increase risk of kidney toxicity.
- colestipol (Colestid) may cause loss of furosemide effectiveness.
- corticosteroids (see Drug Classes) may cause additive loss of potassium.
- cyclosporine (Sandimmune) may cause elevated uric acid levels and lead to gout.
- digitalis preparations (digitoxin, digoxin) requires very careful monitoring and dosage adjustments to prevent fluctuations of blood potassium levels and serious heart rhythm disturbances.
- NSAIDs (see Drug Classes) may blunt the benefits of furosemide.

The following drugs may *decrease* the effects of furosemide

- indomethacin (Indocin) or other NSAIDs.

Driving, Hazardous Activities: Use caution until the possible occurrence of orthostatic hypotension, dizziness, or impaired vision has been determined.

Exposure to Sun: Use caution until your sensitivity has been determined. This drug may cause photosensitivity.

Exposure to Heat: Avoid excessive perspiring, which could cause additional loss of salt and water from the body.

Heavy Exercise or Exertion: Avoid exertion that produces light-headedness, excessive fatigue, or muscle cramping. Isometric exercises—the overload technique for strengthening individual muscles—can raise blood pressure significantly. Ask your doctor for guidance regarding this form of exercise.

Occurrence of Unrelated Illness: Illnesses that cause vomiting or diarrhea can produce a serious imbalance of important body chemistry. Consult your doctor for guidance.

Discontinuation: It may be best to stop this drug 5 to 7 days before major surgery. Ask your doctor, surgeon, and/or anesthesiologist for guidance regarding dosage adjustment or withdrawal.

▷ **Saving Money When Using This Medicine:**

- Other available drugs provide similar effectiveness. Ask your doctor to prescribe the drug that offers the best combination of cost and outcome.
- It may be possible, after significant elimination of fluid, for you to stop taking this medicine. Ask your doctor for help.
- Dose changes are needed for patients with liver or kidney compromise.
- It is important that magnesium also be checked with potassium levels while this medicine is taken.
- Make sure you get your blood pressure checked regularly to make sure your medicines are still helping you. Do this even though you do not have any symptoms, as most cases of high blood pressure do not have symptoms.

GABAPENTIN (gab ah PEN tin)

Prescription Needed: Yes   **Controlled Drug:** No   **Generic:** No

Brand Names: Neurontin

Overview of BENEFITS versus RISKS

Possible Benefits	*Possible Risks*
EFFECTIVE ADD-ON TREATMENT OF DRUG-RESISTANT PARTIAL SEIZURES	Ataxia Dizziness
BENEFICIAL IN GENERALIZED SEIZURES	
VERY USEFUL IN CERTAIN KINDS OF PAIN SYNDROMES	
DOES NOT APPEAR TO INTERACT WITH OTHER ANTICONVULSANTS	

▷ **Illness This Medication Treats:**

(1) Used as part of combination treatment of resistant partial seizures; (2) helps as add-on therapy of generalized seizures.

Other (unlabeled) generally accepted uses: (1) used to help chronic pain (especially radiculopathy); (2) helps nystagmus.

GEMFIBROZIL   (jem FI broh zil)

Prescription Needed: Yes   **Controlled Drug:** No   **Generic:** Yes

Brand Names: Lopid, Gemcor

Overview of BENEFITS versus RISKS	
Possible Benefits	*Possible Risks*
EFFECTIVE REDUCTION OF TRIGLYCERIDE BLOOD LEVELS	Gallstone formation with long-term use
INCREASE IN HDL CHOLESTEROL BLOOD LEVELS	Increased susceptibility to viral and bacterial infections

▷ **Illness This Medication Treats:**
  (1) Abnormally high blood levels of triglycerides in types IV and V blood lipid (fat) disorders; (2) decreases risk of coronary artery disease by decreasing cholesterol.

▷ **Typical Dosage Range:** (Dosage or schedule must be determined by the doctor for each individual.)
  1200 to 1600 mg daily in two divided doses. The average dose is 1200 mg/24 hr. Dose increases should be made gradually over a period of 2 to 3 months.

▷ **Conditions Requiring Dosing Adjustments:**
  Liver function: This drug should not be used by patients with primary biliary cirrhosis and severe liver failure.
  Kidney function: For patients with moderate kidney failure, 50% of the usual dose should be taken at the usual time. Patients with severe kidney compromise should take 25% of the usual dose at the usual dosing interval.

▷ **How Best to Take This Medicine:**   Take 30 minutes before the morning and evening meals. The capsule may be opened for administration.

▷ **How Long This Medicine Is Usually Taken:**   Use on a regular schedule for 4 to 8 weeks usually determines the effectiveness of this drug in reducing blood levels of triglycerides. Long-term use (months to years) requires periodic physician evaluation.

▷ **Tell Your Doctor Before Taking This Medicine If You:**
  • ever had an allergic reaction to it.
  • have biliary cirrhosis of the liver.
  • have impaired liver or kidney function.
  • have gallbladder disease or gallstones.
  • have an underactive thyroid or diabetes.

▷ **Possible Side Effects:**   Moderate increase in blood sugar levels. Tingling of the fingers (paresthesias).

▷ **Possible Adverse Effects:**

If any of the following develop, call your doctor promptly for guidance.

Some Mild Problems Drug Can Cause

Allergic reactions: skin rash, itching.

Headache, dizziness, blurred vision, fatigue, muscle aches and cramps.

Excessive gas, nausea, vomiting, diarrhea.

Some Serious Problems Drug Can Cause

Abnormally low white blood cell count: fever, chills, sore throat.

Liver toxicity.

Formation of gallstones with long-term use.

Rare Raynaud's phenomenon.

Myopathy or rhabdomyolysis.

▷ **Possible Effects on Sex Life:**   Rare decreased libido or impotence.

▷ *CAUTION*

1. This drug should be used only after nondrug methods (primarily diet) have been ineffective in lowering triglyceride levels.
2. If you used the drug clofibrate (Atromid-S) in the past, inform your doctor fully regarding your experience.
3. Comply fully with all recommendations for periodic measurements of blood triglyceride and cholesterol levels. These are essential to the proper management of drug therapy for your disorder.
4. Safety and effectiveness of this drug for those under 12 years old are not established.
5. Those over 60 should watch for any increased tendency to infection; treat all infections promptly.

Advisability of Use During Pregnancy or If Breast-Feeding:

Pregnancy Category: C. Use this drug only if clearly needed. Ask your doctor for guidance. Present in breast milk; avoid taking this drug or refrain from nursing.

▷ **Overdose Symptoms:**   Abdominal pain, nausea, vomiting, diarrhea.

▷ **Suggested Periodic Examinations While Taking This Drug:** (at doctor's discretion)

Complete blood cell counts.

Measurements of blood levels of total cholesterol, HDL and LDL cholesterol fractions, triglycerides, and sugar.

Liver function tests.

▷ **While Taking This Drug the Following Apply:**

Foods: Follow the diet prescribed by your doctor.

Beverages: May be taken with milk.

Other Drugs:

Gemfibrozil may *increase* the effects of

- glyburide and other oral hypoglycemic agents (see Drug Classes).
- lovastatin and may also increase the risk of myopathy.
- warfarin (Coumadin), increasing the risk of bleeding; frequent INR (prothrombin time) measurements and dosage adjustments are necessary.

Gemfibrozil may *decrease* the effects of

- chenodiol (Chenix), reducing its effectiveness for the treatment of gallstones.

Driving, Hazardous Activities: This drug may cause dizziness and blurred vision. Restrict your activities as necessary.

Discontinuation: If adequate reduction of triglycerides does not occur after 3 months of treatment, use of this drug should be discontinued. Following drug withdrawal, blood cholesterol and triglyceride return to pretreatment levels.

▷ **Saving Money When Using This Medicine:**

- A large number of available drugs are similarly effective. Ask your doctor to prescribe the drug that offers the best combination of cost and outcome.
- Make sure you keep follow-up appointments for lab work. If this medicine does not control your cholesterol, an HMG CoA inhibitor may be needed.

GLIMEPIRIDE (GLIM ep ear eyed)

Prescription Needed: Yes   **Controlled Drug:** No   **Generic:** No

Brand Names: Amaryl

Overview of BENEFITS versus RISKS

Possible Benefits	*Possible Risks*
TIGHTER CONTROL OF BLOOD SUGAR	Rare allergic skin reactions
DECREASED RISK OF HEART, KIDNEY, NERVE, OR EYE PROBLEMS BY ATTAINING TIGHTER CONTROL OF BLOOD SUGAR	Potential increased for cardiovascular mortality (as with all oral hypoglycemics; see "Possible Adverse Effects," below)
ONCE-A-DAY DOSING	
DECREASED RISK OF ELEVATED INSULIN LEVELS	
DECREASED RISK OF EXCESSIVELY LOW BLOOD SUGAR	

▷ **Illness This Medication Treats:**

Mild to moderate type II diabetes mellitus (adult-onset) that does not require insulin, but is not adequately controlled by diet or exercise.

▷ **Typical Dosage Range:** (Dosage or schedule must be determined by the doctor for each individual.)

Adult dosing is started with 1 or 2 mg once daily, taken with breakfast or the first meal. Once a dose of 2 mg is reached, any further doses are made as needed or tolerated at 1- to 2-week intervals in steps of no more than 2 mg a day. Usual effective dose is 1–4 mg daily. Some clinicians advocate that type II patients with secondary failure be considered for combined glimepiride and insulin therapy. If the fasting blood sugar is greater than 150 mg/dl and this combination approach is taken, 8 mg is taken with the first main meal. Low-dose insulin is started and adjusted as needed according to ongoing blood sugar measurements.

Over 65 Years of Age: Careful adjustment with lower starting doses and slow increases are recommended because the effects of possible low blood sugar are not well tolerated in this age group.

▷ **Conditions Requiring Dosing Adjustments:**

Liver function: People with mild liver failure should start at 1 mg daily.

Data for patients with moderate to severe liver failure are not available, and this drug should not be used.

Kidney function: Patients with kidney compromise should take 1 mg daily to start. Ongoing dosing MUST be adjusted to blood sugar testing.

▷ **How Best to Take This Medicine:**   Long-term effects of high blood sugar such as nerve damage, kidney disease, blindness, and heart attacks can be delayed or even avoided by tight (mostly in the normal sugar range) blood sugar control. Follow your doctor's advice carefully regarding dosing and diet. If meals are skipped after glimepiride is taken, excessive lowering of the blood sugar (hypoglycemia) may result. Be sure you know the symptoms of hypoglycemia. The tablet may be crushed.

▷ **How Long This Medicine Is Usually Taken:**   Regular use for 1 to 2 weeks determines the effectiveness of this drug in controlling blood sugar. Failure to respond to maximum doses in 1 month constitutes a primary failure. Blood sugars MUST be measured, and your doctor will decide if the drug should be continued.

▷ **Tell Your Doctor Before Taking This Medicine If You:**
- ever had an allergic reaction to it.
- have a severely damaged liver or kidneys.
- have diabetic ketoacidosis.
- do not know how to treat hypoglycemia.
- have a history of congestive heart failure, peptic ulcer disease, liver cirrhosis, or hypothyroidism.
- are pregnant.
- are malnourished, have a high fever, or have a pituitary or adrenal insufficiency.
- currently have an infection.

▷ **Possible Side Effects:**   If drug dose is excessive or meals inadequate, abnormally low blood sugar may result.

▷ **Possible Adverse Effects:**
If any of the following develop, call your doctor promptly for guidance.
Some Mild Problems This Drug Can Cause
   Allergic reactions: hives, itching, rash.
   Headache or dizziness.
   Rare blurred vision or nausea.
Some Serious Problems This Drug Can Cause
   Rare porphyria or lowering of blood sodium (SIADH) reported with medicines in this same class.
   Rare increased risk of cardiovascular mortality based on the University Group Diabetes Program (UGDP). This group looked at long-

term use of tolbutamide and phenformin. Glimepiride was not included in that study.

▷ *CAUTION*

1. **This drug is only part of a total diabetes program.** It is not a substitute for proper diet and regular exercise.
2. Safety and effectiveness of this drug in pediatrics have not been established.
3. For those over 60, this drug should be used with caution; start at 1 mg per day. Slowly increase dose if needed. Repeated hypoglycemia can lead to brain damage in older patients.
4. If you develop an infection, more frequent blood sugar is indicated, and insulin may be required to keep your blood sugar within acceptable limits.

Advisability of Use During Pregnancy or If Breast-Feeding:
Pregnancy Category: C. Most clinicians recommend insulin as the drug of choice for pregnant diabetics. Present in breast milk in animals, unknown in humans; avoid taking this drug or refrain from nursing.

▷ **Overdose Symptoms:** Symptoms of severe hypoglycemia: headache, light-headedness, nervousness, sweating, stupor progressing to coma.

▷ **Suggested Periodical Examinations While Taking This Drug:** (at doctor's discretion)

The American Diabetes Association recommends that EVERY person with diabetes check their blood sugar with a fingerstick blood glucose machine regularly. Most clinicians also recommend periodic hemoglobin A1C (glycosylated hemoglobin); liver function tests; and evaluation of the heart, blood pressure, and circulatory system.

▷ **While Taking This Drug the Following Apply:**
Foods: Follow the diabetic diet prescribed by your doctor.
Beverages: As directed by the diabetic diet.
Alcohol: Use with extreme caution. Alcohol can prolong this medicine's blood sugar–lowering effect. Other medicines in this class have been reported to cause a disulfiramlike reaction (facial sweating, flushing, and vomiting).
Other Drugs:
The following drugs may *increase* the effects of glimepiride
• aspirin or other salicylates.
• cimetidine (Tagamet).
• clofibrate (Atromid-S).
• fenfluramine (Pondimin).
• monoamine oxidase inhibitors (MAOIs—see Drug Classes).
• NSAIDs (see Drug Classes).
• ranitidine (Zantac).
• sulfa drugs, such as Septra.

The following drugs may *decrease* the effects of glimepiride
- beta-blocker drugs (see Drug Classes).
- bumetanide (Bumex).
- conjugated estrogens (Premarin).
- diazoxide (Proglycem).
- ethacrynic acid (Edecrin).
- furosemide (Lasix).
- phenytoin (Dilantin).
- rifampin (Rifadin, others).
- steroids (betamethasone, prednisone, others).
- thiazide diuretics (see Drug Classes).

Glimepiride *taken concurrently* with
- antacids (containing magnesium hydroxide) may result in excessively lowered blood sugar.
- antifungal agents (such as itraconazole or other azoles) may lead to severely lowered blood sugar.
- calcium channel blockers (see Drug Classes) may excessively lower blood sugar.
- cyclosporine (Sandimmune) may lead to cyclosporine toxicity.
- warfarin (Coumadin) can cause an increased lowering of the blood sugar.

Driving, Hazardous Activities: Caution: Dosing schedule, eating, and physical activity must be coordinated to prevent hypoglycemia. Know the symptoms of low blood sugar, so you can avoid hazardous activities and take corrective measures if it occurs.

Exposure to Sun: Caution: Some medicines in this class have caused photosensitivity.

▷ **Saving Money When Using This Medicine:**
- Keeping your blood sugar in the normal range delays or even prevents heart problems, kidney damage, and even blindness.
- Talk with your doctor to make sure that this medicine offers you the best balance of cost and outcomes.
- Call the American Diabetes Association at 1-800-232-3472 to learn more about diabetes. A new book called *The Essential Guide to Chronic Illness* is also an excellent source of information.

GLIPIZIDE   (GLIP i zide)

Prescription Needed: Yes   **Controlled Drug:** No   **Generic:** No

Brand Names: Glucotrol, Glucotrol XL

Overview of BENEFITS versus RISKS	
Possible Benefits	*Possible Risks*
Assistance in regulating blood sugar in noninsulin-dependent diabetes (adjunctive to appropriate diet and weight control)	HYPOGLYCEMIA, severe and prolonged
	Allergic skin reactions (some severe)
	Liver damage (rare)
	Blood cell and bone marrow disorders (rare)

▷ **Illness This Medication Treats:**

Mild to moderate type II diabetes mellitus that does not require insulin, but cannot be adequately controlled by diet alone.

▷ **Typical Dosage Range:** (Dosage or schedule must be determined by the doctor for each individual.)

Initially 5 mg daily with breakfast. At 3- to 7-day intervals the dose may be increased by increments of 2.5 to 5 mg daily, as needed and tolerated. Total daily dosage should not exceed 40 mg. The extended-release form maximum is 20 mg daily.

▷ **Conditions Requiring Dosing Adjustments:**

Liver function: Patients with liver compromise should take a starting dose of 2.5 mg and be closely monitored.

Kidney function: This drug is contraindicated for patients with severe renal compromise. Patients should be monitored closely if this drug is used for patients with mild to moderate renal compromise. It is a rare cause of kidney stones.

▷ **How Best to Take This Medicine:** For daily maintenance doses of 15 mg or more, the total dose should be divided into two equal doses; the first taken with the morning meal, the second with the evening meal. The tablet may be crushed.

▷ **How Long This Medicine Is Usually Taken:** Use on a regular schedule for 1 to 2 weeks determines the effectiveness of this drug in controlling diabetes. Failure to respond to maximal doses within 1 month constitutes a primary failure. Up to 10% of those who respond initially may develop secondary failure. Blood sugars must be measured, and your doctor will then decide if the drug should be stopped or continued.

▷ **Tell Your Doctor Before Taking This Medicine If You:**

- ever had an allergic reaction to it.
- have severe impairment of liver or kidney function.
- are pregnant.
- are allergic to other sulfonylurea or sulfa drugs.
- have diabetes that has been unstable or brittle in the past.

- do not know how to recognize or treat hypoglycemia.
- have a history of congestive heart failure, peptic ulcer disease, cirrhosis of the liver, hypothyroidism, or porphyria.

▷ **Possible Side Effects:**   If drug dosage is excessive or food intake is delayed or inadequate, abnormally low blood sugar is a predictable drug effect.

▷ **Possible Adverse Effects:**
If any of the following develop, call your doctor promptly for guidance.
Some Mild Problems Drug Can Cause
   Allergic reactions: skin rash, itching.
   Headache, drowsiness, dizziness, sweating.
   Nausea, vomiting, diarrhea.
Some Serious Problems Drug Can Cause
   Allergic reactions: hepatitis with jaundice, severe skin reactions.
   Idiosyncratic reaction: hemolytic anemia.
   Disulfiramlike reaction with concurrent use of alcohol.
   Water retention, weight gain.
   Bone marrow depression.

▷ *CAUTION*
   1. This drug is only one part of the total program for managing your diabetes. It is not a substitute for a properly prescribed diet and regular exercise.
   2. Over time (usually several months) this drug may lose its effectiveness in controlling blood sugar levels. Periodic follow-up examinations are necessary to monitor all aspects of response.
   3. This drug is not effective for treating type I insulin-dependent diabetes.
   4. Those over 60 should use this drug with caution. Treatment is started with 2.5 mg/day and increased as needed or tolerated. Repeated episodes of hypoglycemia can cause brain damage.

Advisability of Use During Pregnancy or If Breast-Feeding:
Pregnancy Category: C. Because uncontrolled blood sugar levels during pregnancy are associated with a higher incidence of birth defects, many experts recommend that insulin (instead of an oral agent) be used as necessary to control diabetes during the entire pregnancy. Presence in breast milk is unknown; avoid taking this drug or refrain from nursing.

▷ **Overdose Symptoms:**   Symptoms of mild to severe hypoglycemia: headache, light-headedness, faintness, nervousness, confusion, tremor, sweating, heart palpitation, weakness, hunger, nausea, vomiting, stupor progressing to coma.

▷ **Suggested Periodic Examinations While Taking This Drug:** (at doctor's discretion)

Complete blood cell counts, liver function tests, thyroid function tests, periodic evaluation of heart and circulatory system.

The American Diabetes Association (ADA) recommends that ALL people with diabetes check their blood sugar. Talk with your doctor about getting a machine to do this at home.

▷ **While Taking This Drug the Following Apply:**

Foods: Follow the diabetic diet prescribed by your doctor.

Beverages: As directed in the diabetic diet. This drug may be taken with milk.

Alcohol: Use with extreme caution—alcohol can exaggerate this drug's hypoglycemic effect. This drug infrequently causes a marked intolerance of alcohol, resulting in a disulfiramlike reaction: facial flushing, sweating, palpitation.

Other Drugs:

The following drugs may *increase* the effects of glipizide

• aspirin and other salicylates.
• cimetidine (Tagamet).
• clofibrate (Atromid-S).
• fenfluramine (Pondimin).
• MAO type A inhibitors (see Drug Classes).
• NSAIDs (see Drug Classes).
• ranitidine (Zantac).
• sulfa drugs, such as Septra.

The following drugs may *decrease* the effects of glipizide

• beta-blockers (see Drug Classes).
• bumetanide (Bumex).
• diazoxide (Proglycem).
• ethacrynic acid (Edecrin).
• furosemide (Lasix).
• phenytoin (Dilantin).
• rifampin (Rifadin).
• steroids (prednisone, betamethasone, others).
• thiazide diuretics (see drug profile).

Glipizide *taken concurrently* with

• antacids (containing magnesium hydroxide) may result in increased risk of excessively low blood sugar.
• antifungal agents (such as itraconazole or other azoles) may lead to very low blood sugar.
• calcium channel blockers (see Drug Classes) may cause excessive lowering of blood sugar.
• warfarin (Coumadin) may lead to an excessive blood sugar–lowering (hypoglycemic) effect.

Driving, Hazardous Activities: Carefully regulate your dosage schedule, eating schedule, and physical activities to prevent hypoglycemia. Recognize the early symptoms of hypoglycemia so you can avoid hazardous activities and take corrective measures.

Exposure to Sun: Use caution until your sensitivity has been determined. Some drugs of this class cause photosensitivity.

Occurrence of Unrelated Illness: Acute infections, illnesses causing vomiting or diarrhea, serious injuries, and surgical procedures can interfere with diabetic control and may require the use of insulin. If any of these conditions occur, call your doctor promptly.

Discontinuation: Because of the possibility of secondary failure, it is advisable to evaluate this drug's continued benefit every 6 months.

▷ **Saving Money When Using This Medicine:**
- A large number of available drugs provide similar effectiveness. Ask your doctor to prescribe the drug that offers the best combination of cost and outcome.
- This drug MUST be started at 2.5 mg for patients with liver compromise. Ask your doctor if your liver is compromised enough to warrant this.
- Learn all you can about your disease. The American Diabetes Association (ADA) can help at 1-800-232-3472. A new book called *The Essential Guide to Chronic Illness* is an excellent source of information.

GLYBURIDE (GLI byoor ide)

Other Name: Glibenclamide

Prescription Needed: Yes **Controlled Drug:** No **Generic:** No

Brand Names: DiaBeta, Glubate, Glynase PresTab, Micronase

<table>
<tr><th colspan="2">Overview of BENEFITS versus RISKS</th></tr>
<tr><th>Possible Benefits</th><th>Possible Risks</th></tr>
<tr>
<td>EFFECTIVE CONTROL OF BLOOD SUGAR in noninsulin-dependent diabetes (adjunctive to appropriate diet and weight control)</td>
<td>HYPOGLYCEMIA, severe and prolonged
Allergic skin reactions (some severe)
Rare liver damage
Rare blood cell and bone marrow disorders
Potential risk of increased cardiovascular mortality</td>
</tr>
</table>

▷ **Illness This Medication Treats:**
Mild to moderate type II diabetes mellitus that does not require insulin, but cannot be adequately controlled by diet alone.

▷ **Typical Dosage Range:** Initially 1.25 to 5 mg daily with breakfast. At 7-day intervals the dose may be increased by increments of 2.5 mg daily, as needed and tolerated. Total daily dosage should not exceed 20 mg.

▷ **Conditions Requiring Dosing Adjustments:**
Liver function: Glyburide may cause catastrophic hypoglycemia in patients with liver disease. It is also a rare cause of hepatitis and cholestatic jaundice.
Kidney function: Glyburide should be used with caution by patients with mild renal compromise, with low initial doses and careful patient monitoring. This drug SHOULD NOT be used by patients with moderate or worse kidney failure (creatinine clearance less than 50 ml/min).

▷ **How Best to Take This Medicine:** If the daily maintenance dose is found to be 10 mg or more, the total dose should be divided into two equal doses: the first taken with the morning meal, the second with the evening meal. The tablet may be crushed.

▷ **How Long This Medicine Is Usually Taken:** Use on a regular schedule for 1 to 2 weeks usually determines the effectiveness of this drug in controlling diabetes. Failure to respond to maximal doses within 1 month constitutes a primary failure. Up to 10% of those who respond initially may develop secondary failure. The duration of effective use is determined only by periodic blood sugar measurement.

▷ **Tell Your Doctor Before Taking This Medicine If You:**
- ever had an allergic reaction to it or to other sulfonylurea or sulfa drugs.
- have severe impairment of liver and kidney function.
- are pregnant.
- have diabetes that has been unstable or brittle in the past.
- do not know how to recognize or treat hypoglycemia.
- have a G6PD deficiency.
- have a history of congestive heart failure, peptic ulcer disease, cirrhosis of the liver, problems with blood clotting, hypothyroidism, or porphyria.

▷ **Possible Side Effects:**   If drug dosage is excessive or food intake delayed or inadequate, abnormally low blood sugar is a predictable drug effect.

▷ **Possible Adverse Effects:**
If any of the following develop, call your doctor promptly for guidance.
Some Mild Problems Drug Can Cause
   Allergic reactions: skin rash, itching.
   Headache, drowsiness, dizziness, fatigue.
   Heartburn, nausea.
Some Serious Problems Drug Can Cause
   Allergic reactions: hepatitis with jaundice, severe skin reactions.
   Idiosyncratic reaction: hemolytic anemia.
   Disulfiramlike reaction with concurrent use of alcohol.
   Bone marrow depression.
   Liver toxicity.
   Rare blood clotting defects.
   Rare drug-induced urinary tract stones.
   Rare increased risk of cardiovascular mortality.

▷ *CAUTION*
   1. This drug must be regarded as only one part of the total program for management of your diabetes. It is not a substitute for a properly prescribed diet and regular exercise.
   2. Over time (usually several months) this drug may lose its effectiveness in controlling blood sugar levels. Periodic follow-up examinations are necessary to monitor all aspects of response.
   3. This drug is not effective for treating type I insulin-dependent diabetes.
   4. Those over 60 should use this drug with caution. Therapy is started with 1.25 mg/day; increase dosage cautiously and monitor closely to prevent hypoglycemic reactions. Repeated episodes of hypoglycemia can cause brain damage.

Advisability of Use During Pregnancy or If Breast-Feeding:
Pregnancy Category: C. Because uncontrolled blood sugar levels during pregnancy is associated with a higher incidence of birth defects, many experts recommend using insulin (instead of an oral agent) as necessary to control diabetes during the entire pregnancy. Presence in breast milk is unknown; avoid taking this drug or refrain from nursing.

▷ **Overdose Symptoms:**   Symptoms of mild to severe hypoglycemia: headache, light-headedness, faintness, nervousness, confusion, tremor, sweating, heart palpitation, weakness, hunger, nausea, vomiting, stupor progressing to coma.

▷ **Possible Effects of Long-Term Use:**   Reduced function of the thyroid gland. Reports of increased frequency and severity of heart and blood vessel diseases associated with long-term use of this class of drugs are highly controversial and inconclusive. A direct cause-and-effect relationship is tenuous. Ask your doctor for guidance.

▷ **Suggested Periodic Examinations While Taking This Drug:** (at doctor's discretion)
Complete blood cell counts, liver function tests, thyroid function tests, periodic evaluation of heart and circulatory system.

▷ **While Taking This Drug the Following Apply:**
Foods: Follow the diabetic diet prescribed by your doctor.
Beverages: As directed in the diabetic diet. This drug may be taken with milk.
Alcohol: Alcohol can exaggerate this drug's hypoglycemic effect. This drug infrequently causes a marked intolerance of alcohol, resulting in a disulfiramlike reaction: facial flushing, sweating, palpitation.
Other Drugs:
The following drugs may *increase* the effects of glyburide
• aspirin and other salicylates.
• cimetidine (Tagamet).
• clofibrate (Atromid-S).
• fenfluramine (Pondimin).
• gemfibrozil (Lopid).
• MAO type A inhibitors.
• ranitidine (Zantac).
• sulfa drugs, such as Septra.
The following drugs may *decrease* the effects of glyburide
• beta-blockers.
• bumetanide (Bumex).
• diazoxide (Proglycem).
• ethacrynic acid (Edecrin).
• furosemide (Lasix).
• phenytoin (Dilantin).

- rifampin (Rifadin, others).
- thiazide diuretics (see drug profile).
- thyroid hormones.

Glyburide *taken concurrently* with

- antacids (containing magnesium) may result in risk of excessively lowered blood sugar.
- antifungal agents (such as itraconazole or other azoles) may lead to severe lowering of blood sugar.
- enalapril (Vasotec) may change glucose control.
- steroids (prednisone, others) may result in loss of glucose control.
- warfarin (Coumadin) may lead to bleeding. Increased frequency of INR (prothrombin time) testing is needed.

Driving, Hazardous Activities: Carefully regulate your dosage schedule, eating schedule, and physical activities to prevent hypoglycemia. Recognize the early symptoms of hypoglycemia so you can avoid hazardous activities and take corrective measures.

Exposure to Sun: Use caution until your sensitivity has been determined. Some drugs of this class cause photosensitivity.

Occurrence of Unrelated Illness: Acute infections, illnesses causing vomiting or diarrhea, serious injuries, and surgical procedures can interfere with diabetic control and may require the use of insulin. If any of these conditions occur, call your doctor promptly.

Discontinuation: Because of the possibility of secondary failure, it is advisable to evaluate this drug's continued benefit every 6 months.

▷ **Saving Money When Using This Medicine:**

- A large number of available drugs are similarly effective. Ask your doctor to prescribe the drug that offers the best combination of cost and outcome.
- Dosage of this drug must be adjusted for patients with liver compromise, and it may be contraindicated. The dose must be adjusted for patients with kidney compromise. Ask your doctor if dosing has been appropriately changed.
- Home blood-sugar testing and learning more about diabetes are strongly suggested. Talk with your doctor about fingerstick blood sugar tests and call the American Diabetes Association (ADA) at 1-800-232-3472 for information on your condition. A new book called *The Essential Guide to Chronic Illness* is an excellent source of information.

GRISEOFULVIN (gri see oh FUL vin)

Prescription Needed: Yes   **Controlled Drug:** No   **Generic:** No

Brand Names: Fulvicin P/G, Fulvicin U/F, Grifulvin V, Grisactin, Grisactin Ultra, Gris-PEG, Ultramicrosize Griseofulvin

Overview of BENEFITS versus RISKS	
Possible Benefits	*Possible Risks*
EFFECTIVE TREATMENT OF ALL TYPES OF TINEA INFECTION	Rare drug-induced hepatitis
	Rare peripheral neuritis
	Decreased white blood cell counts
	Disulfiramlike reactions

▷ **Illness This Medication Treats:**

Tinea (ringworm) infections of: the beard (tinea barbae), scalp (tinea capitis), body (tinea corporis), groin (tinea cruris, jock itch), feet (tinea pedis, athlete's foot), fingernails and toenails (tinea unguium).

Note: This drug is effective only against species of fungus that are sensitive to it. It is not effective against yeast organisms, bacteria, or viruses. It should not be used for minor fungus infections that are likely to respond to local treatment with antifungal ointments and lotions.

▷ **Typical Dosage Ranges:** (Dosage or schedule must be determined by the doctor for each individual.)

Children: For ultramicrosize formulations (over 2 years old): 3.3 mg per pound of body weight daily.

12 to 60 Years of Age: For tinea pedis and nail infections: 500 mg/12 hr. For tinea barbae, capitis, corporis, and cruris: 250 mg/12 hr, or 500 mg once daily.

For microsize formulations: 500 to 1000 mg daily, in single or divided doses.

For ultramicrosize formulations: 330 to 375 mg daily, in single or divided doses.

Over 60 Years of Age: Same as for 12 to 60 years of age.

▷ **Conditions Requiring Dosing Adjustments:**

Liver function: This drug is contraindicated for patients with hepatocellular liver failure.

▷ **How Best to Take This Medicine:**   Take with or following meals to reduce stomach irritation; fatty foods increase its absorption. The capsule may be opened and the tablet crushed for administration. Shake the oral suspension well before measuring the dose.

▷ **How Long This Medicine Is Usually Taken:**   To prevent relapse, continual use of this drug on a regular schedule is necessary until the infecting fungus is totally eliminated from infected tissues. Usual treatment periods are as follows: for tinea capitis—10 to 12 weeks; for tinea barbae—4 to 6 weeks; for tinea corporis and cruris—4 to 6 weeks; for tinea pedis—6 to 8 weeks; for tinea unguium—6 to 8 months for fingernails and 8 to 12 months for toenails.

▷ **Tell Your Doctor Before Taking This Medicine If You:**
- ever had an allergic reaction to it.
- have active liver disease.
- have a mild fungus infection that responds to local antifungal treatment.
- are pregnant or planning pregnancy.
- are allergic to any form of penicillin.
- have a history of porphyria.
- have lupus erythematosus.
- are taking oral contraceptives containing estrogen.
- are currently taking an anticoagulant drug.

▷ **Possible Side Effects:**   Mild lowering of blood pressure.
Superinfections: thrush (yeast) infection of the mouth, tongue, or gums.

▷ **Possible Adverse Effects:**
If any of the following develop, call your doctor promptly for guidance.
Some Mild Problems Drug Can Cause
   Allergic reactions: skin rash, hives, itching.
   Headache, dizziness, lethargy, blurred vision, insomnia, confusion.
   Nausea, vomiting, taste disorders, stomach pain, diarrhea.
Some Serious Problems Drug Can Cause
   Allergic reactions: anaphylactic reaction. Severe skin reactions.
   Idiosyncratic reactions: lupuslike syndrome—fever; painful, swollen joints; aching muscles; enlarged lymph glands.
   Rare drug-induced hepatitis: yellow skin and eyes, light-colored stools.
   Peripheral neuritis: numbness and tingling.
   Deficiency of white blood cells.
   Rare hallucinations, liver toxicity, or porphyria.

▷ **Possible Effects on Sex Life:**   Rare enlargement of male breast tissue (gynecomastia).

▷ *CAUTION*
   1. This drug should not be used to treat minor infections that respond to locally applied antifungal preparations.
   2. This drug is not recommended for use during pregnancy. If you

are using an oral contraceptive containing estrogen, you should also use an additional method of contraception while taking this drug and for 1 month after discontinuing it.

3. Troublesome and persistent diarrhea can develop in sensitive individuals. If diarrhea persists more than 24 hours, call your doctor promptly.

4. Safety and effectiveness of this drug for those under 2 years old are not established.

Advisability of Use During Pregnancy or If Breast-Feeding:

Pregnancy Category: C. Use of this drug during any period of pregnancy is not recommended. Presence in breast milk is unknown; avoid taking this drug or refrain from nursing.

▷ **Overdose Symptoms:** Possible nausea, vomiting, diarrhea.

▷ **Suggested Periodic Examinations While Taking This Drug:** (at doctor's discretion)

Complete blood cell counts.

Liver and kidney function tests (during extended use).

▷ **While Taking This Drug the Following Apply:**

Foods: High-fat foods enhance absorption of this drug.

Beverages: This drug should preferably be taken with milk.

Alcohol: Use with caution until combined effect is determined. This drug can increase the intoxicating effects of alcohol. In addition, a disulfiramlike reaction can occur in sensitive individuals.

Other Drugs:

Griseofulvin may *decrease* the effects of

• oral contraceptives (containing estrogen), resulting in breakthrough bleeding and unwanted pregnancy.

• warfarin (Coumadin); monitor INR (prothrombin times) and adjust warfarin dosage as necessary.

The following drugs may *decrease* the effects of griseofulvin

• barbiturates.

• cyclosporine (Sandimmune).

• primidone (Mysoline).

Driving, Hazardous Activities: This drug may cause dizziness, confusion, or impaired vision. Restrict your activities as necessary.

Exposure to Sun: Use caution until your sensitivity is determined. This drug may cause photosensitivity.

Discontinuation: Some fungal infections require long-term treatment. Your doctor should determine when it is appropriate to discontinue this drug.

▷ **Saving Money When Using This Medicine:**

• A large number of drugs are available to treat fungal infections. Ask your doctor to prescribe the drug that offers the best combination of cost and outcome for you.

• Ask your doctor when it is reasonable to discontinue this drug.

GUANFACINE   (GWAHN fa seen)

Prescription Needed: Yes   **Controlled Drug:**   No   **Generic:** No

Brand Name: Tenex

Overview of BENEFITS versus RISKS

Possible Benefits	*Possible Risks*
EFFECTIVE ANTIHYPERTENSIVE in mild to moderate high blood pressure	Amnesia, confusion, mental depression
EFFECTIVE IN HIGH BLOOD PRESSURE OF PREGNANCY	

▷ **Illness This Medication Treats:**

(1) Mild to moderate high blood pressure; generally not to initiate treatment, but added when a first drug proves inadequate; (2) may also be used to treat high blood pressure caused by kidney problems.

▷ **Typical Dosage Range:** (Dosage or schedule must be determined by the doctor for each individual.)

Initially 1 mg once daily, taken at bedtime. The dose may be increased after 3 to 4 weeks to 2 mg daily, as needed and tolerated. If needed, the dose may be increased again to 3 mg daily after 3 to 4 weeks. The total daily requirement may be taken in two divided doses if necessary for stable blood pressure control.

▷ **Conditions Requiring Dosing Adjustments:**

Liver function: Patients with liver compromise should use this drug with caution.

Kidney function: Patients with renal compromise should use this drug with caution; elimination appears to shift to nonrenal elimination mechanisms.

▷ **How Best to Take This Medicine:**   Tablets may be taken without regard to eating. It is recommended that the daily dose be taken at bedtime to reduce the side effect of daytime drowsiness. The tablet may be crushed.

▷ **How Long This Medicine Is Usually Taken:**   Continual use on a regular schedule for 4 to 6 weeks is usually necessary to determine this drug's effectiveness in controlling high blood pressure. Long-term use (months to years) requires physician supervision and help.

▷ **Tell Your Doctor Before Taking This Medicine If You:**

- ever had an allergic reaction to it.
- have a circulatory disorder of the brain.

- have angina or coronary artery disease.
- have or have had serious emotional depression.
- have impaired liver or kidney function.
- are taking any sedative or hypnotic drugs or an antidepressant.
- plan to have surgery under general anesthesia soon.

▷ **Possible Side Effects:**   Drowsiness, dry nose and mouth, constipation, decreased heart rate, mild orthostatic hypotension.

▷ **Possible Adverse Effects:**
If any of the following develop, call your doctor promptly for guidance.
Some Mild Problems Drug Can Cause
  Allergic reactions: skin rash, itching.
  Headache, dizziness, fatigue, insomnia.
  Nausea, diarrhea.
Some Serious Problems Drug Can Cause
  Amnesia, confusion, depression.
  Slow heartbeat.
  Rebound hypertension if abruptly stopped.

▷ **Possible Effects on Sex Life:**   Decreased libido, impotence.

▷ *CAUTION*
  1. ***Do not stop taking this drug suddenly.*** Sudden withdrawal can produce anxiety, nervousness, tremors, fast or irregular heart action, nausea, stomach cramps, vomiting, and rebound hypertension.
  2. Hot weather and the fever associated with infection can reduce blood pressure significantly. Dosage adjustments may be necessary.
  3. Report the development of any tendency to emotional depression.
  4. Safety and effectiveness of this drug for those under 12 years old are not established.
  5. For those over 60, unacceptably high blood pressure should be reduced without the risks associated with excessively low blood pressure. Small doses and frequent blood pressure checks are needed. Watch for light-headedness, dizziness, unsteadiness, fainting, and falling. Sedation and dry mouth are common in elderly users. Report promptly any changes in mood or behavior: depression, delusions, hallucinations.

Advisability of Use During Pregnancy or If Breast-Feeding:
Pregnancy Category: B. Use this drug only if clearly needed. Ask your doctor for guidance. Probably present in breast milk; avoid taking this drug or refrain from nursing.

▷ **Overdose Symptoms:**   Marked drowsiness, weakness, dry mouth, slow pulse, low blood pressure, vomiting, stupor progressing to coma.

▷ **Suggested Periodic Examinations While Taking This Drug:** (at doctor's discretion)
Blood pressure measurements.

▷ **While Taking This Drug the Following Apply:**
Foods: Avoid excessive salt. Ask your doctor for guidance on salt restriction.
Beverages: May be taken with milk.
Alcohol: Use with extreme caution. The combined effects can cause marked drowsiness and exaggerated blood pressure reduction.
Other Drugs:
Guanfacine **taken concurrently** with
- amitriptyline (Elavil) can cause decreased effectiveness as an antihypertensive.
- desipramine and other tricyclic antidepressants may blunt guanfacine's beneficial effects.
- phenobarbital can lead to loss of therapeutic effect of guanfacine.

Driving, Hazardous Activities: Use caution. This drug can cause drowsiness and impair mental alertness, judgment, and coordination.
Exposure to Heat: Use caution. Hot environments may reduce blood pressure significantly; be alert to the possibility of orthostatic hypotension.
Heavy Exercise or Exertion: Use caution. Isometric exercises (overload technique for strengthening individual muscles) can raise blood pressure significantly. This drug may intensify the hypertensive response to isometric exercise. Ask your doctor for guidance.
Occurrence of Unrelated Illness: Fever associated with infections may lower the blood pressure significantly. Repeated vomiting may prevent the regular use of this drug and result in an acute withdrawal reaction. Consult your doctor.
*Discontinuation: **Do not stop taking this drug suddenly.*** A significant withdrawal reaction can occur within 2 to 7 days after the last dose. The dose should be reduced gradually over 3 to 4 days, with periodic blood pressure monitoring.

▷ **Saving Money When Using This Medicine:**
- A large number of drugs are available to treat high blood pressure. Ask your doctor to prescribe the drug that offers the best combination of cost and outcome for you.
- Continue to take your high blood pressure medicine even if you don't have symptoms (high blood pressure usually doesn't). Check

your blood pressure periodically to make sure this medicine is still working for you.

- Ask your doctor about stress management and exercise programs in your community.
- Talk with your doctor about the advisability of taking aspirin every other day.

HALOPERIDOL   (hal oh PER i dohl)

Prescription Needed: Yes   **Controlled Drug:** No   **Generic:** Yes

Brand Names: Haldol, Halperon

Overview of BENEFITS versus RISKS	
Possible Benefits	*Possible Risks*
EFFECTIVE CONTROL OF ACUTE PSYCHOSES	FREQUENT PARKINSON-LIKE SIDE EFFECTS
BENEFICIAL EFFECTS ON THINKING, MOOD, AND BEHAVIOR	SERIOUS TOXIC EFFECTS ON BRAIN with long-term use
EFFECTIVE CONTROL OF SOME TOURETTE'S DISORDERS	Blood cell disorders (rare) Abnormally low white blood cell count
May help some hyperactive children	

▷ **Illness This Medication Treats:**
(1) Psychotic thinking and abnormal behavior associated with acute psychosis of unknown nature, acute schizophrenia, paranoid states, and the manic phase of manic-depressive disorders; (2) helps in controlling outbursts of aggression; (3) Tourette's syndrome.

▷ **Typical Dosage Range:** (Dosage or schedule must be determined by the doctor for each individual.)
Initially 0.5 to 2 mg two or three times daily. Dose may be increased by 0.5 mg/day at 3- to 4-day intervals, as needed and tolerated. The usual dosage range is 0.5 to 30 mg every 24 hours. The total daily dosage should not exceed 100 mg.

▷ **Conditions Requiring Dosing Adjustments:**
Liver function: The dose, dosing interval, and time taken to reach the desired effect should be adjusted for patients with liver compromise.
Kidney function: High doses should be taken with caution by patients with renal compromise.

▷ **How Best to Take This Medicine:**   May be taken with or following food to reduce stomach irritation. The concentrate may be diluted in 2 oz of water or fruit juice; do not add to coffee or tea. The tablet may be crushed.

▷ **How Long This Medicine Is Usually Taken:**   Use on a regular schedule for several weeks usually determines the effectiveness of this drug in controlling the symptoms of psychotic or psychoneurotic behavior. If this treatment is not significantly beneficial within 6 weeks, it should be stopped. Long-term use requires physician supervision.

▷ **Tell Your Doctor Before Taking This Medicine If You:**
- ever had an allergic reaction to it.
- are allergic to the dye tartrazine.
- are experiencing mental depression or have a history of mental depression.
- have any form of Parkinson's disease.
- have cancer of the breast.
- have active liver disease or impaired liver or kidney function.
- currently have a bone marrow or blood cell disorder.
- are allergic or abnormally sensitive to phenothiazines.
- have any type of heart disease.
- have low blood pressure, epilepsy, or glaucoma.
- are taking any drugs with a sedative effect.
- plan to have surgery under general or spinal anesthesia soon.

▷ **Possible Side Effects:**   Mild drowsiness, low blood pressure, blurred vision, dry mouth, constipation, marked and frequent Parkinson-like reactions. Abnormal eye orientations (oculogyric crisis). Abnormal and frequent urination (SIADH).

▷ **Possible Adverse Effects:**
If any of the following develop, call your doctor promptly for guidance.
Some Mild Problems Drug Can Cause
  Allergic reactions: skin rash, hives.
  Dizziness, weakness, agitation, insomnia.
  Loss of appetite, nausea, vomiting, diarrhea.
  Urinary retention.
Some Serious Problems Drug Can Cause
  Allergic reactions: rare liver reaction with jaundice, asthma, spasm of vocal cords.
  Idiosyncratic reaction: neuroleptic malignant syndrome.
  Depression, disorientation, eye damage (deposits in cornea, lens, retina).
  Blood cell disorders: anemia, white blood cell changes.
  Nervous system reactions: rigidity of extremities, tremors, restless-

ness, constant movement, facial grimacing, eye-rolling, spasm of neck muscles, seizures, tardive dyskinesia.

▷ **Possible Effects on Sex Life:**   Decreased libido; impotence; painful ejaculation; priapism. Male breast enlargement and tenderness; female breast enlargement with milk production. Altered timing and pattern of menstruation.

▷ **Adverse Effects That May Mimic Natural Diseases or Disorders:**
Liver reaction may suggest viral hepatitis.
   Nervous system reactions may suggest Parkinson's disease or Reye's syndrome.

▷ *CAUTION*
   1. Use the smallest effective dose for long-term treatment.
   2. Use haloperidol with extreme caution if you have epilepsy; this drug can alter the pattern of seizures.
   3. Individuals with lupus erythematosus and those taking prednisone are more susceptible to nervous system reactions.
   4. Do not use levodopa to treat Parkinson-like reactions; it can cause agitation and worsening of the psychotic disorder.
   5. Obtain prompt evaluation of any change or disturbance in vision.
   6. This drug should not be used for children under 3 years old or 15 kg in weight. Avoid usage in the presence of symptoms suggestive of Reye's syndrome. Children are quite susceptible to nervous system reactions induced by this drug.
   7. This drug can cause significant changes in mood and behavior in those over 60; watch for confusion, agitation, aggression, and paranoia. You may be more susceptible to the development of drowsiness, lethargy, orthostatic hypotension, hypothermia, Parkinson like reactions, and prostatism.

Advisability of Use During Pregnancy or If Breast-Feeding:
Pregnancy Category: C. Avoid using this drug during the first trimester. Use only if clearly needed. Ask your doctor for guidance. Present in breast milk. Monitor the nursing infant closely and discontinue drug or nursing if adverse effects develop.

▷ **Overdose Symptoms:**   Marked drowsiness, weakness, tremor, unsteadiness, agitation, stupor, coma, convulsions.

▷ **Suggested Periodic Examinations While Taking This Drug:** (at doctor's discretion)
Complete blood cell counts, liver function tests, eye examinations, electrocardiograms.
Careful inspection of the tongue for early evidence of fine, involuntary, wavelike movements indicating tardive dyskinesia.

▷ **While Taking This Drug the Following Apply:**
Beverages: May be taken with milk.

Alcohol: Avoid completely. Alcohol can increase this drug's sedative action and accentuate its depressant effects on brain function. Haloperidol can increase the intoxicating effects of alcohol.

Marijuana Smoking: Moderate increase in drowsiness; accentuation of orthostatic hypotension; increased risk of precipitating latent psychosis, confusing interpretation of mental status and drug response.

Other Drugs:

Haloperidol may *increase* the effects of
- all drugs with sedative actions, causing excessive sedation.
- fluvoxamine (Luvox) and result in toxicity.
- some antihypertensive drugs, causing excessive lowering of blood pressure; monitor the combined effects carefully.

Haloperidol may *decrease* the effects of
- guanethidine (Esimil, Ismelin), reducing its antihypertensive effect.

Haloperidol *taken concurrently* with
- anticholinergic medicines may lead to additive dry mouth, sedation, or constipation.
- beta-blockers (see Drug Classes) may cause excessive lowering of blood pressure.
- fluoxetine (Prozac) may pose an increased risk of haloperidol toxicity.
- lithium (Lithobid, others) may cause toxic effects on the brain and nervous system.
- methyldopa (Aldomet) may cause serious dementia.

The following drugs may *decrease* the effects of haloperidol
- antacids containing aluminum and/or magnesium may reduce its absorption.
- barbiturates.
- benztropine (Cogentin).
- carbamazepine (Tegretol).
- phenytoin (Dilantin).
- rifampin (Rifater, others).
- trihexyphenidyl (Artane).

Driving, Hazardous Activities: This drug may impair mental alertness, judgment, and physical coordination. Restrict your activities as necessary.

Exposure to Sun: Use caution until your sensitivity has been determined. This drug can cause photosensitivity.

Exposure to Heat: Use caution in hot environments. This drug may impair the regulation of body temperature and increase the risk of heatstroke.

Exposure to Cold: The elderly are advised to use caution; this drug can increase the risk of hypothermia.

Discontinuation: This drug should not be discontinued abruptly following long-term use. Gradual withdrawal over a period of 2 to 3 weeks is advised. Ask your doctor for guidance.

▷ **Saving Money When Using This Medicine:**
- A large number of drugs are available to treat psychiatric problems. Ask your doctor if this drug offers the best combination of cost and outcome for you.
- It may be possible (after a significant symptom-free period) to stop taking this medicine. Ask your doctor for help.
- A new medicine called olanzapine appears to avoid some of the movement disorder side effects of earlier agents. Discuss this medicine with your doctor.

HISTAMINE (H2) BLOCKING DRUGS

Cimetidine (si MET i deen)
Famotidine (fa MOH te deen)
Nizatidine (ni ZA te deen)
Ranitidine (ra NI te deen)

Prescription Needed: Yes   **Controlled Drug:** No   **Generic:**
No

Brand Names: Tagamet, Tagamet HB (nonprescription form), Zantac, Zantac 75 (nonprescription form), Pepcid, Pepcid AC (nonprescription form), Axid, Axid AR (nonprescription form)

▷ **Warning:** Zantac and Xanax are very different drugs and mistaking one for the other can lead to serious problems. Check the color chart and verify that you are taking the correct drug.

Overview of BENEFITS versus RISKS	
Possible Benefits	*Possible Risks*
EFFECTIVE TREATMENT OF PEPTIC ULCER DISEASE: relief of symptoms, acceleration of healing, prevention of recurrence	Drug-induced hepatitis (rare) Bone marrow depression (rare) Confusion (particularly in compromised elderly) Low blood platelet counts (rare)
CONTROL OF HYPERSECRETORY STOMACH DISORDERS	**Author's note: The nonprescription heartburn forms of these medicines generally have less frequent side effects or adverse effects because of episodic use and lower doses compared to the prescription forms.**
TREATMENT OF REFLUX ESOPHAGITIS	
THE NONPRESCRIPTION FORMS ARE APPROVED TO TREAT HEARTBURN	
Pepcid AC (nonprescription form) is approved for prevention of heartburn	

▷ **Illness This Medication Treats:**
(1) Recurrence of peptic ulcer; (2) cimetidine, famotidine, and ranitidine: both duodenal and gastric ulcers as well as conditions causing extreme production of stomach acid (Zollinger-Ellison syndrome); (3) all four medications: controlling excess acid moving from the stomach into the lower throat (gastroesophageal reflux disease); (4) cimetidine: preventing upper stomach/intestinal bleeding; (5) cimetidine, famotidine, nizatidine, and ranitidine: as combination treatment with antibiotics and bismuth compounds (Pepto-Bismol, etc.) in refractory ulcers where the organism *Helicobacter*

pylori has been found; (6) all four of these medicines are also approved for nonprescription treatment of heartburn. Famotidine (Pepcid AC) and nizatidine (Axid AR) are also approved for prevention of heartburn.

▷ **Typical Dosage Range:** (Dosage or schedule must be determined by the doctor for each individual.)

Infants and Children: Cimetidine: Routine use is not recommended for those under 16 years old.

Famotidine: For those 6 to 15 years old: 0.5 mg per kilogram of body weight twice a day for 8 weeks.

Nizatidine: No data available.

Ranitidine: For those 2 to 18 years old: 1.25 to 2 mg per kilogram of body weight per dose, taken every 12 hours.

16 to 60 Years of Age:

Peptic ulcer and hypersecretory states:

Cimetidine: 300 mg by mouth four times daily, taken with meals and at bedtime. Famotidine: 40 mg by mouth at bedtime for 4 or up to 8 weeks. Maintenance doses of 20 mg at bedtime; up to 640 mg daily for hypersecretory states. Nizatidine: 300 mg by mouth at bedtime; not for hypersecretory states. Ranitidine: 150 mg by mouth twice daily—up to 6 g in hypersecretory states.

Heartburn:

Cimetidine: 100 mg by mouth. Famotidine: 10 mg by mouth before eating foods or drinking liquids that cause you problems, or 10 mg by mouth to treat heartburn. Nizatidine: 75 mg by mouth up to twice a day. Ranitidine: 75 mg by mouth.

Over 60 Years of Age: Cimetidine: Half the usual adult dose to start. Famotidine, nizatidine, and ranitidine: Same dose as for 16 to 60 years of age.

All these drugs pose a risk for formation of masses of undigested vegetable fibers (phytobezoars). Watch for nervousness, confusion, loss of appetite, stomach fullness, nausea, and vomiting.

▷ **Conditions Requiring Dosing Adjustments:**

Liver function: Cimetidine and famotidine are dependent mostly on the liver for elimination. Dose must be decreased for patients with liver failure.

Kidney function: All histamine-blockers are primarily eliminated by the kidneys. Doses MUST be decreased for patients with moderate kidney failure.

▷ **How Best to Take This Medicine:** Cimetidine and ranitidine should be taken immediately after meals for the longest decrease in stomach acid in peptic ulcer treatment. Cimetidine, famotidine, and ranitidine should be taken after meals when used for hypersecretory states.

▷ **How Long This Medicine Is Usually Taken:** Use on a regular schedule for 4 to 6 weeks usually determines the effectiveness of these drugs in healing active peptic ulcer disease. Long-term use (months to years) for prevention requires periodic individualized consideration by your doctor. Continual use for 6 to 12 weeks is needed to heal the esophagus when cimetidine, famotidine, nizatidine, or ranitidine is used in gastroesophageal reflux disease (GERD). Since nonprescription forms are available for heartburn, if heartburn relief has not occurred in 2 hours, or if symptoms worsen, call your doctor.

▷ **Tell Your Doctor Before Taking This Medicine If You:**
- ever had an allergic reaction to it.
- have impaired liver or kidney function.
- have a low sperm count (cimetidine).
- are taking any anticoagulant drug.
- do not tolerate or should not take phenylalanine—ranitidine (Zantac EFFERdose) tablets or granules contain this ingredient.
- have had low white blood cell counts.
- have a history of acute porphyria (ranitidine).
- are taking propranolol or quinidine (cimetidine).

▷ **Possible Adverse Effects:**
If any of the following develop, call your doctor promptly for guidance.
Some Mild Problems Drug Can Cause
Allergic reactions: skin rash and hives.
Rare headache (cimetidine, famotidine, and ranitidine,).
Rare diarrhea (cimetidine, famotidine, nizatidine, and ranitidine).
Rare arthralgia (cimetidine, famotidine, and ranitidine).
Some Serious Problems Drug Can Cause
Allergic reactions: cimetidine and ranitidine are rare causes of pancreatitis and anemia. Cimetidine and nizatidine can cause exfoliative dermatitis.
Idiosyncratic reactions: nervousness, confusion, hallucinations.
Rare liver damage (cimetidine, nizatidine, and ranitidine).
Rare abnormal heart rhythm/arrest (cimetidine, nizatidine, and ranitidine).
Rare bone marrow depression (cimetidine and ranitidine).
Rare decreased platelets (cimetidine, famotidine, nizatidine, and ranitidine).
Rare bronchospasm (cimetidine and famotidine).

▷ **Possible Effects on Sex Life:** Impotence (cimetidine) (rare: famotidine, nizatidine, and ranitidine).
Rare loss of libido (famotidine, nizatidine, and ranitidine).
Male breast enlargement (cimetidine, nizatidine, and ranitidine).

▷ **Possible Delayed Adverse Effects:** Male breast enlargement (cimetidine, nizatidine, and ranitidine).

Famotidine may impair vitamin B12 absorption and lead to deficiency.

▷ *CAUTION*

1. Ulcer rebound or perforation can occur if you stop taking these drugs abruptly.
2. Once usage of this medicine is discontinued, call your doctor promptly if symptoms recur.
3. Some of cimetidine is removed by hemodialysis; redose is needed.
4. Safety and effectiveness of these drugs for children are covered under "Typical Dosage Range," above.
5. Those over 60 face increased risk of masses of partially digested vegetable fibers (phytobezoars), especially people who can't chew well. Watch closely for decreased appetite, stomach fullness, nausea, and vomiting.
6. The nonprescription forms should NOT be used to treat ulcers.

Advisability of Use During Pregnancy or If Breast-Feeding:

Pregnancy Category: B for cimetidine, famotidine, and ranitidine; C for nizatidine. Use cimetidine, famotidine, or ranitidine only if clearly needed. Nizatidine must be avoided during the first 3 months of pregnancy. Ask your doctor for guidance. Present in breast milk; avoid taking these drugs or refrain from nursing.

▷ **Overdose Symptoms:** Confusion, mild slowing of the heart, sweating, drowsiness, muscle twitching, seizures, cardiac arrest, coma.

▷ **Suggested Periodic Examinations While Taking These Drugs:** (at doctor's discretion)

Complete blood counts, liver and kidney function tests, more frequent tests of prothrombin times if an anticoagulant is also taken, and sperm counts (cimetidine).

▷ **While Taking These Drugs the Following Apply:**

Foods: Protein-rich foods increase stomach acid secretion. Ask your doctor for advice.

Nutritional Support: Cimetidine may decrease vitamin B12 over time and requires supplements.

Beverages: Caffeine in caffeine-containing beverages may stay in your body longer than usual with cimetidine. Milk may increase stomach acid secretion.

Alcohol: No interactions; however, stomach acidity is increased by alcohol. Avoid its use.

Tobacco Smoking: Smoking is a clear risk factor for peptic ulcer disease. Stop smoking if possible.

Marijuana Smoking: Possible additive reduction in sperm counts with cimetidine use.

Other Drugs:

Cimetidine may *increase* the effects of

- amiodarone (Cordarone).
- amitriptyline (Elavil) and perhaps other tricyclic antidepressants (see Drug Classes).
- oral anticoagulants, with increased risk of bleeding.
- benzodiazepines (Librium, etc.).
- carbamazepine (Tegretol), causing increased toxicity.
- flecainide (Tambocor) and require dosing changes.
- loratadine (Claritin) by causing a large increase in blood levels. One study DID NOT reveal that this medicine caused adverse heart effects with increased levels, but it appears prudent to lower the dose of loratadine if these medicines are to be combined.
- meperidine (Demerol, others), resulting in toxicity with potential respiratory depression and low blood pressure.
- metoprolol (Lopressor, others), resulting in very slow heartbeat and excessively low blood pressure.
- morphine (MS Contin, MSIR, others), resulting in central nervous system depression and respiratory depression.
- phenytoin (Dilantin).
- procainamide (Procan, Pronestyl).
- propranolol (Inderal).
- quinidine (Quiniglute).
- theophylline (Theo-Dur, etc.).
- venlafaxine (Effexor).
- warfarin (Coumadin).

Ranitidine may *increase* the effects of

- diazepam (Valium).
- procainamide (Procan, Pronestyl).
- glipizide (Glucotrol).
- midazolam (Versed).
- theophylline (Theo-Dur, etc.).
- warfarin (Coumadin).

Famotidine, nizatidine, or ranitidine (prescription forms) may *increase* the effects of

- amoxicillin.
- high-dose aspirin (increased level and toxicity risk).
- pentoxifylline (Trental); however, this reaction has only been documented with cimetidine.
- theophylline (Theo-Dur, others). Ongoing theophylline dosing should be adjusted to symptom control and blood levels.

Cimetidine *taken concurrently* with

- most calcium channel blockers (see Drug Classes) may result in calcium channel toxicity. Doses may need to be reduced if these medicines are to be combined on an ongoing basis.

- carmustine (BiCNU) may cause severe bone marrow depression.
- chloroquine results in toxicity and may cause cardiac arrest.
- cisapride (Propulsid) results in increased cisapride levels and a potentially serious increase in heart rate.
- clozapine (Clozaril) may result in increased blood levels and clozapine toxicity.
- digoxin (Lanoxin) may result in changes in digoxin levels.
- oral hypoglycemic agents such as glipizide (Glucotrol), glyburide (DiaBeta, Micronase), and tolbutamide (Tolinase, others) may result in severe low blood sugars and seizures.
- paroxetine (Paxil) and perhaps other SSRIs (see Drug Classes) may result in increased blood levels of the SSRI and require dosing changes.
- pentoxifylline (Trental) may result in pentoxifylline toxicity.
- zalcitabine (HIVID) may result in zalcitabine toxicity.

Cimetidine, famotidine, nizatidine, or ranitidine **taken concurrently** with

- antacids may result in decreased histamine-blocker levels.

Cimetidine may **decrease** the effects of

- indomethacin, by decreasing absorption.
- iron salts, by decreasing absorption.
- ketoconazole, by decreasing absorption.
- tetracyclines, by decreasing absorption.

Famotidine, nizatidine, or ranitidine may **decrease** the effects of

- indomethacin by decreasing absorption into the body.
- ketoconazole, itraconazole, or fluconazole.
- sucralfate (Carafate).

Driving, Hazardous Activities: Use caution until the degree of confusion, dizziness, or other effects is known.

Occurrence of Unrelated Illness. Idiopathic thrombocytopenic purpura, a rare lowering of blood platelets, contraindicates use of any of these medications. Aplastic anemia, whatever the cause, may be worsened by cimetidine.

Discontinuation: **Do not** suddenly stop taking any of these drugs if used for peptic ulcer disease. Ask your doctor for withdrawal instructions. Be alert to the recurrence of ulcers any time after any of these drugs are stopped.

▷ **Saving Money When Using This Medicine:**
- Ask your doctor to prescribe the drug that offers the best combination of cost and outcome for you.
- It may be possible (after a significant ulcer-free period) to stop taking this medicine. Ask your doctor for help.
- If your duodenal ulcer returns, ask your doctor if *Helicobacter pylori*

should be considered and different treatment (an antibiotic plus a proton pump inhibitor) started.
- Talk with your doctor about using the nonprescription forms to treat heartburn.

HYDRALAZINE (hi DRAL a zeen)

Prescription Needed: Yes   **Controlled Drug:** No   **Generic:** Yes

Brand Names: Alazine, Apresazide [CD], Apresoline, Apresoline-Esidrix [CD], Ser-Ap-Es [CD], Serpasil-Apresoline [CD], Unipres [CD]

Overview of BENEFITS versus RISKS

Possible Benefits	*Possible Risks*
EFFECTIVE ADJUNCT FOR MODERATE TO SEVERE HYPERTENSION	DRUG-INDUCED LUPUS ERYTHEMATOSUSLIKE SYNDROME
Possibly beneficial in managing severe congestive heart failure	May worsen angina pectoris
	Blood cell disorders (rare)
	Liver damage (rare)

▷ **Illness This Medication Treats:**
(1) Moderate to severe high blood pressure in conjunction with other antihypertensives; (2) high blood pressure caused by abnormal kidney blood vessels.

▷ **Typical Dosage Range:** (Dosage or schedule must be determined by the doctor for each individual.)
Initially 10 mg four times daily for 2 to 4 days; then increase to 25 mg four times daily for the balance of the first week. During the second week the dose may be increased to 50 mg four times daily, if needed and tolerated. The total daily dosage should not exceed 300 mg for fast acetylators or 200 mg for slow acetylators. Ask your doctor for guidance.

▷ **Conditions Requiring Dosing Adjustments:**
Liver function: This drug is capable of causing hepatitis, hepatic necrosis, and granulomas (noncancerous growth) and should be used with caution by patients with liver compromise.
Kidney function: For patients with mild to moderate kidney failure, the usual dose can be taken every 8 hours. For patients with severe kidney failure and people who metabolize the drug slowly, the usual dose should be taken every 12 to 24 hours, with 200 mg/day as a

maximum. Patients with renal compromise should use this drug with caution.

▷ **How Best to Take This Medicine:**   Preferably taken with or following meals to enhance absorption and reduce stomach irritation. The tablet may be crushed and the capsule [CD] opened for administration.

▷ **How Long This Medicine Is Usually Taken:**   Use on a regular schedule for several weeks is usually necessary to determine the effectiveness of this drug in lowering blood pressure. Long-term use requires physician supervision.

▷ **Tell Your Doctor Before Taking This Medicine If You:**
 • ever had an allergic reaction to it.
 • have active angina pectoris.
 • have mitral valvular heart disease.
 • have a history of any type of heart disease.
 • have lupus erythematosus.
 • have impaired brain circulation.
 • are subject to migraine headaches.
 • have impaired kidney function.
 • have a history of liver sensitivity to other drugs.
 • plan to have surgery under general anesthesia soon.

▷ **Possible Side Effects:**   Orthostatic hypotension, nasal congestion, constipation, delayed or impaired urination, increased heart rate of 10 to 25 beats/min.

▷ **Possible Adverse Effects:**
 If any of the following develop, call your doctor promptly for guidance.
 Some Mild Problems Drug Can Cause
   Allergic reactions: skin rash, hives, itching, drug fever.
   Headache, dizziness, flushing of face, palpitation.
   Loss of appetite, nausea, vomiting, diarrhea.
   Tremors, muscle cramps.
 Some Serious Problems Drug Can Cause
   Allergic reactions: liver reaction.
   Idiosyncratic reactions: behavioral changes: nervousness, confusion. Bleeding into lung tissue: densities found on X ray. A syndrome resembling rheumatoid arthritis or lupus erythematosus.
   Intensification of coronary artery disease.
   Peripheral neuropathy: weakness, numbness.
   Rare bone marrow depression or congestive heart failure.
   Drug-induced: porphyria, periarteritis nodosa, porphyria, gallstones, or gastrointestinal (stomach or intestinal) bleeding.

▷ **Possible Effects on Sex Life:** Rare reports of impotence and priapism.

▷ **Adverse Effects That May Mimic Natural Diseases or Disorders:** Drug fever may suggest systemic infection. Liver reaction may suggest viral hepatitis. Skin and joint symptoms may suggest lupus erythematosus.

▷ *CAUTION*
1. Toxic reactions are more likely to occur with large doses. Adhere strictly to prescribed dosage schedules. Keep appointments for periodic follow-up examinations.
2. Report the development of any tendency to emotional depression.
3. This drug can cause salt and water retention if no diuretic is taken concurrently.
4. This drug can provoke migraine headache.
5. Dosage is based on age, weight, and kidney function status. Watch for development of a lupus erythematosus–like reaction.
6. In those over 60, low doses are needed. Unacceptably high blood pressure should be reduced without the risks associated with excessively low blood pressure. Sudden, rapid, and excessive reduction of blood pressure can predispose to stroke or heart attack. Watch for dizziness, fainting, or falling. Headache, palpitation, and rapid heart rates are more common in the elderly and can mimic acute anxiety states.

Advisability of Use During Pregnancy or If Breast-Feeding:
Pregnancy Category: C. Avoid use during the first and last 3 months; late in pregnancy, this drug can cause blood platelet deficiency in the newborn infant. Present in breast milk; avoid taking this drug or refrain from nursing.

▷ **Overdose Symptoms:** Marked light-headedness; dizziness; headache; flushing of skin; nausea; vomiting; collapse of circulation: loss of consciousness, cold and sweaty skin, weak and rapid pulse, irregular heart rhythm.

▷ **Suggested Periodic Examinations While Taking This Drug:** (at doctor's discretion)
Complete blood cell counts, liver function tests, blood tests for evidence of lupus erythematosus.

▷ **While Taking This Drug the Following Apply:**
Nutritional Support: Watch for tingling of the hands and feet and take pyridoxine supplements (vitamin B6) as needed. Ask your doctor for guidance.
Beverages: May be taken with milk.
Alcohol: Caution—alcohol can exaggerate this drug's blood pressure–lowering effect and cause excessive reduction.

Tobacco Smoking: Avoid completely. Nicotine can contribute significantly to this drug's ability to intensify angina in susceptible individuals.

Other Drugs:

Hydralazine may *increase* the effects of

- metoprolol (Lopressor).
- oxprenolol (Trasicor).
- propranolol (Inderal).

Hydralazine *taken concurrently* with

- clonidine (Catapres) may additively lower blood pressure.
- furosemide (Lasix) may blunt furosemide's therapeutic benefits.
- nitrates (isosorbide, others) may give increased benefits in patients with heart failure.
- NSAIDs (see Drug Classes) may blunt hydralazine's therapeutic effect.

Driving, Hazardous Activities: This drug may cause light-headedness or dizziness. Restrict your activities as necessary.

Exposure to Heat: Caution is advised. Hot environments may reduce blood pressure significantly.

Exposure to Cold: Caution is advised. Cold environments may increase this drug's ability to cause angina in susceptible individuals.

Heavy Exercise or Exertion: Caution is advised. Excessive exertion can increase this drug's ability to cause angina in susceptible individuals. Also, isometric exercises can raise blood pressure significantly.

▷ **Saving Money When Using This Medicine:**

- A large number of drugs are available to treat hypertension. Ask your doctor if this drug offers the best combination of cost and outcome for you.
- Dosage of this drug must be decreased for people with compromised kidneys. Ask your doctor if your dose has been adjusted.
- A generic form is available and is recommended.
- Have your blood pressure checked in order to make sure this medicine is still working for you.
- Talk with your doctor about stress management and exercise programs available in your community.
- Discuss the benefits versus risks of taking aspirin every other day to help prevent a heart attack.

HYDROCHLOROTHIAZIDE
(hi droh klor oh THI a zide)

Prescription Needed: Yes   **Controlled Drug:** No   **Generic:** Yes

Brand Names: Aldactazide [CD], Aldoril—15/25 [CD], Aldoril D30/D50 [CD], Apresazide [CD], Apresoline-Esidrix [CD], Capozide [CD], Dyazide [CD], Esidrix, HydroDIURIL, Hydropres [CD], Hydro-Z-50, Inderide [CD], Inderide LA [CD], Lopressor HCT [CD], Maxzide [CD], Maxzide-25 [CD], Moduretic [CD], Normozide [CD], Oretic, Oreticyl [CD], Prinzide [CD], Ser-Ap-Es [CD], Serpasil-Esidrix [CD], Thiuretic, Timolide [CD], Trandate HCT [CD], Unipres [CD], Vaseretic [CD], Zestoretic [CD], Ziac, Zide

---

Overview of BENEFITS versus RISKS

Possible Benefits	*Possible Risks*
EFFECTIVE, WELL-TOLERATED DIURETIC	Loss of body potassium
POSSIBLY EFFECTIVE IN MILD HYPERTENSION	Increased blood sugar
ENHANCES EFFECTIVENESS OF OTHER ANTIHYPERTENSIVES	Increased blood uric acid
Beneficial in treatment of diabetes insipidus	Increased blood calcium
	Rare blood cell disorders

See the thiazide diuretics drug profile for further information.

HYDROCODONE (hi droh KOH dohn)

Other Name: hydrocodeinone

Prescription Needed: Yes   **Controlled Drug:** CIII*   **Generic:** Yes

Brand Names: Anexsia [CD], Anexsia 7.5 [CD], Azdone [CD], Dimetane Expectorant-DC [CD], Duocet [CD], Hycodan [CD], Hycomine Compound [CD], Hycomine Pediatric Syrup [CD], Hycomine Syrup [CD], Hycotuss Expectorant [CD], Lorcet-HD [CD], Lorcet Plus [CD], Lortab [CD], Lortab ASA [CD], Norcet 7 [CD], T-Gesic [CD], Triaminic Expectorant DH [CD], Tussend [CD], Tussend Expectorant [CD], Tussionex [CD], Tycolet [CD], Vicodin [CD], Vicodin ES [CD], Zydone [CD]

*See Controlled Drug Schedules inside this book's cover.

```
┌─────────────────────────────────────────────────────────┐
│           Overview of BENEFITS versus RISKS              │
│    Possible Benefits            Possible Risks           │
│  EFFECTIVE RELIEF OF MILD   Potential for habit formation│
│  TO MODERATE PAIN               (dependence)             │
│  EFFECTIVE CONTROL OF       Mild allergic reactions      │
│  COUGH                          (infrequent)             │
│                             Nausea, constipation         │
└─────────────────────────────────────────────────────────┘
```

▷ **Illness This Medication Treats:**
(1) Cough; (2) relief of mild to moderate pain.
As Combination Drug Product [CD]: Hydrocodone is frequently added to cough mixtures containing antihistamines, decongestants, and expectorants to make these "shotgun" preparations more effective in reducing the frequency and severity of cough. It is also combined with milder analgesics, such as acetaminophen and aspirin, to enhance pain relief.

▷ **Typical Dosage Range:** (Dosage or schedule must be determined by the doctor for each individual.)
As analgesic: 5 to 10 mg every 4 to 6 hours as needed. For cough: 5 mg every 4 to 6 hours as needed. Total daily dosage should not exceed 60 mg.

▷ **Conditions Requiring Dosing Adjustments:**
Liver function: Patients with severe liver compromise should use this drug with caution, with decreases in dose or longer dosing intervals.
Kidney function: Patients with kidney compromise should use this drug with caution; dose may need to be decreased. This drug may cause urinary retention; patients with renal (kidney) outflow problems must make a benefit-to-risk decision.

▷ **How Best to Take This Medicine:** May be taken with or following food to reduce stomach irritation or nausea. Tablet may be crushed.

▷ **How Long This Medicine Is Usually Taken:** As required to control pain or cough. Continual use should not exceed 5 to 7 days without interruption and reassessment of need.

▷ **Tell Your Doctor Before Taking This Medicine If You:**
- ever had an allergic reaction to it.
- are having an acute attack of asthma.
- had an unfavorable reaction to any narcotic drug in the past.
- have a history of drug abuse or alcoholism.
- have chronic lung disease with impaired breathing.
- have impaired liver or kidney function.
- have gallbladder disease, a seizure disorder, or an underactive thyroid gland.
- have difficulty emptying the urinary bladder.

- are taking any other drugs that have a sedative effect.
- plan to have surgery under general anesthesia soon.

▷ **Possible Side Effects:**   Drowsiness, light-headedness, dry mouth, urinary retention, constipation.

▷ **Possible Adverse Effects:**

If any of the following develop, call your doctor promptly for guidance.

Some Mild Problems Drug Can Cause

  Allergic reactions: skin rash, hives, itching.

  Dizziness, impaired concentration, sensation of drunkenness, confusion, depression, blurred or double vision, facial flushing, sweating.

  Nausea, vomiting.

Some Serious Problems Drug Can Cause

  Allergic reactions: anaphylaxis (rare), severe skin reactions.

  Idiosyncratic reactions: delirium, hallucinations, excitement, increased sensitivity to pain after the analgesic effect has worn off.

  Seizures (rare), impaired breathing.

  Rare kidney or liver toxicity.

▷ **Adverse Effects That May Mimic Natural Diseases or Disorders:**
  Paradoxical behavioral disturbances may suggest psychotic disorder.

▷ *CAUTION*

1. If you have asthma, chronic bronchitis, or emphysema, the excessive use of this drug may cause significant respiratory difficulty, thickening of bronchial secretions, and suppression of coughing.
2. The concurrent use of this drug with atropinelike drugs can increase the risk of urinary retention and reduced intestinal function.
3. Do not take this drug following acute head injury.
4. Do not use this drug for children under 2 years old, because of their vulnerability to life-threatening respiratory depression.
5. People over 60 should take small doses initially, increasing dosage as needed and tolerated. Limit use to short-term treatment only. There may be increased susceptibility to the development of drowsiness, dizziness, unsteadiness, falling, urinary retention, and constipation (often leading to fecal impaction).
6. This drug MUST be adjusted for patients with liver compromise. Ask your doctor if your dose has been appropriately adjusted.

Advisability of Use During Pregnancy or If Breast-Feeding:

Pregnancy Category: C. Use this drug only if clearly needed and in small, infrequent doses. Presence in breast milk is unknown. Monitor the nursing infant closely and discontinue drug or nursing if adverse effects develop. Ask your doctor for guidance.

▷ **Habit-Forming Potential:** Psychological and/or physical dependence can develop with large doses for an extended period. However, true dependence is infrequent and unlikely with prudent use.

▷ **Overdose Symptoms:** Drowsiness, restlessness, agitation, nausea, vomiting, dry mouth, vertigo, weakness, lethargy, stupor, coma, seizures.

▷ **While Taking This Drug the Following Apply:**

Beverages: No restrictions. May be taken with milk.

Alcohol: Hydrocodone can intensify the intoxicating effects of alcohol, and alcohol can intensify its depressant effects on brain function, breathing, and circulation—NOT RECOMMENDED.

Marijuana Smoking: Increase in drowsiness and pain relief; impairment of mental and physical performance.

Other Drugs:

Hydrocodone may *increase* the effects of
- other drugs with sedative effects.
- atropinelike drugs, increasing the risk of constipation and urinary retention.

Hydrocodone *taken concurrently* with
- cimetidine (Tagamet) may result in increased risk of breathing problems or central nervous system depression.
- MAO inhibitors (see Drug Classes) may result in an increased drug effect and a need to decrease the hydrocodone dose.

Driving, Hazardous Activities: This drug can impair mental alertness, judgment, reaction time, and physical coordination. Avoid hazardous activities accordingly.

Discontinuation: Use of this drug should be limited to short-term use. If it is necessary to use it for an extended time, discontinuation should be gradual to minimize possible withdrawal effects (usually mild).

▷ **Saving Money When Using This Medicine:**
- Pain therapy currently combines medications from several drug classes. Pain should be regularly checked and medicine doses adjusted when needed. Ask your doctor who will assess your pain and make dosing adjustments.

This drug may be combined with a tricyclic antidepressant such as amitriptyline (Elavil) or an NSAID such as ibuprofen (Motrin). Such combinations attack the cause of the pain by several mechanisms and also often allow the opioid dose (such as hydrocodone) to be decreased.
- Many medications are available to treat pain. Ask your doctor if this drug provides the best combination of cost and outcome for you.

HYDROXYCHLOROQUINE   (hi drox ee KLOR oh kwin)

Prescription Needed: Yes   **Controlled Drug:** No   **Generic:** No

Brand Name: Plaquenil

Overview of BENEFITS versus RISKS

Possible Benefits	*Possible Risks*
EFFECTIVE PREVENTION AND TREATMENT OF CERTAIN FORMS OF MALARIA	INFREQUENT DAMAGE OF CORNEAL AND RETINAL EYE TISSUES
Possibly effective in management of acute and chronic rheumatoid arthritis and juvenile arthritis	RARE BUT SERIOUS BONE MARROW DEPRESSION: aplastic anemia, deficient white blood cells and platelets
Possibly effective in management of chronic discoid and systemic lupus erythematosus	Heart muscle damage (rare)
	Ear damage: hearing loss, ringing in ears (rare)

▷ **Illness This Medication Treats:**
 (1) Suppression of development of acute attacks of some types of malarial infection; (2) reduction of disease activity in rheumatoid and juvenile arthritis; (3) suppression of disease activity in chronic discoid and systemic lupus erythematosus.

▷ **Typical Dosage Range:** (Dosage or schedule must be determined by the doctor for each individual.)
 For malaria suppression: 400 mg/7 days.
 For malaria treatment: (1) 800 mg as a single dose; or (2) initially 800 mg, followed by 400 mg in 6 to 8 hours; then 400 mg once a day on the second and third days.
 For rheumatoid arthritis: Up to 6.5 mg per kilogram of lean body weight daily.
 For lupus erythematosus: Up to 6.5 mg per kilogram of lean body weight daily.

▷ **Conditions Requiring Dosing Adjustments:**
 Liver function: This drug should be used with caution based on a benefit-to-risk decision for patients with liver compromise or who are already taking hepatotoxic drugs.
 Kidney function: Patients with renal compromise should use this drug with caution.

▷ **How Best to Take This Medicine:**   Take with food or milk to reduce stomach irritation. The tablet may be crushed and mixed with jam, jelly, or Jell-O for administration. Take full course of treatment as prescribed.

Note: For malaria prevention, begin medication 2 weeks before entering malarious area; continue medication while in the area and for 4 weeks after leaving.

For treating arthritis and lupus, take medication on a regular schedule daily; continual use for 6 months may be necessary to determine maximal benefit.

▷ **How Long This Medicine Is Usually Taken:** Use on a regular schedule for 2 weeks before exposure, during period of exposure, and 4 weeks after exposure is usually necessary to determine the effectiveness of this drug in preventing attacks of malaria. Continual use on a regular schedule for periods up to 6 months may be required to evaluate the potential benefits in reducing the activity of rheumatoid arthritis and lupus erythematosus. If no significant improvement is achieved within this time, this drug should be discontinued. Long-term use (months to years) requires periodic physician evaluation.

▷ **Tell Your Doctor Before Taking This Medicine If You:**
- ever had an allergic reaction to either chloroquine or hydroxychloroquine.
- have an active bone marrow or blood cell disorder or history of these.
- are pregnant or planning pregnancy.
- have a G6PD deficiency.
- have any disorder of the eyes, especially the cornea or retina, or visual field changes.
- have impaired hearing or ringing in the ears.
- have a seizure disorder of any kind.
- have a history of peripheral neuritis.
- have low blood pressure or a heart rhythm disorder.
- have a history of peptic ulcer disease, Crohn's disease, or ulcerative colitis.
- have impaired liver or kidney function.
- have a history of porphyria.
- have any form of psoriasis.
- are taking antacids, cimetidine, digoxin, or penicillamine.

IBUPROFEN (i byu PROH fen)

Prescription Needed: Varies   **Controlled Drug:** No
Generic: Yes

Brand Names: Advil, Children's Advil, Children's Motrin Suspension (nonprescription form), Children's Motrin Drops (nonprescription form), CoAdvil [CD], Dristan Sinus, Haltran, Ibuprohm, IBU-TAB, Junior Strength Motrin Caplets (nonprescription), Medipren, Motrin, Motrin IB, Nuprin, PediaProfen, Rufen

---

Overview of BENEFITS versus RISKS

Possible Benefits	*Possible Risks*
EFFECTIVE RELIEF OF MILD TO MODERATE PAIN AND INFLAMMATION	Gastrointestinal pain, ulceration, bleeding (rare)
	Kidney damage (rare)
	Fluid retention (rare)
	Bone marrow depression

See the propionic acids (NSAIDs) drug profile for further information.

IMIPRAMINE   (im IP ra meen)

Prescription Needed: Yes   **Controlled Drug:**   No   **Generic:** Yes

Brand Names: Antipress, Janimine, Imavate, SK-Pramine, Tipramine, Tofranil, Tofranil-PM

Overview of BENEFITS versus RISKS

Possible Benefits	*Possible Risks*
EFFECTIVE RELIEF OF NEUROTIC AND PSYCHOTIC DEPRESSIVE STATES	ADVERSE BEHAVIORAL EFFECTS: confusion, delirium, disorientation, hallucinations, delusions
EFFECTIVE TREATMENT FOR CHILDHOOD BED-WETTING (enuresis)	CONVERSION OF DEPRESSION TO MANIA in manic-depressive disorders
Additive therapy in chronic, severe pain	Aggravation of schizophrenia and paranoia
Aids cocaine withdrawal	Induction of serious heart rhythm abnormalities
Helps symptoms of attention deficit disorder	Abnormally low white blood cell and platelet counts (rare)
Helps prevent panic attacks	
Helps control binge eating and purging in bulimia	

▷ **Illness This Medication Treats:**
(1) Depression; (2) prevention of childhood bed-wetting in children over 6 years old; (3) may help in various delusional states.

▷ **Typical Dosage Range:** (Dosage or schedule must be determined by the doctor for each individual.)
Initially 75 mg daily, divided into three doses. Dose may be increased cautiously, as needed and tolerated, by 10 to 25 mg daily at intervals of 1 week. The usual maintenance dose is 50 to 150 mg every 24 hours. Total daily dosage should not exceed 200 mg for outpatient therapy. Daily requirement may be taken at bedtime as a single dose.

▷ **Conditions Requiring Dosing Adjustments:**
Liver function: Patients with liver compromise should use this drug with caution and in decreased doses. Imipramine is a rare cause of liver necrosis.

▷ **How Best to Take This Medicine:**   May be taken without regard to meals. If needed, this drug may be taken with food to reduce stomach upset. Capsule may be opened and the tablet crushed. Note: Tofranil-PM capsules should not be used to treat childhood bed-wetting.

▷ **How Long This Medicine Is Usually Taken:**   Continual use on a scheduled basis for 3 to 4 weeks is often needed to determine the effectiveness of this drug in relieving depression; peak response may require 3 or more months of use. Long-term use (months to years) requires evaluation of response and dose changes. See your doctor.

▷ **Tell Your Doctor Before Taking This Medicine If You:**
- ever had an allergic reaction to it or have had an adverse reaction to any other antidepressant.
- are taking, or have taken within the past 14 days, any MAO type A inhibitor.
- have had a recent heart attack (myocardial infarction).
- have narrow-angle glaucoma or increased internal eye pressure.
- have any type of seizure disorder.
- have any type of heart disease, especially coronary artery disease or a heart rhythm disorder.
- are subject to bronchial asthma.
- have impaired liver or kidney function.
- have a thyroid disorder or take thyroid medication.
- have diabetes or sugar intolerance.
- have prostatism.
- have a history of alcoholism.
- plan to have surgery under general anesthesia soon.

▷ **Possible Side Effects:**   Moderate drowsiness, light-headedness (low blood pressure), blurred vision, dry mouth, constipation, impaired urination.

▷ **Possible Adverse Effects:**
If any of the following develop, call your doctor promptly for guidance.
Some Mild Problems Drug Can Cause
Allergic reactions: skin rash, swelling of face or tongue, drug fever.
Headache, dizziness, nervousness, weakness, fainting.
Increased appetite, weight gain.
Irritation of tongue or mouth, altered taste, nausea.
Fluctuations of blood sugar.
Some Serious Problems Drug Can Cause
Allergic reactions: drug-induced hepatitis; anaphylactic reaction.
Idiosyncratic reactions: neuroleptic malignant syndrome.
Adverse behavioral effects: delirium, hallucinations, Tourette's syndrome.
Seizures; reduced control of epilepsy.
Aggravation of paranoid psychoses and schizophrenia.
Heart rhythm disturbances.
Rare liver or kidney toxicity, or myasthenia gravis.

Abnormally low white blood cell and platelet counts: fever, sore throat, infections, abnormal bleeding or bruising.

▷ **Possible Effects on Sex Life:** Decreased libido, increased libido (antidepressant effect), impaired erection, swelling of testicles, impaired ejaculation, impotence, inhibited male orgasm, inhibited female orgasm, male breast enlargement and tenderness, female breast enlargement with milk production.

▷ *CAUTION*

1. Watch for early signs of toxicity or overdose: confusion, agitation, rapid heart rate, heart irregularity. Measuring the blood level will clarify the situation.
2. This drug should be used with caution by patients with depression associated with schizophrenia. Watch closely for any deterioration of thinking or behavior.
3. Drug treatment should be interrupted if electroconvulsive therapy treatment is pending.
4. Safety and effectiveness of this drug for those under 6 years old are not established. Children 6 to 12 years old may be more susceptible than adults to heart toxicity. Therapy should be supervised by a properly trained pediatrician.
5. For people over 60, therapy should start with 25 mg at bedtime. The dose should be increased as needed and tolerated up to 100 mg daily in divided doses. During the first 2 weeks the patient or caregiver should watch for restlessness, agitation, forgetfulness, delusions, instability, or hallucinations. This drug may worsen prostatism.

Advisability of Use During Pregnancy and If Breast-Feeding:
Pregnancy Category: D. Use only if clearly needed. Avoid use of this drug during the first 3 months. Present in breast milk in small amounts. Watch the nursing infant closely and stop drug use or nursing if adverse effects start.

▷ **Habit-Forming Potential:** Psychological or physical dependence is rare and unexpected.

▷ **Overdose Symptoms:** Confusion, hallucinations, drowsiness, tremors, heart irregularity, seizures, stupor; hypothermia early, fever later.

▷ **Suggested Periodic Examinations While Taking This Drug:** (at doctor's discretion)
Monitoring of blood drug levels as appropriate.
Complete blood cell counts; liver and kidney function tests.
Serial blood pressure readings and electrocardiograms.
Measurement of internal eye pressure.

▷ **While Taking This Drug the Following Apply:**

Foods: You may need to limit your food intake to avoid excessive weight gain.

Beverages: May be taken with milk.

Alcohol: Avoid completely. This drug may markedly increase intoxication; the combination can depress brain function significantly.

Tobacco Smoking: May accelerate the elimination of this drug and require increased dosage.

Marijuana Smoking: Increased drowsiness and mouth dryness; may reduce this drug's effect.

Other Drugs:

Imipramine may ***increase*** the effects of

- all drugs with sedative effects; observe for excessive sedation.
- all drugs with atropinelike effects.
- norepinephrine.
- phenytoin (Dilantin).
- warfarin (Coumadin) and require more frequent INR (prothrombin time) testing.

Imipramine may ***decrease*** the effects of

- clonidine (Catapres).
- guanadrel (Hylorel).
- guanethidine (Ismelin, Esimil).
- guanfacine (Tenex).

Imipramine ***taken concurrently*** with

- anticonvulsants may need adjustment of the anticonvulsant dose if seizure pattern changes.
- antihistamines (see Drug Classes) may increase risk of urinary retention, acute glaucoma, or excessive anticholinergic actions.
- clonidine may cause a serious decrease in the antihypertensive effect of clonidine.
- ethchlorvynol (Placidyl) may cause delirium; avoid concurrent use.
- guanfacine results in a serious decrease in antihypertensive benefit from guanfacine.
- MAO type A (see Drug Classes) inhibitors may cause high fever, seizures, and excessive rise in blood pressure; avoid concurrent use and allow a period of 14 days between administration of either drug.
- phenytoin results in increased phenytoin levels. Levels should be checked more frequently if both drugs are continued.
- stimulant drugs (amphetamine, cocaine, epinephrine, phenylpropanolamine, etc.) may cause severe high blood pressure and/or high fever.
- thyroid preparations may increase the risk of heart rhythm disorders.

The following drugs may *increase* the effects of imipramine

- cimetidine (Tagamet).
- estrogens.
- fluoxetine (Prozac).
- fluvoxamine (Luvox).
- labetalol.
- methylphenidate (Ritalin).
- oral contraceptives (birth control pills).
- phenothiazines.
- quinidine.
- ranitidine (Zantac).

The following drugs may *decrease* the effects of imipramine

- barbiturates.
- carbamazepine (Tegretol).
- chloral hydrate (Noctec, Somnos, etc.).
- lithium (Lithobid, Lithotab, etc.).
- reserpine (Serpasil, Ser-Ap-Es, etc.).
- vitamin C (if more than 2 g/day are taken).

Driving, Hazardous Activities: Use caution. This drug may impair alertness, judgment, coordination, and reaction time.

Exposure to Sun: This drug may cause photosensitivity.

Exposure to Heat: Use caution. This drug may inhibit sweating and increase risk of heatstroke. Avoid saunas.

Exposure to Cold: The elderly are at risk for hypothermia.

Exposure to Environmental Chemicals: This drug may hide symptoms of poisoning caused by insecticides (organophosphorous types). Read their labels carefully.

Discontinuation: This drug must be stopped gradually over a period of 3 to 4 weeks. Abrupt withdrawal after prolonged use may cause nausea, vomiting, diarrhea, headache, malaise, disturbed sleep, and vivid dreaming. It may be necessary to adjust the dosages of other drugs taken at the same time.

▷ **Saving Money When Using This Medicine:**

- A large number of available drugs provide similar effectiveness. Ask your doctor to prescribe the drug that offers the best combination of cost and outcome.
- It may be possible (after a significant symptom-free period) to discontinue this medicine. Ask your doctor for help.
- Depression has recently been associated with low bone mineral density (BMD) and possible osteoporosis. Talk with your doctor about risk factors for osteoporosis, your diet, and the amount of exercise you get. BMD testing and calcium supplements may be needed.

INDAPAMIDE (in DAP a mide)

Prescription Needed: Yes   **Controlled Drug:** No   **Generic:** No

Brand Names: Lozol, Lozide

Overview of BENEFITS versus RISKS	
Possible Benefits	*Possible Risks*
EFFECTIVE ONCE-A-DAY TREATMENT OF MILD TO MODERATE HYPERTENSION	Excessive loss of blood potassium
	Increased blood sugar level
	Increased blood uric acid level
EFFECTIVE, MILD DIURETIC	

▷ **Illness This Medication Treats:**
(1) Increases the amount of urine (diuresis) and corrects fluid retention seen in congestive heart failure; (2) initiates treatment for high blood pressure (hypertension).

▷ **Typical Dosage Range:** (Dosage or schedule must be determined by the doctor for each individual.)
Initially 2.5 mg/day, taken as single dose in the morning. If necessary, the dose may be increased to 5 mg/day after 1 week (for diuresis) or after 4 weeks (for hypertension). The total daily dosage should not exceed 5 mg.

▷ **Conditions Requiring Dosing Adjustments:**
Liver function: This drug should be used with caution by patients with liver compromise; electrolytes should be monitored carefully.
Kidney function: This drug should be discontinued if kidney failure progresses once therapy is started.

▷ **How Best to Take This Medicine:** Take with or following food to reduce stomach irritation. Take in the morning to avoid nighttime urination. The tablet may be crushed for administration.

▷ **How Long This Medicine Is Usually Taken:** Continual use on a regular schedule for 2 to 4 weeks is usually needed to see the peak effect of this drug in lowering high blood pressure. Long-term use (months to years) requires careful followup. Use as a diuretic should be intermittent with drug holidays (no drug taken) to reduce the risk of sodium and potassium imbalance. See your doctor regularly.

▷ **Tell Your Doctor Before Taking This Medicine If You:**
- ever had an allergic reaction to it or are allergic to any form of sulfa drug.
- are pregnant or planning pregnancy.
- have a history of kidney or liver disease.

- have diabetes, gout, or lupus erythematosus.
- take any form of cortisone, digitalis, oral antidiabetic, or insulin.
- plan to have surgery under general anesthesia soon.

▷ **Possible Side Effects:** Light-headedness on arising from sitting or lying position.

Increase in blood sugar level, affecting control of diabetes.

Increase in blood uric acid level, affecting control of gout.

Decrease in blood potassium level, causing muscle weakness and cramping.

▷ **Possible Adverse Effects:**

If any of the following develop, call your doctor promptly for guidance.

Some Mild Problems Drug Can Cause

Allergic reactions: skin rashes, hives, itching.

Headache, dizziness, drowsiness, weakness, lethargy, visual disturbance.

Reduced appetite, indigestion, nausea, vomiting, diarrhea.

Some Serious Problems Drug Can Cause

Rare abnormal heartbeats.

Rare liver or kidney toxicity.

Rare serious skin rashes: Stevens-Johnson syndrome or toxic epidermal necrolysis (TEN).

▷ **Possible Effects on Sex Life:** Decreased libido; impotence.

▷ *CAUTION*

1. Increased dosage of this drug can cause excessive loss of sodium and potassium, with loss of appetite, nausea, fatigue, weakness, confusion, and tingling in the extremities.

2. If you are also taking a digitalis preparation (digitoxin, digoxin), ensure proper intake of high-potassium foods to avoid digitalis toxicity.

3. Safety and effectiveness of this drug for those under 12 years old are not established.

4. For people over 60, it's best to start with small doses of this drug. You may be more susceptible to the development of impaired thinking, orthostatic hypotension, potassium loss, and blood sugar increase. Overdosage and extended use of this drug can cause excessive loss of body water, thickening of the blood, and an increased tendency for clotting—predisposing to stroke, heart attack, or thrombophlebitis.

Advisability of Use During Pregnancy and If Breast-Feeding:

Pregnancy Category: B. This drug should not be used during pregnancy unless a very serious complication occurs for which this drug is significantly beneficial. Ask your doctor for guidance. Presence in breast milk is unknown; avoid taking this drug or refrain from nursing.

▷ **Overdose Symptoms:** Dry mouth, thirst, lethargy, weakness, muscle cramping, nausea, vomiting, drowsiness progressing to stupor or coma.

▷ **Suggested Periodic Examinations While Taking This Drug:** (at doctor's discretion)
Measurements of blood levels of sodium, potassium, magnesium chloride, sugar, and uric acid.

▷ **While Taking This Drug the Following Apply:**
Foods: Ask about a high-potassium diet (see Table 11, "High-Potassium Foods," Section Six). Follow your doctor's advice about salt use.
Beverages: This drug may be taken with milk.
Alcohol: Alcohol may exaggerate this drug's blood pressure–lowering effects and cause orthostatic hypotension.
Other Drugs:
Indapamide may *increase* the effects of
- other antihypertensives; dosage adjustments may be necessary to prevent excessive lowering of blood pressure.
- lithium (Lithobid, others), causing lithium toxicity.
Indapamide may *decrease* the effects of
- oral antidiabetics (sulfonylureas—see Drug Classes); dosage adjustments may be necessary for proper control of blood sugar.
Indapamide *taken concurrently* with
- digitalis preparations (digitoxin, digoxin) must be followed closely and dosage adjustments made to prevent fluctuations of blood potassium levels and serious heart rhythm disturbances.
- NSAIDs (see Drug Classes) may blunt the therapeutic effect of indapamide.
The following drugs may *decrease* the effects of indapamide
- cholestyramine (Cuemid, Questran) may interfere with its absorption.
- colestipol (Colestid) may interfere with its absorption.
Take cholestyramine and colestipol 1 hour before any oral diuretic.
Driving, Hazardous Activities: Use caution until the possible occurrence of orthostatic hypotension, drowsiness, dizziness, or impaired vision has been determined.
Exposure to Heat: Excessive perspiring could cause additional loss of salt and water.
Heavy Exercise or Exertion: Isometric exercises (the overload technique for strengthening individual muscles) can raise blood pressure significantly. Ask your doctor for help.
Occurrence of Unrelated Illness: Illnesses that cause vomiting or diarrhea can produce a serious imbalance of important body chemistry. Ask your doctor for guidance.

Discontinuation: Discontinuation of this drug may be advisable 5 to 7 days before major surgery. Ask your doctor, surgeon, and/or anesthesiologist for guidance.

▷ **Saving Money When Using This Medicine:**
- A large number of available drugs provide similar effectiveness. Ask your doctor to prescribe the drug that offers the best combination of cost and outcome.
- It may be possible (after a significant symptom-free period) to discontinue this medicine. Ask your doctor for help.
- Be sure to have your blood pressure checked periodically to confirm that this medicine is still working for you.
- Talk with your doctor about stress management and exercise programs available in your community.
- Find out more about high blood pressure. *The Essential Guide to Chronic Illness* is an excellent source of information.

INDOMETHACIN (in doh METH a sin)

Prescription Needed: Yes   **Controlled Drug:** No   **Generic:** Yes

Brand Names: Indameth, Indocin, Indocin-SR, Zendole

Overview of BENEFITS versus RISKS	
Possible Benefits	*Possible Risks*
EFFECTIVE RELIEF OF MILD TO MODERATE PAIN AND INFLAMMATION	Gastrointestinal pain, ulceration, bleeding (rare)
	Liver or kidney damage (rare)
	Fluid retention (rare)
	Bone marrow depression (rare)
	Mental depression, confusion

See the acetic acids (NSAIDs) drug profile for further information.

INFLUENZA VACCINE (IN flew en za)
Other names: Flu shot or flu vaccine

Prescription Needed: Yes   **Controlled Drug:** No   **Generic:** No

Brand Names: Fluogen, Flu-immune, Flu-Shield, Fluzone

Overview of BENEFITS versus RISKS	
Possible Benefits	*Possible Risks*
PREVENTION OF INFLUENZA CAUSED BY THE VIRUSES TO WHICH IMMUNITY IS CONFERRED	Rare hypersensitivity Very rare Guillain-Barré syndrome (questionable causation)

▷ **Illness This Medication Treats:**
Used to prevent the flu or influenza.

▷ **Typical Dosage Range:** (Dosage or schedule must be determined by the doctor for each individual.)
Infants and Children: Those 6 to 35 months old are given 0.25 ml of a split dose vaccine. If this is the first vaccine, two doses should be given 1 month apart. A split dose is suggested because it tends to cause fewer adverse effects.
For children 3 to 8 years old: 0.5 ml of the selected split virus vaccine. If the child has not been vaccinated, two shots should be given, 1 month apart.
Children 9 years or older should be given 0.5 ml of the split virus vaccine in the deltoid muscle.
13 to 60 Years of Age: 0.5 ml of whole or split virus vaccine in the deltoid muscle.
Over 65 Years of Age: Same as for 13 to 60 years of age.

▷ **How Best to Take This Medicine:** Prior vaccination **does not** mean that you are immune to this year's flu. The best protection comes from a flu shot each year. Some tenderness may occur at the injection site and can be treated with acetaminophen (Tylenol, others).

▷ **How Long This Medicine Is Usually Taken:** Single vaccinations in adults usually give immunity in 2 weeks. It is strongly recommended that you get a flu shot EVERY year.

▷ **Tell Your Doctor Before Taking This Medicine If You:**
  • ever had an allergic reaction to a flu shot.
  • are allergic to eggs, as the virus is grown on eggs.
  • have a sudden illness with fever.
  • have AIDS or an impaired immune system.
  • have had Guillain-Barré syndrome.
  • have a history of seizures.
  • have been receiving cancer chemotherapy.

▷ **Possible Side Effects:** Pain at the vaccination site. Muscle aches, fever, or bothersome tiredness (malaise). This is NOT the flu. The vaccine contains fragments of noninfectious virus, and these symptoms are a reaction to the components of the vaccine.

▷ **Possible Adverse Effects:**
If any of the following develop, call your doctor promptly for guidance.

Some Mild Problems This Drug Can Cause
Allergic reactions: swelling or redness.
Muscle aches or fever.
Nausea or headache.
Rare vasculitis, joint pain, or weakness.

Some Serious Problems This Drug Can Cause
Allergic reactions: rare anaphylactic reactions.
Very rare lowering of blood platelets.
Very rare Guillain-Barré syndrome (only reported during 1976—1977 flu season and of questionable cause).
Very rare vision changes or kidney toxicity.

▷ *CAUTION*

1. The fact that you got a flu shot last year does not mean you will be immune to this year's flu. The vaccine is made differently each year because the virus strains differ each year, and so the side effects or adverse effects may change each year.
2. Although the flu vaccine may confer immunity to other viruses, there may still be viral strains capable of causing a flu-like syndrome that may effect you.
3. If you develop muscle aches or fever, acetaminophen (Tylenol, others) will help. DO NOT take aspirin to help such symptoms.
4. Call your doctor immediately if you develop hives. facial swelling, or difficult breathing after getting this vaccination.
5. Safety and effectiveness of this vaccine are not established for infants less than 6 months old.
6. This vaccine may be especially valuable for people over 60 years old.

Advisability of Use During Pregnancy and If Breast-Feeding:
Pregnancy Category: C. Use this vaccine only if clearly needed. Ask your doctor. Presence in breast milk is unknown. Watch the nursing infant closely, and call your doctor if adverse effects develop.

▷ **Overdose Symptoms:** No specific cases reported. Treatment would be consistent with symptoms that developed.

▷ **While Taking This Drug the Following Apply:**
Alcohol: An interaction is not expected, but excessive alcohol may blunt the immune response.
Other Drugs:
Influenza vaccine may *increase* the effects of
• carbamazepine (Tegretol) by decreasing removal from the body.
• phenobarbital.
• theophylline (Theo-Dur, others).

- warfarin (Coumadin) and pose increased bleeding risk. More INR (prothrombin time) testing is needed.

Influenza vaccine *taken concurrently* with

- cyclosporine (Sandimmune) may blunt the response to the vaccine.
- immunosupressive agents (chemotherapy, corticosteroids) may lessen the protective effect of the vaccine.
- methotrexate can blunt the vaccine's benefits.
- phenytoin (Dilantin) can change the blood levels of phenytoin.

Author's note: There is now a Vaccine Adverse Event Reporting System (VAERS). The toll-free number is 1-800-822-7967.

Driving, Hazardous Activities: Caution: This vaccine may make you feel lethargic for a few days.

▷ **Saving Money When Using This Medicine:**
- A *New England Journal of Medicine* article clearly demonstrated the benefits of healthy young adults getting a flu shot. Preventing the flu saves money by decreasing lost time from work, avoiding complications from influenza for people over 60, and avoiding secondary infections.

INSULIN   (IN suh lin)

Prescription Needed: No   **Controlled Drug:** No   **Generic:** Yes

Brand Names: Humalog, Humulin L, Humulin N, Humulin R, Humulin U, Humulin U Ultralente, Humulin 70/30, Iletin I NPH, Insulatard NPH, Lente Iletin I, Lente Iletin II Beef, Lente Iletin II Pork, Lente Insulin, Mixtard, Mixtard Human 70/30, Novolin L, Novolin N, NovolinPen, Novolin R, NPH Iletin I, NPH Iletin II Beef, NPH Iletin II Pork, NPH Insulin, NPH Purified Pork, Protamine, Zinc & Iletin I, Protamine, Zinc & Iletin II Beef, Protamine, Zinc & Iletin II Pork, Regular Iletin I, Regular Iletin II Beef, Regular Iletin II Pork, Regular Iletin II U-500, Regular Insulin, Regular Purified Pork Insulin, Semilente Iletin I, Semilente Insulin, Semilente Purified Pork, Ultralente Iletin I, Ultralente Insulin, Ultralente Purified Beef, Velosulin

---

Overview of BENEFITS versus RISKS

Possible Benefits	*Possible Risks*
EFFECTIVE CONTROL OF TYPE I (INSULIN-DEPENDENT) DIABETES MELLITUS	HYPOGLYCEMIA WITH EXCESSIVE DOSAGE
EFFECTIVE CONTROL OF HIGH BLOOD SUGAR DURING PREGNANCY	Infrequent allergic reactions

---

▷ **Illness This Medication Treats:**

(1) Control of insulin-dependent diabetes mellitus and for those not usually insulin-dependent who are presently ill; (2) control of blood sugar in critically ill patients being fed by intravenous nutrient mixtures or total parenteral nutrition (TPN).

Other (unlabeled) generally accepted use: control of blood sugar that is out of control during pregnancy.

▷ **Typical Dosage Range:** (Dosage or schedule must be determined by the doctor for each individual.)

According to individual requirements for the optimal regulation of blood sugar on a 24-hour basis.

▷ **Conditions Requiring Dosing Adjustments:**

Kidney function: Patients with compromised kidneys should use insulin with caution.

▷ **How Best to Take This Medicine:** Inject insulin subcutaneously according to the schedule your doctor prescribes. The timing and frequency of injections varies with the type of insulin. The following table of insulin actions (according to type) will help you understand your treatment schedule.

Insulin Type	Action Onset	Peak	Duration
Regular	0.5–1 hr	2–4 hr	5–7 hr
Isophane (NPH)	3–4 hr	6–12 hr	18–28 hr
Regular 30%/NPH 70%	0.5 hr	4–8 hr	24 hr
Semilente	1–3 hr	2–8 hr	12–16 hr
Lente	1–3 hr	8–12 hr	18–28 hr
Ultralente	4–6 hr	18–24 hr	36 hr
Protamine Zinc	4–6 hr	14–24 hr	36 hr

▷ **How Long This Medicine Is Usually Taken:** Type I insulin-dependent diabetes mellitus usually requires insulin treatment for life. Type II noninsulin-dependent diabetes is usually controlled by oral antidiabetics and/or diet but may require insulin for adequate control with serious infections, injuries, burns, surgical procedures, and other forms of physical stress. Insulin is used as needed on a temporary basis to regulate and normalize the body's use of sugar until recovery is complete and basic health is restored. EFFECTIVE CONTROL OF BLOOD SUGAR can help you totally avoid the kidney failure, heart problems, high blood pressure, nerve damage, or blindness that goes along with long-standing, poorly controlled blood sugar. See your doctor regularly.

▷ **Tell Your Doctor Before Taking This Medicine If You:**

- have a need for it and its correct dosage schedule have not been established by a properly qualified physician.
- have a history of allergic reaction to any form of insulin.
- do not know how to recognize and treat abnormally low blood sugar.
- are taking any aspirin, beta-blockers, fenfluramine (Pondimin), or monoamine oxidase type A inhibitors (MAOIs).

▷ **Possible Side Effects:** In management of stable diabetes, no side effects occur when insulin dose, diet, and physical activity are correctly balanced and maintained.

In management of unstable (brittle) diabetes, unexpected drops in blood sugar levels can occur, resulting in periods of hypoglycemia.

▷ **Possible Adverse Effects:**

If any of the following develop, call your doctor promptly for guidance.

Some Mild Problems Drug Can Cause

Allergic reactions: local redness, swelling, and itching at site of injection; occasional hives.

Thinning of subcutaneous tissue at sites of injection.

Some Serious Problems Drug Can Cause

Allergic reaction: anaphylactic reactions.

Severe, prolonged hypoglycemia.

Rare hemolytic anemia or porphyria.

▷ **Adverse Effects That May Mimic Natural Diseases or Disorders:**

The early signs of hypoglycemia may be mistaken for alcoholic intoxication.

▷ *CAUTION*

1. It is most important that you carry with you a personal identification card noting that you have diabetes and are taking insulin.
2. Recognize the onset of hypoglycemia and know how to treat it. Always carry a readily available form of sugar, such as hard candy or sugar cubes. Report all episodes of hypoglycemia to your doctor.
3. Improvement in vision may occur during the first several weeks of insulin treatment. Defer any examination for glasses for 6 weeks after starting insulin.

4. The rates of insulin absorption vary significantly from one body site to another. Absorption is 80% greater from the abdominal wall than from the leg, and 30% greater than from the arm. People with unstable diabetes may have better control of blood sugar levels by rotating the injection site within the same body region rather than from one site to another.

5. Insulin dosages and schedules are modified according to patient size. Adhere strictly to the doctor's prescribed routine.

6. For people over 60, insulin requirements may change with aging. Periodic evaluation of individual status is necessary to determine correct insulin dosage and scheduling. The aging brain adapts well to higher blood sugar levels. Attempts to maintain strictly normal blood sugar levels may result in unrecognized hypoglycemia that shows as confusion and abnormal behavior. Repeated episodes of hypoglycemia (especially if severe) may cause brain damage.

Advisability of Use During Pregnancy and If Breast-Feeding:

Pregnancy Category: B. Insulin is the drug of choice for managing diabetes during pregnancy. To preserve the health of the mother and fetus, every effort must be made to establish the best dose of insulin necessary for good control and to prevent episodes of hypoglycemia. Not present in breast milk. Insulin treatment of the mother has no adverse effect on the nursing infant. Breast-feeding may decrease insulin requirements; dosage adjustment may be necessary.

▷ **Overdose Symptoms:** Hypoglycemia: fatigue, weakness, headache, nervousness, irritability, sweating, tremors, hunger, confusion, delirium, abnormal behavior (resembling alcoholic intoxication), loss of consciousness, seizures.

▷ **Suggested Periodic Examinations While Taking This Drug:** (at doctor's discretion)
Checking of urine sugar content when you are ill. Measurement of blood sugar levels at intervals recommended by your doctor.

▷ **While Taking This Drug the Following Apply:**
Foods: Follow your diabetic diet conscientiously. Do not omit snack foods in mid-afternoon or at bedtime if they help prevent hypoglycemia.
Beverages: According to prescribed diabetic diet.
Alcohol: Excessive use can induce severe hypoglycemia, resulting in brain damage.
Tobacco Smoking: Regular smoking decreases insulin absorption and increases insulin requirements by 30%.
Marijuana Smoking: Possible increase in blood sugar levels.

Other Drugs:
The following drugs may ***increase*** the effects of insulin

- aspirin and other salicylates.
- some beta-blockers (especially the nonselective ones); may prolong insulin-induced hypoglycemia.
- clofibrate (Atromid-S).
- fenfluramine (Pondimin).
- MAO type A inhibitors (MAOIs).
- oral hypoglycemic agents (see Drug Classes); may result in additive hypoglycemia.

The following drugs may ***decrease*** the effects of insulin (by raising blood sugar levels)

- chlorthalidone (Hygroton).
- cortisonelike drugs.
- furosemide (Lasix).
- oral contraceptives (birth control pills).
- phenytoin (Dilantin, etc.).
- thiazide diuretics.
- thyroid preparations.

Driving, Hazardous Activities: Be prepared to stop and take corrective action when indications of impending hypoglycemia occur.

Exposure to Heat: Use caution. Sauna baths can significantly increase the rate of insulin absorption and cause hypoglycemia.

Heavy Exercise or Exertion: Use caution. Periods of unusual or unplanned heavy physical activity will hasten blood sugar utilization and predispose to hypoglycemia.

Occurrence of Unrelated Illness: Report all illnesses that prevent regular eating. The omission of meals as a result of nausea, vomiting, or injury may lead to hypoglycemia. Untreated infections can increase insulin requirements. Consult your doctor for help.

Discontinuation: Do not stop taking insulin without consulting your doctor. Insulin-dependent diabetes requires continual treatment on a regular basis. Omission of insulin may result in life-threatening coma.

Special Storage Instructions: Keep insulin in a cool place, preferably the refrigerator. Protect it from freezing; protect it from strong light and high temperatures when not refrigerated.

Observe the Following Expiration Times: Do not use insulin if it is older than the expiration date on the vial.

▷ **Saving Money When Using This Medicine:**
- Ask your doctor if insulin offers the best combination of cost and outcome for the condition being treated.
- It may be possible (after a significant period of normal glucoses) to stop taking insulin if it was used under certain conditions. Ask your doctor for help.

- Many kinds of insulin are available. The best long-term outcome happens when blood glucose levels are maintained in the normal range. Talk with your doctor about regular fingerstick blood sugar testing if you are not presently doing this.
- Often different kinds of insulin must be combined for the best glucose control. Human insulin is the least likely to cause insulin antibodies to form.
- Find out as much as possible about your condition. *The Essential Guide to Chronic Illness* is an excellent source of information.

IODOQUINOL (i oh doh KWIN ohl)

Other Name: Di-iodohydroxyquin

Prescription Needed: Yes   **Controlled Drug:** No   **Generic:** Yes

Brand Names: Diquinol, Yodoxin

Overview of BENEFITS versus RISKS	
Possible Benefits	*Possible Risks*
EFFECTIVE TREATMENT OF CARRIERS OF INTESTINAL AMEBA (cyst passers)	OPTIC NERVE DAMAGE Peripheral neuritis Drug-induced goiter
Effective adjunctive treatment of invasive amebic infections	

▷ **Illness This Medication Treats:**
(1) Carriers of amebic cysts who have no symptoms of infection;
(2) resistant skin conditions such as seborrhea

▷ **Typical Dosage Range:** (Dosage or schedule must be determined by the doctor for each individual.)
Infants and Children: Less than 6 years old: 210 mg per 15 lb of body weight, three times a day for 20 days. Maximum daily dose is 1.95 g.
6 to 12 years old: Two 210 mg tablets three times daily for 20 days.
12 to 60 Years of Age: 630 or 650 mg three times a day for 20 days. The total daily dose should not exceed 2 g.
Over 60 Years of Age: Same as for 12 to 60 years of age.
Note: If necessary, the course of treatment may be repeated after a drug-free interval of 2 to 3 weeks.

IPRATROPIUM (i pra TROH pee um)

Prescription Needed: Yes   **Controlled Drug:** No   **Generic:** No

Brand Names: Atrovent, Atrovent nasal spray, Combivent

Overview of BENEFITS versus RISKS	
Possible Benefits	*Possible Risks*
EFFECTIVE BRONCHODILATOR FOR TREATMENT OF CHRONIC BRONCHITIS AND EMPHYSEMA Possibly effective as adjunctive treatment in some cases of bronchial asthma	Mild and infrequent adverse effects

▷ **Illness This Medication Treats:**
(1) Difficult breathing episodes in chronic bronchitis and emphysema. Should not be used to treat acute attacks of asthma because it takes a while to work. (2) Nasal spray form helps runny nose (rhinorrhea) from allergic or nonallergic perennial rhinitis (including the common cold) in adults and children over 12 years old.

▷ **Typical Dosage Range:** (Dosage or schedule must be determined by the doctor for each individual.)
Initially two inhalations (36 mcg) four times a day, 4 hours apart. If necessary, the dose may be increased to four inhalations (80 mcg) at one time to obtain optimal relief. Maintain 4-hour intervals between doses. Total daily dosage should not exceed 12 inhalations (216 mcg).
Nasal spray: 0.03% formula: two sprays (21 mcg each) in each nostril two to three times a day for up to 4 days. The 0.06% formula is used as two sprays (42 mcg each) in each nostril three to four times a day, also up to 4 days.

▷ **Conditions Requiring Dosing Adjustments:**
Kidney function: Patients with bladder neck obstructions should use this drug with caution.

▷ **How Best to Take This Medicine:** Carefully follow the patient instructions provided with the inhaler. Shake well before using.

▷ **How Long This Medicine Is Usually Taken:** Continual use on a regular schedule for 48 to 72 hours is usually necessary to determine the effectiveness of this drug. Long-term use (months to years) requires checking response and adjusting dosage. See your doctor.

▷ **Tell Your Doctor Before Taking This Medicine If You:**
- ever had an allergic reaction to it or atropine or aerosol propellants (fluorocarbons).
- had a previous adverse reaction to any belladonna derivative or from benzalkonium chloride/edetate sodium (nasal spray).
- have a history of glaucoma.
- have any form of urinary retention or prostatism.

▷ **Possible Side Effects:** Throat dryness, cough, irritation from aerosol, blurred vision, dry mouth, impaired urination. Nosebleeds with the nasal spray form.

▷ **Possible Adverse Effects:**
If any of the following develop, call your doctor promptly for guidance.
Some Mild Problems Drug Can Cause
Allergic reactions: skin rash, hives.
Headache, dizziness, nervousness.
Lip and mouth ulcers, unpleasant taste, nausea.
Some Serious Problems Drug Can Cause
Allergic reactions: RARE first-dose angioedema or bronchospasm.

▷ *CAUTION*
1. Ipratropium won't start to work for 5 to 15 minutes. It should **not** be used alone to treat acute asthma attacks, which need a fast result.
2. When used as an adjunct to beta-adrenergic antiasthmatic drugs (albuterol, terbutaline, metaproterenol, etc.), the beta-adrenergic aerosol should be used approximately 5 minutes before ipratropium, to prevent fluorocarbon toxicity.
3. When used as an adjunct to steroid or cromolyn aerosols (beclomethasone, Intal), ipratropium should be used approximately 5 minutes before the steroid or cromolyn aerosol to prevent fluorocarbon toxicity.
4. Avoid the accidental spraying of this aerosol into the eyes, which could cause temporary blurring of vision.
5. Safety and effectiveness of this drug for those under 12 years old are not established.
6. For people over 60, prostatism may worsen; the dose must be adjusted as needed.
7. Call your doctor if, while you are using the nasal spray, your runny nose continues and you develop a fever.

Advisability of Use During Pregnancy and If Breast-Feeding:
Pregnancy Category: B. Use this drug only if clearly needed. Probably present in breast milk in very small amounts. Watch the nursing infant closely and stop taking this drug or nursing if adverse effects start.

▷ **Overdose Symptoms:** The drug taken by aerosol inhalation is not well absorbed into the circulation. No systemic effects of overdose are expected.

▷ **Suggested Periodic Examinations While Taking This Drug:** (at doctor's discretion)
Internal eye pressure measurements if appropriate.

▷ **While Taking This Drug the Following Apply:**
Tobacco Smoking: No interactions are expected. However, smoking should be avoided completely if you have chronic bronchitis or emphysema.
Other Drugs:
Ipratropium may *increase* the effects of
- albuterol (Proventil, others).
- other atropinelike drugs.
- tricyclic antidepressants—their anticholinergic side effects.
Driving, Hazardous Activities: This drug may cause dizziness or blurred vision. Restrict your activities as necessary.
Exposure to Cold: Inhaling cold air may cause bronchospasm and induce asthmatic breathing and cough; dosage adjustment of this drug may be necessary.
Heavy Exercise or Exertion: This drug is not considered consistently effective in preventing or treating exercise-induced asthma.
Discontinuation: Consult your doctor for guidance. Substitute medication may be advisable.

▷ **Saving Money When Using This Medicine:**
- A large number of available drugs help asthma. Ask your doctor to prescribe the drug that offers the best combination of cost and outcome. Talk with your doctor about nebulized lidocaine's benefits. Discuss the use of nedocromil or cromolyn to prevent asthma attacks.
- It may be possible (after a significant asthma-free period) to stop taking this medicine. Ask your doctor for help.
- Find out as much as possible about your condition. *The Essential Guide to Chronic Illness* is an excellent source of information.

ISONIAZID (i soh NI a zid)

Other Names: Isonicotinic acid hydrazide, INH
Prescription Needed: Yes   **Controlled Drug:** No   **Generic:** Yes
Brand Names: Laniazid, Nydrazid, P-I-N Forte [CD], Rifamate [CD], Rifater [CD], Rimactane/INH Dual Pack [CD], Teebaconin, Teebaconin and Vitamin B6 [CD]

Overview of BENEFITS versus RISKS

Possible Benefits

EFFECTIVE PREVENTION
AND TREATMENT OF
ACTIVE TUBERCULOSIS

Possible Risks

ALLERGIC LIVER REACTION
Peripheral neuropathy
Bone marrow depression
Mental and behavioral
disturbances

▷ **Illness This Medication Treats:**

(1) Prevents active tuberculous infection in people at high risk due to exposure to infection or recent conversion of a negative tuberculin skin test to positive; (2) combined with other drugs for treatment of tuberculosis.

As Combination Drug Product [CD]: Available in combination with rifampin, another antitubercular drug, which is more effective than either drug alone. Isoniazid can cause low pyridoxine (vitamin B6); for this reason, a combination of the two drugs is available in tablet form.

▷ **Typical Dosage Range:** (Dosage or schedule must be determined by the doctor for each individual.)

For prevention: 300 mg once daily. For treatment: 5 mg per kilogram of body weight, daily. The total daily dosage should not exceed 300 mg.

▷ **Conditions Requiring Dosing Adjustments:**

Liver function: This drug should NOT be used by patients with acute liver disease. Discontinue if the liver function tests increase to three times the normal value.

Kidney function: Patients with renal compromise should use this drug with caution—it is a rare cause of nephrosis. For patients with severe kidney compromise (creatinine clearance <10 ml/min), the daily dose should be decreased by 50%.

▷ **How Best to Take This Medicine:** May be taken with food to prevent stomach irritation. The tablet may be crushed for administration.

▷ **How Long This Medicine Is Usually Taken:** Continual use of this drug on a regular schedule for many months is often necessary, depending on the nature of the infection. Shorter courses of intermittent high dosage may be adequate in some cases. See your doctor regularly.

▷ **Tell Your Doctor Before Taking This Medicine If You:**

- ever had an allergic reaction to it.
- have active liver disease or serious impairment of liver or kidney function.

- drink an alcoholic beverage daily.
- have a seizure disorder.
- take other drugs on a long-term basis, especially phenytoin (Dilantin).
- plan to have surgery under general anesthesia soon.
- are pregnant or nursing your baby.

▷ **Possible Adverse Effects:**
If any of the following develop, call your doctor promptly for guidance.
Some Mild Problems Drug Can Cause
Allergic reactions: skin rash, fever, swollen glands, painful muscles and joints.
Dizziness, indigestion, nausea, vomiting.
Some Serious Problems Drug Can Cause
Allergic reactions: drug-induced hepatitis—loss of appetite, nausea, fatigue, fever, itching, yellow discoloration of eyes and skin.
Peripheral neuritis: numbness, tingling.
Acute mental and behavioral disturbances, impaired vision, increase in epileptic seizures.
Bone marrow depression: fatigue, fever, sore throat, abnormal bleeding or bruising.
Severe skin reactions (Stevens-Johnson syndrome, pellagra).
Rare porphyria, lupus erythematosus–like syndrome.
Very rare kidney toxicity or muscle damage (rhabdomyolysis).

▷ **Possible Effects on Sex Life:**   Male breast enlargement and tenderness (gynecomastia).

▷ **Possible Delayed Adverse Effects:**   An increase in the frequency of liver cirrhosis has been reported.

▷ **Adverse Effects That May Mimic Natural Diseases or Disorders:**
Drug-induced hepatitis may suggest viral hepatitis.

▷ *CAUTION*
1. Ask your doctor about determining whether you are a slow or rapid inactivator (acetylator). This has a bearing on your predisposition to developing adverse effects.
2. Copper sulfate tests for urine sugar may give a false-positive test result (diabetics, please note).
3. Use this drug with caution in children with seizure disorders. Slow acetylators are more prone to adverse drug effects. It is advisable to give supplemental pyridoxine (vitamin B6).
4. Those over 60 may have a greater incidence of liver damage, and their liver status should be monitored carefully. Watch for any indications of an acute brain syndrome consisting of confusion, delirium, and seizures.

Advisability of Use During Pregnancy and If Breast-Feeding:
Pregnancy Category: C. If clearly needed, isoniazid is used now at any time during pregnancy. Ask your doctor for guidance. Present in breast milk; avoid taking this drug or refrain from nursing.

▷ **Overdose Symptoms:** Nausea, vomiting, dizziness, blurred vision, hallucinations, slurred speech, stupor, coma, seizures.

▷ **Suggested Periodic Examinations While Taking This Drug:** (at doctor's discretion)
Complete blood cell counts, liver function tests, complete eye examinations.

▷ **While Taking This Drug the Following Apply:**
Foods: Eat the following foods cautiously until your tolerance is determined: Swiss and Cheshire cheeses, tuna fish, skipjack fish and *Sardinella* species. These may interact with this drug to produce skin rash, itching, sweating, chills, headache, light-headedness, or rapid heart rate.

Nutritional Support: It is advisable to take a pyridoxine (vitamin B6) supplement to prevent peripheral neuritis. Ask your doctor for the dosage.

Beverages: May be taken with milk.

Alcohol: Alcohol may reduce the effectiveness of this drug and increase the risk of liver toxicity.

Other Drugs:
Isoniazid may **increase** the effects of
- carbamazepine (Tegretol), causing toxicity.
- phenytoin (Dilantin), causing toxicity.

The following drugs may **decrease** the effects of isoniazid
- cortisonelike drugs.

Isoniazid **taken concurrently** with
- acetaminophen (Tylenol, others) may increase risk of liver damage.
- antacids may decrease isoniazid absorption and blunt its benefits. Separate the dosings by 2 hours.
- BCG vaccine will decrease BCG's effectiveness.
- diazepam and perhaps other benzodiazepines (see Drug Classes) may result in increased blood levels and toxicity.
- ketoconazole, itraconazole, or related compounds may blunt antifungal benefits.
- meperidine (Demerol) may lead to excessive lowering of blood pressure.
- oral hypoglycemic agents (see Drug Classes) may lead to loss of control of blood glucose.
- rifampin (Rifadin, others) may increase risk of liver toxicity.
- theophylline (Theo-Dur, others) may lead to theophylline toxicity.

- valproic acid (Depakene) may lead to isoniazid or valproic acid toxicity.
- warfarin (Coumadin) may increase risk of bleeding. Increased INR (prothrombin time) tests are needed.

Driving, Hazardous Activities: This drug may cause dizziness. Restrict your activities as necessary.

Discontinuation: Long-term treatment is required. Do not stop taking this drug without consulting your doctor.

▷ **Saving Money When Using This Medicine:**
- There is currently an epidemic of multidrug-resistant tuberculosis (TB) in this country. If you live in an area where this form is endemic, you may need to take three or four antituberculosis drugs at the same time. Ask your doctor to prescribe the drug regimen that offers the best combination of cost and outcome.

ISOSORBIDE DINITRATE   (i soh SOHR bide di NI trayt)

Other Name: Sorbide nitrate

Prescription Needed: Yes   **Controlled Drug:** No   **Generic:** Yes

Brand Names: Dilatrate-SR, Isonate, Isordil, Isordil Tembids, Isordil Titradose, Sorbitrate SA, Sorbitrate

▷ **Warning:** The brand names Isordil and Isuprel can be mistaken for each other, leading to serious medication errors. These names represent very different drugs. Isordil (white, yellow, blue, or green tablets), the generic drug isosorbide dinitrate, is used to treat angina. Isuprel (a sublingual tablet for dissolving in the mouth), the generic drug isoproterenol, is a bronchodilator used to treat asthma. Verify that you are taking the correct drug.

Overview of BENEFITS versus RISKS

Possible Benefits	*Possible Risks*
EFFECTIVE RELIEF AND PREVENTION OF ANGINA	Orthostatic hypotension
EFFECTIVE ADJUNCTIVE TREATMENT IN SELECTED CASES OF CONGESTIVE HEART FAILURE	Rare skin reactions (severe peeling)

▷ **Illness This Medication Treats:**
(1) Acute attacks of anginal pain in sublingual (under-the-tongue) and chewable tablet forms; (2) prevention of angina by longer-acting tablets and capsules; not effective in relieving acute anginal pain.

▷ **Typical Dosage Range:** (Dosage or schedule must be determined by the doctor for each individual.)

Infants and Children: Dosage not established.

12 to 60 Years of Age: Sublingual tablets: 5 to 10 mg dissolved under the tongue every 2 to 3 hours; use for relief of acute attack and prevention of anticipated attack.

Chewable tablets: Initially 5 mg chewed, to evaluate tolerance; increase dose to 5 or 10 mg every 2 to 3 hours as needed and tolerated. Use for relief of acute attack and prevention of anticipated attack.

Tablets: 5 to 30 mg four times daily to prevent acute attack; usual dose is 10 to 20 mg four times a day.

Prolonged-action capsules and tablets: 40 mg every 6 to 12 hours as needed to prevent acute attacks.

The total daily dosage should not exceed 120 mg.

Over 60 Years of Age: Same as for 12 to 60 years of age.

▷ **Conditions Requiring Dosing Adjustments:**

Liver function: Patients with liver compromise should use this drug with caution, as increased blood levels will occur. The dose should be decreased for patients with liver compromise.

Kidney function: No specific dosing changes are needed for patients with compromised kidneys. This drug can discolor (brown to black) urine.

▷ **How Best to Take This Medicine:** Capsules and tablets to be swallowed are best taken on an empty stomach to achieve maximal blood levels. Regular tablets may be crushed for administration; prolonged-action capsules and tablets should be taken whole and not altered.

▷ **How Long This Medicine Is Usually Taken:** Continual use on a regular schedule for 3 to 7 days is usually necessary to (1) determine this drug's effectiveness in preventing or relieving acute anginal pain, and (2) establish the optimal dosage schedule. Long-term use (months to years) requires physician supervision.

▷ **Tell Your Doctor Before Taking This Medicine If You:**
- ever had an allergic reaction to it.
- have had a very recent heart attack (myocardial infarction).
- are pregnant or are planning pregnancy.
- are allergic to the dye tartrazine.
- have an overactive thyroid gland.
- had an unfavorable response to other nitrate drugs or vasodilators in the past.
- have a history of low blood pressure.
- have any form of glaucoma.

▷ **Possible Side Effects:** Flushing of face, throbbing in head, palpitation, rapid heart rate, abnormal lowering of blood pressure on standing (orthostatic hypotension).

▷ **Possible Adverse Effects:**
If any of the following develop, call your doctor promptly for guidance.
Some Mild Problems Drug Can Cause
  Allergic reaction: skin rash.
  Headache (may be severe and persistent), dizziness, fainting.
  Nausea, vomiting.
Some Serious Problems Drug Can Cause
  Allergic reaction: severe dermatitis with peeling of skin.
  Transient ischemic attacks (TIAs) in people with impaired circulation in the brain: dizziness, fainting, impaired vision or speech, localized numbness or weakness.
  Anemia (if you have a G6PD deficiency).

▷ **Adverse Effects That May Mimic Natural Diseases or Disorders:**
Spells of low blood pressure (due to this drug) may be mistaken for late-onset epilepsy.

▷ *CAUTION*
  1. Development of tolerance to long-acting nitrates may render the sublingual tablets of nitroglycerin less effective in relieving acute anginal attacks. Antianginal effectiveness is restored after 1 week of abstinence from long-acting nitrates. Talk with your doctor about a nitrate-free period.
  2. Many over-the-counter (OTC) medications for allergies, colds, and coughs contain drugs that may counteract the desired effects of this drug. Ask your doctor or pharmacist for guidance before using such medications.
  3. People over 60 should take small doses until their tolerance has been determined. They may be more susceptible to the development of low blood pressure and associated blackout spells, fainting, and falling. Throbbing headaches and flushing may be more apparent.

Advisability of Use During Pregnancy and If Breast-Feeding:
Pregnancy Category: C. Use this drug only if clearly needed. Presence in breast milk is unknown. If the drug is necessary, monitor the nursing infant for low blood pressure and poor feeding.

▷ **Overdose Symptoms:** Headache, dizziness, marked flushing of face and skin, vomiting, weakness, fainting, difficult breathing, coma.

▷ **Suggested Periodic Examinations While Taking This Drug:** (at doctor's discretion)

Measurement of internal eye pressure. Red blood cell counts and hemoglobin evaluation.

▷ **While Taking This Drug the Following Apply:**

Beverages: May be taken with milk.

Alcohol: Avoid alcohol completely in the presence of any side effects or adverse effects. Alcohol may exaggerate the blood pressure–lowering effect of this drug.

Tobacco Smoking: Nicotine can reduce the effectiveness of this drug. Avoid all forms of tobacco.

Marijuana Smoking: Possible reduced effectiveness of this drug; mild to moderate increase in angina; possible changes in electrocardiogram, confusing interpretation.

Other Drugs:

Isosorbide dinitrate *taken concurrently* with

- antihypertensive drugs may cause excessive lowering of blood pressure; dosage adjustments may be necessary.
- hydralazine (Apresoline) may work well in helping control angina.
- propranolol (Inderal) can help improve exercise time without angina.

Driving, Hazardous Activities: Usually no restrictions. This drug may cause dizziness or spells of low blood pressure. Restrict your activities as necessary.

Exposure to Heat: Use caution. Hot environments can cause a significant drop in blood pressure.

Exposure to Cold: Cold environments can increase the need for this drug and limit its effectiveness.

Heavy Exercise or Exertion: This drug may allow you to be more active without anginal pain. Use caution and avoid excessive exertion.

Discontinuation: Withdraw this drug gradually after long-term use; reduce dosage and frequency of prolonged-action dosage forms gradually over a period of 4 to 6 weeks.

▷ **Saving Money When Using This Medicine:**

- Many medications are available to treat anginal pain. Ask your doctor if this drug provides the best combination of cost and outcome for you.
- Ask your doctor how long this drug is usually taken to treat your condition.
- Acceptable generic forms of this drug are available.
- Talk with your doctor about the use of aspirin every other day in order to help prevent a heart attack.

ISOSORBIDE MONONITRATE
(i soh SOHR bide mon oh NI trayt)

Prescription Needed: Yes   **Controlled Drug:** No   **Generic:** No

Brand Names: Elantan, Imdur, Ismo, Monoket

Overview of BENEFITS versus RISKS

Possible Benefits	*Possible Risks*
EFFECTIVE PREVENTION OF ANGINA	Orthostatic hypotension Headache

---

▷ **Illness This Medication Treats:**
The frequency and severity of recurrent angina; not effective in relieving acute episodes of anginal pain.

▷ **Typical Dosage Range:** (Dosage or schedule must be determined by the doctor for each individual.)
Infants and Children: Dosage not established.
12 to 60 Years of Age: 20 mg (one tablet), taken twice daily: take the first tablet on arising; take the second tablet 7 hours later. Do not take additional doses during the balance of the day. The total daily dosage should not exceed 40 mg.
Over 60 Years of Age: Same as for 12 to 60 years of age.

▷ **Conditions Requiring Dosing Adjustments:**
Liver function: This drug should be used with caution by patients with liver compromise; however, no specific guidelines for dosage reduction are available.
Kidney function: No dosing changes are recommended for patients with renal compromise. Isosorbide mononitrate may turn the urine brown to black in color.

▷ **How Best to Take This Medicine:**   This drug should preferably be taken on an empty stomach to achieve maximal blood levels. The tablet may be crushed for administration.

▷ **How Long This Medicine Is Usually Taken:**   Use on a regular schedule for 3 to 7 days is usually necessary to determine this drug's effectiveness in preventing episodes of acute anginal pain. Long-term use (months to years) requires your doctor's supervision.

▷ **Tell Your Doctor Before Taking This Medicine If You:**
• ever had an allergic reaction to it.
• have had a very recent heart attack (myocardial infarction).
• currently have congestive heart failure.
• had an unfavorable response to other nitrate drugs or vasodilators in the past.

- have severe anemia or an overactive thyroid.
- have a history of low blood pressure.
- have any form of glaucoma.

▷ **Possible Side Effects:** Flushing of face, throbbing in head, palpitation, rapid heart rate, orthostatic hypotension. Excessive lowering of blood pressure.

▷ **Possible Adverse Effects:**
If any of the following develop, call your doctor promptly for guidance.
Some Mild Problems Drug Can Cause
   Allergic reactions: skin rash, itching.
   Headache, dizziness, fainting.
   Nausea, vomiting. Bad breath.
Some Serious Problems Drug Can Cause
   Transient ischemic attacks (TIAs) in presence of impaired circulation within the brain: dizziness, fainting, impaired vision or speech, localized numbness or weakness.
   Bone marrow depression.
   Anemia (in those with G6PD deficiency)
   Rare abnormal heartbeat.

▷ **Possible Effects on Sex Life:** Impotence.

▷ *CAUTION*
   1. Adhere strictly to the dosage schedule outlined above. If headaches are frequent or troublesome, tell your doctor. Aspirin or acetaminophen may be taken to relieve them.
   2. Many over-the-counter (OTC) medications for allergies, colds, and coughs contain drugs that may counteract the desired effects of this drug. Ask your doctor or pharmacist for guidance before using such medications.
   3. People over 60 should take small doses until tolerance has been determined. They may be more susceptible to low blood pressure and associated blackout spells, fainting, and falling. Throbbing headaches and flushing may be more apparent.

Advisability of Use During Pregnancy and If Breast-Feeding:
Pregnancy Category: B for Imdur, C for Ismo. Use this drug only if clearly needed. Ask your doctor for guidance. Presence in breast milk is unknown. If this drug is thought to be necessary, monitor the nursing infant for low blood pressure and poor feeding.

▷ **Overdose Symptoms:** Headache, dizziness, marked flushing of face and skin, vomiting, weakness, fainting, difficult breathing, coma.

▷ **Suggested Periodic Examinations While Taking This Drug:** (at doctor's discretion)
Measurement of internal eye pressure.

▷ **While Taking This Drug the Following Apply:**

Beverages: May be taken with milk.

Alcohol: Avoid alcohol completely in the presence of any side effects or adverse effects of this drug. Alcohol may exaggerate the drug's blood pressure–lowering effect.

Tobacco Smoking: Nicotine can reduce the effectiveness of this drug. Avoid all forms of tobacco.

Marijuana Smoking: May cause reduced effectiveness of this drug; mild to moderate increase in angina; possible changes in electrocardiogram, confusing interpretation.

Other Drugs:

Isosorbide mononitrate **taken concurrently** with

- antihypertensives may cause excessive lowering of blood pressure; dosage adjustments may be necessary.
- calcium channel blockers (see Drug Classes) may cause marked orthostatic hypotension.
- hydralazine (Apresoline) may help control angina.
- propranolol (Inderal) can help improve exercise time without angina.

Driving, Hazardous Activities: Usually no restrictions. This drug may cause dizziness or spells of low blood pressure. Restrict your activities as necessary.

Exposure to Heat: Use caution. Hot environments can cause significant drops in blood pressure.

Exposure to Cold: Cold environments can increase the need for this drug and limit its effectiveness.

Heavy Exercise or Exertion: This drug may allow you to be more active without anginal pain. Use caution and avoid excessive exertion.

Discontinuation: It is advisable to withdraw this drug gradually (2 to 4 weeks) after long-term use.

▷ **Saving Money When Using This Medicine:**

- Many medications are available to treat anginal pain. Ask your doctor if this drug provides the best combination of cost and outcomes for you.
- Talk with your doctor about the benefits versus risks of taking aspirin every other day in order to prevent a heart attack. Also ask about taking an additional aspirin should symptoms of a heart attack begin.

ISOTRETINOIN (i soh TRET i noin)

Prescription Needed: Yes   **Controlled Drug:** No   **Generic:** No

Brand Name: Accutane

Overview of BENEFITS versus RISKS

Possible Benefits	*Possible Risks*
EFFECTIVE TREATMENT OF SEVERE CYSTIC ACNE	MAJOR BIRTH DEFECTS
	Initial worsening of acne (transient)
	Inflammation of lips
	Dry skin, nose, and mouth
	Musculoskeletal discomfort
	Corneal opacities (rare)

▷ **Illness This Medication Treats:**

Severe, disfiguring nodular and cystic acne that has failed to respond to all other forms of standard therapy. *It should not be used to treat mild forms of acne.* It is also used to treat some less common conditions of the skin due to keratin production disorders.

▷ **Typical Dosage Range:** (Dosage or schedule must be determined by the doctor for each individual.)

Initial dosage is individualized according to the patient's weight and the severity of the acne; the usual dose is 0.5 to 2 mg per kilogram of body weight daily, taken in two divided doses for 15 to 20 weeks. After weeks of treatment, the dose should be adjusted according to the response and the development of adverse effects.

▷ **Conditions Requiring Dosing Adjustments:**

Liver function: The dose should be empirically decreased when used by patients with compromised livers.

Kidney function: The drug is eliminated via the urine and feces. Patients with renal compromise should use this drug with caution.

▷ **How Best to Take This Medicine:** Begin treatment only on the second or third day of your next normal menstrual period. Take with meals (morning and evening) to achieve optimal blood levels. The capsule should not be opened for administration.

▷ **How Long This Medicine Is Usually Taken:** Use on a regular schedule for 15 to 20 weeks usually determines the effectiveness of this drug in clearing or improving severe cystic acne. This drug may be discontinued earlier if the total cyst count is reduced by more than 70%. If a repeat course is necessary, it should not be started until 2 months after discontinuing this drug. Long-term use (months to years) requires supervision and periodic evaluation by your doctor.

▷ **Tell Your Doctor Before Taking This Medicine If You:**
- ever had an allergic reaction to it or are allergic to parabens (the additives used to preserve the drug.)
- are pregnant or planning pregnancy.
- ever had an allergic reaction to any form of vitamin A.
- are considering donating blood (you will NOT be eligible for 1 month after the last isotretinoin dose).
- have diabetes mellitus.
- have a cholesterol or triglyceride disorder.
- have a history of liver or kidney disease.

▷ **Possible Side Effects:**   Dryness of the nose and mouth, inflammation of the lips, dryness of the skin with itching, peeling of the palms and soles.

▷ **Possible Adverse Effects:**
If any of the following develop, call your doctor promptly for guidance.
Some Mild Problems Drug Can Cause
   Allergic reaction: skin rash.
   Thinning of hair, conjunctivitis, intolerance of contact lenses, decreased night vision, muscular and joint aches, headache, fatigue, indigestion.
Some Serious Problems Drug Can Cause
   Skin infections, worsening of arthritis, inflammatory bowel disorders.
   Abnormal acceleration of bone development in children.
   Development of opacities in the cornea.
   Reduced red and white blood cell counts; increased platelet count.
   Increased pressure in the head with associated headache, visual disturbances, nausea, and vomiting. Seizures.
   Drug-induced hepatitis.
   Rare kidney toxicity, pancreatitis, or hepatitis.

▷ **Possible Effects on Sex Life:**   Decreased male and female libido, beginning after 1 month.
   Impotence, beginning after 3 months of use.
   Decreased vaginal secretions.
   Altered timing and pattern of menstruation.
   Female breast discharge.

▷ *CAUTION*
   1. This drug should not be used to treat mild forms of acne.
   2. A transient worsening of your acne may occur during the first few weeks of treatment; this subsides with continued use of this drug.
   3. Do not take any other form of vitamin A with this drug. (Check the contents of multiple vitamin preparations.)
   4. Women with the potential for pregnancy should have a *blood* pregnancy test within 2 weeks before taking this drug and should

use two effective forms of contraception simultaneously during its use. It is recommended that contraception be continued until normal menstruation resumes after this drug is discontinued.

5. This drug may cause increased blood levels of cholesterol and tri-glycerides.

6. If repeated courses of this drug are prescribed, wait a minimum of 2 months between courses before resuming medication.

7. In children, long-term use (6 to 12 months) may cause abnormal acceleration of bone growth and development. Your doctor can monitor this possibility by periodic X-ray examination of long bones.

Advisability of Use During Pregnancy and If Breast-Feeding:
Pregnancy Category: X. Avoid using this drug completely during entire pregnancy. Presence in breast milk is unknown; avoid using this drug or refrain from nursing.

▷ **Overdose Symptoms:**   No experience with overdosage in humans to date.

▷ **Suggested Periodic Examinations While Taking This Drug:** (at doctor's discretion)
Complete blood cell counts, including platelet counts.
Measurements of blood cholesterol and triglyceride levels.
Complete eye examinations.
Liver and kidney function tests.

▷ **While Taking This Drug the Following Apply:**
Other Drugs:
Isotretinoin *taken concurrently* with
• carbamazepine (Tegretol) may blunt carbamazepine's therapeutic benefits and require dosing changes.
• minocycline may increase risk of severe headache, visual changes, or papilledema.
• tetracyclines (see Drug Classes) may increase risk of pseudotumor cerebri.
Exposure to Sun: This drug can cause photosensitivity. Avoid excessive exposure to the sun until your sensitivity is determined.

▷ **Saving Money When Using This Medicine:**
• Many medications are available to treat acne. Ask your doctor if this drug provides the best combination of cost and outcome for you. Ask your doctor how long this drug is usually taken to treat your condition.
• Find out as much as possible about your condition. *The Essential Guide to Chronic Illness* is an excellent source of information.

ISRADIPINE (is RA di peen)

Prescription Needed: Yes   **Controlled Drug:** No   **Generic:** No

Brand Names: DynaCirc

Controversies in Medicine: Results of several studies have indicated that medicines in this chemical family should NOT be used in some patients with extremely compromised hearts. Amlodipine (Norvasc) is the only calcium channel blocker that presently has data to show that it is SAFE, even in the most severely ill congestive heart failure patients. Amlodipine is the only calcium channel blocker to be FDA-approved as safe for use in treating hypertension or angina in patients who also have congestive heart failure. There have been several FDA hearings on calcium channel blockers in general.

One retrospective chart review yielded data showing that there was increased risk if nifedipine immediate-release forms were used for treating conditions other than angina in those over 71. There was a caution advised, but the form of nifedipine in question was not approved for uses other than angina. A recent FDA panel found medicines in this class to be safe and effective. A study of nearly 6,000 patients at Tel Aviv Medical Center found that there was no statistically significant risk of death in patients who took calcium channel blockers versus those who did not take these medicines.

Overview of BENEFITS versus RISKS

Possible Benefits	*Possible Risks*
EFFECTIVE TREATMENT OF MILD TO MODERATE HYPERTENSION	Headache Dizziness Fluid retention Palpitations

---

▷ **Illness This Medication Treats:**
  Mild to moderate hypertension, alone or concurrently with thiazide-type diuretics.

▷ **Typical Dosage Range:** (Dosage or schedule must be determined by the doctor for each individual.)
  Initially 2.5 mg two times daily, 12 hours apart, for a trial period of 2 to 4 weeks. If necessary, the dose may be increased by 5 mg/day at intervals of 2 to 4 weeks. The usual maintenance dose is 5 to 10 mg daily. The total daily dosage should not exceed 20 mg.

▷ **Conditions Requiring Dosing Adjustments:**
  Liver function: No specific guidelines for dosage reduction are available, yet empirical decreases in dosing are prudent for patients with compromised livers.

Kidney function: Patients with kidney compromise should use this drug with caution.

▷ **How Best to Take This Medicine:** May be taken with or following food to reduce stomach irritation. The capsule may be opened for administration; mix the contents with food and swallow promptly.

▷ **How Long This Medicine Is Usually Taken:** Continual use on a regular schedule for 2 to 4 weeks is usually necessary to determine this drug's effectiveness. The smallest effective dose should be used in long-term treatment (months to years). Physician supervision and periodic evaluation are essential.

▷ **Tell Your Doctor Before Taking This Medicine If You:**
- ever had an allergic reaction to it.
- had an unfavorable response to any calcium blocker in the past.
- are currently taking any beta-blocker.
- are taking any drugs that lower blood pressure.
- have a history of congestive heart failure, heart attack, narrowing of the aorta, or stroke.
- have muscular dystrophy or myasthenia gravis.
- are subject to disturbances of heart rhythm.
- have impaired liver or kidney function.
- plan to have surgery under general anesthesia soon.

▷ **Possible Side Effects:** Rapid heart rate, swelling of the feet and ankles, flushing and sensation of warmth. Abnormal growth of gums (gingival hyperplasia).

▷ **Possible Adverse Effects:**
If any of the following develop, call your doctor promptly for guidance.
Some Mild Problems Drug Can Cause
   Allergic reactions: skin rash, itching.
   Headache, dizziness, weakness, nervousness, blurred vision.
   Palpitation, shortness of breath.
   Nausea, vomiting, constipation.
   Cramps in legs and feet.
Some Serious Problems Drug Can Cause
   Rare heart rhythm disturbances.
   Increased frequency or severity of angina on initiation of treatment or following an increase in dose.
   Marked drop in blood pressure with fainting.
   Very rare lowering of white blood cell counts.

▷ **Possible Effects on Sex Life:** Decreased libido, impotence.

▷ *CAUTION*
  1. If you are monitoring your own blood pressure, make your measurements just before each dose and 2 to 3 hours after each dose

to obtain an accurate picture of this drug's effect. This will detect excessive fluctuations between high and low readings.

2. Be sure to tell all doctors and dentists that you are taking this drug. Note its use on your personal identification card.

3. You may use nitroglycerin and other nitrate drugs as needed to relieve acute episodes of angina pain. However, if your angina attacks are becoming more frequent or intense, notify your doctor promptly.

4. Safety and effectiveness of this drug for those under 18 years old are not established.

5. People over 60 should watch for development of weakness, dizziness, fainting, and falling. Take necessary precautions to prevent injury.

Advisability of Use During Pregnancy and If Breast-Feeding:

Pregnancy Category: C. Avoid using this drug during the first 3 months. Use during the last 6 months only if clearly needed. Ask your doctor for guidance. Presence in breast milk is unknown; avoid taking this drug or refrain from nursing.

▷ **Overdose Symptoms:** Weakness, light-headedness, fainting, fast pulse, low blood pressure, shortness of breath, flushed and warm skin, tremors.

▷ **Suggested Periodic Examinations While Taking This Drug:** (at doctor's discretion)

Evaluations of heart function, including electrocardiograms; measurements of blood pressure in supine, sitting, and standing positions.

▷ **While Taking This Drug the Following Apply:**

Foods: Avoid excessive salt intake.

Beverages: May be taken with milk.

Alcohol: Alcohol may exaggerate the drop in blood pressure some people experience.

Tobacco Smoking: Nicotine may reduce this drug's effectiveness.

Marijuana Smoking: Possible reduced effectiveness of this drug; mild to moderate increase in angina; possible changes in electrocardiogram, confusing interpretation.

Other Drugs:

Isradipine **taken concurrently** with

- beta-blockers or digitalis preparations may affect heart rate and rhythm adversely. Careful monitoring by your doctor is necessary if these drugs are taken concurrently.
- carbamazepine (Tegretol) has resulted in decreased carbamazepine blood levels with other calcium channel blockers. Increased checking of blood levels is advised.
- digoxin (Lanoxin, others) may lead to an increased blood level.

- magnesium, especially in higher doses, may lead to abnormally low blood pressure.
- phenytoin (Dilantin) may result in loss of isradipine's effectiveness.
- rifampin (Rifadin, others) may blunt the benefits of isradipine.

Driving, Hazardous Activities: Usually no restrictions. This drug may cause drowsiness or dizziness. Restrict your activities as necessary.

Exposure to Heat: Caution is advised. Hot environments can exaggerate the blood pressure–lowering effects of this drug. Observe for light-headedness or weakness.

Heavy Exercise or Exertion: This drug may allow you to be more active without resulting angina pain. Use caution and avoid excessive exercise that could impair heart function in the absence of warning pain.

Discontinuation: Do not discontinue this drug abruptly. Consult your doctor regarding gradual withdrawal. Observe for the possible development of rebound angina.

▷ **Saving Money When Using This Medicine:**

- Therapy of hypertension often combines medications from several drug classes. Ask your doctor if this drug provides the best combination of cost and outcome for you.
- Ask your doctor how long this drug is usually taken to treat your condition, and how often he or she would like you to get your blood pressure checked.
- Talk with your doctor about the benefits versus risks of taking aspirin every other day in order to prevent a heart attack.
- Ask your doctor about the benefits of stress management and exercise programs in your community.
- Read more about your condition. *The Essential Guide to Chronic Illness* is an excellent source of information.

KETOCONAZOLE   (kee toh KOHN a zohl)

Prescription: Yes   **Controlled Drug:** No   **Generic:** No
Brand Names: Nizoral

Overview of BENEFITS versus RISKS

Possible Benefits	*Possible Risks*
EFFECTIVE TREATMENT OF THE FOLLOWING FUNGUS INFECTIONS: blastomycosis, candidiasis, chromomycosis, coccidioidomycosis, histoplasmosis, paracoccidioidomycosis, tinea (ringworm)	RARE SERIOUS DRUG-INDUCED LIVER DAMAGE
	Rare but serious allergic reactions
	Rare low blood platelets or anemia
Beneficial treatment of advanced prostate cancer	
Beneficial auxiliary treatment of Cushing's syndrome	

▷ **Illness This Medication Treats:**

(1) Lung and systemic blastomycosis; (2) *Candida* (yeast) infections of the skin, mouth, throat, and esophagus (may be AIDS-related); (3) systemic *Candida* infections—pneumonia, peritonitis, urinary tract infections (may be AIDS-related); (4) auxiliary treatment of chromomycosis; (5) lung and systemic coccidioidomycosis; (6) lung and systemic histoplasmosis; (7) paracoccidioidomycosis; (8) treatment of tinea infections of the body, groin (jock itch), and feet (athlete's foot).

▷ **Typical Dosage Range:** (Dosage or schedule must be determined by the doctor for each individual.)

Infants and Children: Up to 2 years old: Dosage not established.

Over 2 years old: 3.3 to 10 mg per kilogram of body weight, once daily; the dosage depends on the nature of the infection.

12 to 60 Years of Age: For fungus infections: 200 to 400 mg once daily; total daily dosage should not exceed 1 g (1000 mg).

For prostate cancer: 400 mg three times daily; total daily dosage should not exceed 1200 mg.

For Cushing's syndrome: 600 to 1200 mg once daily; total daily dosage should not exceed 1200 mg.

Over 60 Years of Age: Same as for 12 to 60 years. Dosage adjustment for patients with reduced kidney function is not necessary.

▷ **Conditions Requiring Dosing Adjustments:**

Liver function: No specific guidelines for dosage decreases are available; however, the dose should be empirically decreased in patients with liver compromise.

Achlorhydria: This medicine requires an acid environment to get into your body. Talk with your doctor if your stomach acid is low.

▷ **How Best to Take This Medicine:** Preferably taken with or after food to enhance absorption and reduce stomach irritation. Do not take with antacids. The tablet may be crushed. Take the full course prescribed.

▷ **How Long This Medicine Is Usually Taken:** Use on a regular schedule for 2 to 4 weeks usually determines the effectiveness of this drug in controlling fungal infections. Actual cures or long-term suppression often require continual treatment for many months. Periodic physician evaluation of response is essential.

▷ **Tell Your Doctor Before Taking This Medicine If You:**
- ever had an allergic reaction to it.
- have active liver disease.
- are allergic to related antifungal drugs: clotrimazole, fluconazole, itraconazole, miconazole.
- have a history of liver disease or impaired liver function.
- are taking a nonsedating antihistamine.
- have a history of low blood platelets or anemia.
- have a history of alcoholism.
- have a deficiency of stomach hydrochloric acid.
- are currently taking any other drugs.

▷ **Possible Side Effects:** Suppression of testosterone and adrenal corticosteroid hormone production (more pronounced with high drug doses). Ringing in the ears. Hair loss.

▷ **Possible Adverse Effects:**
If any of the following develop, call your doctor promptly for guidance.
Some Mild Problems Drug Can Cause
Allergic reactions: skin rash, itching.
Headache, dizziness, drowsiness, photophobia.
Nausea and vomiting, diarrhea.
Some Serious Problems Drug Can Cause
Allergic reactions: anaphylactic reaction.
Severe liver toxicity (very rare): loss of appetite, fatigue, yellow skin and eyes, light-colored stools.
Rare mental depression.
Abnormally low blood platelet counts: abnormal bruising or bleeding.
Rare low thyroid gland function or suppression of the adrenal gland.

▷ **Possible Effects on Sex Life:**   Decreased testosterone blood levels: reduced sperm counts, decreased libido, impotence, male breast enlargement and tenderness.
Altered menstrual patterns.

▷ **Possible Delayed Adverse Effects:**   Deficiency of adrenal corticosteroid hormones (cortisone-related); this could be serious during stress resulting from illness or injury.

▷ *CAUTION*
   1. Safety and effectiveness for those under 2 years old are not established.
   2. Call your doctor immediately if you start to develop yellow eyes or skin or dark urine with light-colored stools.
   3. No information is available for use by people over 60. It is advisable to avoid high doses.
   Advisability of Use During Pregnancy and If Breast-Feeding:
   Pregnancy Category: C. Use this drug only if clearly needed. Ask your doctor for guidance. Present in breast milk; avoid drug or refrain from nursing.

▷ **Overdose Symptoms:**   Possible nausea, vomiting, diarrhea.

▷ **Suggested Periodic Examinations While Taking This Drug:** (at doctor's discretion)
Liver function tests should be performed before long-term treatment is started and monthly during treatment.
Sperm counts.

▷ **While Taking This Drug the Following Apply:**
Beverages: May be taken with milk.
Alcohol: Avoid completely. Alcohol can cause a disulfiramlike reaction. Alcohol may also cause liver toxicity.
Other Drugs:
Ketoconazole may *increase* the effects of
• nonsedating antihistamines such as astemizole (Hismanal) and terfenadine (Seldane), causing serious heart rhythm problems. DO NOT COMBINE.
• cortisonelike drugs (prednisone, etc.).
• cyclosporine (Sandimmune).
• loratadine (Claritin) is also a nonsedating antihistamine, but HAS NOT been associated with serious heart problems when combined with ketoconazole. Since loratadine blood levels do increase if it is taken with ketoconazole, it is prudent to decrease the loratadine dose if the medicines are to be combined.
• quinidine (Quinaglute, others) may lead to quinidine toxicity.
• sucralfate (Carafate) may blunt the therapeutic benefits of ketoconazole.

- warfarin (Coumadin), causing unwanted bleeding; monitor prothrombin times as necessary.

Ketoconazole may **decrease** the effects of

- theophyllines (aminophylline, Theo-Dur, etc.).
- didanosine (Videx).

The following drugs may **decrease** the effects of ketoconazole

- antacids; if needed, take antacids 2 hours after ketoconazole.
- histamine (H2) blocking drugs: cimetidine, famotidine, nizatidine, ranitidine; if needed, take 2 hours after ketoconazole.
- isoniazid (Laniazid, Nydrazid, etc.).
- rifampin (Rifadin, Rimactane, etc.).

Ketoconazole **taken concurrently** with

- cisapride (Propulsid) may result in altered blood levels.
- miconazole (Monistat) may increase blood levels of either drug.
- phenytoin (Dilantin) may change blood levels of both medicines.

Driving, Hazardous Activities: May cause dizziness or drowsiness. Restrict your activities as necessary.

Exposure to Sun: May cause photophobia; wear sunglasses if appropriate.

Discontinuation: Take the full course prescribed. Continual treatment for several months may be necessary. Ask your doctor about the appropriate time to consider discontinuation.

▷ **Saving Money When Using This Medicine:**

- Many medications are available for fungal infections. Ask your doctor if this drug provides the best combination of cost and outcome for you.
- If your condition does not improve or becomes systemic, talk with your doctor about lipid-associated antifungals such as Abelcet.

KETOPROFEN (kee toh PROH fen)

Prescription: Yes   **Controlled Drug:** No   **Generic:** No

Brand Names: Actron (nonprescription form), Orudis, Orudis SR, Oruvail ER

Overview of BENEFITS versus RISKS	
Possible Benefits	*Possible Risks*
EFFECTIVE RELIEF OF MILD TO MODERATE PAIN AND INFLAMMATION	Gastrointestinal pain, ulceration, bleeding (rare)
	Liver or kidney damage (rare)
	Fluid retention (rare)
	Bone marrow depression (rare)

See the propionic acids (NSAIDs) drug profile for further information.

LABETALOL   (la BET a lohl)

Prescription: Yes   **Controlled Drug:** No   **Generic:** No

Brand Names: Normodyne, Normozide [CD], Trandate, Trandate HCT [CD]

```
┌──────────────────────────────────────────────────────────┐
│            Overview of BENEFITS versus RISKS               │
│    Possible Benefits            Possible Risks             │
│  EFFECTIVE,                 CONGESTIVE HEART               │
│    WELL-TOLERATED             FAILURE in advanced heart    │
│    ANTIHYPERTENSIVE in        disease                      │
│    mild to moderate high blood   Worsening of angina in    │
│    pressure                   coronary heart disease (if   │
│  PROLONGS LIFE AFTER          drug is abruptly withdrawn)  │
│    HEART ATTACKS            Masking of low blood sugar in  │
│                               drug-treated diabetes        │
│                            Liver toxicity                  │
└──────────────────────────────────────────────────────────┘
```

▷ **Illness This Medication Treats:**

(1) Mild to moderate high blood pressure; used alone or concurrently with other antihypertensive drugs, such as diuretics; (2) therapy of hypertension and angina; (3) when used after heart attacks as part of combination therapy, beta-blockers have been shown to decrease the risk of repeat heart attacks, limit the size of the initial heart attack, and help control arrhythmia.

▷ **Typical Dosage Range:** (Dosage or schedule must be determined by the doctor for each individual.)

Initially 100 mg twice daily, 12 hours apart; the dose may be increased by 100 mg twice daily every 2 to 3 days as required to reduce blood pressure. The usual maintenance dose is 200 to 400 mg twice daily. The total dose should not exceed 2400 mg/24 hr, taken as 800 mg three times daily.

▷ **Conditions Requiring Dosing Adjustments:**

Liver function: Patients with liver compromise should use this drug with caution, and decrease the usual dose. It is a rare cause of severe liver damage.

Kidney function: Dosing changes are not thought to be required for any degree of renal compromise. Patients with urine outflow problems should use this drug with caution.

▷ **How Best to Take This Medicine:** Take at the same times each day, preferably following the morning and evening meals. The tablet may be crushed for administration. Do not discontinue abruptly.

▷ **How Long This Medicine Is Usually Taken:** Use on a regular schedule for 10 to 14 days usually determines the effectiveness of this drug in lowering blood pressure. The long-term use (months to years) is determined by the course of your blood pressure over time and your response to the overall treatment program (weight reduction, salt restriction, smoking cessation, etc.). See your doctor regularly.

▷ **Tell Your Doctor Before Taking This Medicine If You:**
- ever had an allergic reaction to it.
- have active bronchial asthma.
- have congestive heart failure.
- have an abnormally slow heart rate or a serious form of heart block.
- had an adverse reaction to any beta-blocker drug in the past.
- have a history of serious heart disease, with or without episodes of heart failure.
- have a history of hay fever (allergic rhinitis), asthma, chronic bronchitis, or emphysema.
- have a history of overactive thyroid function.
- have a history of low blood sugar.
- have impaired liver or kidney function.
- have diabetes or myasthenia gravis.
- are currently taking any form of digitalis, quinidine, or reserpine, or any calcium blocker.
- have intermittent claudication.
- plan to have surgery under general anesthesia soon.

▷ **Possible Side Effects:** Lethargy and fatigability, light-headedness in upright position.

▷ **Possible Adverse Effects:**
If any of the following develop, call your doctor promptly for guidance.
Some Mild Problems Drug Can Cause
    Allergic reactions: skin rash, itching.
    Headache, drowsiness, dizziness, scalp tingling (during early treatment)
    Vivid dreams, nightmares, or depression.
    Nausea, diarrhea.
    Joint and muscle discomfort, fluid retention (edema).
Some Serious Problems Drug Can Cause
    Chest pain, shortness of breath, precipitation of congestive heart failure.
    Muscle toxicity, worsening of intermittent claudication.
    Induction of bronchial asthma (in asthmatics).
    Aggravation of myasthenia gravis.
    Liver damage with jaundice (rare).
    Difficult urination (urinary bladder retention).

▷ **Possible Effects on Sex Life:** Impotence, inhibited ejaculation, prolonged erection following orgasm (with higher doses), Peyronie's disease.

Decreased vaginal secretions (with low doses), inhibited female orgasm (with higher doses).

▷ *CAUTION*

1. ***Do not stop taking this drug suddenly*** without the knowledge and guidance of your doctor. Carry an identification card that states you are taking this drug.

2. Ask your doctor or pharmacist before using nasal decongestants in over-the-counter cold preparations and nose drops. These can cause sudden increases in blood pressure when taken concurrently with beta-blockers.

3. Report any tendency to emotional depression.

4. Safety and effectiveness of this drug for those under 12 years old are not established. However, if this drug is used, watch for low blood sugar during periods of reduced food intake.

5. Therapy in people over 60 should proceed ***cautiously*** with all antihypertensives. Unacceptably high blood pressure should be reduced without creating the risks associated with excessively low blood pressure. Start treatment with small doses and monitor the blood pressure response frequently. Sudden, rapid, and excessive reduction of blood pressure can predispose to stroke or heart attack. Observe for dizziness, unsteadiness, tendency to fall, confusion, hallucinations, depression, or urinary frequency.

Advisability of Use During Pregnancy and If Breast-Feeding:

Pregnancy Category: C. Use this drug only if clearly needed. Ask your doctor for guidance. Present in breast milk in very small amounts; avoid using this drug or refrain from nursing.

▷ **Overdose Symptoms:** Weakness, slow pulse, low blood pressure, fainting, cold and sweaty skin, congestive heart failure, possible coma and convulsions.

▷ **Suggested Periodic Examinations While Taking This Drug:** (at doctor's discretion)

Measurements of blood pressure, evaluation of heart function.

▷ **While Taking This Drug the Following Apply:**

Foods: Avoid excessive salt intake.

Beverages: May be taken with milk.

Alcohol: Alcohol may exaggerate this drug's ability to lower blood pressure and increase its mild sedative effect.

Tobacco Smoking: Nicotine may reduce this drug's effectiveness in treating high blood pressure. In addition, high doses of this drug may potentiate the constriction of the bronchial tubes caused by regular smoking.

Other Drugs:

Labetalol may ***increase*** the effects of

- oral hypoglycemic agents and could prolong the recovery of any hypoglycemia that may occur.

- other antihypertensives causing excessive lowering of blood pressure. Dosage adjustments may be necessary.

Labetalol *taken concurrently* with

- amiodarone (Cordarone) may result in extremely low heart rates or cardiac arrest.
- cimetidine (Tagamet) may elevate labetalol blood levels and result in very low blood pressure or heart rate.
- clonidine (Catapres) requires close monitoring for rebound high blood pressure if clonidine is withdrawn while labetalol is still being taken.
- epinephrine may result in severe increases in blood pressure.
- fluvoxamine (Luvox) may lead to excessive slowing of the heart or very low blood pressure.
- imipramine and perhaps other tricyclic antidepressants (see Drug Classes) may result in antidepressant toxicity.
- insulin requires close monitoring to avoid undetected hypoglycemia.
- NSAIDs (see Drug Classes) may blunt the benefits of labetalol.
- phenothiazines (see Drug Classes) may cause additive lowering of blood pressure.
- ritodrine (Yutopar) may blunt beneficial effects of labetalol.

Driving, Hazardous Activities: Use caution until the full extent of fatigue, dizziness, and blood pressure change have been determined.

Exposure to Heat: Caution is advised. Hot environments can lower the blood pressure and exaggerate the effects of this drug.

Exposure to Cold: Caution is advised. Cold environments can enhance the circulatory deficiency in the extremities that may occur with some beta-blockers. The elderly should take precautions to prevent hypothermia.

Heavy Exercise or Exertion: Avoid exertion that produces lightheadedness, excessive fatigue, or muscle cramping. This drug may intensify the hypertensive response to isometric exercise.

Occurrence of Unrelated Illness: The fever that accompanies systemic infections can lower the blood pressure and require adjustment of dosage. Illnesses that cause nausea or vomiting may interrupt the regular dosage schedule. Ask your doctor for guidance.

Discontinuation: Avoid sudden discontinuation of this drug in all situations. Gradual reduction of dose over a period of 2 to 3 weeks is recommended. Ask your doctor for specific guidance if possible.

▷ **Saving Money When Using This Medicine:**

- Many medications are available to treat high blood pressure. Ask your doctor if this drug provides the best combination of cost and outcome for you. Ask your doctor how long this drug is usually taken to treat your condition.

- Ask your doctor about the benefits of taking aspirin every other day, as well as stress management or exercise programs in your community.

LEVODOPA (lee voh DOH pa)

Prescription: Yes   **Controlled Drug:** No   **Generic:** Yes

Brand Names: Bendopa, Dopar, Larodopa, Sinemet [CD], Sinemet CR [CD]

Overview of BENEFITS versus RISKS

Possible Benefits	*Possible Risks*
EFFECTIVE RELIEF OF SYMPTOMS IN IDIOPATHIC PARKINSON'S DISEASE	Emotional depression, confusion, abnormal thinking and behavior Abnormal involuntary movements Heart rhythm disturbance Urinary bladder retention Induction of peptic ulcer (rare) Rare blood cell abnormalities: hemolytic anemia, reduced white blood cell count

---

▷ **Illness This Medication Treats:**

Major types of Parkinson's disease: paralysis agitans ("shaking palsy" of unknown cause) following encephalitis, parkinsonism of aging, and forms following carbon monoxide or manganese poisoning.

As Combination Drug Product [CD]: In combination with carbidopa, a chemical that prevents the decomposition of levodopa before it reaches its site of action in the brain; reduces the amount of levodopa required by 75%. This combination is more effective in smaller doses and reduces the frequency and severity of adverse effects.

▷ **Typical Dosage Range:** (Dosage or schedule must be determined by the doctor for each individual.)

Initially 250 mg two to four times a day. The dose may be increased cautiously by increments of 100 to 750 mg at 3- to 7-day intervals as needed and tolerated. The total dosage should not exceed 8000 mg/24 hr; with the combination drug Sinemet the total levodopa requirement will be considerably less.

Levodopa naive: One 25/100 tablet three times daily. Increased as needed and tolerated to a maximum of eight tablets daily.

▷ **Conditions Requiring Dosing Adjustments:**

Kidney function: Dosage changes are not required. The drug can cause urine retention, and patients with urine outflow problems should be closely watched.

Intestinal parasites: A recent report of large increases in dose requirements in a patient with *Strongyloides stercoralis* has been filed.

▷ **How Best to Take This Medicine:** This drug should preferably be taken with or following carbohydrate foods to reduce stomach irritation; when possible, avoid taking concurrently with high-protein foods. The regular tablet may be crushed. The sustained-release tablet (Sinemet CR) may be cut in half, but should not be crushed or chewed.

▷ **How Long This Medicine Is Usually Taken:** Up to 3 to 6 weeks of regular use may be needed to realize this drug's effectiveness in relieving symptoms of parkinsonism. Determining maximal effectiveness may require continual use for 6 months. Long-term use (months to years) requires physician supervision.

▷ **Tell Your Doctor Before Taking This Medicine If You:**

- ever had an allergic reaction to it.
- have inadequately controlled narrow-angle glaucoma.
- are taking, or have taken within the past 14 days, any MAO type A inhibitor.
- have diabetes, epilepsy, heart disease, high blood pressure, or chronic lung disease.
- have impaired liver or kidney function.
- have a history of peptic ulcer disease or malignant melanoma.
- plan to have surgery under general anesthesia soon.

▷ **Possible Side Effects:** Fatigue, lethargy, altered taste, offensive body odor, orthostatic hypotension.

Pink to red coloration of urine, turning black on exposure to air (of no significance).

▷ **Possible Adverse Effects:**

If any of the following develop, call your doctor promptly for guidance.

Some Mild Problems Drug Can Cause

Allergic reactions: skin rash, itching.

Headache, dizziness, numbness, insomnia, nightmares, blurred vision, double vision.

Loss of appetite, nausea, vomiting, dry mouth, difficult swallowing, excessive gas, diarrhea, constipation.

Loss of hair (rare).

Some Serious Problems Drug Can Cause

Idiosyncratic reactions: hemolytic anemia; neuroleptic malignant syndrome.

Confusion, delusions, hallucinations, agitation, paranoia, depression, psychotic episodes, seizures.

Congestive heart failure.

Abnormal involuntary movements of the head, face, and extremities.

Disturbances of heart rhythm, high blood pressure (rare).

Peptic ulcer, gastrointestinal bleeding.

Urinary bladder retention.

Abnormally low white blood cell count—lowered resistance to infection, fever, sore throat.

▷ **Possible Effects on Sex Life:** Increased libido reported by both males and females; inhibited ejaculation (rare); priapism. Postmenopausal bleeding.

▷ **Adverse Effects That May Mimic Natural Diseases or Disorders:** Mental reactions may resemble idiopathic psychosis.

▷ *CAUTION*

1. To reduce the high frequency of serious adverse effects, begin treatment with small doses, and increase dosage gradually until the desired response is achieved.

2. As improvement occurs, avoid excessive and hurried activity (which often causes falls and injury).

3. This drug can cause precocious puberty in prepubertal boys. Observe closely for hypersexual behavior and premature growth of the genital organs.

4. For people over 60, treatment should begin with half the usual adult dose; dosage should be increased cautiously, in small increments as needed and tolerated. Observe for possible significant behavioral changes: depression or inappropriate elation, acute confusion, agitation, paranoia, dementia, nightmares, and hallucinations. Abnormal involuntary movements may also occur.

Advisability of Use During Pregnancy and If Breast-Feeding:
Pregnancy Category: C. Avoid using this drug during the first 3 months. Use only if clearly needed during the last 6 months. Present in breast milk; avoid using this drug or refrain from nursing.

▷ **Overdose Symptoms:** Muscle twitching, spastic closure of eyelids, nausea, vomiting, diarrhea, weakness, fainting, confusion, agitation, hallucinations.

▷ **Suggested Periodic Examinations While Taking This Drug:** (at doctor's discretion)
Complete blood cell counts; measurements of internal eye pressure; blood pressure measurements in lying, sitting, and standing positions.

▷ **While Taking This Drug the Following Apply:**

Foods: Insofar as possible, do not take concurrently with protein foods; proteins compete with this drug for absorption.

Nutritional Support: If levodopa is taken alone (without carbidopa), monitor for peripheral neuritis and take small supplements of pyridoxine (vitamin B6) if needed: 10 mg or less (larger doses can decrease the effectiveness of levodopa). When levodopa is combined with carbidopa (Sinemet), supplemental pyridoxine is not required.

Beverages: May be taken with milk.

Marijuana Smoking: Increased fatigue and lethargy; possible accentuation of orthostatic hypotension.

Other Drugs:

Levodopa *taken concurrently* with

- MAO type A inhibitors may cause a dangerous rise in blood pressure and body temperature; do not use concurrently.
- phenothiazines (see Drug Classes) may blunt the therapeutic benefits of levodopa.
- reserpine (Naquival, others) may blunt levodopa's therapeutic effects.
- risperidone (Risperdal) may blunt levodopa's therapeutic effects.
- tricyclic antidepressants (see Drug Classes) may decrease levodopa absorption and blunt the therapeutic effects of levodopa.

The following drugs may *decrease* the effects of levodopa

- benzodiazepines (see Drug Classes); may blunt the therapeutic effect of levodopa.
- bromocriptine (Parlodel); may blunt the therapeutic effect of bromocriptine.
- clonidine (Catapres); may blunt the therapeutic effect of levodopa.
- fentanyl/droperidol (Innovar); can cause muscular rigidity.
- iron salts.
- isoniazid (INH); may cause flushing, worsening of Parkinson's symptoms, and increased blood pressure. DO NOT combine.
- monoamine oxidase (MAO) type A inhibitors (see Drug Class); can lead to a dangerous increase in blood pressure and body temperature. DO NOT combine.
- papaverine (Cerespan, Pavabid, Vasospan, etc.).
- phenytoin (Dilantin, etc.).
- pyridoxine (vitamin B6).

Driving, Hazardous Activities: May cause dizziness, impaired vision, and orthostatic hypotension. Restrict your activities as necessary.

Exposure to Heat: Use caution. This drug can cause flushing and excessive sweating and predispose to heat exhaustion.

Occurrence of Unrelated Illness: Suspicious dark-colored skin lesions should be evaluated carefully to rule out the possibility of malignant melanoma. During the course of any intercurrent infection, monitor the white blood cell count carefully for normal response.

▷ **Saving Money When Using This Medicine:**
- Many medications are available to treat Parkinson's disease. Ask your doctor if this drug provides the best combination of cost and outcomes for you. A generic form is available.

LEVOTHYROXINE (lee voh thi ROX een)

Other Names: L-thyroxine, thyroxine, T4

Prescription: Yes   **Controlled Drug:** No   **Generic:** Yes

Brand Names: Armour Thyroid, Euthroid [CD], Levothroid, Levoxine, Synthroid, Thyroid USP, Thyrolar [CD]

Overview of BENEFITS versus RISKS	
Possible Benefits	*Possible Risks*
EFFECTIVE REPLACEMENT THERAPY WITH THYROID HORMONE DEFICIENCY	Intensification of angina in presence of coronary artery disease
EFFECTIVE TREATMENT OF SIMPLE GOITER AND CHRONIC THYROIDITIS	Drug-induced hyperthyroidism (with excessive dosage)
EFFECTIVE TREATMENT OF THYROID GLAND CANCER	Rare spasm of coronary vessels

▷ **Illness This Medication Treats:**
(1) Replacement therapy to correct thyroid deficiency; (2) treats simple (nonendemic) goiter and benign thyroid nodules; (3) treatment of Hashimoto's thyroiditis; (4) adjunctive prevention and treatment of thyroid cancer.

As Combination Drug Product [CD]: This hormone is available in combination with the other principal thyroid hormone, liothyronine, in a preparation (generic name: liotrix) that resembles the natural hormone.

▷ **Typical Dosage Range:** (Dosage or schedule must be determined by the doctor for each individual.)

Infants and Children: Up to 6 months: 8 to 10 mcg per kilogram of body weight, in a single daily dose.

6 to 12 months: 6 to 8 mcg per kilogram of body weight, in a single daily dose.

1 to 5 years: 5 to 6 mcg per kilogram of body weight, in a single daily dose.

6 to 10 years: 4 to 5 mcg per kilogram of body weight, in a single daily dose.

Over 10 years: 2 to 3 mcg per kilogram of body weight, in a single daily dose, until the usual adult daily dose is reached: 150 to 200 mcg.

12 to 60 Years of Age: Initially 0.05 mg as a single daily dose; increase by 0.025 to 0.05 mg at intervals of 2 to 3 weeks, as needed and tolerated. The usual maintenance dose is 0.075 to 0.125 mg per day. The total daily dosage should not exceed 0.3 mg.

Over 60 Years of Age: Initially 0.0125 to 0.025 mg as a single daily dose; increase gradually at intervals of 3 to 4 weeks, as needed and tolerated. The usual maintenance dose is approximately 0.075 mg daily.

▷ **How Best to Take This Medicine:** This drug should preferably be taken in the morning on an empty stomach to ensure maximal absorption and uniform results. The tablets may be crushed.

▷ **How Long This Medicine Is Usually Taken:** Use on a regular schedule for 4 to 6 weeks usually determines the effectiveness of this drug in correcting the symptoms of thyroid deficiency. Long-term use (months to years, possibly for life) requires physician supervision.

▷ **Tell Your Doctor Before Taking This Medicine If You:**
- ever had an allergic reaction to it.
- are recovering from a recent heart attack.
- are using it to lose weight and your thyroid function is normal.
- have high blood pressure, any form of heart disease, or diabetes.
- have a history of Addison's disease or adrenal gland deficiency.
- are taking any antiasthmatic medications.
- are taking an anticoagulant.

▷ **Possible Adverse Effects:**
If any of the following develop, call your doctor promptly for guidance.
Some Mild Problems Drug Can Cause
Allergic reactions: skin rash, hives.
Headache in sensitive individuals, even with proper dosage adjustment.
Some Serious Problems Drug Can Cause
Increased frequency or intensity of angina in the presence of coronary artery disease.
Rare porphyria, decreased IgA, or myasthenia gravis.
May be a risk factor for osteoporosis
Note: Other adverse effects are manifestations of excessive dosage.

▷ **Possible Effects on Sex Life:** Altered menstrual pattern during dosage adjustments.
Possibly beneficial in treating impaired sexual function associated with true hypothyroidism.

▷ *CAUTION*
1. The need for and response to thyroid hormone treatment varies greatly from person to person. Do not change your dosage schedule without consulting your doctor.

2. In the absence of verified thyroid deficiency, the use of this drug for nonspecific fatigue, obesity, infertility, or slow growth is inappropriate and could be harmful.

3. To facilitate normal growth and development, the thyroid-deficient child often requires higher dosage than the adult. A transient loss of hair may occur during the early months of treatment. Monitor the child's response to thyroid therapy by periodic measurements of bone age, growth, and mental and physical development.

4. People over 60 should use this drug with caution. Thyroid hormone replacement requirements for this population are usually about 25% lower than in younger adults. Observe closely for any indications that suggest overdosage.

Advisability of Use During Pregnancy and If Breast-Feeding:

Pregnancy Category: A. Use this drug only if clearly needed and with carefully adjusted dosage. Present in breast milk in minimal amounts. Breast-feeding is considered safe with correctly adjusted dosage.

▷ **Overdose Symptoms:**   Headache, sense of increased body heat, nervousness, increased sweating, hand tremors, insomnia, rapid and irregular heart action, diarrhea, muscle cramping, weight loss.

▷ **Suggested Periodic Examinations While Taking This Drug:** (at doctor's discretion)

Measurement of thyroid hormone levels in blood. DEXA testing to check bone mineral density and risk of osteoporosis.

▷ **While Taking This Drug the Following Apply:**

Other Drugs:

Levothyroxine may *increase* the effects of

- warfarin (Coumadin), increasing the risk of bleeding; reduction in anticoagulant dosage is usually necessary. Have INR (prothrombin time) checked more often.

Levothyroxine may *decrease* the effects of

- digoxin (Lanoxin) when correcting hypothyroidism; a larger dose of digoxin may be needed.

Levothyroxine *taken concurrently* with

- antacids may cause a decreased therapeutic benefit of levothyroxine.

- all antidiabetics (insulin and oral hypoglycemic agents—see Drug Classes) may require an increase in the antidiabetic dosage to obtain proper control of blood sugar levels. After correct doses of both drugs have been determined, a reduction in thyroid dose may require a simultaneous reduction of the antidiabetic to prevent hypoglycemia.

- benzodiazepines (see Drug Classes) may enhance the therapeutic effects of both medicines. Dose reductions may be needed.

- conjugated estrogens (Premarin, others) may require an increased levothyroxine dose.
- tricyclic antidepressants may cause an increase in the activity of both drugs; monitor for indications of overdosage of each drug.

The following drug may ***decrease*** the effects of levothyroxine

- cholestyramine (Cuemid, Questran) may reduce its absorption; intake of the two drugs should be separated by 5 hours.
- colestipol (Colestid).
- iron salts (by decreasing levothyroxine absorption).
- lovastatin (Mevacor).
- phenytoin (Dilantin); may increase removal of levothyroxine from the body and require increased doses to get the same therapeutic benefit.
- sodium polystyrene sulfonate (Kayexalate).
- sucralfate (Carafate).

Exposure to Heat: May decrease individual tolerance to warm environments, increasing discomfort from heat. Call your doctor if you develop symptoms of overdosage during the warm months.

Heavy Exercise or Exertion: Use caution if you have angina (coronary artery disease). This drug may increase its frequency or severity during physical activity.

Discontinuation: This drug must be taken continually on a regular schedule to correct thyroid deficiency. Do not stop taking it without talking to your doctor.

▷ **Saving Money When Using This Medicine:**

- Few medications are available to treat low thyroid function. Ask your doctor if this drug provides the best combination of cost and outcome for you.
- Ask your doctor how long this drug is usually taken to treat your condition.
- Thyroid testing and levels are expensive. Frequent testing is usually not needed. Ask your doctor if any ordered tests can be delayed or eliminated.
- Talk with your doctor about the need for calcium replacement, exercise, and bone mineral density testing for osteoporosis.

LIDOCAINE AND PRILOCAINE CREAM (LIE do kane) (PRY low kane)

Prescription: Yes   **Controlled Drug:** No   **Generic:** No
Brand Names: Emla cream [CD]

▷ **Warning:** This cream should NOT be used by patients with congenital methemoglobinemia.
The maximum application area should NOT be exceeded.

Overview of BENEFITS versus RISKS

Possible Benefits	*Possible Risks*
EFFECTIVE PAIN CONTROL	Systemic absorption and possible adverse effects Methemoglobinemia

---

▷ **Illness This Medication Treats:**

As Combination Drug Product [CD]: Use currently included in FDA-approved labeling: on normal skin as a topical anesthetic for local pain relief. Often used in pediatric units in hospitals before intravenous lines are placed.

▷ **Typical Dosage Range:** (Dosage or schedule must be determined by the doctor for each individual.)

Infants and Children: For body weight up to 10 kg: Maximum application area in square centimeters is 100. For body weight of 10 to 20 kg: Maximum application area in square centimeters is 600. For body weight above 20 kg: Maximum application area in square centimeters is 2000.

12 to 60 Years of Age: Estimated mean lidocaine absorption is 0.045 mg per square centimeter per hour.

Estimated mean absorption of prilocaine is 0.077 mg per square centimeter per hour.

Over 60 Years of Age: Same as for 12 to 60 years of age, except for patients with liver or kidney compromise.

▷ **Conditions Requiring Dosing Adjustments:**

Liver function: Consideration must be given to reduced application area for patients with liver compromise.

LIOTHYRONINE (li oh THI roh neen)

Other Names: Triiodothyronine, T3

Prescription: Yes   **Controlled Drug:** No   **Generic:** Yes

Brand Names: Armour Thyroid, Cyronine, Cytomel, Euthroid [CD], Thyrolar [CD], Triostat

Overview of BENEFITS versus RISKS	
Possible Benefits	*Possible Risks*
EFFECTIVE REPLACEMENT THERAPY WITH THYROID HORMONE DEFICIENCY (HYPOTHYROIDISM) EFFECTIVE TREATMENT OF SIMPLE GOITER AND CHRONIC THYROIDITIS EFFECTIVE TREATMENT OF THYROID GLAND CANCER	Intensification of angina in presence of coronary artery disease Drug-induced hyperthyroidism (with excessive dosage) Rapid heartbeat Heart attack

▷ **Illness This Medication Treats:**

(1) Hypothyroidism: a replacement therapy to correct thyroid deficiency; (2) simple (nonendemic) goiter and benign thyroid nodules; (3) Hashimoto's thyroiditis; (4) adjunctive prevention and treatment of thyroid cancer; (5) cretinism; (6) can help diagnose various thyroid problems.

As Combination Drug Product [CD]: This hormone is available in combination with the other principal thyroid hormone, levothyroxine, in a preparation (generic name: liotrix) that resembles the natural hormone.

▷ **Typical Dosage Range:** (Dosage or schedule must be determined by the doctor for each individual.)

Infants and Children: Use of this drug is not recommended.

12 to 60 Years of Age: For mild hypothyroidism: Initially 25 mcg daily; increase by 12.5 to 25 mcg at intervals of 1 to 2 weeks as needed and tolerated. The usual maintenance dose is 25 to 50 mcg daily.

For severe hypothyroidism. Initially 2.5 to 5 mcg daily, increase by 5 to 10 mcg at intervals of 1 to 2 weeks. When a dose of 25 mcg is reached, increase by 12.5 to 25 mcg at intervals of 1 to 2 weeks, as needed and tolerated. The usual maintenance dose is 25 to 50 mcg daily.

For simple goiter. Initially 5 mcg daily; increase by 5 to 10 mcg at intervals of 1 to 2 weeks. When a dose of 25 mcg is reached, increase by 12.5 to 25 mcg at intervals of 1 week, as needed and tolerated. The usual maintenance dose is 50 to 100 mcg daily.

Over 60 Years of Age: Initially 5 mcg as a single daily dose; increase by 5 mcg at intervals of 2 weeks, as needed and tolerated. The usual maintenance dose is 12.5 to 37.5 mcg daily.

▷ **How Best to Take This Medicine:**   This drug should preferably be taken in the morning on an empty stomach to ensure maximal absorption and uniform results. The tablets may be crushed.

▷ **How Long This Medicine Is Usually Taken:** Use on a regular schedule for 2 to 4 days is usually necessary to determine the effectiveness of this drug in correcting the symptoms of thyroid deficiency. Long-term use (months to years, possibly for life) requires supervision and periodic evaluation by your doctor. See your doctor regularly.

▷ **Tell Your Doctor Before Taking This Medicine If You:**
- ever had an allergic reaction to it.
- are recovering from a recent heart attack.
- are using it to lose weight and your thyroid function is normal.
- have high blood pressure, any form of heart disease, or diabetes.
- have a history of Addison's disease or adrenal gland deficiency.
- are taking any antiasthmatic medications.
- are taking an anticoagulant.

▷ **Possible Side Effects:** Tachycardia, hair loss.

▷ **Possible Adverse Effects:**
If any of the following develop, call your doctor promptly for guidance.
Some Mild Problems Drug Can Cause
Allergic reactions: skin rash, hives.
Headache in some people, even with proper dosage adjustment.
Some Serious Problems Drug Can Cause
Worsening of angina in the presence of coronary artery disease.
Heart attack.
Osteoporosis.
Drug-induced myasthenia gravis.
Note: Other adverse effects are manifestations of excessive dosage.

▷ **Possible Effects on Sex Life:** Altered menstrual pattern during dosage adjustments.
Possibly beneficial in treating impaired sexual function associated with true hypothyroidism.

▷ *CAUTION*
1. The need for and response to thyroid hormone treatment varies greatly from person to person. Careful supervision of individual response is necessary to determine correct dosage. Do not change your dosage schedule without consulting your doctor.
2. In the absence of verified thyroid deficiency, the use of liothyronine to treat nonspecific fatigue, obesity, infertility, or slow growth is inappropriate and could be harmful.
3. This drug is not recommended for children. Its ability to reach the brain and nervous system is uncertain. Levothyroxine is the drug of choice for thyroid deficiency in infants and children.
4. People over 60 should use this drug with caution. Usually the thy-

roid hormone replacement requirements for this population are about 25% lower than in younger adults. Watch closely for any indications that suggest possible overdosage.

Advisability of Use During Pregnancy and If Breast-Feeding:
Pregnancy Category: A. Use only if clearly needed and with carefully adjusted dosage. Present in breast milk in minimal amounts. Breast-feeding is considered safe with correctly adjusted dosage.

▷ **Overdose Symptoms:** Headache, sense of increased body heat, nervousness, increased sweating, hand tremors, insomnia, rapid and irregular heart action, diarrhea, muscle cramping, weight loss.

▷ **Suggested Periodic Examinations While Taking This Drug:** (at doctor's discretion)
Measurement of thyroid hormone levels in blood.

▷ **While Taking This Drug the Following Apply:**
Other Drugs:
Liothyronine may *increase* the effects of
- warfarin (Coumadin), increasing the risk of bleeding; reduction in the anticoagulant dosage is usually necessary. Monitor prothrombin times as necessary.

Liothyronine may *decrease* the effects of
- digoxin (Lanoxin) when correcting hypothyroidism; a larger dose of digoxin may be needed.

Liothyronine *taken concurrently* with
- all antidiabetics (insulin and oral hypoglycemic agents—see Drug Classes) may require an increase in the antidiabetic dosage to obtain proper control of blood sugar levels. After correct doses of both drugs have been determined, a reduction in thyroid dose may require a simultaneous reduction in the antidiabetic dose to prevent hypoglycemia.
- estrogens (including birth control pills and Premarin) may result in a need for increased liothyronine dosing.
- monoamine oxidase (MAO) type A inhibitors (see Drug Classes) may increase the therapeutic benefits of the antidepressant.
- tricyclic antidepressants may increase the activity of both drugs; monitor for indications of overdosage of each drug.

The following drug may *decrease* the effects of liothyronine
- cholestyramine (Cuemid, Questran); may reduce its absorption. Intake of the two drugs should be separated by 5 hours.

Exposure to Heat: May decrease individual tolerance to warm environments, increasing discomfort with heat. Call your doctor if you develop symptoms of overdosage during the warm months.

Heavy Exercise or Exertion: Use caution if you have angina (coronary artery disease). This drug may increase its frequency or severity during physical activity.

Discontinuation: This drug must be taken continually on a regular schedule to correct thyroid deficiency. Do not stop taking it without talking to your doctor.

▷ **Saving Money When Using This Medicine:**
- Ask your doctor if this drug provides the best combination of cost and outcome for you, and how long this drug is usually taken to treat your condition.
- Thyroid function tests are expensive. Ask your doctor if the tests ordered can be done less frequently.
- Talk with your doctor about osteoporosis testing and prevention.

LISINOPRIL (li SIN oh pril)

Prescription: Yes   **Controlled Drug:** No   **Generic:** No
Brand Names: Prinivil, Prinzide [CD], Zestoretic [CD], Zestril

Overview of BENEFITS versus RISKS	
Possible Benefits	*Possible Risks*
EFFECTIVE CONTROL OF MILD TO SEVERE HIGH BLOOD PRESSURE IMPROVES PATIENT SURVIVAL AFTER A HEART ATTACK	Headache, dizziness, fatigue Low blood pressure Allergic swelling of face, tongue, throat, vocal cords Kidney compromise Rare lowering of white blood cell counts

▷ **Illness This Medication Treats:**
(1) Mild to moderate high blood pressure usually responds to low doses; severe high blood pressure may require higher doses and the concurrent use of a thiazide or other class of antihypertensive. (2) Helps improve survival in congestive heart failure; (3) increases chances of survival after a heart attack and decreases heart attack symptoms.
As Combination Drug Product [CD]: Combination with the diuretic hydrochlorothiazide enhances antihypertensive action.

▷ **Typical Dosage Range:** (Dosage or schedule must be determined by the doctor for each individual.)
Infants and Children: Dosage not established.
12 to 60 Years of Age: Initially 10 mg once daily for those not taking a diuretic; 5 mg once daily for those taking a diuretic. Usual maintenance dose is 20 to 40 mg/day, taken in a single dose. Total daily dosage should not exceed 80 mg.
After a heart attack: 5 mg may be given within 24 hours after symptoms start. If this dose is tolerated, a repeat dose is given 24 hours

later, and then increased to 10 mg a day. Therapy continues for at least 6 weeks.

Over 60 Years of Age: Exercise tolerance has been improved by 2.5 to 20 mg daily. A longer period of adjustment should be taken in between any needed dosage changes.

▷ **Conditions Requiring Dosing Adjustments:**

Kidney function: Patients with moderate kidney failure should start with 5 mg daily. For patients with severe kidney failure, the starting dose is 2.5 mg of lisinopril daily. This drug is contraindicated for patients with renal artery stenosis.

▷ **How Best to Take This Medicine:** Take on an empty stomach or with food, at same time each day. The tablet may be crushed.

▷ **How Long This Medicine Is Usually Taken:** Continual use on a regular schedule for several weeks is usually necessary to determine this drug's effectiveness in controlling high blood pressure. The proper treatment of high blood pressure usually requires the long-term use of effective medications. See your doctor regularly.

▷ **Tell Your Doctor Before Taking This Medicine If You:**

- ever had an allergic reaction to it.
- currently have a blood cell or bone marrow disorder.
- have an abnormally high level of blood potassium.
- have a history of kidney disease or impaired kidney function.
- have scleroderma or systemic lupus erythematosus.
- have cerebral artery disease.
- have any form of heart disease.
- are breast-feeding your infant.
- have myasthenia gravis or another autoimmune disease.
- are taking any other antihypertensives, diuretics, nitrates, or potassium supplements.
- plan to have surgery under general anesthesia soon.

▷ **Possible Side Effects:** Dizziness, orthostatic hypotension, increased blood potassium level.

▷ **Possible Adverse Effects:**

If any of the following develop, call your doctor promptly for guidance.

Some Mild Problems Drug Can Cause

Allergic reactions: skin rash, itching.
Headache, fatigue, numbness, and tingling.
Chest pain, palpitation, cough.
Nausea, vomiting, diarrhea.
Rare blurred vision or psoriasis.

Some Serious Problems Drug Can Cause

Allergic reactions: swelling (angioedema) of face, tongue, and/or vocal cords, which can be life-threatening.

Impairment of kidney function.

Rare bone marrow depression, hepatitis, positive ANA titer with joint changes or pancreatitis.

▷ **Possible Effects on Sex Life:**   Decreased libido, impotence.

▷ *CAUTION*

1. Ask your doctor about the advisability of discontinuing other antihypertensive drugs (especially diuretics) for 1 week before starting this drug.
2. **Report promptly** any indications of infection (fever, sore throat), or water retention (weight gain, puffiness, swollen feet or ankles).
3. Do not use a salt substitute without your doctor's knowledge and approval (many contain potassium).
4. Obtain blood cell counts and urine analyses **before** starting this drug.
5. Safety and effectiveness of this drug for infants and children are not established.
6. For people over 60, small doses are advisable until tolerance has been determined. Sudden and excessive lowering of blood pressure can predispose to stroke or heart attack in those with impaired brain circulation or coronary artery heart disease.
7. Call your doctor immediately if you develop swelling of the face or tongue while you are taking this medicine.

Advisability of Use During Pregnancy and If Breast-Feeding:
Pregnancy Category: D during the first 3 months of pregnancy. Avoid use of this drug during pregnancy. D during the last 6 months of pregnancy. Presence in breast milk is unknown; avoid taking this drug or refrain from nursing.

▷ **Overdose Symptoms:**   Excessive drop in blood pressure, lightheadedness, dizziness, fainting.

▷ **Suggested Periodic Examinations While Taking This Drug:** (at doctor's discretion)
Before starting drug: complete blood cell counts; urine analysis with measurement of protein content; blood potassium level.
During use of drug: blood cell counts; measurements of blood potassium.

▷ **While Taking This Drug the Following Apply:**
Foods: Ask your doctor about salt intake.
Nutritional Support: Do not take potassium supplements unless directed by your doctor.
Beverages: May be taken with milk.
Alcohol: Use caution until combined effect has been determined. Alcohol may enhance the blood pressure–lowering effect of this drug.

Other Drugs:

Lisinopril *taken concurrently* with

- acetaminophen may lead to increased blood pressure.
- allopurinol (Zyloprim) may increase risk of hypersensitivity reactions.
- chlorpromazine (Thorazine) may lead to excessively low blood pressure.
- cyclosporine (Sandimmune) can cause acute kidney failure.
- lithium (Lithobid, others) may lead to lithium toxicity.
- loop diuretics such as bumetanide (Bumex) or furosemide (Lasix) may lead to increased blood pressure effects.
- NSAIDs (see Drug Classes) may blunt the therapeutic effect of lisinopril.
- potassium preparations (K-Lyte, Slow-K, etc.) may cause increased blood levels of potassium, with risk of serious heart rhythm disturbances.
- potassium-sparing diuretics—amiloride (Moduretic), spironolactone (Aldactazide), triamterene (Dyazide)—may cause increased blood levels of potassium, with risk of serious heart rhythm disturbances.

Driving, Hazardous Activities: Usually no restrictions. Be aware of possible drops in blood pressure, with resultant dizziness or faintness.

Exposure to Sun: Caution is advised. A similar drug of this class can cause photosensitivity.

Exposure to Heat: Caution is advised. Avoid excessive perspiring with resultant loss of body water and drop in blood pressure.

Occurrence of Unrelated Illness: Report promptly any disorder that causes nausea, vomiting, or diarrhea. Fluid and chemical imbalances must be corrected as soon as possible.

Discontinuation: This drug may be stopped abruptly without a sudden increase in blood pressure. However, you should talk to your doctor about its withdrawal for any reason.

▷ **Saving Money When Using This Medicine:**

- Many medications are available to treat high blood pressure. Ask your doctor if this drug provides the best combination of cost and outcome for you, and how long this drug is usually taken to treat your condition.
- If you are taking a diuretic at the same time, ask about checking magnesium and potassium levels.
- Talk with your doctor about stress management and exercise programs in your community.
- Find out more about your condition. *The Essential Guide to Chronic Illness* is an excellent source of information.

LITHIUM (LITH i um)

Prescription: Yes   **Controlled Drug:** No   **Generic:** Yes

Brand Names: Cibalith-S, Eskalith, Eskalith CR, Lithane, Lithobid, Lithonate, Lithotabs

---

Overview of BENEFITS versus RISKS

Possible Benefits	*Possible Risks*
RAPID REVERSAL OF ACUTE MANIA	VERY NARROW MARGIN BETWEEN TREATMENT AND TOXIC BLOOD LEVELS
STABILIZATION OF MOOD	
Prevention of recurrent depression in responders	POTENTIALLY FATAL TOXICITY with inadequate monitoring
	Infrequent induction of diabetes mellitus, hypothyroidism
	Diabetes-insipiduslike syndrome (excessive dilute urine without sugar)

▷ **Illness This Medication Treats:**

(1) Manic-depressive disorders. Reduces the frequency and severity of mood swings; also treats the depression phase in people who do not experience the manic phase. (2) Eases and controls mania.

▷ **Typical Dosage Range:** (Dosage or schedule must be determined by the doctor for each individual.)

First day: 300 mg taken three times, 6 hours apart; second day and thereafter: increase dose to 1200 mg/24 hr and later to 1800 mg/24 hr if needed and tolerated. Usually blood levels are kept at 1 to 1.5 mmol/L and relate to benefits versus toxic effects. The usual maintenance dose is 600 to 1200 mg every 24 hours taken in three divided doses. Total daily dose should not exceed 3600 mg.

▷ **Conditions Requiring Dosing Adjustments:**

Kidney function: Almost all of a lithium dose is removed by the kidneys. Use of this drug by people with compromised kidneys requires a benefit-to-risk decision. If the decision is made to use lithium, frequent and careful monitoring and decreased dosing must be provided.

▷ **How Best to Take This Medicine:**   May be taken with or after meals to reduce stomach irritation. The capsules may be opened and the regular tablets crushed for administration; the prolonged-action tablets should be swallowed whole and not altered.

▷ **How Long This Medicine Is Usually Taken:** Use on a regular schedule for 1 to 3 weeks usually determines the effectiveness of this drug in correcting acute mania; several months of continual treatment may be required to correct depression. Long-term use (months to years) requires supervision and periodic physician evaluation.

▷ **Tell Your Doctor Before Taking This Medicine If You:**
- ever had an allergic reaction to it.
- have uncontrolled diabetes or uncorrected hypothyroidism.
- will be unable to comply with the need for regular monitoring of blood levels.
- have a history of a schizophreniclike thought disorder.
- have any type of organic brain disease or a history of grand mal epilepsy.
- have diabetes, heart disease, hypothyroidism, or impaired kidney function.
- are on a salt-restricted diet.
- are pregnant, planning pregnancy, or breast-feeding your infant.
- are taking any diuretic drug or a cortisonelike steroid preparation.
- have kidney failure.
- plan to have surgery under general anesthesia soon.

▷ **Possible Side Effects:** Increased thirst and urine volume may occur in 60% of initial users and in 20% of long-term maintenance users. Weight gain may occur in first few months of use. Drowsiness and lethargy may occur in sensitive individuals.

▷ **Possible Adverse Effects**
If any of the following develop, call your doctor promptly for guidance.
Some Mild Problems Drug Can Cause
Allergic reactions: skin rashes, generalized itching.
Skin dryness, loss of hair.
Headache, dizziness, weakness, blurred vision, ringing in ears, fine hand tremor.
Metallic taste, stomach irritation, nausea, vomiting, incontinence, diarrhea.
Some Serious Problems Drug Can Cause
Blackout spells, stupor, slurred speech, spasmodic movements of extremities, epilepticlike seizures.
Loss of bladder or rectal control.
Diabetes-insipiduslike syndrome: excessive dilute urine.
Rare inflammation of the heart or abnormal heart rhythms, porphyria, or neuroleptic malignant syndrome.
Drug-induced myasthenia gravis or systemic lupus erythematosus.

▷ **Possible Effects on Sex Life:** Decreased libido (blood level of 0.7—0.9 mEq/L); inhibited erection (0.6—0.8 mEq/L); male infertility; female breast swelling with milk production.

▷ **Adverse Effects That May Mimic Natural Diseases or Disorders:** Painful discoloration and coldness of the hands and feet may resemble Raynaud's syndrome.

▷ *CAUTION*

1. This drug has a very narrow margin of safe use. The blood level of drug required to be effective is quite close to the toxic level. Periodic measurement of blood lithium levels is mandatory for appropriate dosage adjustments. Follow instructions exactly regarding drug dosage and periodic blood examinations.

2. Lithium should be discontinued at the first signs of toxicity: drowsiness, sluggishness, unsteadiness, tremor, muscle twitching, vomiting, or diarrhea.

3. The major causes of lithium toxicity are accidental overdose (sometimes due to inadequate blood level monitoring); impaired kidney function; salt restriction; inadequate fluid intake, dehydration; concurrent use of diuretics; intercurrent illness; childbirth (rapid decrease in kidney clearance of lithium); initiation of treatment with a new drug.

4. Over-the-counter preparations that contain iodides (some cough products and vitamin-mineral supplements) should be avoided because of the added antithyroid effect when taken with lithium.

5. Safety and effectiveness of this drug for those under 12 years old are not established. Follow your doctor's instructions exactly.

6. People over 60 should take initial and maintenance doses smaller than standard doses for younger adults; treatment should start with a test dose of 75 to 150 mg daily. Watch closely for early indications of toxic effects, especially if you are on a low-salt diet and using diuretics. Parkinsonian reactions (abnormal gait and movements) occur with greater frequency; coma can develop without warning symptoms.

Advisability of Use During Pregnancy and If Breast-Feeding:
Pregnancy Category: D. Avoid use of this drug during the first 3 months. Use only if clearly necessary during the last 6 months. Monitor the mother's blood lithium levels carefully to avoid possible toxicity. Present in breast milk; avoid taking this drug or refrain from nursing.

▷ **Overdose Symptoms:** Drowsiness, weakness, lack of coordination, nausea, vomiting, diarrhea, muscle spasms, blurred vision, dizziness, staggering gait, slurred speech, confusion, stupor, coma, seizures.

▷ **Suggested Periodic Examinations While Taking This Drug:** (at doctor's discretion)

Regular determinations of blood lithium levels are absolutely essential to safe and effective use.

Time to sample blood for lithium level: 12 hours after evening dose, or just before next dose.

Recommended therapeutic range: 0.8–1.2 mEq/L.

Periodic evaluation of thyroid gland size and function.

Complete blood cell counts; kidney function tests.

▷ **While Taking This Drug the Following Apply:**

Foods: Maintain a normal diet; **do not** restrict your use of salt.

Beverages: No restrictions. Drink at least 8 to 12 glasses of liquids every 24 hours. This drug may be taken with milk.

Alcohol: Use with caution until the combined effects have been determined—expect a greater effect with fewer drinks. Avoid alcohol completely if any symptoms of lithium toxicity develop.

Marijuana Smoking: Possible increase in apathy, lethargy, drowsiness, or sluggishness; accentuation of lithium-induced tremor; increased risk of precipitating psychotic behavior.

Other Drugs:

Lithium may *increase* the effects of

- tricyclic antidepressants.

Lithium *taken concurrently* with

- ACE inhibitors such as captopril (Capoten) may increase lithium levels as much as 3 times.
- calcium channel blockers (see Drug Classes) may lead to nerve toxicity.
- carbamazepine (Tegretol), chlorpromazine (Thorazine, etc.) and other phenothiazines, fluoxetine (Prozac), haloperidol (Haldol), or methyldopa (Aldomet, etc.) is usually well tolerated; however, it may cause a severe neurotoxic reaction in susceptible individuals. Use these combinations very cautiously.
- clozapine (Clozaril) may result in serious agranulocytosis, delirium, or neuroleptic malignant syndrome.
- diazepam (Valium) may cause hypothermia.
- fludrocortisone (Florinef) may result in loss of mineralocorticoid benefits of fludrocortisone.
- fluvoxamine (Luvox) may result in increased lithium levels and toxicity.
- methyldopa (Aldomet) is usually well tolerated, but may cause severe nerve toxicity (neurotoxicity) in some people.
- methyldopa (Flagyl) may result in lithium toxicity.
- monoamine oxidase (MAO) type A inhibitors may result in the serotonin syndrome and serious illness.

- nicotine (Nicorette gum or nicotine patches) may lead to supersensitivity to nicotine.
- verapamil (Calan, Isoptin) may cause unpredictable effects; both lithium toxicity and decreased lithium blood levels have been reported.

The following drugs may *increase* the effects of lithium

- bumetanide (Bumex).
- ethacrynic acid (Edecrin).
- fluoxetine (Prozac).
- furosemide (Lasix, etc.).
- indomethacin (Indocin).
- piroxicam (Feldene) and perhaps other NSAIDs (see Drug Classes).
- thiazide diuretics (see drug profile).

The following drugs may *decrease* the effects of lithium

- acetazolamide (Diamox, etc.).
- sodium bicarbonate.
- theophylline (Theo-Dur, etc.) and related drugs.

Driving, Hazardous Activities: May impair mental alertness, judgment, physical coordination, and reaction time. Restrict your activities as necessary.

Exposure to Heat: Excessive sweating can cause significant salt and water depletion and resultant lithium toxicity. Avoid sauna baths.

Occurrence of Unrelated Illness: Any illness that causes fever, sweating, vomiting, or diarrhea can result in significant alterations of blood and tissue concentrations. Close monitoring of your physical condition and blood levels is necessary to prevent serious toxicity.

Discontinuation: Sudden discontinuation does not cause withdrawal symptoms. Avoid premature discontinuation of this drug; some individuals may require continual treatment for up to a year to achieve maximal response. Discontinuation by "responders" may result in recurrence of either mania or depression. Lithium should be discontinued with symptoms of brain toxicity or an uncorrectable diabetes-insipiduslike syndrome.

▷ **Saving Money When Using This Medicine:**

- Ask your doctor if this drug provides the best combination of cost and outcome for you, and how long this drug is usually taken to treat your condition.
- Find out more about your condition. *The Essential Guide to Chronic Illness* is an excellent source of information.

LOMEFLOXACIN (loh me FLOX a sin)

Prescription: Yes   **Controlled Drug:** No   **Generic:** No
Brand Name: Maxaquin

▷ **Warning:**   This drug may cause tendon rupture. If it is prescribed for
you, ask your doctor if you should limit exercise or exertion during
therapy. Call your doctor immediately if pain or inflammation
appears while you are taking this medicine. A rare idiosyncratic reaction has also been reported for medicines in this class: mental
confusion and disorientation. Talk with your doctor if you or a loved
one become confused or disoriented after taking this medicine.

Overview of BENEFITS versus RISKS

Possible Benefits	*Possible Risks*
HIGHLY EFFECTIVE TREATMENT FOR SOME INFECTIONS OF THE LOWER RESPIRATORY TRACT and URINARY TRACT	Rare but serious allergic reactions
	Rare seizures
	Headache, dizziness
	Nausea, diarrhea
Effective prevention of postoperative lower urinary tract infection	Rare tendon rupture
	Rare neurologic reactions

▷ **Illness This Medication Treats:**
Responsive infections (in adults) of (1) the lower respiratory tract
(lungs and bronchial tubes); (2) the urinary tract (kidneys, bladder,
urethra). (3) Prevents postoperative infection following transure-
thral surgical procedures.

▷ **Typical Dosage Range:** (Dosage or schedule must be determined by
the doctor for each individual.)
Infants and Children: Use of this drug is not recommended.
18 to 60 Years of Age: For bronchitis: 400 mg daily for 10 days.
For bladder infections (cystitis): 400 mg daily for 10 days.
For complicated urinary tract infections: 400 mg daily for 14 days.
For preoperative prevention of urinary tract infection: 400 mg (single
dose) taken 2 to 6 hours before surgery.
Over 60 Years of Age: Same as for 18 to 60 years of age.

▷ **Conditions Requiring Dosing Adjustments:**
Kidney function: Patients with mild to moderate kidney failure can
take a 400 mg loading dose followed by 200 mg daily. For patients
with severe failure, 200 mg may be taken less frequently.

▷ **How Best to Take This Medicine:**   May be taken without regard to
food. Drink fluids liberally during the entire course of treatment.

Avoid antacids containing aluminum or magnesium and supplements containing iron or zinc for 2 hours before and after dosing. The tablet may be crushed.

▷ **How Long This Medicine Is Usually Taken:**   Continual use on a regular schedule for up to 10 days is usually necessary to determine the effectiveness of this drug in eradicating infection. The drug should be continued for at least 2 days after all indications of infection have disappeared.

▷ **Tell Your Doctor Before Taking This Medicine If You:**
- ever had an allergic reaction to it.
- are pregnant or breast-feeding.
- have a seizure disorder that is not adequately controlled.
- are given a prescription for a person under 18 years old.
- are allergic to cinoxacin (Cinobac), nalidixic acid (NegGram), ciprofloxacin (Cipro), norfloxacin (Noroxin), ofloxacin (Floxin), or related quinolone drugs.
- have a history of a seizure disorder or circulatory disorder of the brain.
- have a history of tendon disease.
- develop tendon pain or confusion and disorientation while taking this medicine.
- have impaired kidney function.
- are taking any form of probenecid, sucralfate, antacids, or warfarin.

▷ **Possible Side Effects:**   Superinfections: yeast vaginitis.

▷ **Possible Adverse Effects:**
If any of the following develop, call your doctor promptly for guidance.
Some Mild Problems Drug Can Cause
Allergic reactions: rash, itching.
Headache, dizziness, weakness, insomnia, visual disturbances.
Nausea, vomiting, diarrhea.
Some Serious Problems Drug Can Cause
Allergic reactions: anaphylactic reactions.
Idiosyncratic reactions: rare and unpredictable central nervous system problems ranging from sleep disorders to extreme confusion have been reported with medicines in this class.
Rare tendon rupture.

▷ **Possible Effects on Sex Life:**   Intermenstrual bleeding.

▷ *CAUTION*
1. High doses or prolonged use of other drugs of this class may cause crystal formation in the kidney. Drinking copious amounts of water, up to 2 qt/24 hr, can prevent this.
2. Drugs of this class may decrease the formation of saliva and pre-

dispose to the development of dental cavities or gum disease. Consult your dentist if dry mouth persists.

3. If a skin rash, hives, or other indications of allergy develops, discontinue this drug and call your doctor promptly.
4. Avoid iron and mineral supplements while taking this drug.
5. Safety and effectiveness of this drug for those under 18 years old are not established. Avoid using this drug completely; it can impair normal bone growth and development in immature animals.
6. People over 60 may have an age-related decrease in kidney function and require dosage reduction.
7. You should talk with your doctor immediately if confusion, changes in thinking, or tendon pain starts once you begin taking this medicine.

Advisability of Use During Pregnancy and If Breast-Feeding:

Pregnancy Category: C. The potential for adverse effects on fetal bone development contraindicates use of this drug during entire pregnancy. Presence in breast milk is unknown; avoid taking this drug or refrain from nursing.

▷ **Overdose Symptoms:** Nausea, vomiting, diarrhea. Delirium, hallucinations, and seizures.

▷ **Possible Effects of Long-Term Use:** Superinfections.

▷ **While Taking This Drug the Following Apply:**

Beverages: May be taken with milk.

Other Drugs:

Lomefloxacin may *increase* the effects of
• warfarin (Coumadin), increasing the risk of bleeding; more frequent INR (prothrombin time) testing is necessary.

The following drugs may *increase* the effects of lomefloxacin
• furosemide (Lasix).
• probenecid (Benemid).

The following drugs may *decrease* the effects of lomefloxacin
• antacids containing aluminum or magnesium; can reduce the absorption of lomefloxacin and lessen its effectiveness.
• iron salts.
• sucralfate (Carafate); can impair absorption of lomefloxacin.

Take antacids or sucralfate 4 hours before or 2 hours after taking lomefloxacin.

Driving, Hazardous Activities: May cause drowsiness, dizziness, and impaired vision. Restrict your activities as necessary.

Exposure to Sun: This drug may rarely cause photosensitivity. Sunglasses are advised if your eyes are overly sensitive to bright light.

Discontinuation: If you experience no adverse effects, take the full course prescribed for maximal results. Ask your doctor about stopping treatment.

▷ **Saving Money When Using This Medicine:**
- Many medications are available to treat infections. Ask your doctor if this drug provides the best combination of cost and outcome for you, and how long this drug is usually taken to treat your condition.

LOPERAMIDE (loh PER a mide)

Prescription: Yes   **Controlled Drug:** No   **Generic:** No

Brand Names: Imodium, Imodium AD, Kaopectate 1-D, Maalox-AD, Pepto Diarrhea Control

Overview of BENEFITS versus RISKS	
Possible Benefits	*Possible Risks*
EFFECTIVE RELIEF OF INTESTINAL CRAMPING AND DIARRHEA	Drowsiness Constipation Induction of toxic megacolon

▷ **Illness This Medication Treats:**
(1) Controls cramping and diarrhea associated with acute gastroenteritis and chronic enteritis and colitis; (2) decreases amount of discharge from ileostomies.

▷ **Typical Dosage Range:** (Dosage or schedule must be determined by the doctor for each individual.)
For acute diarrhea: 4 mg initially, then 2 mg after each unformed stool until diarrhea is controlled. For chronic diarrhea: 4 to 8 mg every day in divided doses, taken 8 to 12 hours apart. Total daily dosage should not exceed 16 mg.

▷ **How Best to Take This Medicine:** May be taken on an empty stomach or with food if stomach irritation occurs. The capsule may be opened for administration.

▷ **How Long This Medicine Is Usually Taken:** 48 hours of scheduled use usually determines the effectiveness of this drug in controlling acute diarrhea; continual use for 10 days may be needed to evaluate its effectiveness in controlling chronic diarrhea. If diarrhea persists, call your doctor.

▷ **Tell Your Doctor Before Taking This Medicine If You:**
- ever had an allergic reaction to it.
- are given a prescription for a child under 2 years old.
- have a history of liver disease or impaired liver function.
- have acute dysentery or develop swelling (distention) of the abdomen while taking this medicine.
- have regional enteritis or ulcerative colitis.

▷ **Possible Side Effects:**   Drowsiness, constipation.

▷ **Possible Adverse Effects:**

If any of the following develop, call your doctor promptly for guidance.

Some Mild Problems Drug Can Cause

Allergic reaction: skin rash.

Fatigue, dizziness.

Reduced appetite, dry mouth, nausea, vomiting, bloating.

Some Serious Problems Drug Can Cause

Toxic megacolon (distended, immobile colon with fluid retention) may develop.

Rare necrotizing enterocolitis or paralytic ileus.

▷ *CAUTION*

1. Do not exceed recommended doses.
2. If this drug is used to treat chronic diarrhea, report promptly any bloating, abdominal distention, nausea, vomiting, constipation, or abdominal pain.
3. This drug is not for use in those under 2 years old. Follow your doctor's instructions exactly regarding dosage. Observe for drowsiness, irritability, personality changes, and altered behavior.
4. People over 60 should receive small doses. You may be more sensitive to the drug's sedative and constipating effects.

Advisability of Use During Pregnancy and If Breast-Feeding:

Pregnancy Category: B. Use this drug sparingly and only if clearly needed. Ask doctor for guidance. Presence in breast milk is small, usually in clinically insignificant amounts. Talk with your doctor about the benefits versus risks of nursing.

▷ **Overdose Symptoms:**   Drowsiness, lethargy, depression, dry mouth.

▷ **While Taking This Drug the Following Apply:**

Foods: Follow prescribed diet.

Beverages: May be taken with milk.

Alcohol: Use with caution until combined effects have been determined. This drug may increase the depressant action of alcohol on the brain.

Driving, Hazardous Activities: This drug may cause drowsiness or dizziness. Restrict your activities as necessary.

▷ **Saving Money When Using This Medicine:**

• Many medications are available to treat diarrhea. Ask your doctor if this drug provides the best combination of cost and outcome for you, and how long this drug is usually taken to treat your condition.

• Ask when this medicine should control your diarrhea and what to do if it does not. Tests of blood electrolytes may be needed.

LORAZEPAM   (lor A za pam)

Prescription: Yes   **Controlled Drug:**   C-IV*   **Generic:**
Yes

Brand Names: Ativan, Lorazepam Intensol

Overview of BENEFITS versus RISKS

Possible Benefits	*Possible Risks*
RELIEF OF ANXIETY AND NERVOUS TENSION	Habit-forming potential with prolonged use
NOT CHANGED SIGNIFICANTLY INTO ACTIVE DRUG FORMS IN THE LIVER	Minor impairment of mental functions
	Very rare blood cell disorders
	Very rare movement disorders
Wide margin of safety with therapeutic doses	Very rare liver disorders
	Dose-related respiratory depression
	Withdrawal symptoms if abruptly stopped

▷ **Illness This Medication Treats:**
   (1) Anxiety; (2) relief of insomnia; (3) in surgical cases, delivering effective anesthesia; (4) intravenously as a sedative.
   Other (unlabeled) generally accepted uses: (1) eases severe symptoms of alcohol detoxification (delirium tremens or DTs); (2) administered under the tongue for treatment of serial seizures in children; (3) can be used to promote a beneficial amnesia in some patients who have suffered severe vomiting from chemotherapy, or in some chronic pain patients.

▷ **Typical Dosage Range:** (Dosage or schedule must be determined by the doctor for each individual.)
   Infants and Children: Safety and effectiveness of this drug for those under 18 years old are not established. This drug has been used in 1- to 4-mg doses under the tongue for treatment of serial seizures in children.
   18 to 60 Years of Age: Sedation and anxiety: Therapy is started with 1 mg/day in two to three divided doses. Doses may be increased as needed and tolerated to the usual maintenance dose of 2 to 6 mg daily in divided doses. The maximum dose is 10 mg daily.
   Insomnia: 2 to 4 mg at bedtime.
   Over 60 Years of Age: Sedation and anxiety: Therapy is started with 0.5 to 1 mg in divided doses. Initial dose should NOT exceed 2 mg daily.
   Insomnia: 0.5 to 1 mg at bedtime.

*See Controlled Drug Schedules inside this book's cover.

▷ **Conditions Requiring Dosing Adjustments:**
Liver function: The dose MUST be decreased for patients with liver compromise and should NOT be used by patients with liver failure.
Kidney function: This drug should NOT be used by patients with kidney failure. For patients with mild to moderate kidney compromise the dose MUST be decreased.

▷ **How Best to Take This Medicine:** The tablet may be crushed and taken on an empty stomach or with milk or food. Do NOT stop taking this drug abruptly if it has been taken for more than 4 weeks.

▷ **How Long This Medicine Is Usually Taken:** Use on a regular schedule for 3 to 5 days usually determines the effectiveness of this drug in relieving moderate anxiety or insomnia. Continual use should be limited to 1 to 3 weeks. See your doctor regularly.

▷ **Tell Your Doctor Before Taking This Medicine If You:**
- ever had an allergic reaction to it.
- have a primary depression or psychosis.
- have excessively low blood pressure.
- have narrow-angle glaucoma.
- are allergic to any benzodiazepine.
- have a history of alcoholism or drug abuse.
- are pregnant or planning pregnancy.
- have impaired liver or kidney function.
- have a history of low white blood cell counts.
- have asthma, emphysema, epilepsy, or myasthenia gravis.
- take other prescription or nonprescription medicines that were not discussed with your doctor when lorazepam was prescribed.

▷ **Possible Side Effects:** Sedation, dizziness, unsteadiness, "hangover" effects on the day following bedtime use.

▷ **Possible Adverse Effects:**
If any of the following develop, call your doctor promptly for guidance.
Some Mild Problems Drug Can Cause
Allergic reactions: rashes (rare), hives.
Dizziness, fainting, blurred vision, slurred speech, constipation, and sweating.
Insomnia or confusion.
Some Serious Problems Drug Can Cause
Allergic reactions: liver damage with jaundice (rare).
Low white blood cell counts (rare).
Paradoxical excitement and rage (rare).
Respiratory depression (dose-related).
Rare abnormal body movements, porphyria, or seizures.

▷ **Possible Effects on Sex Life:** Extremely rare decreased male libido or impotence.

▷ **Possible Effects on Laboratory Tests:** White blood cell counts: decreased.
Liver function tests: increased SGPT, SGOT, and LDH.

▷ *CAUTION*
1. This drug should NOT be stopped abruptly if it has been taken continually for more then 4 weeks.
2. Some over-the-counter medications containing antihistamines can cause excessive sedation if taken with lorazepam.
3. Lorazepam should NOT be combined with alcohol; the combination worsens adverse mental effects, decreases coordination, and increases lorazepam levels.
4. Safety and effectiveness of this drug for those under 18 years old are not established. This drug has been used under the tongue in children with serial seizures.
5. Small doses are indicated for those over 60. Watch for lethargy, fatigue, weakness, and paradoxical agitation, anger, hostility, and rage.

Advisability of Use During Pregnancy and If Breast-Feeding:
Pregnancy Category: D. Frequent use of this drug in late pregnancy can result in floppy infant syndrome in the newborn: weakness, lethargy, depressed breathing, and low body temperature. Avoid use during the entire pregnancy. Present in breast milk; avoid taking this drug or refrain from nursing.

▷ **Habit-Forming Potential:** This drug can cause psychological and/or physical dependence if taken in large doses for an extended period.

▷ **Overdose Symptoms:** Marked drowsiness, weakness, feeling of drunkenness, staggering gait, depression of breathing, stupor progressing to coma.

▷ **Suggested Periodic Examinations While Taking This Drug:** (at doctor's discretion)
Liver function tests and complete blood cell counts.

▷ **While Taking This Drug the Following Apply:**
Beverages: Avoid excessive caffeine-containing beverages: coffee, tea, cola, and chocolate.
Alcohol: Avoid this combination. Alcohol increases depression of mental function, worsens coordination, and causes increased lorazepam levels.
Tobacco Smoking: Heavy smoking may reduce this drug's calming action.

Marijuana Smoking: Additive drowsiness and impaired physical performance.

Other Drugs:

Lorazepam *taken concurrently* with

- clozapine (Clozaril) may lead to marked sedation and incoordination.
- heparin can lead to increased and unexpectedly magnified effects of lorazepam.
- lithium (Lithobid, others) may result in lowered body temperature (hypothermic reaction).
- oxycodone (Percocet, others) and other central nervous system depressants may result in additive central nervous system (CNS) or respiratory depression.
- phenytoin (Dilantin) may result in altered phenytoin or lorazepam levels.

The following drugs may *increase* the effects of lorazepam

- probenecid; increases lorazepam level by 50%.
- valproic acid (Depakene).

The following drugs may *decrease* the effects of lorazepam

- oral contraceptives (birth control pills).
- caffeine, amphetamines, or other stimulants.
- theophylline (Theo-Dur, others).

Driving, Hazardous Activities: This drug can impair alertness and coordination. Restrict your activities as necessary.

Discontinuation: Do NOT stop taking this drug suddenly if it has been taken for over 4 weeks. Consult your doctor about gradually tapering the dosage.

▷ **Saving Money When Using This Medicine:**

- Many medications are available to treat anxiety. Ask your doctor if this drug provides the best combination of cost and outcome for you, and how long this drug is usually taken to treat your condition.
- Generic forms are acceptable.
- Ask your doctor about stress management and exercise programs available in your community.

LOVASTATIN (loh vah STA tin)

Prescription: Yes   **Controlled Drug:** No   **Generic:** No

Brand Name: Mevacor

Overview of BENEFITS versus RISKS

Possible Benefits	*Possible Risks*
EFFECTIVE REDUCTION OF TOTAL BLOOD CHOLESTEROL	Drug-induced hepatitis without jaundice
	Rare drug-induced myositis, muscle inflammation
	Rare drug-induced stomach ulceration

▷ **Illness This Medication Treats:**
(1) Abnormally high total blood cholesterol levels in people with types IIa and IIb hypercholesterolemia; used in conjunction with a cholesterol-lowering diet. Lovastatin should not be used until a trial of nondrug methods for lowering cholesterol has proved to be inadequate. (2) Slows the progression of atherosclerosis in people with coronary heart disease and also reduces the number of heart attacks.

▷ **Typical Dosage Range:** (Dosage or schedule must be determined by the doctor for each individual.)
Initially 20 mg once a day; dose may be increased up to 40 mg twice a day, as needed and tolerated. Dosage adjustments should be made at 4-week intervals. The total daily dosage should not exceed 80 mg.

▷ **Conditions Requiring Dosing Adjustments:**
Liver function: Patients with liver compromise should use this drug with caution and in decreased doses.
Kidney function: Many clinicians consider 20 mg/day as a maximum dose for people with severe kidney damage (creatinine clearance less than 30 ml/min).

▷ **How Best to Take This Medicine:** Take this drug with food, preferably with the evening meal, for maximal effectiveness (the highest rates of cholesterol production occur between midnight and 5 A.M.). The tablet may be crushed.

▷ **How Long This Medicine Is Usually Taken:** 4 to 6 weeks is usually necessary to determine this drug's effectiveness in reducing blood levels of total and LDL cholesterol. Long-term use (months to years) requires periodic physician evaluation.

▷ **Tell Your Doctor Before Taking This Medicine If You:**
- ever had an allergic reaction to it.
- have active liver disease or have a history of liver disease or impaired liver function.
- have active peptic ulcer disease or a history of peptic ulcer disease or upper gastrointestinal bleeding.
- are not using any method of birth control, are planning pregnancy, or are pregnant or breast-feeding.
- have any chronic muscle disorder.
- regularly consume substantial amounts of alcohol.
- have cataracts or impaired vision.
- have any type of chronic muscular disorder.

▷ **Possible Side Effects:** Abnormal liver function tests without associated symptoms.

▷ **Possible Adverse Effects:**
If any of the following develop, call your doctor promptly for guidance.
Some Mild Problems Drug Can Cause
Allergic reactions: skin rash, itching.
Headache, dizziness, blurred vision, altered taste.
Stomach pain, nausea, excessive gas, constipation, diarrhea.
Muscle cramps and/or pain.
Some Serious Problems Drug Can Cause
Rare occurrence of marked and persistent abnormal liver function tests with focal hepatitis (without jaundice) after 1 year of use.
Rare sudden muscle damage (acute myopathy) during long-term use.
Cataracts were a concern based on some early data, but longer term data did not show lens problems.
Rare neuropathy or systemic lupus erythematosus–like syndrome.

▷ *CAUTION*
1. If pregnancy occurs while you are taking this drug, discontinue using it immediately and call your doctor.
2. Report promptly any muscle pain or tenderness, especially if accompanied by fever or malaise.
3. Report promptly the development of altered or impaired vision so that an appropriate evaluation can be made.
4. Safety and effectiveness of this drug for those under 20 years old are not established.
5. People over 60 should tell their doctor about any personal or family history of cataracts. Comply with all recommendations regarding periodic eye examinations. Report promptly any alterations in vision.

Advisability of Use During Pregnancy and If Breast-Feeding:
Pregnancy Category: X. Avoid using this drug during entire pregnancy. Probably present in breast milk. Avoid taking this drug or refrain from nursing.

▷ **Possible Effects of Long-Term Use:**   Abnormal liver function with focal hepatitis.

▷ **Suggested Periodic Examinations While Taking This Drug:** (at doctor's discretion).
Blood cholesterol studies: total cholesterol, HDL and LDL fractions.
Liver function tests every 4 to 6 weeks during the first 15 months of use and periodically thereafter.
Complete eye examination at beginning of treatment and periodically thereafter. Ask your doctor for guidance.

▷ **While Taking This Drug the Following Apply:**
Foods: Follow a standard low-cholesterol diet.
Beverages: No restrictions. This drug may be taken with milk.
Alcohol: No interactions expected. Use sparingly.
Other Drugs
Lovastatin *taken concurrently* with
• clofibrate (Atromid-S) may result in severe muscle damage.
• cyclosporine (Sandimmune) may lead to severe muscle damage.
• erythromycin (E.E.S.) and perhaps other macrolide antibiotics (see Drug Classes) may result in severe muscle damage.
• gemfibrozil (Lopid) may lead to muscle damage.
• niacin can lead to muscle damage.
• warfarin may result in bleeding. Increased frequency of INR (prothrombin time) testing is needed.
Driving, Hazardous Activities: May cause dizziness or impaired vision. Restrict your activities as necessary.
Discontinuation: Do not stop taking this drug without your doctor's knowledge and guidance.

▷ **Saving Money When Using This Medicine:**
• Many medications are available to treat elevated cholesterol. Ask your doctor if this drug provides the best combination of cost and outcome for you.
• Ask your doctor if taking aspirin every other day to help prevent a heart attack is a good idea for you.

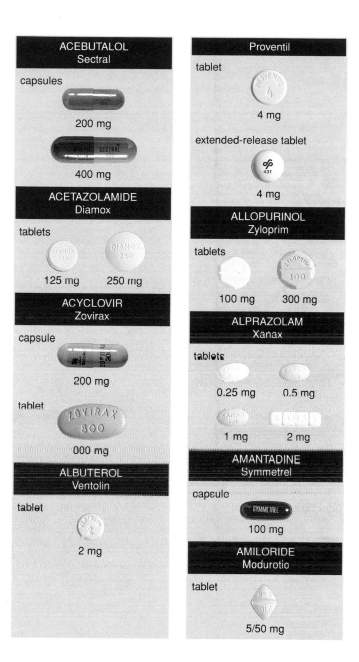

ACEBUTALOL Sectral	Proventil
capsules	**tablet**
200 mg	4 mg
400 mg	**extended-release tablet**
	4 mg
ACETAZOLAMIDE Diamox	ALLOPURINOL Zyloprim
tablets	**tablets**
125 mg 250 mg	100 mg 300 mg
ACYCLOVIR Zovirax	ALPRAZOLAM Xanax
capsule	**tablets**
200 mg	0.25 mg 0.5 mg
tablet	1 mg 2 mg
000 mg	AMANTADINE Symmetrel
ALBUTEROL Ventolin	**capsule**
tablet	100 mg
2 mg	AMILORIDE Moduretic
	tablet
	5/50 mg

AMINOPHYLLINE
Aminophylline Generic

tablet

100 mg

AMITRIPTYLINE
Elavil

tablets

10 mg

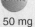

25 mg

50 mg

75 mg

100 mg   150 mg

AMLODIPINE
Norvasc

tablet

5 mg

AMOXAPINE
Asendin

tablets

25 mg   50 mg   100 mg

AMOXICILLIN
Amoxil

capsules

250 mg

500 mg

tablets, chewable

125 mg   250 mg

Polymox

capsules

250 mg

500 mg

AMOXICILLIN/CLAVULANATE
Augmentin

tablets

250/125 mg

500/125 mg

AMOXICILLIN/CLAVULANATE
Augmentin

tablet, chewable

250/62.50 mg

AMPICILLIN
Omnipen

capsule

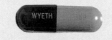

500 mg

Polycillin

capsules

250 mg

500 mg

ASTEMIZOLE
Hismanal

tablet

10 mg

ATENOLOL
Tenormin

tablets

25 mg   50 mg   100 mg

AZATHIOPRINE
Imuran

tablet

50 mg

AZITHROMYCIN
Zithromax

capsule

250 mg

BECLOMETHASONE
Beclovent

inhaler

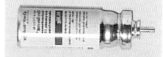

Vanceril

inhaler

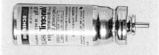

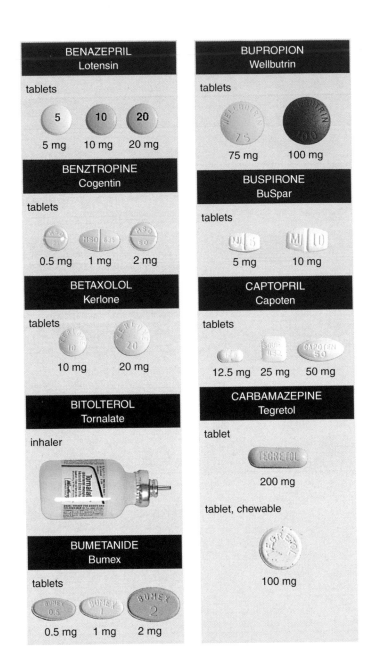

BENAZEPRIL
Lotensin

tablets

5 mg   10 mg   20 mg

BENZTROPINE
Cogentin

tablets

0.5 mg   1 mg   2 mg

BETAXOLOL
Kerlone

tablets

10 mg   20 mg

BITOLTEROL
Tornalate

inhaler

BUMETANIDE
Bumex

tablets

0.5 mg   1 mg   2 mg

BUPROPION
Wellbutrin

tablets

75 mg   100 mg

BUSPIRONE
BuSpar

tablets

5 mg   10 mg

CAPTOPRIL
Capoten

tablets

12.5 mg   25 mg   50 mg

CARBAMAZEPINE
Tegretol

tablet

200 mg

tablet, chewable

100 mg

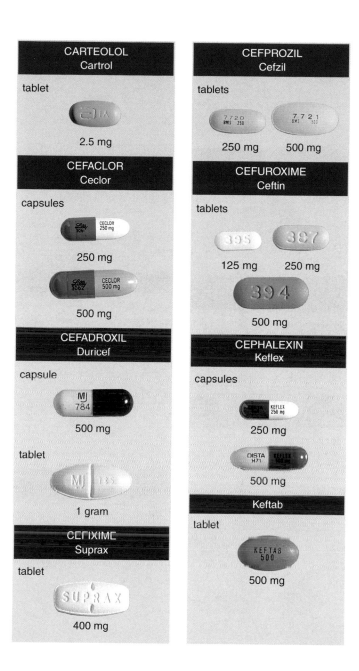

CARTEOLOL
Cartrol

tablet

2.5 mg

CEFACLOR
Ceclor

capsules

CECLOR 250 mg

250 mg

CECLOR 500 mg

500 mg

CEFADROXIL
Duricef

capsule

MJ 784

500 mg

tablet

MJ 735

1 gram

CEFIXIME
Suprax

tablet

SUPRAX

400 mg

CEFPROZIL
Cefzil

tablets

7720 BMS 250

250 mg

7721 BMS 500

500 mg

CEFUROXIME
Ceftin

tablets

395

125 mg

387

250 mg

394

500 mg

CEPHALEXIN
Keflex

capsules

KEFLEX 250 mg

250 mg

DISTA H71 KEFLEX 500 mg

500 mg

Keftab

tablet

KEFTAB 500

500 mg

| CHLORAMBUCIL | CHLORPROPAMIDE |
| Leukeran | Diabinese |

tablet

2 mg

250 mg

CHLOROQUINE
Aralen

tablet

500 mg

CHLORTHALIDONE
Hygroton

tablets

25 mg   50 mg

CHLOROTHIAZIDE
Diuril

tablets

250 mg   500 mg

CHOLESTYRAMINE

Questran Light

Questran Powder

CHLORPROMAZINE
Thorazine

capsules, extended-release

75 mg

150 mg

tablets

100 mg   200 mg

CIMETIDINE
Tagamet

tablets

200 mg   300 mg

400 mg   800 mg

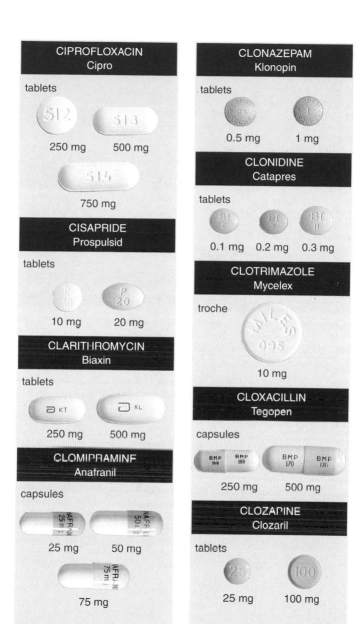

CIPROFLOXACIN
Cipro

tablets

250 mg   500 mg

750 mg

CISAPRIDE
Prospulsid

tablets

10 mg   20 mg

CLARITHROMYCIN
Biaxin

tablets

250 mg   500 mg

CLOMIPRAMINE
Anafranil

capsules

25 mg   50 mg

75 mg

CLONAZEPAM
Klonopin

tablets

0.5 mg   1 mg

CLONIDINE
Catapres

tablets

0.1 mg   0.2 mg   0.3 mg

CLOTRIMAZOLE
Mycelex

troche

10 mg

CLOXACILLIN
Tegopen

capsules

250 mg   500 mg

CLOZAPINE
Clozaril

tablets

25 mg   100 mg

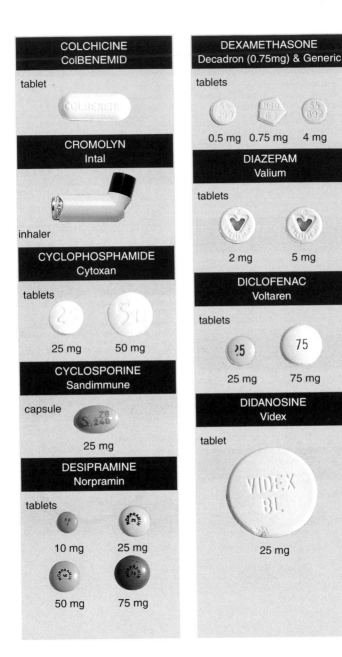

COLCHICINE
ColBENEMID

tablet

CROMOLYN
Intal

inhaler

CYCLOPHOSPHAMIDE
Cytoxan

tablets

25 mg   50 mg

CYCLOSPORINE
Sandimmune

capsule

25 mg

DESIPRAMINE
Norpramin

tablets

10 mg   25 mg

50 mg   75 mg

DEXAMETHASONE
Decadron (0.75mg) & Generic

tablets

0.5 mg   0.75 mg   4 mg

DIAZEPAM
Valium

tablets

2 mg   5 mg

DICLOFENAC
Voltaren

tablets

25 mg   75 mg

DIDANOSINE
Videx

tablet

25 mg

| DIFLUNISAL | Cardizem CD |
| Dolobid | capsules |

tablets

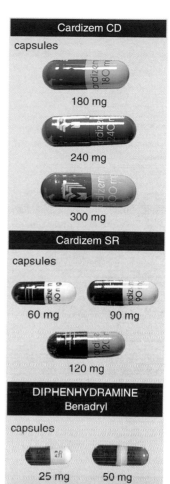

DOLOBID 250 mg   DOLOBID 500 mg

DIGOXIN
Lanoxicaps

capsules

0.1 mg   0.2 mg

Lanoxin

tablets

0.125 mg   0.25 mg   0.5 mg

DILTIAZEM
Cardizem

tablets

30 mg   60 mg

90 mg

120 mg

Cardizem CD

capsules

180 mg

240 mg

300 mg

Cardizem SR

capsules

60 mg   90 mg

120 mg

DIPHENHYDRAMINE
Benadryl

capsules

25 mg   50 mg

DIPYRIDAMOLE
Persantine

tablets

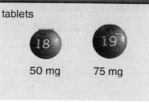

50 mg   75 mg

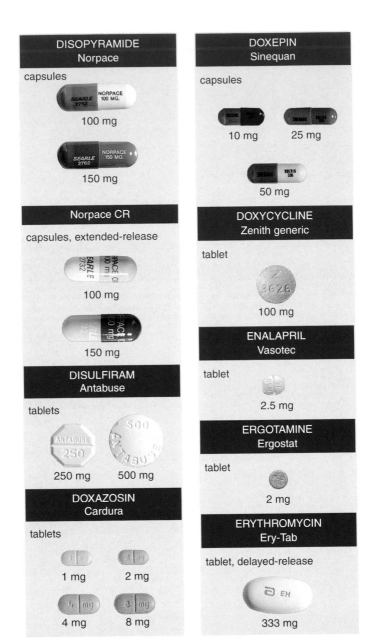

DISOPYRAMIDE
Norpace

capsules

100 mg

150 mg

Norpace CR

capsules, extended-release

100 mg

150 mg

DISULFIRAM
Antabuse

tablets

250 mg   500 mg

DOXAZOSIN
Cardura

tablets

1 mg   2 mg

4 mg   8 mg

DOXEPIN
Sinequan

capsules

10 mg   25 mg

50 mg

DOXYCYCLINE
Zenith generic

tablet

100 mg

ENALAPRIL
Vasotec

tablet

2.5 mg

ERGOTAMINE
Ergostat

tablet

2 mg

ERYTHROMYCIN
Ery-Tab

tablet, delayed-release

333 mg

E-Mycin

tablets, delayed-release

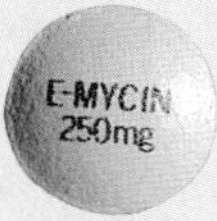

250 mg 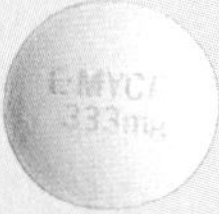   333 mg

Eryc

capsule, delayed-release

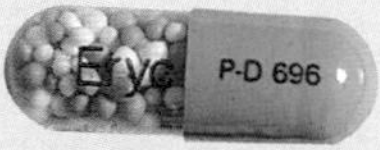

250 mg

Erythrocin

tablets

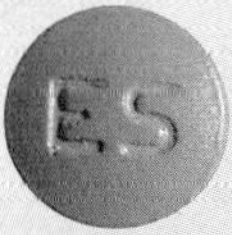

250 mg 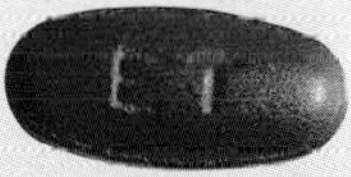   500 mg

ESTROGENS
Estrace

tablets

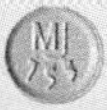

1 mg 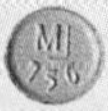   2 mg

Ogen

tablets

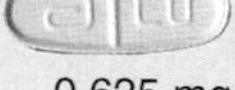

0.625 mg 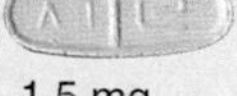   1.5 mg

Premarin

tablets

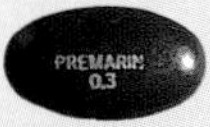

0.3 mg 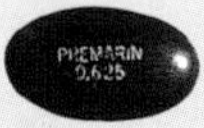   0.625 mg

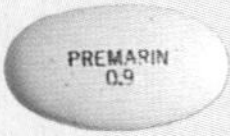

0.9 mg 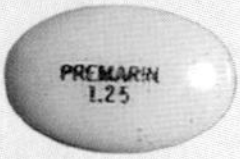   1.25 mg

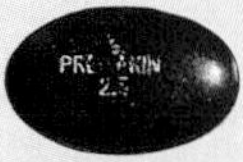

2.5 mg

ETHAMBUTOL
Myambutol

tablet

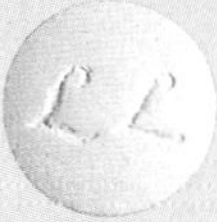

400 mg

ETHOSUXIMIDE
Zarontin

capsule

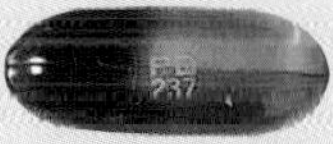

250 mg

ETRETINATE
Tegison

capsule

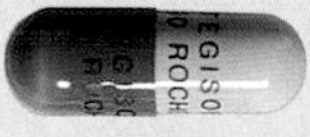

10 mg

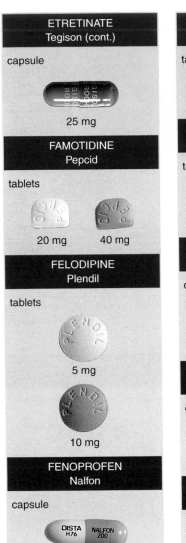

ETRETINATE
Tegison (cont.)

capsule

25 mg

FAMOTIDINE
Pepcid

tablets

20 mg   40 mg

FELODIPINE
Plendil

tablets

5 mg

10 mg

FENOPROFEN
Nalfon

capsule

200 mg

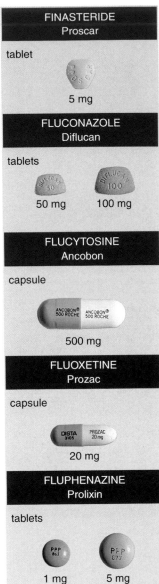

FINASTERIDE
Proscar

tablet

5 mg

FLUCONAZOLE
Diflucan

tablets

50 mg   100 mg

FLUCYTOSINE
Ancobon

capsule

500 mg

FLUOXETINE
Prozac

capsule

20 mg

FLUPHENAZINE
Prolixin

tablets

1 mg   5 mg

FLURAZEPAM
Dalmane

capsules

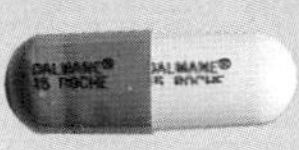

15 mg

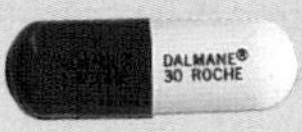

30 mg

FLURBIPROFEN
Ansaid

tablets

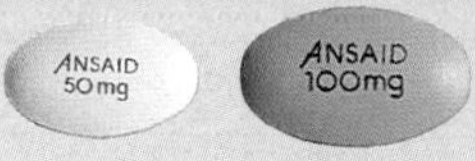

50 mg   100 mg

FLUTAMIDE
Eulexin

capsule

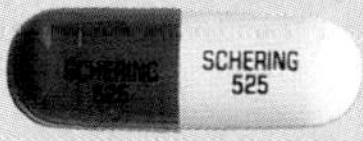

125 mg

FOSINOPRIL
Monopril

tablets

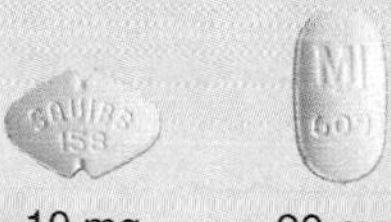

10 mg   20 mg

FUROSEMIDE
Lasix

tablets

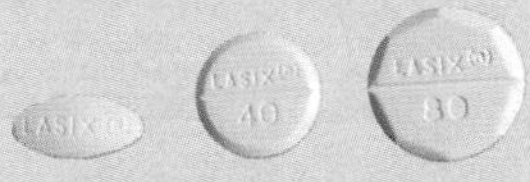

20 mg   40 mg   80 mg

GEMFIBROZIL
Lopid

tablet

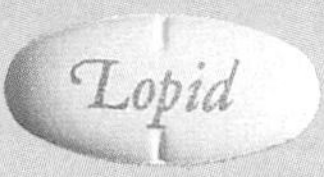

600 mg

GLIPIZIDE
Glucotrol

tablets

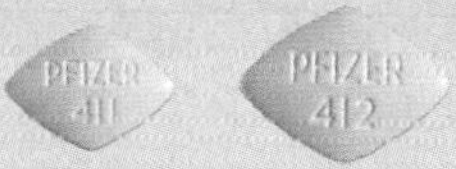

5 mg   10 mg

GLYBURIDE
DiaBeta

tablets

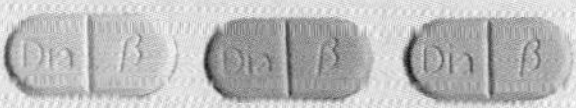

1.25 mg   2.5 mg   5 mg

Micronase

tablets

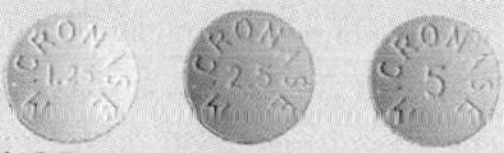

1.25 mg   2.5 mg   5 mg

GRISEOFULVIN
Fulvicin P/G

tablets

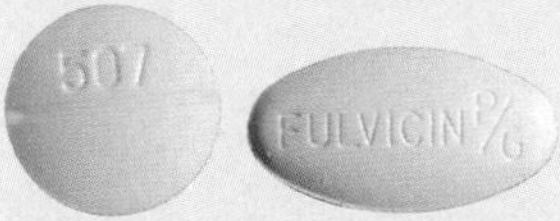

250 mg   330 mg

GUANFACINE
Tenex

tablets

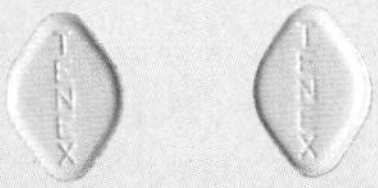

1 mg   2 mg

HALOPERIDOL
Haldol

tablets

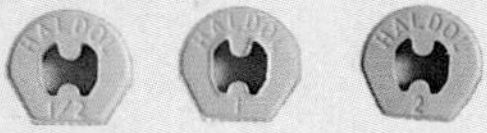

0.5 mg   1 mg   2 mg

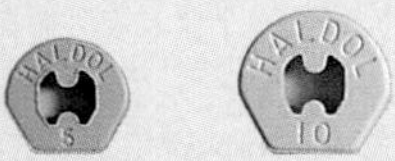

5 mg   10 mg

HYDRALAZINE
Apresoline

tablet

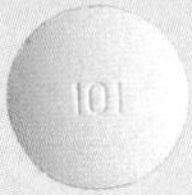

100 mg

HYDROCHLOROTHIAZIDE
Esidrix

tablets

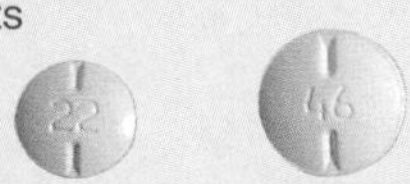

25 mg   50 mg

HYDROCODONE
(& acetaminophen)
Vicodin

tablet

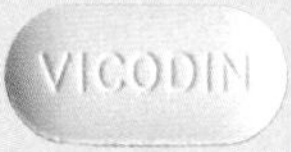

5/500 mg

Vicodin ES

tablet

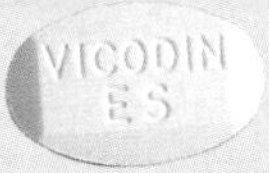

7.5/750 mg

HYDROXYCHLOROQUINE
Plaquenil

tablet

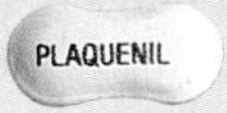

200 mg

IBUPROFEN
Motrin

tablets

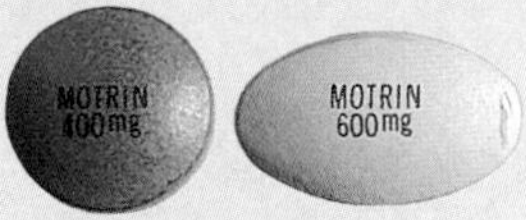

400 mg   600 mg

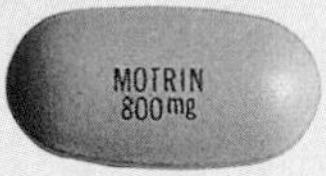

800 mg

IMIPRAMINE
Tofranil

tablets

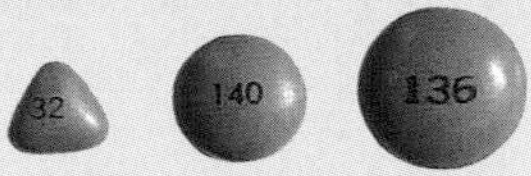

10 mg   25 mg   50 mg

Tofranil-PM

capsule

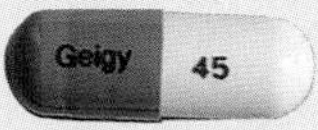

125 mg

INDAPAMIDE
Lozol

tablet

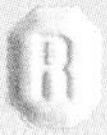

2.5 mg

INDOMETHACIN
Indocin

capsules

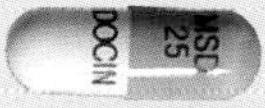

25 mg

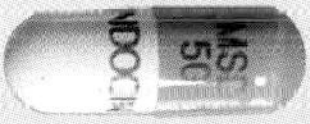

50 mg

Indocin SR

capsule

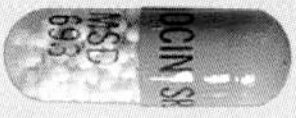

75 mg

ISONIAZID
INH

tablet

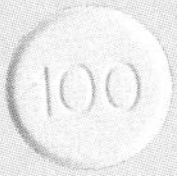

100 mg

ISOSORBIDE DINITRATE
Isordil

tablets

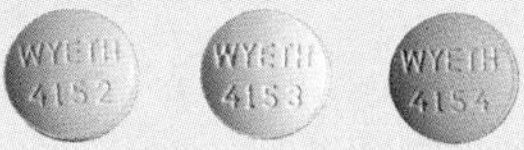

5 mg   10 mg   20 mg

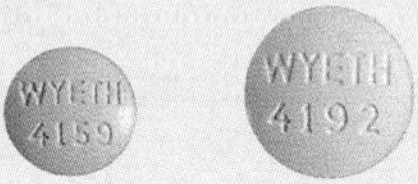

30 mg   40 mg

tablet, extended-release

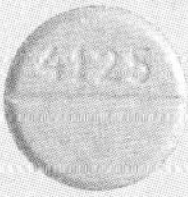

40 mg

tablet, sublingual

5 mg

ISOSORBIDE MONONITRATE
Ismo

tablet

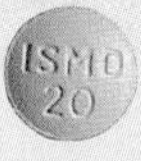

20 mg

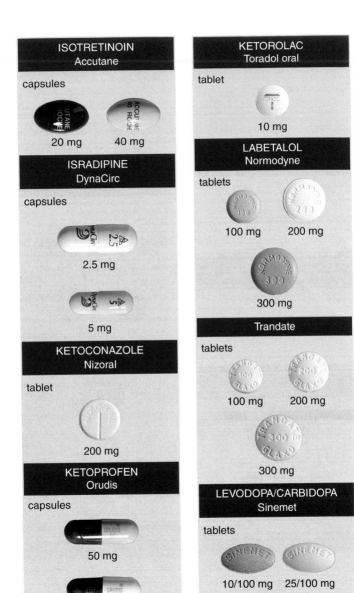

ISOTRETINOIN
Accutane

capsules

20 mg   40 mg

ISRADIPINE
DynaCirc

capsules

2.5 mg

5 mg

KETOCONAZOLE
Nizoral

tablet

200 mg

KETOPROFEN
Orudis

capsules

50 mg

75 mg

KETOROLAC
Toradol oral

tablet

10 mg

LABETALOL
Normodyne

tablets

100 mg   200 mg

300 mg

Trandate

tablets

100 mg   200 mg

300 mg

LEVODOPA/CARBIDOPA
Sinemet

tablets

10/100 mg   25/100 mg

Sinemet (cont.)

tablet

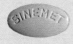

25/250 mg

Sinemet CR

tablet, sustained-release

50/200 mg

LEVOTHYROXINE
Synthroid

tablets

0.025 mg 0.05 mg 0.075 mg

0.1 mg 0.112 mg 0.125 mg

0.15 mg 0.175 mg

LIOTHYRONINE
Cytomel

tablets

5 mcg 25 mcg

LISINOPRIL
Prinivil

tablets

5 mg 10 mg 20 mg

Zestril

tablets

5 mg 10 mg 20 mg

LITHIUM
Eskalith CR

tablet, controlled-release

450 mg

Lithobid

tablet

300 mg

LOMEFLOXACIN
Maxaquin

tablet

400 mg

LOVASTATIN
Mevacor

tablets

20 mg   40 mg

MAPROTILINE
Ludiomil

tablets

25 mg   50 mg

MECLOFENAMATE
Meclomen

capsule

100 mg

MEDROXYPROGESTERONE
Provera

tablets

2.5 mg   5 mg   10 mg

MEPERIDINE
Demerol

tablets

50 mg   100 mg

MERCAPTOPURINE
Purinethol

tablet

50 mg

MESALAMINE
Asacol

tablet

400 mg

METAPROTERENOL
Alupent

tablet

20 mg

METFORMIN
Glucophage

tablets

500 mg   850 mg

METHOTREXATE
Lederle generic

tablet

2.5 mg

METHYLPHENIDATE
Ritalin

tablets

5 mg   10 mg   20 mg

METHYLPREDNISOLONE
Medrol

tablet

4 mg

METOCLOPRAMIDE
Reglan

tablets

5 mg   10 mg

METOLAZONE
Zaroxolyn

tablets

2.5 mg   5 mg

METOPROLOL
Lopressor

tablets

50 mg   100 mg

Toprol XL

tablets, extended-release

50 mg   100 mg

METRONIDAZOLE
Flagyl

tablets

250 mg   500 mg

MEXILETINE
Mexitil

capsules

150 mg

200 mg

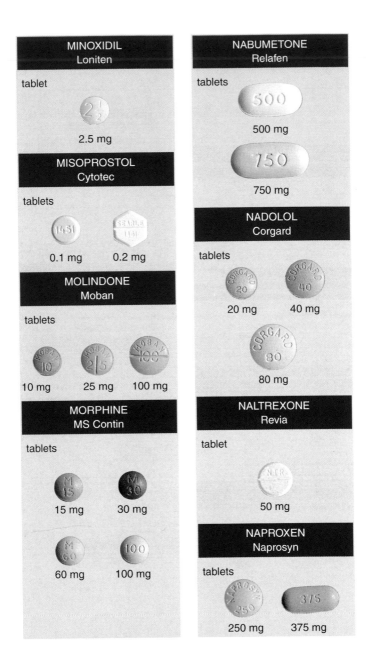

MINOXIDIL
Loniten

tablet

2.5 mg

MISOPROSTOL
Cytotec

tablets

0.1 mg   0.2 mg

MOLINDONE
Moban

tablets

10 mg   25 mg   100 mg

MORPHINE
MS Contin

tablets

15 mg   30 mg

60 mg   100 mg

NABUMETONE
Relafen

tablets

500 mg

750 mg

NADOLOL
Corgard

tablets

20 mg   40 mg

80 mg

NALTREXONE
Revia

tablet

50 mg

NAPROXEN
Naprosyn

tablets

250 mg   375 mg

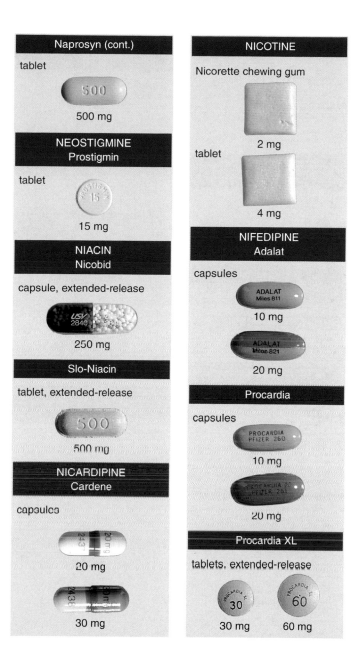

Naprosyn (cont.)	**NICOTINE**
tablet	Nicorette chewing gum
500 mg	2 mg
NEOSTIGMINE Prostigmin	tablet
tablet	4 mg
15 mg	**NIFEDIPINE** Adalat
NIACIN Nicobid	capsules
capsule, extended-release	ADALAT Miles 811 10 mg
250 mg	ADALAT Miles 821 20 mg
Slo-Niacin	**Procardia**
tablet, extended-release	capsules
500 mg	PROCARDIA PFIZER 260 10 mg
NICARDIPINE Cardene	PROCARDIA 20 PFIZER 261 20 mg
capsules	**Procardia XL**
20 mg	tablets, extended-release
30 mg	30 mg 60 mg

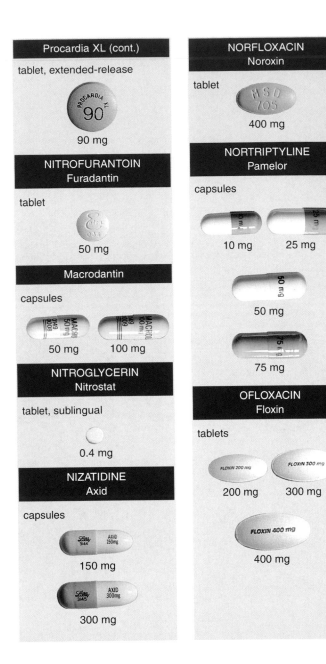

Procardia XL (cont.)

tablet, extended-release

PROCARDIA XL
90

90 mg

NITROFURANTOIN
Furadantin

tablet

50 mg

Macrodantin

capsules

50 mg   100 mg

NITROGLYCERIN
Nitrostat

tablet, sublingual

0.4 mg

NIZATIDINE
Axid

capsules

AXID
150mg

150 mg

AXID
300mg

300 mg

NORFLOXACIN
Noroxin

tablet

MSD
705

400 mg

NORTRIPTYLINE
Pamelor

capsules

10 mg   25 mg

50 mg

75 mg

OFLOXACIN
Floxin

tablets

FLOXIN 200 mg   FLOXIN 300 mg

200 mg   300 mg

FLOXIN 400 mg

400 mg

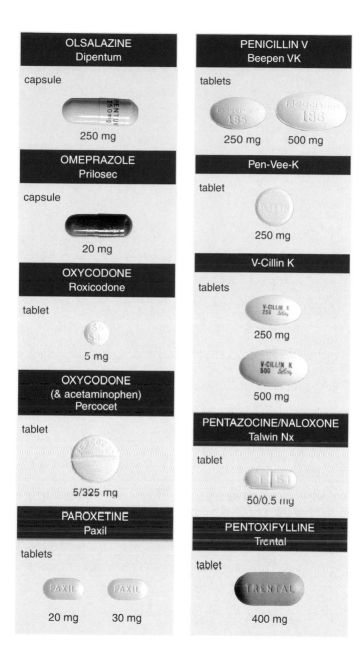

OLSALAZINE
Dipentum

capsule

250 mg

OMEPRAZOLE
Prilosec

capsule

20 mg

OXYCODONE
Roxicodone

tablet

5 mg

OXYCODONE
(& acetaminophen)
Percocet

tablet

5/325 mg

PAROXETINE
Paxil

tablets

20 mg   30 mg

PENICILLIN V
Beepen VK

tablets

250 mg   500 mg

Pen-Vee-K

tablet

250 mg

V-Cillin K

tablets

250 mg

500 mg

PENTAZOCINE/NALOXONE
Talwin Nx

tablet

50/0.5 mg

PENTOXIFYLLINE
Trental

tablet

400 mg

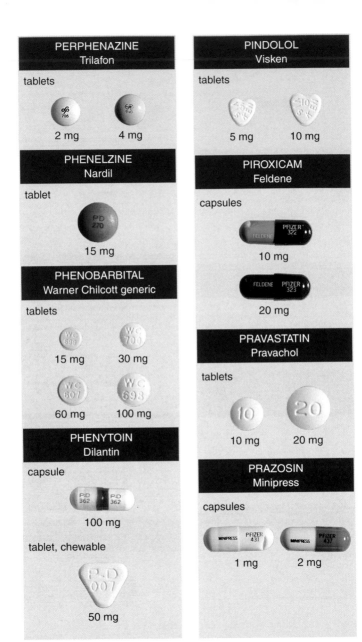

PERPHENAZINE
Trilafon

tablets

2 mg   4 mg

PHENELZINE
Nardil

tablet

PD
270

15 mg

PHENOBARBITAL
Warner Chilcott generic

tablets

WC
699
15 mg

WC
700
30 mg

WC
607
60 mg

WC
698
100 mg

PHENYTOIN
Dilantin

capsule

P-D
362   P-D
362
100 mg

tablet, chewable

P-D
007
50 mg

PINDOLOL
Visken

tablets

5 mg   10 mg

PIROXICAM
Feldene

capsules

FELDENE   PFIZER
322
10 mg

FELDENE   PFIZER
323
20 mg

PRAVASTATIN
Pravachol

tablets

10   20
10 mg   20 mg

PRAZOSIN
Minipress

capsules

MINIPRESS   PFIZER
431
1 mg

MINIPRESS   PFIZER
437
2 mg

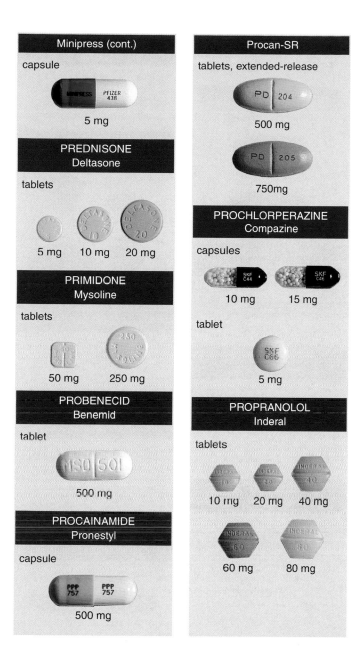

Minipress (cont.)

capsule

5 mg

PREDNISONE
Deltasone

tablets

5 mg   10 mg   20 mg

PRIMIDONE
Mysoline

tablets

50 mg   250 mg

PROBENECID
Benemid

tablet

500 mg

PROCAINAMIDE
Pronestyl

capsule

500 mg

Procan-SR

tablets, extended-release

500 mg

750mg

PROCHLORPERAZINE
Compazine

capsules

10 mg   15 mg

tablet

5 mg

PROPRANOLOL
Inderal

tablets

10 mg   20 mg   40 mg

60 mg   80 mg

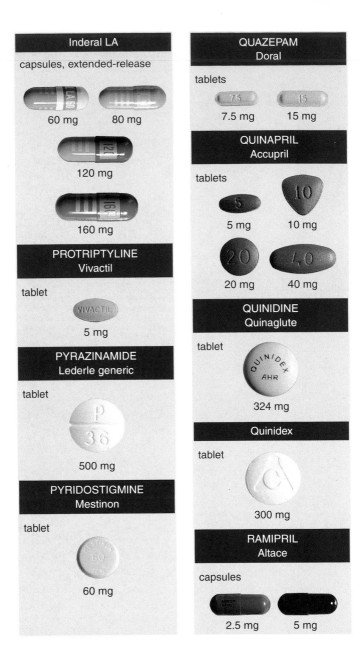

Inderal LA capsules, extended-release 60 mg 80 mg 120 mg 160 mg	**QUAZEPAM** Doral tablets 7.5 mg 15 mg
PROTRIPTYLINE Vivactil tablet VIVACTIL 5 mg	**QUINAPRIL** Accupril tablets 5 10 5 mg 10 mg 20 40 20 mg 40 mg
PYRAZINAMIDE Lederle generic tablet P 36 500 mg	**QUINIDINE** Quinaglute tablet QUINIDEX AHR 324 mg
PYRIDOSTIGMINE Mestinon tablet 60 60 mg	**Quinidex** tablet 300 mg
	RAMIPRIL Altace capsules 2.5 mg 5 mg

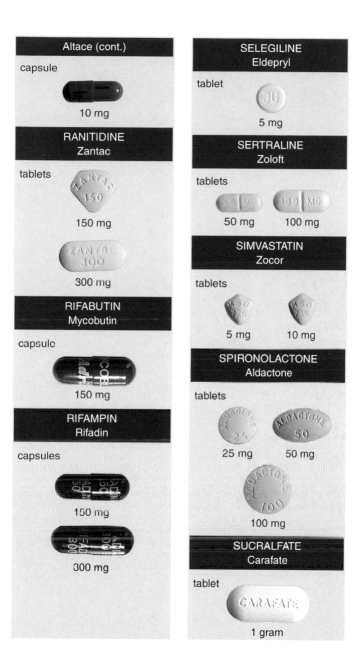

Altace (cont.)

capsule

10 mg

RANITIDINE
Zantac

tablets

ZANTAC 150

150 mg

ZANTAC 300

300 mg

RIFABUTIN
Mycobutin

capsule

150 mg

RIFAMPIN
Rifadin

capsules

150 mg

300 mg

SELEGILINE
Eldepryl

tablet

JU

5 mg

SERTRALINE
Zoloft

tablets

50 mg   100 mg

SIMVASTATIN
Zocor

tablets

5 mg   10 mg

SPIRONOLACTONE
Aldactone

tablets

ALDACTONE 25   ALDACTONE 50

25 mg   50 mg

ALDACTONE 100

100 mg

SUCRALFATE
Carafate

tablet

CARAFATE

1 gram

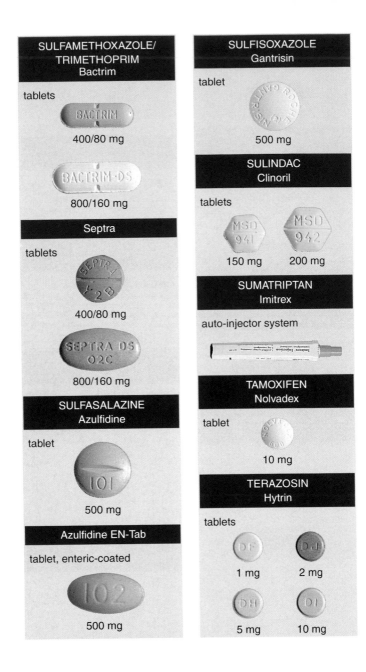

SULFAMETHOXAZOLE/ TRIMETHOPRIM
Bactrim

tablets

BACTRIM

400/80 mg

BACTRIM-DS

800/160 mg

Septra

tablets

SEPTRA Y 2 B

400/80 mg

SEPTRA DS O2C

800/160 mg

SULFASALAZINE
Azulfidine

tablet

101

500 mg

Azulfidine EN-Tab

tablet, enteric-coated

102

500 mg

SULFISOXAZOLE
Gantrisin

tablet

GANTRISIN ROCHE

500 mg

SULINDAC
Clinoril

tablets

MSD 941

150 mg

MSD 942

200 mg

SUMATRIPTAN
Imitrex

auto-injector system

TAMOXIFEN
Nolvadex

tablet

NOLVA 600

10 mg

TERAZOSIN
Hytrin

tablets

DF

1 mg

DJ

2 mg

DH

5 mg

DI

10 mg

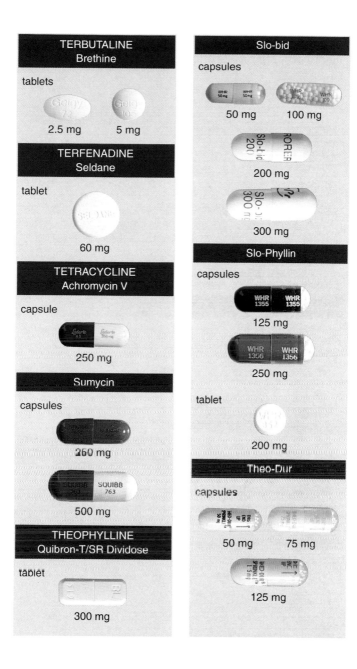

TERBUTALINE
Brethine

tablets

2.5 mg   5 mg

TERFENADINE
Seldane

tablet

60 mg

TETRACYCLINE
Achromycin V

capsule

250 mg

Sumycin

capsules

250 mg

500 mg

THEOPHYLLINE
Quibron-T/SR Dividose

tablet

300 mg

Slo-bid

capsules

50 mg   100 mg

200 mg

300 mg

Slo-Phyllin

capsules

125 mg

250 mg

tablet

200 mg

Theo-Dur

capsules

50 mg   75 mg

125 mg

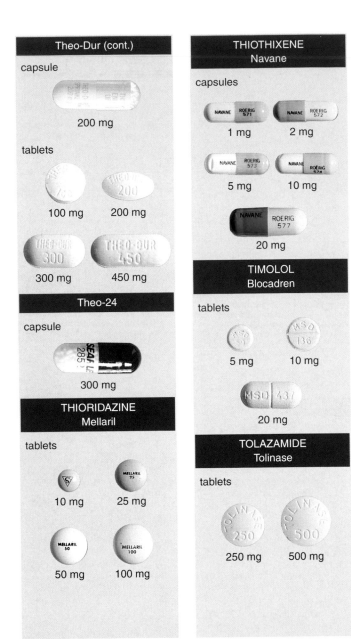

Theo-Dur (cont.)

capsule

200 mg

tablets

100 mg

200 mg

300 mg

450 mg

Theo-24

capsule

300 mg

THIORIDAZINE
Mellaril

tablets

10 mg

25 mg

50 mg

100 mg

THIOTHIXENE
Navane

capsules

1 mg

2 mg

5 mg

10 mg

20 mg

TIMOLOL
Blocadren

tablets

5 mg

10 mg

20 mg

TOLAZAMIDE
Tolinase

tablets

250 mg

500 mg

TOLBUTAMIDE	TRIAMTERENE/
Orinase	HYDROCHLOROTHIAZIDE
	Dyazide

TOLBUTAMIDE
Orinase

tablet

500 mg

TOLMETIN
Tolectin

tablet

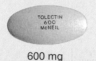

600 mg

Tolectin DS

capsule

400 mg

TRAZODONE
Desyrel

tablets

50 mg   100 mg

150 mg

TRIAMTERENE/ HYDROCHLOROTHIAZIDE
Dyazide

capsule

50/25 mg

Maxzide

tablets

37.5/25 mg   75/50 mg

TRIFLUOPERAZINE
Stelazine

tablets

1 mg   2 mg   5 mg

TRIMETHOPRIM
Trimpox

tablet

100 mg

VALPROIC ACID
Depakote Sprinkle

capsule

125 mg

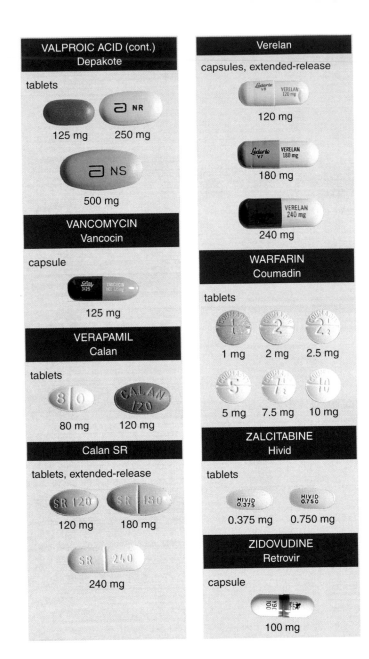

VALPROIC ACID (cont.)
Depakote

tablets

125 mg   250 mg

500 mg

VANCOMYCIN
Vancocin

capsule

125 mg

VERAPAMIL
Calan

tablets

80 mg   120 mg

Calan SR

tablets, extended-release

120 mg   180 mg

240 mg

Verelan

capsules, extended-release

120 mg

180 mg

240 mg

WARFARIN
Coumadin

tablets

1 mg   2 mg   2.5 mg

5 mg   7.5 mg   10 mg

ZALCITABINE
Hivid

tablets

0.375 mg   0.750 mg

ZIDOVUDINE
Retrovir

capsule

100 mg

MAPROTILINE (ma PROH ti leen)

Prescription: Yes **Controlled Drug:** No **Generic:** No
Brand Name: Ludiomil

Overview of BENEFITS versus RISKS	
Possible Benefits	*Possible Risks*
EFFECTIVE RELIEF OF ALL TYPES OF DEPRESSION	ADVERSE BEHAVIORAL EFFECTS
	CONVERSION OF DEPRESSION TO MANIA in manic-depressive disorders
	Irregular heart rhythms
	Rare liver toxicity with jaundice
	Rare seizures with therapeutic doses
	Rare lowered white blood cells

▷ **Illness This Medication Treats:**

Symptoms of spontaneous (endogenous) depression and reactive depressions. This drug is used only when a diagnosis of true depression of significant degree has been established; not for mild and transient despondency associated with many life situations.

Other (unlabeled) generally accepted uses: used to help bed-wetting in children.

▷ **Typical Dosage Range:** (Dosage or schedule must be determined by the doctor for each individual.)

Initially 25 mg three times daily. Dose may be increased cautiously, as needed and tolerated, by 10 to 25 mg daily at intervals of 1 week. Usual maintenance dose is 50 to 100 mg every 24 hours. The total daily dose should not exceed 150 mg. When the optimal requirement is determined, it may be taken at bedtime as one dose.

Bed-wetting (children 6 to 14 years old): Start at 10 mg/day and slowly increase as needed and tolerated.

▷ **Conditions Requiring Dosing Adjustments:**

Liver function: This drug should be used with caution, and the dose empirically decreased, by patients with liver compromise.

Kidney function: Dosage adjustments are not indicated for patients with kidney compromise. Patients with urine outflow problems should use this drug with caution, as maprotiline may worsen the problem.

▷ **How Best to Take This Medicine:** Tablet may be crushed and taken without regard to meals.

▷ **How Long This Medicine Is Usually Taken:**   Some benefit may be apparent within 2 weeks, but adequate response may require continual use of this drug for 4 to 6 weeks or longer. Long-term use should not exceed 6 months without evaluation regarding the need for continuation. See your doctor regularly.

▷ **Tell Your Doctor Before Taking This Medicine If You:**
- ever had an allergic reaction to it.
- are taking, or have taken within the past 14 days, any MAO type A inhibitor.
- are recovering from a recent heart attack.
- are allergic or overly sensitive to any tricyclic antidepressant.
- are nursing your infant.
- have a history of any of the following: alcoholism, asthma, epilepsy, glaucoma, heart disease, paranoia, prostate gland enlargement, schizophrenia, or overactive thyroid function.
- have impaired liver function.
- plan to have surgery under general anesthesia soon.

▷ **Possible Side Effects:**   Drowsiness, blurred vision, dry mouth, constipation, impaired urination.

▷ **Possible Adverse Effects:**
If any of the following develop, call your doctor promptly for guidance.
Some Mild Problems Drug Can Cause
   Allergic reactions: skin rash, itching.
   Insomnia, nervousness, palpitations, dizziness, tremors, fainting, weakness.
   Nausea, vomiting, acid indigestion, diarrhea.
   Increased sweating.
Some Serious Problems Drug Can Cause
   Behavioral effects: anxiety, confusion, hallucinations.
   Aggravation of paranoid psychosis and schizophrenia.
   Aggravation of seizure disorders (epilepsy).
   Liver toxicity with jaundice.
   Rare decreased white blood cells or myoclonus.

▷ **Possible Effects on Sex Life:**   Decreased libido, increased libido (antidepressant effect), impotence, male breast enlargement and tenderness, female breast enlargement with milk production, swelling of testicles.

▷ *CAUTION*
   1. Dosage must be adjusted for each person individually. Report for follow-up evaluation and laboratory tests as directed by your doctor.

2. Watch for early indications of toxicity: confusion, agitation, rapid heartbeat.

3. Maprotiline should be withheld if electroconvulsive therapy is to be used to treat your depression.

4. Safety and effectiveness of this drug for those under 18 years old are not established.

5. For those over 60, during the first 2 weeks of treatment look for confusion, agitation, forgetfulness, disorientation, delusions, and hallucinations; reduction of dosage or discontinuation may be necessary. Unsteadiness may predispose to falling and injury. This drug can increase the degree of impaired urination associated with prostate gland enlargement.

Advisability of Use During Pregnancy and If Breast-Feeding:

Pregnancy Category: B. Avoid use during first 3 months. Use this drug during the last 6 months only if clearly needed. Present in breast milk. Monitor the nursing infant closely for drowsiness or failure to feed properly; discontinue drug or nursing if adverse effects develop.

▷ **Overdose Symptoms:** Confusion, hallucinations, marked drowsiness, heart palpitations, dilated pupils, tremors, stupor, deep sleep, coma, convulsions.

▷ **Suggested Periodic Examinations While Taking This Drug:** (at doctor's discretion)

Complete blood cell counts, liver function tests, serial blood pressure readings, and electrocardiograms.

▷ **While Taking This Drug the Following Apply:**

Beverages: May be taken with milk.

Alcohol: Avoid completely. This drug can markedly increase the intoxicating effects of alcohol and accentuate its depressant action on brain function.

Marijuana Smoking: Increased drowsiness and dryness of mouth; possible reduced effectiveness of this drug.

Other Drugs:

Maprotiline may *increase* the effects of

• atropinelike drugs.

• all drugs with sedative effects, causing excessive sedation.

Maprotiline may *decrease* the effects of

• clonidine (Catapres).

• guanethidine (Ismelin).

• methyldopa (Aldomet).

• reserpine (Serpasil, Ser-Ap-Es, etc.).

Maprotiline *taken concurrently* with

• amphetaminelike drugs may cause severe high blood pressure and/or high fever.

- antiseizure drugs requires careful monitoring for change in seizure patterns; dosage adjustments may be necessary.
- carbamazepine (Tegretol) may increase the carbamazepine level, causing potential carbamazepine toxicity and also blunting the therapeutic benefits of maprotiline.
- ethchlorvynol (Placidyl) may cause delirium; avoid concurrent use.
- MAO type A inhibitors may cause high fever, delirium, and convulsions.
- quinidine (Quinaglute, others) may lead to maprotiline toxicity. Doses may need to be reduced.
- thyroid preparations may impair heart rhythm and function.
- tricyclic antidepressants (TCAs) may result in increased antidepressant levels and maprotiline toxicity.

Ask your doctor for guidance regarding adjustment of thyroid dose.

The following drugs may **decrease** the effects of maprotiline

- estrogens.
- oral contraceptives (birth control pills).

Driving, Hazardous Activities: This drug may impair mental alertness, judgment, physical coordination, and reaction time. Avoid hazardous activities.

Exposure to Sun: Use caution until your sensitivity to the sun has been determined. This drug may cause photosensitivity.

Exposure to Heat: This drug can inhibit sweating and impair the body's adaptation to hot environments, increasing the risk of heatstroke. Avoid saunas.

Exposure to Cold: The elderly should use caution and avoid conditions conducive to hypothermia.

Discontinuation: It is advisable to discontinue this drug gradually. Abrupt withdrawal after long-term use may cause headache, malaise, and nausea.

▷ **Saving Money When Using This Medicine:**

- Many medications are available to treat depression. Ask your doctor if this drug provides the best combination of cost and outcome for you.
- Depression has recently been associated with osteoporosis. Ask your doctor about calcium supplements, exercise, and risk factors. Bone mineral density testing may also be needed.

MECLOFENAMATE (me kloh fen AM ayt)

Prescription: Yes   **Controlled Drug:** No   **Generic:** Yes

Brand Names: Meclodium, Meclomen

Overview of BENEFITS versus RISKS	
Possible Benefits	*Possible Risks*
EFFECTIVE RELIEF OF MILD TO MODERATE PAIN AND INFLAMMATION	Gastrointestinal pain, ulceration, bleeding (rare)
	Kidney damage (rare)
	Fluid retention (rare)
	Bone marrow depression (rare)

See the fenamate (NSAIDs) drug profile for further information.

MEDROXYPROGESTERONE (me DROX ee proh JESS te rohn)

Prescription: Yes   **Controlled Drug:** No   **Generic:** Yes

Brand Names: Amen, Curretab, Depo-Provera, Premphase, Prempro, Provera

Overview of BENEFITS versus RISKS	
Possible Benefits	*Possible Risks*
EFFECTIVE TREATMENT OF ABSENT OR ABNORMAL MENSTRUATION due to hormone imbalance	Thrombophlebitis (rare)
	Pulmonary embolism (rare)
	Liver reaction with jaundice (rare)
EFFECTIVE CONTRACEPTION when taken by injection	Drug-induced birth defects
Useful adjunctive therapy in selected cases of uterine and kidney cancer	

▷ **Illness This Medication Treats:**

(1) Initiation and regulation of menstruation and correction of abnormal patterns of bleeding caused by hormonal imbalance (not organic disease); (2) metastatic, inoperable, or recurrent endometrial cancer; (3) kidney cancer; (4) as a contraceptive injected into the muscle once every 3 months: (5) helps dysfunctional uterine bleeding.

▷ **Typical Dosage Range:** (Dosage or schedule must be determined by the doctor for each individual.)

To initiate menstruation: 5 to 10 mg every day for 5 to 10 days, started at any time. To correct abnormal bleeding: 5 to 10 mg every day for 5 to 10 days, started on the 16th or 21st day of the menstrual cycle. Withdrawal bleeding usually begins within 3 to 7 days after the drug is stopped.

As a contraceptive: Intramuscular injections of 150 mg every 3 months.

▷ **Conditions Requiring Dosing Adjustments:**

Liver function: This drug should be used with caution, and the dose empirically decreased, by patients with liver compromise.

▷ **How Best to Take This Medicine:** Take this drug on an empty stomach or with food to prevent nausea. The tablet may be crushed.

▷ **How Long This Medicine Is Usually Taken:** Continual use on a regular schedule for two or three menstrual cycles is usually necessary to determine the effectiveness of this drug in correcting abnormal patterns of menstrual bleeding. See your doctor regularly.

▷ **Tell Your Doctor Before Taking This Medicine If You:**
- ever had an allergic reaction to it.
- are pregnant.
- have seriously impaired liver function.
- have a history of cancer of the breast or reproductive organs.
- have a history of thrombophlebitis, embolism, or stroke.
- have abnormal and unexplained vaginal bleeding.
- have impaired kidney function.
- have asthma, diabetes, emotional depression, epilepsy, heart disease, or migraine headaches.

▷ **Possible Side Effects:** Fluid retention, weight gain, changes in menstrual timing and flow, spotting between periods.

▷ **Possible Adverse Effects:**

If any of the following develop, call your doctor promptly for guidance.

Some Mild Problems Drug Can Cause

Allergic reactions: skin rash, itching.

Fatigue, weakness, nausea.

Acne, excessive hair growth.

Some Serious Problems Drug Can Cause

Liver toxicity with jaundice: yellow eyes and skin, dark-colored urine, light-colored stools.

Thrombophlebitis: pain or tenderness in thigh or leg.

Pulmonary embolism: sudden shortness of breath, chest pain, cough, bloody sputum.

Stroke: sudden headache, blackouts, sudden weakness or paralysis of any part of the body, inability to speak.

Retinal thrombosis: sudden impairment or loss of vision.

Pneumonitis, especially in patients who have had radiation therapy.

▷ **Possible Effects on Sex Life:** Altered timing and pattern of menstruation.

Female breast tenderness and secretion.

Decreased vaginal secretions, infertility.

▷ *CAUTION*

1. Children whose mothers take this drug during the first 4 months of pregnancy have an increased risk of birth defects.
2. Inform your doctor promptly if you think you may be pregnant.
3. This drug should not be used as a test for pregnancy.
4. This drug should not be used in infants or children.
5. This drug may be used selectively by those over 60 as adjunctive therapy for cancer of the breast, uterus, and kidney. Observe for excessive fluid retention.

Advisability of Use During Pregnancy and If Breast-Feeding:

Pregnancy Category: D. Use of this drug is a benefit-to-risk decision during the first 3 months of pregnancy; this drug should NOT be used during the last 6 months of pregnancy. Present in breast milk; avoid taking this drug or refrain from nursing.

▷ **Overdose Symptoms:** Nausea, vomiting, fluid retention, breast enlargement and discomfort, abnormal vaginal bleeding.

▷ **Suggested Periodic Examinations While Taking This Drug:** (at doctor's discretion)

Regular examinations (every 6–12 months) of the breasts and reproductive organs (pelvic examination of the uterus and ovaries, including Pap smear).

▷ **While Taking This Drug the Following Apply:**

Other Drugs:

The following drugs may *decrease* the effects of medroxyprogesterone

- rifampin (Rifadin, Rimactane, etc.); may hasten its elimination.

Medroxyprogesterone *taken concurrently* with

- digitoxin may result in higher than expected digitoxin levels.
- tamoxifen (Nolvadex) may blunt the therapeutic effects of tamoxifen.
- warfarin (Coumadin) may lengthen the time it takes to remove warfarin from the body. More frequent INR (prothrombin time) testing is needed.

Driving, Hazardous Activities: Usually no restrictions. See your doctor for assessment of individual risk and guidance about specific restrictions.

▷ **Saving Money When Using This Medicine:**
- Ask your doctor if this drug provides the best combination of cost and outcome for you.
- Acceptable generics are available for therapy.

MEFENAMIC ACID (me FEN am ik a sid)

Prescription: Yes   **Controlled Drug:** No   **Generic:** No
Brand Name: Ponstel

▷ **Warning:** The use of mefenamic acid beyond 1 week is NOT recommended.

Overview of BENEFITS versus RISKS	
Possible Benefits	*Possible Risks*
Effective relief of mild to moderate pain and inflammation	Hemolytic anemia
	Low white blood cell counts (rare)
	Gastrointestinal pain, ulceration, and bleeding (rare)
	Rare kidney damage
	Rare systemic lupus erythematosus
	Rare pancreatitis

See the fenamates (NSAIDs) drug profile for further information.

MEPERIDINE (me PER i deen)

Other Name: Pethidine

Prescription: Yes   **Controlled Drug:** C-II*   **Generic:** Yes

Brand Names: Demerol, Demerol APAP [CD], Mepergan, Pethadol

Overview of BENEFITS versus RISKS

Possible Benefits	*Possible Risks*
EFFECTIVE RELIEF OF MODERATE TO SEVERE PAIN	POTENTIAL FOR HABIT FORMATION (DEPENDENCE)
	Weakness, fainting
	Disorientation, hallucinations
	Interference with urination

▷ **Illness This Medication Treats:**
Moderate to severe pain of any cause.

▷ **Typical Dosage Range:** (Dosage or schedule must be determined by the doctor for each individual.)
Taken by mouth: 50 to 150 mg every 3 to 4 hours to relieve pain; the usual dose is 100 mg. The total daily dosage should not exceed 900 mg. Current pain theory considers regular use of medicine, rather than as-needed dosing, as a more effective approach.

▷ **Conditions Requiring Dosing Adjustments:**
Liver function: The initial dose should be the same; however, subsequent doses should be decreased by 50% or the dosing interval doubled for patients with compromised livers.
Kidney function: Patients with mild to moderate kidney failure should take 75% of the usual dose at the usual interval. People with severe kidney failure should take 50% of the usual dose at the usual interval. **Multiple doses should be avoided,** as the normeperidine metabolite may accumulate and can cause severe central nervous system reactions (seizures).

▷ **How Best to Take This Medicine:**   May be taken with or following food to reduce stomach irritation or nausea. The tablet may be crushed. The syrup may be diluted in 4 oz of water to reduce the numbing effect on the tongue and mouth.

▷ **How Long This Medicine Is Usually Taken:**   As required to control pain. Current pain theory favors scheduled and regular use rather than the as-needed approach. Continual use should not exceed 5 to 7 days without interruption and reassessment of need.

*See Controlled Drug Schedules inside this book's cover.

▷ **Tell Your Doctor Before Taking This Medicine If You:**
- ever had an allergic reaction to it.
- are having an acute attack of asthma.
- are taking, or have taken within the past 14 days, any MAO type A inhibitor.
- have a history of drug abuse or alcoholism.
- have impaired liver or kidney function.
- have a history of asthma, epilepsy, or glaucoma.
- are taking any other drugs that have a sedative effect.
- plan to have surgery under general anesthesia soon.

▷ **Possible Side Effects:**   Drowsiness, light-headedness, weakness, euphoria, dry mouth, urinary retention, constipation.

▷ **Possible Adverse Effects:**
If any of the following develop, call your doctor promptly for guidance.
Some Mild Problems Drug Can Cause
Allergic reactions: skin rash, itching.
Headache, dizziness, sensation of drunkenness, depression, blurred or double vision.
Facial flushing, sweating, heart palpitation.
Nausea, vomiting.
Some Serious Problems Drug Can Cause
Allergic reactions: anaphylactic reactions.
Drop in blood pressure, causing severe weakness and fainting.
Disorientation, hallucinations, unstable gait, tremor, muscle twitching.
Respiratory depression.
Rare kidney failure.
Seizures, especially in patients with kidney failure who are taking multiple doses.

▷ **Possible Effects on Sex Life:**   Blunting of the sexual response. Retrograde ejaculation.

▷ **Adverse Effects That May Mimic Natural Diseases or Disorders:**
Paradoxical behavioral disturbances may suggest psychotic disorder.

▷ *CAUTION*
1. If you have asthma, chronic bronchitis, or emphysema, excessive use of this drug may cause significant respiratory difficulty, thickening of bronchial secretions, and suppression of coughing.
2. Concurrent use of this drug with atropinelike drugs can increase the risk of urinary retention and reduced intestinal function.
3. Do not take this drug following acute head injury.
4. This drug should NOT be used in infants less than 1 year old, who are very vulnerable to respiratory depression.

5. For people over 60 small doses and slow increases, as needed and tolerated, are prudent. There may be an increased risk of drowsiness, dizziness, falling, urinary retention, and constipation.

Advisability of Use During Pregnancy and If Breast-Feeding:

Pregnancy Category: B, D if used in higher doses and for a longer period of time, especially when the baby is due to be born. Avoid using this drug during the first 3 months. Use sparingly and in small doses during the last 6 months, only if clearly needed. Present in breast milk; avoid taking this drug or refrain from nursing.

▷ **Habit-Forming Potential:** This drug can cause psychological and physical dependence.

▷ **Overdose Symptoms:** Marked drowsiness, confusion, tremors, convulsions, stupor progressing to coma.

▷ **While Taking This Drug the Following Apply:**

Beverages: May be taken with milk.

Alcohol: Opioid analgesics can intensify the intoxicating effects of alcohol, and alcohol can intensify the depressant effects of opioids on brain function, breathing, and circulation. Alcohol is best avoided.

Marijuana Smoking: Increase in drowsiness and pain relief; impairment of mental and physical performance.

Other Drugs:

Meperidine may **increase** the effects of
- other drugs with sedative effects.
- atropinelike drugs, increasing the risk of constipation and urinary retention.

Meperidine **taken concurrently** with
- cimetidine (Tagamet), famotidine (Pepcid), nizatidine (Axid), omeprazole (Prilosec), and other medicines that increase the alkalinity of the stomach, may lead to increased meperidine levels and toxicity.
- intravenous acyclovir (Zovirax) may lead to kidney or nerve problems.
- MAO type A inhibitors can cause the equivalent of an acute narcotic overdose: unconsciousness; severe depression of breathing, heart action, and circulation. A variation of this reaction is excitability, convulsions, high fever, and rapid heart action.
- phenothiazines can cause excessive and prolonged depression of brain functions, breathing, and circulation.
- phenytoin (Dilantin) may blunt the benefits of meperidine.
- tricyclic antidepressants (see Drug Classes) may result in worsening of meperidine's respiratory depressant effect.

Driving, Hazardous Activities: This drug can impair mental alertness, judgment, reaction time, and physical coordination. Avoid hazardous activities.

Discontinuation: It is best to limit this drug to short-term use. If used for extended periods, it is necessary for discontinuation to be gradual to minimize possible effects of withdrawal.

▷ **Saving Money When Using This Medicine:**
- Pain therapy currently combines medications from several drug classes. This drug may be combined with a tricyclic antidepressant such as amitriptyline (Elavil) or an NSAID such as ibuprofen (Motrin) to attack the cause of the pain from several mechanisms; such combinations also often allow the opioid dose (such as fentanyl) to be decreased.
- Many medications are available to treat pain. Ask your doctor if this drug provides the best combination of cost and outcome for you, and how long this drug is usually taken to treat your condition.
- Talk with your doctor to see if visiting a chronic pain center is appropriate.

MERCAPTOPURINE   (mer kap toh PYUR een)

Other Names: 6-mercaptopurine, 6-MP

Prescription: Yes   **Controlled Drug:** No   **Generic:** No

Brand Name: Purinethol

Overview of BENEFITS versus RISKS	
Possible Benefits	*Possible Risks*
EFFECTIVE TREATMENT OF CERTAIN ACUTE AND CHRONIC LEUKEMIAS AND LYMPHOMAS	BONE MARROW DEPRESSION DRUG-INDUCED LIVER DAMAGE
Effective treatment of polycythemia vera	Rare gastrointestinal ulceration
Possible effective treatment of Crohn's disease and ulcerative colitis	
Possible effective treatment of severe psoriatic arthritis	

▷ **Illness This Medication Treats:**
(1) Acute lymphocytic leukemia; (2) acute nonlymphocytic leukemia.

▷ **Typical Dosage Range:** (Dosage or schedule must be determined by the doctor for each individual.)
Infants and Children: For leukemia: 2.5 mg per kilogram of body weight (to the nearest 25 mg) daily, in single or divided doses. Some centers follow the same dose increase as adults if response is not acceptable, and then increase to 75 mg per square meter of body

area on days 29 to 42; they also combine mercaptopurine with vincristine, prednisone, and methotrexate. Maintenance doses continue as for adults.

12 to 60 Years of Age: For leukemia: Initially 2.5 mg per kilogram of body weight (to the nearest 25 mg) daily, in single or divided doses, for 4 weeks. If white blood cell or platelet counts do not fall and there is no clinical improvement, the dose may be increased as needed and tolerated to 5 mg per kilogram of body weight daily. For maintenance: 1.5 to 2.5 mg per kilogram of body weight daily.

For inflammatory bowel disease: 1.5 mg per kilogram of body weight daily, for 2 to 3 months. The dose is then adjusted to keep the platelet count above 100,000 and the white blood cell count above 4,500.

Over 60 Years of Age: Same as for 12 to 60 years of age.

▷ **Conditions Requiring Dosing Adjustments:**

Liver function: Patients with liver compromise should use this drug with caution and in decreased doses. Mercaptopurine is also a rare cause of liver toxicity.

Kidney function: Patients with renal compromise should use a decreased dose to avoid accumulation of this drug; it is a rare cause of crystals in the urine.

TMPT negatives: Some patients do not have an enzyme called thiopurine methyltransferase. Doses will need to be decreased by 10% for these patients.

▷ **How Best to Take This Medicine:** May be taken with or following food to reduce stomach irritation. The tablet may be crushed for administration.

▷ **How Long This Medicine Is Usually Taken:** Continual use on a regular schedule for 4 to 6 weeks is usually necessary to determine this drug's effectiveness in inducing remission in leukemia; continual use for 2 to 3 months is necessary to determine its benefit in treating inflammatory bowel disease. Long-term use (months to years) requires periodic physician evaluation.

▷ **Tell Your Doctor Before Taking This Medicine If You:**

- ever had an allergic reaction to it.
- are pregnant.
- have a history of drug-induced bone marrow depression.
- have impaired liver or kidney function.
- have a solid tumor or lymphoma.
- are not using any contraception.
- have leukemia that has spread to the central nervous system.
- have gout.
- have been exposed recently to chickenpox or herpes zoster (shingles).
- are taking any allopurinol, probenecid, sulfinpyrazone, anticoagulants, or immunosuppressants.

▷ **Possible Side Effects:**   Bone marrow depression.
Abnormally increased blood uric acid levels; possible urate kidney stones.

▷ **Possible Adverse Effects:**
If any of the following develop, call your doctor promptly for guidance.
Some Mild Problems Drug Can Cause
   Allergic reactions: skin rash, itching.
   Headache, weakness.
   Loss of appetite, mouth and lip sores, nausea, vomiting, diarrhea.
Some Serious Problems Drug Can Cause
   Liver damage with jaundice.
   Kidney damage: fever, cloudy urine.
   Gastrointestinal ulceration: stomach pain, bloody or black stools.
   Pancreatitis.

▷ **Possible Effects on Sex Life:**   Suppression of sperm production; cessation of menstruation.

▷ **Possible Delayed Adverse Effects:**   Bone marrow depression may not be apparent during early treatment.

▷ *CAUTION*
   1. Comply fully with all requests for periodic laboratory tests.
   2. Report promptly any indications of infection or abnormal bleeding or bruising.
   3. Tell your doctor promptly if you become pregnant.
   4. Avoid immunizations while taking this drug. Also, avoid contact with people who have recently taken oral poliovirus vaccine.
   5. People over 60 may be more susceptible to bone marrow depression. Periodic blood counts are mandatory.

Advisability of Use During Pregnancy and If Breast-Feeding:
Pregnancy Category: D. Avoid using this drug during entire pregnancy if possible. Use a nonhormonal method of contraception. Presence in breast milk is unknown; avoid taking this drug or refrain from nursing.

▷ **Overdose Symptoms:**   Headache, dizziness, abdominal pain, nausea.

▷ **Suggested Periodic Examinations While Taking This Drug:** (at doctor's discretion)
Complete blood cell counts.
Blood uric acid levels.
Liver and kidney function tests.

▷ **While Taking This Drug the Following Apply:**
Beverages: Drink liquids liberally, up to 2 qt daily.
Alcohol: Avoid completely.

Other Drugs:

Mercaptopurine may *decrease* the effects of
- warfarin (Coumadin); monitor INR (prothrombin times) more frequently.

The following drugs may *increase* the effects of mercaptopurine
- allopurinol (Zyloprim).
- methotrexate (Mexate); may lead to mercaptopurine toxicity.

Discontinuation: To be determined by your doctor.

▷ **Saving Money When Using This Medicine:**
- Many medications are available to treat leukemia. Ask your doctor if this drug provides the best combination of cost and outcome for you. Also discuss investigational medicines.
- Ask your doctor how long this drug is usually taken to treat your condition.

MESALAMINE (me SAL a meen)

Other Names: Mesalazine, 5-aminosalicylic acid, 5-ASA

Prescription: Yes **Controlled Drug:** No **Generic:** No

Brand Names: Asacol, Pentasa, Rowasa

Overview of BENEFITS versus RISKS	
Possible Benefits	*Possible Risks*
EFFECTIVE SUPPRESSION OF INFLAMMATORY BOWEL DISEASE	Allergic reactions: acute intolerance syndrome Drug-induced kidney damage (very rare)

▷ **Illness This Medication Treats:**
(1) Active mild to moderate ulcerative colitis, proctosigmoiditis, and proctitis; (2) maintains remission in chronic ulcerative colitis and proctitis.

▷ **Typical Dosage Range:** (Dosage or schedule must be determined by the doctor for each individual.)
Infants and Children: Dosage not established.
12 to 60 Years of Age: Rectal suspension: 4 g (as a retention enema) every night for 3 to 6 weeks.
Suppositories: 500 mg (inserted into rectum) two or three times daily.
Tablets: 400 to 800 mg (one or two tablets by mouth) three times daily for 6 weeks. The total daily dose should not exceed 2400 mg.
Over 60 Years of Age: Same as for 12 to 60 years of age.

▷ **Conditions Requiring Dosing Adjustments:**
  Kidney function: Patients with renal compromise should use this drug with caution.

▷ **How Best to Take This Medicine:**   Rectal suspension: Use as a retention enema at bedtime; if possible, empty the rectum before instilling the suspension. Try to retain the suspension all night.
  Tablets: Preferably taken with 8 oz of water on an empty stomach, 1 hour before or 2 hours after eating. However, it may be taken with or following food to reduce stomach irritation. The sustained-release tablet should be swallowed whole without alteration.

▷ **How Long This Medicine Is Usually Taken:**   Continual use on a regular schedule for 1 to 3 weeks is usually necessary to determine this drug's effectiveness in controlling ulcerative colitis symptoms. Long-term use (months to years) requires supervision and periodic physician evaluation.

▷ **Tell Your Doctor Before Taking This Medicine If You:**
  • ever had an allergic reaction to it.
  • have severely impaired kidney function.
  • are allergic to aspirin (or other salicylates), olsalazine, or sulfasalazine.
  • are allergic by nature: history of hay fever, asthma, hives, eczema.
  • are allergic to sulfites.
  • have active ulcer disease.
  • have a history of blood clotting problems.
  • are taking other medicines that effect the bone marrow.
  • have impaired liver or kidney function.
  • are currently taking sulfasalazine (Azulfidine).

▷ **Possible Side Effects:**   Anal irritation (with use of rectal suspension or suppositories).

▷ **Possible Adverse Effects:**
  If any of the following develop, call your doctor promptly for guidance.
  Some Mild Problems Drug Can Cause
    Allergic reactions: skin rash.
    Headache, hair loss (rare).
    Ringing in the ears.
    Nausea, stomach pain, excessive gas.
  Some Serious Problems Drug Can Cause
    Allergic reactions: acute intolerance syndrome—fever, skin rash, severe headache, severe stomach pain, bloody diarrhea.
    Rare kidney damage (nephrosis).
    Rare pancreatitis, peptic ulcers, or peripheral neuropathy.
    Rare liver damage or heart problems.
    Rare low white blood cells or platelets, or anemia.

▷ *CAUTION*

1. Report promptly any early indications of acute intolerance syndrome, and discontinue taking this drug.
2. Shake the rectal suspension dosage form thoroughly before administering.
3. Safety and effectiveness of this drug for those under 12 years old are not established.

Advisability of Use During Pregnancy and If Breast-Feeding:

Pregnancy Category: B. Use this drug only if clearly needed. Ask your doctor for guidance. Present in breast milk; avoid taking this drug or refrain from nursing.

▷ **Overdose Symptoms:** Headache, dizziness, nausea, vomiting, abdominal cramping.

▷ **Suggested Periodic Examinations While Taking This Drug:** (at doctor's discretion)

Kidney function tests, urinalysis.

▷ **While Taking This Drug the Following Apply:**

Foods: Decreases mesalamine levels. Follow prescribed diet.

Beverages: May be taken with milk.

Other Drugs·

Mesalamine *taken concurrently* with

• varicella virus vaccine (Varivax) may result in Reye's syndrome. Avoid taking this medicine for 6 weeks after taking varicella vaccine.

▷ **Saving Money When Using This Medicine:**

• Several medications are available to treat ulcerative colitis. Ask your doctor if this drug provides the best combination of cost and outcome for you.

METAPROTERENOL (met a proh TER e nohl)

Other Name: Orciprenaline

Prescription: Yes   **Controlled Drug:** No   **Generic:** Yes

Brand Names: Alupent, Arm-a-Med, Dey-Dose, Metaprel, Prometa

Overview of BENEFITS versus RISKS	
Possible Benefits	*Possible Risks*
VERY EFFECTIVE RELIEF OF BRONCHOSPASM	Increased blood pressure
	Fine hand tremor
	Irregular heart rhythm (with excessive use)

▷ **Illness This Medication Treats:**

(1) Acute bronchial asthma and reduction of the frequency and severity of chronic, recurrent asthmatic attacks; (2) relief of reversible

bronchospasm associated with chronic bronchitis and emphysema; (3) eases symptoms of obstructive bronchial disease.

▷ **Typical Dosage Range:**
Inhaler: Two or three inhalations every 3 to 4 hours; do not exceed 12 inhalations/day. Hand nebulizer: 5 to 15 inhalations every 4 hours; do not exceed 40 inhalations/day. Syrup and tablets: 20 mg every 6 to 8 hours.

▷ **Conditions Requiring Dosing Adjustments:**
Liver function: Specific guidelines for dosing adjustment for patients with liver compromise (particularly because of the drug's episodic nature) are usually not indicated.

▷ **How Best to Take This Medicine:**   May be taken on empty stomach or with food or milk. Tablets should not be crushed for administration. For aerosol and nebulizer, follow the written instructions carefully. Do not overuse.

▷ **How Long This Medicine Is Usually Taken:**   According to individual requirements. Do not use beyond the time necessary to terminate episodes of asthma.

▷ **Tell Your Doctor Before Taking This Medicine If You:**
- ever had an allergic reaction to it.
- currently have an irregular heart rhythm.
- are taking, or have taken within the past 2 weeks, any MAO type A inhibitor.
- are overly sensitive to other drugs that stimulate the sympathetic nervous system.
- are currently using epinephrine (Adrenalin, Primatene Mist, etc.) to relieve asthmatic breathing.
- have any type of heart or circulatory disorder, especially high blood pressure or coronary heart disease.
- have diabetes or an overactive thyroid gland.
- are taking any form of digitalis or any stimulant drug.

▷ **Possible Side Effects:**   Aerosol: Dryness or irritation of mouth or throat, altered taste.
Tablet: Nervousness, palpitation.

▷ **Possible Adverse Effects:**
If any of the following develop, call your doctor promptly for guidance.
Some Mild Problems Drug Can Cause
Headache, dizziness, insomnia, fine tremor of hands.
Rapid, pounding heartbeat; increased sweating; muscle cramps.
Nausea, heartburn, vomiting.
Some Serious Problems Drug Can Cause
Rapid or irregular heart rhythm, intensification of angina, increased blood pressure.

Rare hallucinations.

Rare paradoxical spasm of the bronchi.

▷ **CAUTION**

1. Concurrent use of the aerosol inhalation of this drug with beclomethasone aerosol (Beclovent, Vanceril) may increase the risk of toxicity due to fluorocarbon propellants. It is advisable to use this aerosol 20 to 30 minutes *before* beclomethasone aerosol to reduce the risk of toxicity and enhance beclomethasone penetration.

2. *Avoid excessive use of aerosol inhalation.* The excessive or prolonged use by inhalation can reduce its effectiveness and cause serious heart rhythm disturbances, including cardiac arrest.

3. Do not use this drug concurrently with epinephrine. These two drugs may be used alternately with an interval of 4 hours between doses.

4. If you do not respond to your usual effective dose, ask your doctor for guidance. Do not increase the size or frequency of the dose without your doctor's approval.

5. Safety and effectiveness of use of the aerosol and nebulized solution have not been established for children under 12 years old. Safety and effectiveness of use of the syrup and tablet have not been established for children under 6 years old.

6. People over 60 should avoid excessive and continual use. If acute asthma is not relieved promptly, other drugs will have to be tried. Observe for nervousness, palpitations, irregular heart rhythm, and muscle tremors. Use this drug with extreme caution if you have hardening of the arteries, heart disease, or high blood pressure.

Advisability of Use During Pregnancy and If Breast-Feeding:

Pregnancy Category: C. Avoid use of this drug during first 3 months. Use during the last 6 months only if clearly needed. Presence in breast milk is unknown; avoid taking this drug or refrain from nursing.

▷ **Overdose Symptoms:** Nervousness, palpitation, rapid heart rate, sweating, headache, tremor, vomiting, chest pain.

▷ **Suggested Periodic Examinations While Taking This Drug:** (at doctor's discretion)

Blood pressure measurements, evaluation of heart status.

▷ **While Taking This Drug the Following Apply:**

Beverages: Avoid excessive use of caffeine-containing beverages: coffee, tea, cola, chocolate.

Other Drugs:

Metaproterenol *taken concurrently* with

- albuterol (Proventil, others) may increase risk of heart (cardiovascular) side effects.

- MAO type A inhibitors may cause excessive increase in blood pressure and undesirable heart stimulation.
- phenothiazines (see Drug Classes) may blunt the central effects of this medicine.

Driving, Hazardous Activities: Usually no restrictions. Use caution if excessive nervousness or dizziness occurs.

Heavy Exercise or Exertion: Use caution. Excessive exercise can induce asthma in sensitive individuals.

▷ **Saving Money When Using This Medicine:**
- Many medications are available to treat asthma. Ask your doctor if this drug provides the best combination of cost and outcome for you, and how long this drug is usually taken to treat your condition.
- Ask your doctor if using nedocromil or cromolyn could help prevent some attacks of asthma for you.
- Discuss using nebulized lidocaine as an agent to decrease asthmatic attacks for you.

METHADONE (METH a dohn)

Prescription: Yes   **Controlled Drug:** C-II*   **Generic:** Yes
Brand Names: Dolophine, Diskets

Overview of BENEFITS versus RISKS	
Possible Benefits	*Possible Risks*
EFFECTIVE RELIEF OF MODERATE TO SEVERE PAIN	POTENTIAL FOR HABIT FORMATION (DEPENDENCE)
SUBSTITUTION AND WITHDRAWAL FROM HEROIN ADDICTION	Weakness, fainting
	Disorientation, hallucinations
	Interference with urination

▷ **Illness This Medication Treats:**
(1) Moderate to severe pain of any cause; (2) a primary provision of an appropriate substitute for heroin in treatment programs for drug addiction.

▷ **Typical Dosage Range:** (Dosage or schedule must be determined by the doctor for each individual.)
Taken by mouth: 2.5 to 10 mg every 3 to 4 hours. Timed dosing is often used when starting to treat pain; later the best strategy to prevent pain is used. Total daily dosage should not exceed 80 mg. (Dosage schedules for maintenance treatment during heroin withdrawal must be individualized.)

*See Controlled Drug Schedules inside this book's cover.

▷ **Conditions Requiring Dosing Adjustments:**

Liver function: Patients with liver compromise should use this drug with caution, giving consideration to decreased dosages.

Kidney function: Patients with mild kidney failure should take the usual dose every 6 hours. People with moderate to severe kidney failure should take the usual dose every 8 hours. Patients with severe failure should take the usual dose every 8 to 12 hours.

▷ **Saving Money When Using This Medicine:**

- Pain therapy currently combines medications from several drug classes. Methadone combined with a tricyclic antidepressant such as amitriptyline (Elavil) or an NSAID such as ibuprofen (Motrin) attacks the cause of the pain from several mechanisms, often allowing the opioid dose (such as fentanyl) to be decreased.
- Many medications are available to treat pain, and there are two medicines to help those addicted to heroin. Ask your doctor if this drug provides the best combination of cost and outcome for you.
- Ask your doctor how long this drug is usually taken to treat your condition.

METHOTREXATE (meth oh TREX ayt)

Other Names: Amethopterin, MTX

Prescription Needed: Yes   **Controlled Drug:** No   **Generic:** Yes

Brand Names: Ambitrex, Folex, Mexate, Rheumatrex Dose Pack

Overview of BENEFITS versus RISKS	
Possible Benefits	*Possible Risks*
EFFECTIVE TREATMENT OF SOME CASES OF SEVERE DISABLING PSORIASIS	GASTROINTESTINAL ULCERATION AND BLEEDING
EFFECTIVE TREATMENT OF CERTAIN ADULT AND CHILDHOOD CANCERS	MOUTH AND THROAT ULCERATION
PREVENTION OF BONE MARROW TRANSPLANT REJECTION	SEVERE BONE MARROW DEPRESSION
	DAMAGE TO LUNGS, LIVER, AND KIDNEYS
Helpful adjunctive therapy for severe, refractory rheumatoid arthritis and related disorders	Loss of hair

▷ **Illness This Medication Treats:**

(1) Severe forms of disabling psoriasis that have failed to respond to all standard treatment procedures; (2) combination therapy of acute

lymphocytic leukemia; (3) combination therapy of various kinds of adult and childhood cancer; (4) prevention of transplanted bone marrow rejection; (5) treatment of connective tissue disorders such as rheumatoid arthritis, scleroderma, and related conditions. Methotrexate's use in rheumatoid arthritis is restricted to selected adults with severe active disease that has failed to respond to conventional therapy.

▷ **Typical Dosage Range:** (Dosage or schedule must be determined by the doctor for each individual.)

For psoriasis (alternate schedules): (1) 10 to 50 mg once a week; (2) 2.5 to 5 mg every 12 hours for three doses, or every 8 hours for four doses, once a week up to a maximum of 30 mg/week; (3) 2.5 mg/day for 5 days, followed by 2 days without the drug, with gradual increase in dosage to a maximum of 6.25 mg/day.

For rheumatoid arthritis (alternate schedules): (1) A single oral dose of 7.5 mg once weekly; (2) divided doses of 2.5 mg every 12 hours for 3 doses/week. Dosage may be increased gradually as needed and tolerated. Do not exceed a weekly dose of 20 mg.

For acute lymphocytic leukemia (ALL): An induction of 3.3 mg per square meter of body area in combination with a corticosteroid is usually given daily for 4 to 6 weeks. Maintenance: A total weekly dose of 30 mg per square meter of body area is given as two divided oral or intramuscular injections. Some centers also use 2.5 mg per kilogram of body weight intravenously every 14 days.

▷ **Conditions Requiring Dosing Adjustments:**

Liver Function: Patients with liver compromise should use this drug with caution and in decreased doses. For patients with a bilirubin of less than 3.0 mg% and SGOT less than 180 IU, 100% of the usual dose may be taken at the usual interval. For patients with bilirubin values of 3.1 to 5.0 and SGOT of greater than 180, 75% of the usual dose can be taken at the usual interval. If the bilirubin is greater than 5.0, the dose should not be taken until the value lowers.

Kidney function: Use of this drug is a benefit-to-risk decision, as increased systemic effects may occur in patients with compromised kidneys. This drug should NOT be given to patients with severe kidney failure (creatinine clearances less than 10 ml/min). For patients with mild to moderate kidney compromise (creatinine clearances of 40–80 ml/min), 50% of the usual dose should be taken at the usual dosing intervals.

▷ **How Best to Take This Medicine:**   May be taken with food to reduce stomach irritation. Drink at least 2 to 3 qt of liquids daily. The tablet may be crushed.

▷ **How Long This Medicine Is Usually Taken:**   Use on a regular schedule for several weeks usually determines the effectiveness of this drug in reducing the severity and extent of psoriasis. Response in rheumatoid arthritis usually begins after 3 to 6 weeks. When a favorable response has been achieved, the dosage should be reduced to the smallest amount that maintains acceptable improvement. Long-term use (months to years) requires your doctor's supervision.

▷ **Tell Your Doctor Before Taking This Medicine If You:**
- ever had an allergic reaction to it.
- currently have, or have had, a recent exposure to either chickenpox or shingles (herpes zoster).
- are pregnant or planning pregnancy, and you are taking this drug to treat psoriasis or rheumatoid arthritis.
- have active liver disease, peptic ulcer, regional enteritis, or ulcerative colitis, or a history of these conditions or gout.
- currently have a blood cell or bone marrow disorder or a history of bone marrow impairment of any kind, especially drug-induced bone marrow depression.
- have a white blood cell count less than 3,000 or your platelet count is less than 100,000.
- have a chronic infection of any kind.
- have impaired liver or kidney function.

▷ **Possible Side Effects:**   The following are due to the pharmacologic actions of this drug. **Report such developments to your doctor promptly.**
Sores on the lips or in the mouth or throat; vomiting; intestinal cramping; diarrhea (may be bloody); painful urination; bloody urine.
Reduced resistance to infection, fatigue, weakness, fever, abnormal bleeding or bruising (bone marrow depression).

▷ **Possible Adverse Effects:**
If any of the following develop, call your doctor promptly for guidance.
Some Mild Problems Drug Can Cause
  Allergic reactions: skin rash, itching.
  Headache, drowsiness, blurred vision.
  Loss of appetite, nausea, vomiting.
  Loss of hair, loss of skin pigmentation, acne.
Some Serious Problems Drug Can Cause
  Allergic reactions: drug-induced pneumonia—cough, shortness of breath.
  Nervous system toxicity: speech disturbances, paralysis, seizures.
  Liver toxicity with jaundice
  Kidney toxicity: reduced urine volume, kidney failure.
  Bone marrow depression and possible *Pneumocystis carinii* pneumonia.
  Fluid buildup in the lung.

Severe skin reactions (toxic epidermal necrolysis, or TEN).
Possible chromosomal damage (from occupational exposure).

▷ **Possible Effects on Sex Life:**   Altered timing and pattern of menstruation. Swelling and tenderness of male breast tissue (gynecomastia). Decreased sperm count.

▷ **Possible Delayed Adverse Effects:**   Some reports suggest that methotrexate therapy may contribute to secondary cancers; other studies have not confirmed this.

▷ *CAUTION*

1. This drug has a high potential for serious toxicity. Its use must be monitored carefully and continually by a doctor skilled in its proper administration. Request the Patient Package Insert that is available with this drug (Rheumatrex Dose Pack) and read it thoroughly.
2. Appropriate laboratory examinations, performed before and during the use of this drug, are mandatory. Comply fully with your doctor's instructions regarding periodic studies.
3. Women with the potential for pregnancy should have a pregnancy test before taking this drug and use effective contraception during its use and for 8 weeks following its discontinuation.
4. Vaccination by live virus vaccines should be avoided during the use of this drug. Because immune functions are suppressed by this drug, live virus vaccines could actually produce infection rather than stimulate an immune response.
5. People over 60 should have a careful evaluation of kidney function both before starting treatment and during the entire course of therapy.

Advisability of Use During Pregnancy or If Breast-Feeding:
Pregnancy Category: X. Use of this drug during pregnancy to treat psoriasis or rheumatoid arthritis cannot be justified. Present in breast milk; avoid taking this drug or refrain from nursing.

▷ **Overdose Symptoms:**   The side effects and adverse effects listed above develop earlier and with greater severity.

▷ **Suggested Periodic Examinations While Taking This Drug:** (at doctor's discretion)
Complete blood cell counts (MCV especially), liver and kidney function tests, blood uric acid levels, chest X-ray examinations.

▷ **While Taking This Drug the Following Apply:**
Foods: Avoid highly seasoned foods that could be irritating. Between courses of treatment, eat liberally of the following foods: beef, chicken, lamb and pork liver, asparagus, navy beans, kale, and spinach. For patients being treated for rheumatoid arthritis, many clini-

cians give folic acid in a dose of 1 mg a day in order to help decrease side effects.

Beverages: No restrictions. This drug may be taken with milk.

Alcohol: Avoid completely.

Other Drugs:

Methotrexate may **decrease** the effects of
- digoxin (Lanoxin).
- phenytoin (Dilantin).

The following drugs may **increase** the effects of methotrexate and enhance its toxicity
- aspirin and other salicylates.
- NSAIDs (see Drug Classes).
- probenecid (Benemid).

Methotrexate **taken concurrently** with
- bismuth subsalicylate (Pepto-Bismol, others) may lead to methotrexate toxicity.
- carbenicillin (Geocillin, others) may lead to methotrexate toxicity.
- cholestyramine (Questran, others) and other cholesterol-lowering resins may result in decreased methotrexate effectiveness.
- co-trimoxazole (Bactrim) may lead to abnormal lowering of all blood cells (pancytopenia).
- cyclosporine (Sandimmune) may result in increased toxicity from both medicines.
- etretinate (Tegison) can lead to increased liver toxicity.
- pneumococcal, yellow fever, or smallpox—and perhaps other—vaccines may blunt the therapeutic response to the vaccine.
- sulfa drugs such as sulfamethoxazole can result in increased blood toxicity.
- thiazide diuretics (see Drug Classes) may increase risk of myelosuppression.

Driving, Hazardous Activities: May cause drowsiness, dizziness, or blurred vision. Restrict your activities as necessary.

Exposure to Sun: Use caution until skin sensitivity has been determined; this drug can cause photosensitivity. Avoid ultraviolet lamps.

▷ **Saving Money When Using This Medicine:**
- Many new drugs are available to treat cancer. Ask your doctor if this medicine offers the best balance of cost and outcomes for you.
- A generic form can be substituted for the brand name.
- When used for rheumatoid arthritis, methotrexate combined with 1 mg of folic acid a day can help decrease side effects. Discuss this with your doctor.

METHYLPHENIDATE (meth il FEN i dayt)

Prescription Needed: Yes   **Controlled Drug:** C-II*   **Generic:** Yes

Brand Names: Ritalin, Ritalin-SR

Overview of BENEFITS versus RISKS	
Possible Benefits	*Possible Risks*
EFFECTIVE CONTROL OF NARCOLEPSY	POTENTIAL FOR SERIOUS PSYCHOLOGICAL DEPENDENCE
USEFUL AS ADJUNCTIVE TREATMENT FOR ATTENTION DEFICIT DISORDERS OF CHILDHOOD	SUPPRESSION OF GROWTH IN CHILDHOOD
Useful in treatment of mild to moderate depression	Abnormal behavior
Helps some cases of emotional withdrawal in the elderly	Rare blood cell disorders

▷ **Illness This Medication Treats:**
  (1) Narcolepsy, recurrent spells of uncontrollable drowsiness and sleep; and (2) attention deficit hyperactivity disorders of childhood, formerly known as the hyperactive child syndrome, minimal brain damage, and minimal brain dysfunction.
  Other (unlabeled) generally accepted uses:(1) treats apathetic and withdrawal states in the elderly; (2) used as part of combination therapy for chronic pain.

▷ **Typical Dosage Range:** (Dosage or schedule must be determined by the doctor for each individual.)
  5 to 20 mg two or three times per day.

▷ **Conditions Requiring Dosing Adjustments:**
  Liver function: Patients with liver compromise should use this drug with caution and consider decreased doses.

▷ **How Best to Take This Medicine:** Take the tablet 30 to 45 minutes before meals. The regular tablet may be crushed; the prolonged-action tablet should be taken whole, not crushed.

▷ **How Long This Medicine Is Usually Taken:** Use on a regular schedule for 3 to 4 weeks is usually needed to see the effectiveness of this drug in controlling the symptoms of narcolepsy or improving the behavior of attention deficit children. If there is no improvement, the original diagnosis may be in question, and the medicine

*See Controlled Drug Schedules inside this book's cover.

should be stopped and the child reevaluated. Long-term use (months to years) requires physician supervision.

▷ **Tell Your Doctor Before Taking This Medicine If You:**
- ever had an allergic reaction to it.
- have inadequately treated glaucoma.
- are experiencing a period of severe anxiety, nervous tension, or emotional depression.
- have Tourette's syndrome.
- have high blood pressure, angina, or epilepsy.
- are taking, or have taken within the past 14 days, any MAO type A inhibitor.

▷ **Possible Side Effects:** Nervousness, insomnia. Suppression of growth in children (this medicine is often stopped in the summer to allow a "catch-up" period).

▷ **Possible Adverse Effects:**
If any of the following develop, call your doctor promptly for guidance.
Some Mild Problems Drug Can Cause
Allergic reactions: skin rash, drug fever, joint pains.
Headache, dizziness, rapid and forceful heart palpitation.
Reduced appetite, nausea, abdominal discomfort.
Some Serious Problems Drug Can Cause
Allergic reactions: severe skin reactions, extensive bruising due to allergic destruction of blood platelets.
Idiosyncratic reaction: abnormal patterns of behavior.
Rare and questionable abnormally low red blood cell or white blood cell counts.
Rare porphyria or muscle damage.

▷ *CAUTION*
1. Careful dosage adjustments on an individual basis are mandatory.
2. Paradoxical reactions can occur, aggravating initial symptoms.
3. Safety and effectiveness of this drug for those under 6 years old have not been established. Discontinue giving this drug if it is not beneficial in managing an attention deficit disorder after a trial of 1 month. During long-term use, monitor the child for normal growth and development.
4. For those over 60, small starting doses are indicated. The elderly may be more susceptible to nervousness, agitation, insomnia, high blood pressure, angina, or heart rhythm disturbance.
5. This drug should only be used to treat attention deficit disorder or attention deficit hyperactivity disorder after a detailed assessment by a qualified specialist is made.
6. This medicine SHOULD NOT be casually prescribed for routine

behavior challenges (as a chemical restraint). Methylphenidate is properly prescribed for children after an extensive and sometimes repeat evaluation by a specially trained professional.

Advisability of Use During Pregnancy or If Breast-Feeding:

Pregnancy Category: B. Use only if clearly needed. Ask your doctor for guidance. Presence in breast milk is unknown; avoid taking this drug or refrain from nursing.

▷ **Habit-Forming Potential:** This drug can produce tolerance and cause serious psychological dependence, a potentially dangerous characteristic of amphetaminelike drugs.

▷ **Overdose Symptoms:** Headache, vomiting, agitation, tremors, muscle twitching, dry mouth, sweating, fever, confusion, hallucinations, seizures, coma.

▷ **Suggested Periodic Examinations While Taking This Drug:** (at doctor's discretion)
Complete blood cell counts, blood pressure measurements.

▷ **While Taking This Drug the Following Apply:**

Foods: Avoid foods rich in tyramine; combined with tyramine, this drug may cause an excessive rise in blood pressure.

Beverages: Avoid beverages prepared from meat or meat extracts. This drug may be taken with milk.

Alcohol: Avoid beer, Chianti wines, and vermouth.

Other Drugs:

Methylphenidate may *increase* the effects of
• tricyclic antidepressants, enhancing their toxic effects.

Methylphenidate may *decrease* the effects of
• guanethidine (Ismelin), impairing its ability to lower blood pressure.

Methylphenidate *taken concurrently* with
• anticonvulsants may cause a significant change in the pattern of epileptic seizures; dosage adjustments may be necessary for proper control.
• MAO type A inhibitors may significantly increase blood pressure. Avoid concurrent use.
• tricyclic antidepressants (TCAs) may lead to undesirable increases in blood pressure.

Driving, Hazardous Activities: May cause dizziness or drowsiness. Restrict your activities as necessary.

Discontinuation: If it has been necessary to use this drug for an extended period of time, do not discontinue it abruptly. Careful supervision is necessary during withdrawal to prevent severe depression and erratic behavior.

▷ **Saving Money When Using This Medicine:**
- Ask your doctor if this medicine offers the best balance of cost and outcome for you or your child.
- If your child's response has been good during the first 6 months, ask your doctor if a medication-free summer would help with growth.
- An acceptable generic form is available.

METHYLPREDNISOLONE (meth il pred NIS oh lohn)

Prescription Needed: Yes **Controlled Drug:** No **Generic:** Yes

Brand Names: A-Methapred, Medrol, Medrol Enpak, Solu-Medrol

Overview of BENEFITS versus RISKS	
Possible Benefits	*Possible Risks*
EFFECTIVE RELIEF OF SYMPTOMS FOR A WIDE VARIETY OF INFLAMMATORY AND ALLERGIC DISORDERS EFFECTIVE IMMUNOSUPPRESSION in selected benign and malignant disorders	Short-term use (up to 10 days) is usually well tolerated Long-term use (exceeding 2 weeks) is associated with many possible adverse effects: ALTERED MOOD AND PERSONALITY; CATARACTS, GLAUCOMA; HYPERTENSION; OSTEOPOROSIS; ASEPTIC BONE NECROSIS; INCREASED SUSCEPTIBILITY TO INFECTIONS

▷ **Illness This Medication Treats:**
(1) A wide variety of allergic and inflammatory conditions: serious skin disorders, asthma, regional enteritis, ulcerative colitis, and all types of major rheumatic disorders including bursitis, tendinitis, and most forms of arthritis; (2) low platelet counts of unknown cause; (3) part of combination treatment of anaphylactic shock; (4) shock due to adrenal gland insufficiency.

▷ **Typical Dosage Range:** (Dosage or schedule must be determined by the doctor for each individual.)
4 to 48 mg daily as a single dose or in divided doses.

▷ **Conditions Requiring Dosing Adjustments:**
Kidney function: This drug can worsen existing kidney compromise. These patients require a benefit-to-risk decision.

Obesity: The amount of time that this medicine stays in the body can be extended in obese patients. Dosing MUST be based on ideal body weight.

▷ **How Best to Take This Medicine:**   Take with or following food to prevent stomach irritation, preferably in the morning. The tablet may be crushed.

▷ **How Long This Medicine Is Usually Taken:**   For acute disorders: 4 to 10 days. For chronic disorders: according to individual requirements. The duration of use should not exceed the time necessary to obtain adequate symptomatic relief in acute self-limiting conditions, or the time required to stabilize a chronic condition and permit gradual withdrawal. Because of its intermediate duration of action, this drug is appropriate for alternate-day administration. See your doctor regularly.

▷ **Tell Your Doctor Before Taking This Medicine If You:**
- ever had an allergic reaction to it.
- have active peptic ulcer disease.
- have an active infection of the eye caused by the herpes simplex virus.
- have active tuberculosis—it blunts the immune response.
- had an unfavorable reaction to any cortisonelike drug in the past.
- have liver compromise.
- have been exposed to measles or chickenpox.
- have a history of peptic ulcer disease, thrombophlebitis, or tuberculosis.
- have diabetes, glaucoma, high blood pressure, deficient thyroid function, or myasthenia gravis.
- plan to have surgery of any kind in the near future.

▷ **Possible Side Effects:**   Increased appetite, weight gain, retention of salt and water, excretion of potassium, increased susceptibility to infection. Cushing's syndrome (abdominal obesity, buffalo hump, and moon-shaped face).

▷ **Possible Adverse Effects:**
If any of the following develop, call your doctor promptly for guidance.
Some Mild Problems Drug Can Cause
Allergic reaction: skin rash.
Headache, dizziness, insomnia.
Abdominal distention.
Muscle cramping and weakness.
Acne, excessive growth of facial hair.
Some Serious Problems Drug Can Cause
Serious mental and emotional disturbances.
Reactivation of latent tuberculosis.

Development of peptic ulcer.

Increased blood pressure.

Decreased ability to heal wounds.

Cataracts.

Osteonecrosis.

Inflammation of the pancreas.

Thrombophlebitis—pain or tenderness in thigh or leg, with or without swelling.

Increased osteoporosis risk (with long-term use).

Pulmonary embolism—sudden shortness of breath, pain in the chest, coughing, bloody sputum.

▷ **Possible Effects on Sex Life:** Altered timing and pattern of menstruation.

▷ **Adverse Effects That May Mimic Natural Diseases or Disorders:**
Pattern of symptoms and signs resembling Cushing's syndrome.

▷ *CAUTION*

1. Carry a personal identification card that states you are taking this drug, if your course of treatment is to exceed 1 week.

2. Do not discontinue this drug abruptly if you are using it for long-term treatment.

3. If vaccination against measles, rabies, smallpox, or yellow fever is required, discontinue this drug 72 hours before vaccination and do not resume it for at least 14 days after vaccination.

4. Avoid prolonged use of this drug if possible in infants or children. During long-term use, observe for suppression of normal growth and the possibility of increased intracranial pressure. Following long-term use, the child may be at risk for adrenal deficiency during stress for as long as 18 months after the drug is stopped.

5. Cortisonelike drugs should be used very sparingly after the age of 60 and only when the disorder under treatment is unresponsive to adequate trials of unrelated drugs. Avoid prolonged use. Continual use (even in small doses) can increase the severity of diabetes, enhance fluid retention, raise blood pressure, weaken resistance to infection, induce stomach ulcer and accelerate the development of cataract and osteoporosis.

6. You are at increased risk for viral illnesses such as measles or chickenpox. Call your doctor if you are exposed to these illnesses.

7. Dermatitis may occur around the mouth. Talk to the doctor if this happens.

Advisability of Use During Pregnancy or If Breast-Feeding:

Pregnancy Category: C. Avoid completely during the first 3 months. Limit use of this drug during the last 6 months as much as possible. If used, examine the infant for possible deficiency of adrenal function. Present in breast milk; avoid taking this drug or refrain from nursing.

▷ **Habit-Forming Potential:** Use of this drug to suppress symptoms over an extended period of time may produce functional dependence. In treating conditions such as asthma and rheumatoid arthritis, it is advisable to keep the dose as small as possible and attempt drug withdrawal after periods of reasonable improvement. Such procedures may reduce the degree of steroid rebound—the return of symptoms as the drug is withdrawn.

▷ **Overdose Symptoms:** Fatigue, muscle weakness, stomach irritation, acid indigestion, excessive sweating, facial flushing, fluid retention, swelling of extremities, increased blood pressure.

▷ **Suggested Periodic Examinations While Taking This Drug:** (at doctor's discretion)
Measurements of blood pressure, blood sugar, and potassium levels.
Complete eye examinations at regular intervals.
Chest X ray if there is a history of tuberculosis.
Determination of the development rate of the growing child to detect growth retardation.

▷ **While Taking This Drug the Following Apply:**
Foods: Ask your doctor regarding the need to restrict your salt intake or eat potassium-rich foods. During long-term use of this drug, a high-protein diet is advisable.
Nutritional Support: During long-term use, take a vitamin supplement. During wound repair, take a zinc supplement.
Beverages: Drink all forms of milk liberally.
Alcohol: Use caution if you are prone to peptic ulcer disease.
Tobacco Smoking: Nicotine increases the blood levels of naturally produced cortisone and related hormones. Heavy smoking may add to the drug's expected actions and requires close observation for excessive effects.
Marijuana Smoking: May cause additional impairment of immunity.
Other Drugs:
Methylprednisolone may *decrease* the effects of
• insulin or oral hypoglycemic agents (see Drug Classes) and require dosing changes.
• isoniazid (INH, Niconyl, etc.).
• salicylates (aspirin, sodium salicylate, etc.).
Methylprednisolone *taken concurrently* with
• amphotericin B (Fungizone) may result in increased potassium loss.
• carbamazepine (Tegretol) may decrease methylprednisolone's effectiveness.

- cholestyramine (Questran) may decrease the amount of methylprednisolone that gets into your body and blunt its therapeutic effects.
- cyclosporine (Sandimmune) may result in increased steroid levels and cyclosporine toxicity.
- ketoconazole (Nizoral) may increase blood levels of methylprednisolone and result in ketoconazole toxicity.
- loop diuretics such as furosemide (Lasix) or bumetanide (Bumex) may lead to increased potassium loss.
- NSAIDs (see Drug Classes) may cause increased risk of ulceration of the stomach or intestines.
- oral anticoagulants may either increase or decrease their effectiveness; consult your doctor regarding the need for prothrombin time testing and dosage adjustment.
- primidone (Mysoline) may lead to increased metabolism of methylprednisolone and decreased therapeutic benefit of methylprednisolone.
- rifampin (Rifadin, others) may cause increased methylprednisolone metabolism and blunted beneficial effects.
- thiazide diuretics (see Drug Classes) may lead to additive potassium loss.
- theophylline (Theo-Dur, others) changes blood levels. More frequent blood level testing is needed.
- vaccines (such as flu, pneumococcal, or others) may blunt the therapeutic effect of the vaccine.

The following drugs may **decrease** the effects of methylprednisolone
- antacids may reduce its absorption.
- barbiturates (Amytal, Butisol, phenobarbital, etc.).
- phenytoin (Dilantin, etc.).
- rifampin (Rifadin, Rimactane, etc.).

Driving, Hazardous Activities: Usually no restrictions. Be alert to the rare occurrence of dizziness.

Occurrence of Unrelated Illness: May decrease resistance to infection. Tell your doctor if you develop an infection of any kind. This drug may also reduce your body's ability to respond to the stress of acute illness, injury, or surgery. Keep your doctor fully informed of any significant changes in your state of health.

Discontinuation: Do not stop this drug abruptly after taking it for an extended period. Ask your doctor for guidance regarding gradual withdrawal. In the event of illness, injury, or surgery for 2 years after discontinuing this drug, it is essential to tell attending medical personnel that you have used this drug. Impaired response to stress following the use of cortisonelike drugs may last for 1 to 2 years.

▷ **Saving Money When Using This Medicine:**
- Many new drugs are available to treat inflammation. Ask your doctor if this medicine offers the best balance of cost and outcome for you. A generic form can be substituted for the brand name.
- Ask your doctor how long this medicine is typically used to treat your condition.
- If long-term use is contemplated, talk with your doctor about specific risk factors, exercise, calcium supplements, and bone mineral density testing.

METHYSERGIDE (meth i SER jide)

Prescription Needed: Yes   **Controlled Drug:** No   **Generic:** No

Brand Name: Sansert

Overview of BENEFITS versus RISKS	
Possible Benefits	*Possible Risks*
EFFECTIVE PREVENTION OF MIGRAINE AND CLUSTER HEADACHES	FIBROSIS (SCARRING) INSIDE CHEST AND ABDOMINAL CAVITIES, OF HEART AND LUNG TISSUES ADJACENT TO MAJOR BLOOD VESSELS AND INTERNAL ORGANS
	Aggravation of hypertension, coronary artery disease, and peripheral vascular disease

▷ **Illness This Medication Treats:**
Prevention of frequent and/or disabling vascular headaches (migraine, cluster, etc.) that have not responded to other conventional treatment.

▷ **Typical Dosage Range:** (Dosage or schedule must be determined by the doctor for each individual.)
Infants and Children: Not recommended.
12 to 60 Years of Age: 2 to 6 mg daily, in divided doses. A medicine-free period of 3 to 4 weeks after every 6-month course of methysergide must occur.
Over 60 Years of Age: 2 to 4 mg daily, in divided doses. Use this drug very cautiously, with frequent monitoring for adverse effects.

▷ **Conditions Requiring Dosing Adjustments:**
Liver function: This drug should not be used by patients with liver compromise.
Kidney function: This drug should not be used by patients with kidney compromise.

▷ **How Best to Take This Medicine:** Take with food or milk to reduce stomach irritation. The tablet may be crushed. Limit continual use to 6 months; avoid this drug completely for a period of 4 weeks between courses.

▷ **How Long This Medicine Is Usually Taken:** Use on a regular schedule for 3 weeks is usually necessary to determine the effectiveness of this drug in prevention recurrence of vascular headache. If significant benefit does not occur during this trial, this drug should be stopped. Long-term use (months to years) requires periodic physician evaluation.

▷ **Tell Your Doctor Before Taking This Medicine If You:**
- ever had an allergic reaction to it.
- are pregnant.
- currently have a severe infection.
- have angina pectoris; Buerger's disease; chronic lung disease; connective tissue (collagen) disease; coronary artery disease; hardening of the arteries; heart valve disease; high blood pressure (significant hypertension); kidney disease or significantly impaired kidney function; liver disease or significantly impaired liver function; active peptic ulcer disease; peripheral vascular disease; phlebitis of any kind; Raynaud's disease or phenomenon.
- had an adverse reaction to *any other form of ergot*.
- have a history of peptic ulcer disease.

▷ **Possible Side Effects:** Fluid retention, weight gain (in some people).

▷ **Possible Adverse Effects:**
If any of the following develop, call your doctor promptly for guidance.
Some Mild Problems Drug Can Cause
Allergic reactions: skin rashes, flushing of the face, transient loss of scalp hair.
Dizziness, drowsiness, unsteadiness, altered vision.
Nausea, vomiting, diarrhea.
Transient muscle and joint pains.
Some Serious Problems Drug Can Cause
Idiosyncratic reactions: nightmares, hallucinations, acute mental disturbances.
Fibrosis involving the chest and/or abdominal cavities, heart valves, lungs, kidneys, major blood vessels.

Spasm and narrowing of coronary and peripheral arteries: anginal chest pain; cold and painful extremities; leg cramps while walking.

Hemolytic anemia.

Abnormally low white blood cell counts.

Very rare heart attack.

▷ **Possible Effects on Sex Life:**   Fibrosis of penile tissues.

▷ **Adverse Effects That May Mimic Natural Diseases or Disorders:**
Swelling of the hands, lower legs, feet, and ankles (peripheral edema) may suggest heart or kidney dysfunction.

▷ *CAUTION*
   1. Continual use of this drug without interruption must not exceed 6 months. Gradual reduction of dose is advised during the last 2 to 3 weeks of each course to prevent withdrawal headache rebound. Do not use this drug for a period of 4 to 6 weeks before resuming. This drug-free period is mandatory to reduce the risk of developing fibrosis of internal tissues.
   2. Report promptly the development of any symptoms that may indicate fibrosis: fatigue, fever, chest pain, difficult breathing, stomach or flank pain, changes in urination pattern.
   3. This drug is useful only for prevention of recurring vascular headaches; it is not recommended for acute attacks of headache. It is ineffective and should not be used for tension headaches.
   4. Use of this drug is not recommended in infants or children.
   5. The age-related changes in blood vessels and circulatory and kidney function makes people over 60 more susceptible to serious adverse effects of this drug. See the list of diseases and disorders that are contraindications to its use above. Ask your doctor for guidance.

Advisability of Use During Pregnancy or If Breast-Feeding:
Pregnancy Category: X. The manufacturer states that this drug is contraindicated during entire pregnancy. Present in breast milk; avoid taking this drug or refrain from nursing.

▷ **Overdose Symptoms:**   Nausea, vomiting, stomach pain, diarrhea, dizziness, excitement, cold hands and feet.

▷ **Suggested Periodic Examinations While Taking This Drug:** (at doctor's discretion)
Careful examination at regular intervals (6 to 12 months) for scar tissue formation or circulatory complications.

Complete blood cell counts.

Kidney function tests.

▷ **While Taking This Drug the Following Apply:**

Foods: No restrictions other than foods to which you are allergic. Some vascular headaches are due to food allergy.

Alcohol: No interactions expected. Observe closely to determine if alcoholic beverages initiate a migrainelike headache.

Tobacco Smoking: Avoid completely.

Other Drugs:

Methysergide *taken concurrently* with

- beta-blockers may result in hazardous constriction of peripheral arteries; monitor the combined effects on circulation in the extremities.

Driving, Hazardous Activities: May cause dizziness, drowsiness, or impaired vision. Restrict your activities as necessary.

Exposure to Cold: Use caution. Cold environments may increase the occurrence of reduced circulation to the extremities.

Discontinuation: Do not stop abruptly if this drug has been taken for an extended period. Gradual withdrawal over 2 to 3 weeks can prevent the development of rebound vascular headaches.

▷ **Saving Money When Using This Medicine:**

- Several new drugs are available to treat migraines. Ask your doctor if this medicine offers the best balance of cost and outcome for you.
- Talk with your doctor about using a medicine that works to help prevent migraine headaches.
- Learn as much as possible about your condition. *The Essential Guide to Chronic Illness* is an excellent resource.

METOCLOPRAMIDE (met oh kloh PRA mide)

Prescription Needed: Yes   **Controlled Drug:** No   **Generic:** Yes

Brand Names: Maxolon, Octamide, Reclomide, Reglan

Overview of BENEFITS versus RISKS

Possible Benefits	*Possible Risks*
EFFECTIVE STOMACH STIMULANT FOR CORRECTING DELAYED EMPTYING	Sedation and fatigue
	Parkinson-like reactions
	Rare tardive dyskinesia
Symptomatic relief in reflux esophagitis	
Relief of nausea and vomiting associated with migraine headache	

▷ **Illness This Medication Treats:**
(1) Stomach retention (gastroparesis) seen in diabetes; (2) acid reflux from the stomach into the esophagus (esophagitis); (3) nausea and vomiting associated with migraine headaches; (4) nausea and vomiting induced by anticancer drugs; (5) may be helpful when a tube needs to be placed in the stomach.

▷ **Typical Dosage Range:** (Dosage or schedule must be determined by the doctor for each individual.)
10 mg taken 30 minutes before breakfast, lunch, and dinner, and at bedtime (four times a day). The total daily dose should not exceed 0.5 mg per kilogram of body weight.

▷ **Conditions Requiring Dosing Adjustments:**
Kidney function: For patients with moderate kidney failure, 75% of the usual dose can be taken at the usual dosing interval. For patients with severe kidney failure, 50% of the usual dose can be taken at the usual dosing interval. For these patients a benefit-to-risk decision is required.

▷ **How Best to Take This Medicine:**   Take tablet or syrup 30 minutes before each meal and at bedtime. The tablet may be crushed.

▷ **How Long This Medicine Is Usually Taken:**   Continual use on a regular schedule for 5 to 7 days is usually necessary to determine the effectiveness of this drug in accelerating stomach emptying and relieving symptoms of heartburn, fullness, and belching. Long-term use (months to years) requires supervision and periodic evaluation. See your doctor regularly.

▷ **Tell Your Doctor Before Taking This Medicine If You:**
- ever had an allergic reaction to it.
- have a seizure disorder of any kind.
- have active gastrointestinal bleeding.
- have a pheochromocytoma.
- are allergic or overly sensitive to procaine or procainamide.
- are taking tricyclic antidepressants or have taken an MAO inhibitor (see Drug Classes) within the past 14 days.
- have impaired liver or kidney function.
- have Parkinson's disease.
- have high blood pressure or a history of depression.
- are taking any atropinelike drugs, antipsychotic drugs, or opioid analgesics.

▷ **Possible Side Effects:**   Drowsiness and lethargy, breast tenderness and swelling, milk production.

▷ **Possible Adverse Effects:**
If any of the following develop, call your doctor promptly for guidance.
Some Mild Problems Drug Can Cause
Allergic reaction: skin rash.
Headache, dizziness, restlessness, depression, insomnia.
Dry mouth, nausea, diarrhea, constipation.
Urinary retention or incontinence.
Some Serious Problems Drug Can Cause
Idiosyncratic reactions: neuroleptic malignant syndrome.
Parkinson-like reactions.
Rare tardive dyskinesia.
Very rare decreased white blood cells.
Rare severe increases in blood pressure (hypertensive crisis).
Rare drug-induced porphyria.
Rare abnormal heartbeats.
Rare abnormal fixed positioning of the eyes (oculogyric crisis).

▷ **Possible Effects on Sex Life:**   Decreased libido, impaired erection, decreased sperm count. Abnormally sustained erection (priapism). Altered timing and pattern of menstruation, galactorrhea.

▷ *CAUTION*
1. Watch for early development of Parkinson-like reactions in infants and children soon after starting treatment with this drug. Use of the smallest effective dose can minimize these reactions in this population.
2. For those over 60 years of age, Parkinson-like reactions and tardive dyskinesia are more likely with the use of high doses over an extended period. Determine the smallest effective dose and use only when clearly needed.

Advisability of Use During Pregnancy or If Breast-Feeding:

Pregnancy Category: B. Use only if clearly needed. Present in breast milk; avoid taking this drug or refrain from nursing.

▷ **Overdose Symptoms:** Marked drowsiness, confusion, muscle spasms, jerking movements of head and face, tremors, shuffling gait.

▷ **Suggested Periodic Examinations While Taking This Drug:** (at doctor's discretion)

During long-term use, look for fine, wormlike movements on the surface of the tongue; these may be the first indications of an emerging tardive dyskinesia.

▷ **While Taking This Drug the Following Apply:**

Beverages: May be taken with milk.

Alcohol: Use with extreme caution or avoid. Combined effects can result in excessive sedation and marked intoxication.

Other Drugs:

Metoclopramide may *decrease* the effects of

- cimetidine (Tagamet).
- digoxin (slow-dissolving dosage forms), reducing its effectiveness.

Metoclopramide *taken concurrently* with

- acetaminophen may increase metoclopramide absorption. Decreased metoclopramide doses may be needed.
- cyclosporine (Sandimmune) may lead to cyclosporine toxicity.
- major antipsychotic drugs (phenothiazines, thiothixenes, haloperidol, etc.) may increase the risk of developing Parkinson-like reactions.
- morphine (slow-release) may result in a faster start of medicine effects and sedation.
- penicillin may blunt the therapeutic effects of the antibiotic.
- quinidine (Quinaglute, others) may blunt quinidine's therapeutic benefits.

The following drugs may *decrease* the effects of metoclopramide

- atropinelike drugs.
- opioid analgesics (see Drug Classes).

Driving, Hazardous Activities: May cause drowsiness and dizziness. Restrict your activities as necessary.

▷ **Saving Money When Using This Medicine:**

- A new drug is available to treat many of the same conditions for which this drug is used. Ask your doctor if this medicine offers the best balance of cost and outcome for you.
- A generic form can be substituted for the brand name.
- Ask your doctor how long this medicine is usually taken to treat your condition.
- If this medicine is being used for diabetic gastroparesis, remember

that many diabetic complications arise from blood sugar that is poorly controlled. Talk with your doctor about regular fingerstick blood sugar testing. Also ask if taking aspirin every other day makes sense for you.

METOLAZONE   (me TOHL a zohn)

Prescription Needed: Yes   **Controlled Drug:** No   **Generic:** No

Brand Names: Diulo, Mykrox, Zaroxolyn

Overview of BENEFITS versus RISKS	
Possible Benefits	*Possible Risks*
EFFECTIVE, WELL-TOLERATED DIURETIC	Loss of body potassium
	Increased blood sugar
	Increased blood uric acid
POSSIBLY EFFECTIVE IN MILD HYPERTENSION	Liver damage, jaundice (rare)
ENHANCES EFFECTIVENESS OF OTHER ANTIHYPERTENSIVES	Blood cell disorder: abnormally low white blood cell count (rare)

See the thiazide diuretics drug profile for further information.

METOPROLOL   (me TOH proh lohl)

Prescription Needed: Yes   **Controlled Drug:** No   **Generic:** No

Brand Names: Lopressor, Lopressor HCT [CD], Lopressor OROS, Lopressor Slow-Release, Toprol, Toprol-XL

Overview of BENEFITS versus RISKS

Possible Benefits	*Possible Risks*
EFFECTIVE, WELL-TOLERATED ANTIHYPERTENSIVE for mild to moderate high blood pressure	CONGESTIVE HEART FAILURE in advanced heart disease
	Worsening of angina in coronary heart disease (abrupt withdrawal)
	Masking of low blood sugar (hypoglycemia) in drug-treated diabetes
	Provocation of asthma (with high doses)

▷ **Illness This Medication Treats:**
   (1) Mild to moderate high blood pressure; may be used alone or concurrently with other antihypertensive drugs, such as diuretics; (2) helps in reduction of frequency and severity of angina; (3) helps reduce the risk of a second heart attack.

▷ **Typical Dosage Range:** (Dosage or schedule must be determined by the doctor for each individual.)
   Initially 50 mg twice daily (12 hours apart). The dose may be increased gradually at intervals of 7 to 10 days, as needed and tolerated, up to 300 mg/day. For maintenance: 100 mg twice per day. The total daily dose should not exceed 450 mg.

▷ **Conditions Requiring Dosing Adjustments:**
   Liver function: Patients with liver compromise should use this drug with caution.

▷ **How Best to Take This Medicine:**   May be taken without regard to eating. The regular tablet may be crushed for administration. The prolonged-action tablet should be swallowed whole (not altered). Do not stop taking this drug abruptly.

▷ **How Long This Medicine Is Usually Taken:**   Up to 14 days of regular use may be needed to determine the effectiveness of this drug in lowering blood pressure. Long-term use of this drug (months to years) is determined by the course of your blood pressure over time and your response to the overall treatment program (weight reduction, salt restriction, smoking cessation, etc.). See your doctor regularly.

▷ **Tell Your Doctor Before Taking This Medicine If You:**
- ever had an allergic reaction to it.
- have congestive heart failure.
- have an abnormally slow heart rate or serious form of heart block.
- are taking, or have taken within the past 14 days, any monoamine oxidase (MAO) type A inhibitor.
- had an adverse reaction to any beta-blocker in the past.
- have a history of serious heart disease, with or without episodes of heart failure.
- have a history of hay fever, asthma, chronic bronchitis, or emphysema.
- have a history of overactive thyroid function.
- have a history of low blood sugar.
- have impaired liver or kidney function.
- have diabetes or myasthenia gravis.
- take any form of digitalis, quinidine, or reserpine, or any calcium blocker.
- plan to have surgery under general anesthesia soon.

▷ **Possible Side Effects:**   Lethargy and fatigability, cold extremities, slow heart rate, light-headedness in upright position.

▷ **Possible Adverse Effects:**
If any of the following develop, call your doctor promptly for guidance.
Some Mild Problems Drug Can Cause
Allergic reactions: skin rash, itching.
Headache, dizziness, insomnia, abnormal dreams.
Nausea, vomiting, constipation, diarrhea.
Joint and muscle discomfort, fluid retention.
Some Serious Problems Drug Can Cause
Mental depression, anxiety.
Chest pain, shortness of breath, precipitation of congestive heart failure.
Hallucinations.
Rare liver compromise or carpal tunnel syndrome.
Precipitation of myasthenia gravis.
Induction of bronchial asthma (in asthmatic individuals).

▷ **Possible Effects on Sex Life:** Decreased libido (four times more common in men); impaired erection (less common than with most beta-blockers); Peyronie's disease.

▷ *CAUTION*

1. *Do not stop taking this drug suddenly* without the knowledge and guidance of your doctor. Carry a notation stating that you are taking this drug.

2. Ask your doctor or pharmacist before using nasal decongestants, usually present in over-the-counter cold preparations and nose drops. These can cause sudden increases in blood pressure when taken concurrently with a beta-blocker.

3. Report the development of any tendency to emotional depression.

4. Safety and effectiveness of this drug for those under 12 years have not been established. However, if this drug is used, observe for low blood sugar during periods of reduced food intake.

5. Those over 60 should proceed *cautiously* with all antihypertensives. Unacceptably high blood pressure should be reduced without the risks associated with excessively low blood pressure. Start treatment with small doses, and monitor the blood pressure response frequently. Sudden, rapid, and excessive reduction of blood pressure can predispose to stroke or heart attack. Observe for dizziness, unsteadiness, tendency to fall, confusion, hallucinations, depression, or urinary frequency.

6. This drug should NOT be used by people with a creatinine clearance less than 40 ml/min.

Advisability of Use During Pregnancy or If Breast-Feeding:

Pregnancy Category: C. Use only if clearly needed. Ask your doctor for guidance. Present in breast milk in large amounts. Avoid using this drug or refrain from nursing.

▷ **Overdose Symptoms:**   Weakness, slow pulse, low blood pressure, fainting, cold and sweaty skin, congestive heart failure, possible coma and convulsions.

▷ **Suggested Periodic Examinations While Taking This Drug:** (at doctor's discretion)

Measurements of blood pressure, evaluation of heart function.

▷ **While Taking This Drug the Following Apply:**

Foods: Avoid excessive salt intake.

Beverages: May be taken with milk.

Alcohol: Alcohol may exaggerate this drug's ability to lower the blood pressure and increase its mild sedative effect.

Tobacco Smoking: Nicotine may reduce this drug's effectiveness in treating high blood pressure. In addition, high doses may potentiate the constriction of the bronchial tubes caused by regular smoking.

Other Drugs:

Metoprolol may *increase* the effects of

- other antihypertensive drugs, causing excessive lowering of the blood pressure. Dosage adjustments may be necessary.

- reserpine (Ser-Ap-Es, etc.), causing sedation, depression, slowing of the heart rate, and lowering of blood pressure.
- verapamil (Calan, Isoptin), causing excessive depression of heart function; monitor this combination closely.

Metoprolol *taken concurrently* with

- amiodarone (Cordarone) may lead to an extremely slow heartbeat and cardiac arrest.
- clonidine (Catapres) requires close monitoring for rebound high blood pressure if clonidine is withdrawn while metoprolol is still being taken.
- fluoxetine (Prozac) may lead to metoprolol toxicity.
- fluvoxamine (Luvox) can cause metoprolol toxicity.
- insulin requires close monitoring to avoid undetected hypoglycemia.
- lidocaine can lead to lidocaine toxicity.
- nifedipine (Adalat, others) may lead to heart failure.
- oral hypoglycemic agents (see Drug Classes) can prolong hypoglycemia if it occurs.
- phenothiazines (see Drug Classes) may lead to low blood pressure or phenothiazine toxicity.
- quinidine (Quinaglute) can cause an abnormally slow heartbeat.
- tocainide (Tonocard) may lead to depressed ability of the heart to beat.
- venlafaxine (Effexor) may lead to metabolic changes and toxic blood levels of both medicines.

The following drugs may *increase* the effects of metoprolol

- cimetidine (Tagamet).
- diltiazem (Cardizem).
- methimazole (Tapazole).
- MAO inhibitors (see Drug Classes).
- oral contraceptives (birth control pills).
- propylthiouracil (Propacil).

The following drugs may *decrease* the effects of metoprolol

- barbiturates (phenobarbital, etc.).
- indomethacin (Indocin), and possibly other NSAID aspirin substitutes, may impair metoprolol's antihypertensive effect.
- rifampin (Rifadin, Rimactane).

Driving, Hazardous Activities: Use caution until the full extent of drowsiness, lethargy, and blood pressure change has been determined.

Exposure to Heat: Caution is advised. Hot environments can lower the blood pressure and exaggerate the effects of this drug.

Exposure to Cold: Caution is advised. Cold environments enhance the circulatory deficiency in the extremities that may occur. The elderly should take precautions to prevent hypothermia.

Heavy Exercise or Exertion: It is best to avoid exertion that produces light-headedness, excessive fatigue, or muscle cramping. This drug may intensify the hypertensive response to isometric exercise.

Occurrence of Unrelated Illness: The fever that accompanies systemic infections can lower blood pressure and require dosage adjustment. Illnesses that cause nausea or vomiting may interrupt the regular dosage schedule. Ask your doctor for guidance.

Discontinuation: It is advisable to avoid sudden discontinuation of this drug in all situations. If possible, gradual reduction of dose over a period of 2 to 3 weeks is recommended. Ask your doctor for specific guidance.

▷ **Saving Money When Using This Medicine:**
- Many beta-blockers are available to treat high blood pressure. Ask your doctor if this medicine offers the best balance of cost and outcome for you.
- A once-a-day form is available and may actually be less expensive than the immediate-release form. Ask your doctor if this is true for you.
- Have your blood pressure checked regularly, to make sure this medicine is still working for you.
- Talk with your doctor to see if taking aspirin every other day makes sense for you.

METRONIDAZOLE (me troh NI da zohl)

Prescription Needed: Yes **Controlled Drug:** No **Generic:** Yes

Brand Names: Flagyl, Metizol, MetroGel, Metryl, Protostat, SK Metronidazole

---

Overview of BENEFITS versus RISKS

Possible Benefits	*Possible Risks*
EFFECTIVE TREATMENT FOR *TRICHOMONAS* INFECTIONS, AMEBIC DYSENTERY, AND GIARDIASIS	Superinfection with yeast organisms
Effective treatment for some anaerobic bacterial infections	Peripheral neuropathy
	Abnormally low white blood cell count (transient)
Effective local treatment for rosacea	Aggravation of epilepsy
	Colitis

▷ **Illness This Medication Treats:**

(1) *Trichomonas* infections of the vaginal canal, cervix, or male urethra; (2) amebic dysentery, *Giardia* infections of the intestine, and serious infections caused by certain strains of anaerobic bacteria; (3) *Gardnerella* infections of the vagina; (4) rosacea with local application of a gel dosage form; (5) pseudomembranous colitis; (6) bedsores; (7) prevention of some surgical infections.

Other (unlabeled) generally accepted uses: (1) combination antibiotic treatment of duodenal ulcers caused by *Helicobacter pylori*; (2) help lesions heal in Crohn's disease.

▷ **Typical Dosage Range:** (Dosage or schedule must be determined by the doctor for each individual.)

Varies with infection to be treated.

For trichomoniasis: 1-day course: 2 g as a single dose, or 1 g for two doses 12 hours apart. 7-day course: 250 mg three times each day for 7 consecutive days (7-day course preferred).

For amebiasis: 500 to 750 mg three times each day for 5 to 10 consecutive days.

For giardiasis: 2 g once a day for 3 days; or 250 to 500 mg three times each day for 5 to 7 days.

The total daily dosage should not exceed 4 g (4000 mg).

▷ **Conditions Requiring Dosing Adjustments:**

Liver function: The dose should be decreased by one-third for patients with mild to moderate liver compromise. Metronidazole should NOT be used by patients with severe liver compromise.

Kidney function: For patients with severe kidney failure, 50% of the normal dose can be taken at the usual dosing interval. Use of metronidazole by these patients requires a benefit-to-risk decision because of the risk of systemic lupus erythematosus (SLE) from this drug's metabolites.

▷ **How Best to Take This Medicine:**   May be taken with or following food to reduce stomach irritation. The tablet may be crushed for administration.

▷ **How Long This Medicine Is Usually Taken:**   Continual use on a regular schedule, as outlined, is necessary to ensure effectiveness. Do not repeat the course of treatment without your doctor's approval.

▷ **Tell Your Doctor Before Taking This Medicine If You:**
  • ever had an allergic reaction to it.
  • currently have a bone marrow or blood cell disorder.
  • have any type of central nervous system disorder, including epilepsy.
  • have a history of any type of blood cell disorder, especially drug-induced.
  • have impaired liver or kidney function.
  • are pregnant or breast-feeding.

▷ **Possible Side Effects:**   A sharp, metallic, unpleasant taste.
Dark discoloration of the urine (of no significance).
Superinfection by yeast organisms in the mouth or vagina.

▷ **Possible Adverse Effects:**
If any of the following develop, call your doctor promptly for guidance.
Some Mild Problems Drug Can Cause
  Allergic reactions: skin rash, flushing, itching.
  Headache, dizziness, incoordination, unsteadiness.
  Loss of appetite, nausea, vomiting, diarrhea.
  Irritation of mouth and tongue, possibly due to yeast infection.
Some Serious Problems Drug Can Cause
  Idiosyncratic reactions: abnormal behavior, confusion, depression.
  Peripheral neuropathy.
  Abnormally low white blood cell count (transient): fever, sore throat, infections.
  Rare pneumonitis, pancreatitis, or porphyria.

▷ **Possible Effects on Sex Life:**   Decreased libido; decreased vaginal secretions (difficult or painful intercourse).

▷ **Possible Delayed Adverse Effects:**   Studies have shown that this drug can cause cancer in mice and possibly rats. No evidence to date shows that it causes cancer in humans when used in specified dosages. Follow your doctor's instructions exactly. Avoid unnecessary or prolonged use.

▷ **CAUTION**

1. Troublesome and persistent diarrhea can develop in sensitive individuals. If diarrhea persists for more than 24 hours, discontinue this drug and call your doctor.
2. Discontinue this drug immediately if you develop any indications of toxic effects on the brain or nervous system: confusion, irritability, dizziness, incoordination, unsteady stance or gait, muscle jerking or twitching, numbness or weakness in the extremities.
3. Avoid use of this drug in infants and children with a history of bone marrow or blood cell disorders.
4. Those over 60 may have natural changes in the skin that predispose to yeast infections in the genital and anal regions. Report the development of rashes and itching promptly.

Advisability of Use During Pregnancy or If Breast-Feeding:

Pregnancy Category: B. The manufacturer advises against use of this drug during the first 3 months. Use during the last 6 months is not advised unless it is absolutely essential to the mother's health. Present in breast milk; avoid taking this drug or refrain from nursing.

▷ **Overdose Symptoms:**   Weakness, stomach irritation, nausea, vomiting, confusion, disorientation.

▷ **Suggested Periodic Examinations While Taking This Drug:** (at doctor's discretion)

Complete blood cell counts.

▷ **While Taking This Drug the Following Apply:**

Beverages: May be taken with milk.

Alcohol: A disulfiramlike reaction has been reported. DO NOT DRINK alcohol.

Other Drugs.

Metronidazole may *increase* the effects of

- warfarin (Coumadin, etc.), causing abnormal bleeding. The INR (prothrombin time) should be monitored closely, especially during the first 10 days of concurrent use.

Metronidazole *taken concurrently* with

- antacids may blunt the therapeutic benefits of metronidazole.
- oral contraceptives (birth control pills) may block their effectiveness and result in unwanted pregnancy.
- cholestyramine (Questran) or other cholesterol-lowering resins may blunt metronidazole's benefits.
- co-trimoxazole or other sulfa drugs may result in a disulfiramlike reaction.
- disulfiram (Antabuse) may cause severe emotional and behavioral disturbances.

- lithium (Lithobid, others) can lead to lithium toxicity.
- phenytoin (Dilantin) may result in increased blood levels of phenytoin. Lab testing of phenytoin levels and adjustment of phenytoin dosing to lab results is prudent.

Driving, Hazardous Activities: May cause dizziness or incoordination. Restrict your activities as necessary.

▷ **Saving Money When Using This Medicine:**
- Many new drugs are available to treat infections. Ask your doctor if this medicine offers the best balance of cost and outcome for you.
- A generic form can be substituted for the brand name.
- Ask your doctor how long this medicine is usually taken to treat your condition.
- If you have an anaerobic infection, you can shorten your length of stay in the hospital by changing from an intravenous drug to metronidazole taken by mouth.

MEXILETINE (mex IL e teen)

Prescription Needed: Yes   **Controlled Drug:** No   **Generic:** No

Brand Name: Mexitil

Overview of BENEFITS versus RISKS	
Possible Benefits	*Possible Risks*
EFFECTIVE TREATMENT FOR SELECTED HEART RHYTHM DISORDERS	NARROW TREATMENT RANGE
	FREQUENT ADVERSE EFFECTS
	WORSENING OF SOME ARRHYTHMIAS
	Rare seizures, liver injury, and reduced white blood cell count

▷ **Illness This Medication Treats:**
Correction of premature heartbeats formed in the ventricles (lower heart chambers) that have not been helped by other agents.

▷ **Typical Dosage Range:** (Dosage or schedule must be determined by the doctor for each individual.)
The loading dose is 400 mg, followed by 200 mg/8 hr. At intervals of 2 to 3 days, increase dose by 50 to 100 mg, as needed and tolerated. The total daily dosage should not exceed 1200 mg. Measurement of

drug blood levels are prudent to determine optimal dose and schedule.

▷ **Conditions Requiring Dosing Adjustments:**
Liver function: The dose should be decreased by one-fourth to one-third for patients with compromised livers. Blood levels should be obtained at prudent intervals.
Kidney function: The dose should be decreased for patients with severe kidney compromise; however, no specific guidelines are available. Use of mexiletine by these patients requires a benefit-to-risk decision.

▷ **How Best to Take This Medicine:** Take this drug with food or antacid to reduce stomach irritation, and take it at the same times each day to obtain uniform results. The capsule may be opened for administration.

▷ **How Long This Medicine Is Usually Taken:** Continual use on a regular schedule for 1 to 2 weeks is usually necessary to determine the effectiveness of this drug in correcting or preventing responsive rhythm disorders. Long-term use requires supervision and periodic evaluation. See your doctor regularly.

▷ **Tell Your Doctor Before Taking This Medicine If You:**
- ever had an allergic reaction to it.
- have second- or third-degree heart block (determined by electrocardiogram), uncorrected by a pacemaker.
- have had any unfavorable reactions to other antiarrhythmics in the past.
- have a history of heart disease of any kind, especially heart block or heart failure.
- have impaired liver function.
- have a seizure disorder of any kind.
- are taking any form of digitalis, a potassium supplement, or a diuretic that can cause excessive loss of body potassium (ask your doctor).

▷ **Possible Side Effects:** Nervousness, light-headedness

▷ **Possible Adverse Effects:**
If any of the following develop, call your doctor promptly for guidance.
Some Mild Problems Drug Can Cause
Allergic reaction: skin rash.
Headache, dizziness, visual disturbance, weakness, tremor.
Loss of appetite, nausea, vomiting, constipation, diarrhea, abdominal pain.

Some Serious Problems Drug Can Cause

Idiosyncratic reactions: depression, amnesia, hallucinations, seizures.

Drug-induced heart rhythm disorders, shortness of breath, palpitations, chest pain, swelling of feet.

Urinary retention.

Liver damage with jaundice.

Rare seizures, myelofibrosis, ataxia, or systemic lupus erythematosus.

Abnormally low white blood cell and blood platelet counts (rare): fever, sore throat, abnormal bleeding or bruising.

▷ **Possible Effects on Sex Life:**   Decreased libido, impotence (rare).

▷ *CAUTION*

1. Thorough evaluation of your heart function (including electrocardiograms) is necessary before using this drug.

2. Periodic evaluation of your heart function is necessary to determine your response. Some individuals may experience worsening of their heart rhythm disorder and/or deterioration of heart function. Close monitoring of heart rate, rhythm, and overall performance is essential.

3. Dosage must be adjusted carefully for each individual. Do not change your dosage without the knowledge and supervision of your doctor.

4. Do not take any other antiarrhythmic while taking this drug unless directed by your doctor.

5. Carry a personal identification card that states you are taking this drug. Inform all attending medical personnel that you are taking this drug, especially if you require surgery.

6. Safety and effectiveness of this drug for those under 12 years have not been established. Mexiletine's initial use requires hospitalization and supervision by a qualified cardiologist.

7. Those over 60 with reduced liver function may require a decreased dose. Watch carefully for light-headedness, dizziness, unsteadiness, and a tendency to fall.

Advisability of Use During Pregnancy or If Breast-Feeding:

Pregnancy Category: C. Avoid using this drug during the first 3 months. Use this drug only if clearly needed. Ask your doctor for guidance. Present in breast milk; avoid taking this drug or refrain from nursing.

▷ **Overdose Symptoms:**   Impaired urination, constipation, marked drop in blood pressure, abnormal heart rhythms, congestive heart failure, dizziness, incoordination, seizures.

▷ **Suggested Periodic Examinations While Taking This Drug:** (at doctor's discretion)

Electrocardiograms, complete blood cell counts, liver function tests.

▷ **While Taking This Drug the Following Apply:**

Foods: Ask your doctor regarding any need for salt restriction.

Beverages: May be taken with milk.

Alcohol: Alcohol can increase the blood pressure–lowering effects of this drug.

Tobacco Smoking: Nicotine can cause irritability of the heart and reduce this drug's effectiveness.

Other Drugs:

Mexiletine may *increase* the effects of

• antihypertensive drugs, causing excessive lowering of blood pressure.

• beta-blockers (see Drug Classes).

• disopyramide (Norpace).

• theophylline (Theo-Dur, others), leading to theophylline toxicity.

The following drugs may *decrease* the effects of mexiletine

• phenytoin (Dilantin, etc.).

• rifampin (Rifadin, Rimactane).

Driving, Hazardous Activities: May cause weakness, dizziness, or blurred vision. Restrict your activities as necessary.

Occurrence of Unrelated Illness: Disorders that cause vomiting, diarrhea, or dehydration can affect this drug's action adversely. Report such developments promptly.

Discontinuation: This drug should not be discontinued abruptly following long-term use. Ask your doctor for guidance regarding gradual dose reduction.

▷ **Saving Money When Using This Medicine:**

• Ask your doctor if this medicine offers the best balance of cost and outcome for you

• Doses must be decreased for patients with liver or kidney compromise.

• Talk with your doctor to see if taking aspirin every other day makes sense for you.

MINOXIDIL (min OX i dil)

Prescription Needed: Yes **Controlled Drug:** No **Generic:** Yes

Brand Names: Loniten, Minodyl, Minoximen, Rogaine

Author's note: Rogaine treatment for baldness is now available without a prescription.

```
┌─────────────────────────────────────────────────────────┐
│              Overview of BENEFITS versus RISKS           │
│        Possible Benefits            Possible Risks        │
│     A POTENT, LONG-ACTING        EXCESSIVE BODY HAIR      │
│       ANTIHYPERTENSIVE             GROWTH                 │
│     EFFECTIVE FOR SEVERE         SALT AND WATER           │
│       HYPERTENSION                 RETENTION              │
│     EFFECTIVE FOR                Excessively rapid heart rate │
│       ACCELERATED AND           Aggravation of angina     │
│       MALIGNANT                 Local scalp irritation (topical │
│       HYPERTENSION                 use)                   │
│     Moderately effective in treating                     │
│       male-pattern baldness                              │
└─────────────────────────────────────────────────────────┘
```

▷ **Illness This Medication Treats:**
  (1) Severe high blood pressure that cannot be controlled by conventional therapy; (2) male-pattern baldness or female androgenic baldness, with topical application to the scalp; (3) effective for people with kidney failure and high blood pressure.

▷ **Typical Dosage Range:**   For hypertension: Initially 5 mg/24 hr in one dose. Gradually increase dose to 10, 20, then 40 mg every 24 hours, taken in one or two divided doses daily, as needed and tolerated. The usual maintenance dose is 10 to 40 mg every 24 hours. The total daily dosage should not exceed 50 mg. For male-pattern baldness: Apply thinly 1 ml of topical solution to the balding area of the scalp twice daily. The total daily dosage should not exceed 2 ml.

▷ **Conditions Requiring Dosing Adjustments:**
  Liver function: This drug is metabolized (90%) in the liver. Patients with liver compromise should use this drug with caution.
  Kidney function: For patients with moderate kidney failure, the dose should be decreased empirically.

▷ **How Best to Take This Medicine:**   For hypertension: Tablets may be taken with or following food to prevent nausea. Take at the same time each day. The tablet may be crushed for administration. For baldness: *The topical solution is for external, local use only; do not swallow.* Begin application at the center of the bald area; apply thinly on dry scalp and hair to cover the entire area. Carefully follow the instructions with the applicator.

▷ **How Long This Medicine Is Usually Taken:**   Use on a regular schedule for 3 to 7 days is usually necessary to determine the effectiveness of this drug in controlling severe hypertension. Continual use of the topical solution for at least 4 months is necessary to determine its ability to promote hair growth. Long-term use (months to years) of both dosage forms requires physician supervision.

▷ **Tell Your Doctor Before Taking This Medicine If You:**
- ever had an allergic reaction to it.
- have a pheochromocytoma.
- have pulmonary hypertension due to mitral valve stenosis.
- are pregnant or planning pregnancy.
- have a history of coronary artery disease or impaired heart function.
- have a history of stroke or impaired brain circulation.
- have impaired liver or kidney function.

▷ **Possible Side Effects:** Increased heart rate; fluid retention with weight gain; excessive hair growth on face, arms, legs, and back.

▷ **Possible Adverse Effects:**
If any of the following develop, call your doctor promptly for guidance.
Some Mild Problems Drug Can Cause
Allergic reactions: skin rash. Localized dermatitis at site of application of topical solution.
Headache, dizziness, fainting.
Nausea, increased thirst.
Some Serious Problems Drug Can Cause
Idiosyncratic reaction: fluid formation around the heart.
Development of angina pectoris; development of high blood pressure in the lung circulation.
Rare systemic lupus erythematosus or lowering of white blood cells or platelets (white blood cell and platelet effect is rare and transitory).

▷ **Possible Effects on Sex Life:** Male breast tenderness. Some data state that this medicine may help ejaculation and sex drive in men who have had this blunted by other medicines.

▷ *CAUTION*
1. Long-term use of this drug for hypertension usually requires the concurrent use of an effective diuretic to counteract salt and water retention.
2. Long-term use of this drug for hypertension often requires the concurrent use of a beta-blocker to control excessive acceleration of the heart rate.
3. It is best to avoid the concurrent use of this drug with guanethidine; the combination can cause severe orthostatic hypotension.
4. Ask your doctor about the advisability of a no-salt-added diet.
5. Only very small amounts are absorbed into the general circulation when the topical solution is applied to the scalp. However, some systemic effects have been reported. Tell your doctor promptly if you experience any unusual symptoms.
6. Dosage schedules for infants and children should be determined

by a qualified pediatrician. Monitor closely for salt and water retention.

7. People over 60 should use this drug very cautiously. Small doses and a maximum total daily dose of 75 mg is indicated. Headache, palpitation, and rapid heart rate due to this drug are more common in this age group and can mimic acute anxiety states. Observe for dizziness, unsteadiness, fainting, and falling.

Advisability of Use During Pregnancy or If Breast-Feeding:

Pregnancy Category: C. Avoid using this drug during the first 3 months. Use only if clearly needed during the last 6 months. Present in breast milk; avoid taking this drug or refrain from nursing.

▷ **Overdose Symptoms:** Headache, dizziness, weakness, nausea, marked low blood pressure, weak and rapid pulse, loss of consciousness.

▷ **Suggested Periodic Examinations While Taking This Drug:** (at doctor's discretion)

Body weight measurement for insidious gain due to water retention. Electrocardiographic and echocardiographic heart examinations.

▷ **While Taking This Drug the Following Apply:**

Foods: Avoid excessive salt and heavily salted foods.

Beverages: No restrictions. This drug may be taken with milk.

Alcohol: Use with extreme caution until combined effects have been determined. Alcohol can exaggerate the blood pressure–lowering effects of this drug.

Tobacco Smoking: Best avoided. Nicotine can contribute significantly to angina in susceptible individuals.

Other Drugs:

Minoxidil may *increase* the effects of

• all other antihypertensive drugs; careful dosage adjustments are mandatory.

Minoxidil *taken concurrently* with

• guanethidine (Ismelin, Esimil) may cause severe orthostatic hypotension; avoid this combination.

• NSAIDs (see Drug Classes) may blunt the therapeutic effect of minoxidil in helping control blood pressure.

• vitamin E may reverse hair growth.

Driving, Hazardous Activities: May cause dizziness and fatigue. Restrict your activities as necessary.

Discontinuation: This drug should not be stopped abruptly. If it is to be discontinued, ask your doctor about gradual reduction in dosage and appropriate replacement with other drugs for hypertension. Following the discontinuation of the topical solution, the pretreatment pattern of baldness may return within 3 to 4 months.

▷ **Saving Money When Using This Medicine:**
- Many new drugs are available to treat high blood pressure. Ask your doctor if this medicine offers the best balance of cost and outcome for you. Also ask how often he or she wants you to check your blood pressure.
- Another drug, finasteride (Proscar), has been found to help male-pattern baldness. Ask your doctor which drug delivers the best balance of cost and outcome for you.
- The dose should be decreased for patients with liver or kidney compromise. Ask your doctor whether the dose decrease is proportionate to the degree of your compromise.
- A generic form can be substituted for the brand name.
- Ask your doctor if taking aspirin every day makes sense for you.

MISOPROSTOL (mi soh PROH stohl)

Prescription Needed: Yes   **Controlled Drug:** No   **Generic:** No

Brand Names: Arthrotec, Cytotec

Overview of BENEFITS versus RISKS	
Possible Benefits	*Possible Risks*
EFFECTIVE PREVENTION OF STOMACH ULCERATION WHILE TAKING ANTI-INFLAMMATORY DRUGS	ABORTION Diarrhea (transient) Rare neuropathy
Effective treatment of duodenal ulcer	

▷ **Illness This Medication Treats:**
Prevents stomach ulcers during long-term use of anti-inflammatory drugs for arthritis and related conditions.

▷ **Typical Dosage Range:** (Dosage or schedule must be determined by the doctor for each individual.)
For prevention of stomach ulcer: 100 to 200 mcg four times daily, taken concurrently during the use of any anti-inflammatory drug (see Antiarthritic/Anti-Inflammatory Agents Drug Class).
For treatment of duodenal ulcer: 200 mcg four times daily for 4 to 8 weeks.

▷ **Conditions Requiring Dosing Adjustments:**
Kidney function: The dose should be decreased for patients with compromised kidneys, or when the drug is not well tolerated.

▷ **How Best to Take This Medicine:** Take the prescribed dose with each of three daily meals; take the last (fourth) dose of the day with food at bedtime. The tablet may be crushed.

▷ **How Long This Medicine Is Usually Taken:** For prevention of stomach ulcer, continual use on a regular schedule is recommended for the entire period of anti-inflammatory drug use. For treatment of duodenal ulcer, continual use on a regular schedule for 4 weeks is recommended; if ulcer healing is not complete, a second course of 4 weeks is advised. Long-term use (months to years) requires periodic evaluation of response and dosage adjustment. See your doctor regularly.

▷ **Tell Your Doctor Before Taking This Medicine If You:**
- ever had an allergic reaction to it.
- are allergic to any type of prostaglandin.
- are pregnant or breast-feeding.
- are not able or willing to use effective contraception while taking this drug.
- have a history of peptic ulcer disease or Crohn's disease.
- have impaired kidney function.
- have a seizure disorder.

▷ **Possible Side Effects:** Diarrhea, usually beginning after 13 days of use and subsiding spontaneously after 8 days.

Abortion (miscarriage); this is often incomplete and accompanied by serious uterine bleeding that may require hospitalization and urgent treatment.

▷ **Possible Adverse Effects:**
If any of the following develop, call your doctor promptly for guidance.
Mild Problems Drug Can Cause
Allergic reaction: skin rash.
Headache, dizziness.
Abdominal pain, nausea, vomiting, flatulence, constipation.
Ringing in the ears.
Rare passing out (syncope).
Serious Problems Drug Can Cause
Allergic reactions: rare anaphylaxis.
Postmenopausal vaginal bleeding; this may require further evaluation.
Rare anemia, low blood platelets, or blood in the urine.
Rare spasm of the bronchi or neuropathy.

▷ **Possible Effects on Sex Life:** Reduced libido and impotence reported rarely, but causal relationship is not established. Menstrual irregularity, menstrual cramps, heavy menstrual flow, spotting between periods.

▷ *CAUTION*

1. This drug can cause abortion; do not take this drug if you are pregnant, or make it available to others who may be or who may become pregnant.
2. If your doctor prescribes this drug, you should have a negative serum pregnancy test within 2 weeks before starting treatment.
3. Start taking this drug only on the second or third day of your next normal menstrual period.
4. Also initiate effective contraceptive measures when you begin this drug. Discuss the use of oral contraceptives or intrauterine devices with your doctor.
5. Should pregnancy occur while you are taking this drug, discontinue it immediately and tell your doctor.
6. Safety and effectiveness of this drug for those under 18 years old have not been established.
7. People over 60 usually tolerate this drug well. If you experience some light-headedness or faintness, call your doctor.

Advisability of Use During Pregnancy or If Breast-Feeding:

Pregnancy Category: X. Avoid using this drug completely. Present in breast milk is unknown; avoid taking this drug or refrain from nursing.

▷ **Overdose Symptoms:** Abdominal pain, diarrhea, fever, drowsiness, weakness, tremor, convulsions, difficult breathing.

▷ **Suggested Periodic Examinations While Taking This Drug:** (at doctor's discretion)
Monitoring for accidental pregnancy.

▷ **While Taking This Drug the Following Apply:**
Beverages: May be taken with milk.
Alcohol: No interactions are expected. However, use alcohol sparingly if at all; it can promote the development of stomach ulcer and reduce this drug's effectiveness.
Tobacco Smoking: No interactions are expected. However, nicotine is conducive to stomach ulcer.
Other Drugs:
Misoprostol *taken concurrently* with
• antacids that contain magnesium may increase the risk of diarrhea; avoid this combination.
• indomethacin and some other NSAIDs (see Drug Classes) may result in decreased NSAID blood levels and decrease their benefits.
Driving, Hazardous Activities: May cause dizziness, light-headedness, stomach pain, or diarrhea. Restrict your activities as necessary.

Discontinuation: This drug should be taken concurrently with antiarthritic or anti-inflammatory drugs, which can induce stomach ulceration. See your doctor if you have reason to discontinue it prematurely.

▷ **Saving Money When Using This Medicine:**
- Histamine (H2) blockers can also be used to treat or prevent the conditions for which this drug is used. Ask your doctor if this medicine offers the best balance of cost and outcome for you.
- If your kidneys are compromised, this drug is usually not well tolerated. Ask your doctor if an H2-blocker would be a better choice.
- If the condition for which you take the NSAID resolves, this drug may be stopped as well.

MOLINDONE (moh LIN dohn)

Prescription Needed: Yes   **Controlled Drug:** No   **Generic:** No

Brand Name: Moban

Overview of BENEFITS versus RISKS	
Possible Benefits	*Possible Risks*
EFFECTIVE TREATMENT OF SOME CASES OF SCHIZOPHRENIA	NARROW TREATMENT MARGIN
May be effective for schizophrenia that has not responded to other drugs	SERIOUS TOXIC EFFECTS ON BRAIN: PARKINSON-LIKE REACTIONS; SEVERE RESTLESSNESS; ABNORMAL INVOLUNTARY MOVEMENTS; TARDIVE DYSKINESIAS
	Liver toxicity, jaundice
	Atropinelike side effects

▷ **Illness This Medication Treats:**
(1) Helps acute and chronic schizophrenia to control abnormal thoughts, confusion, hallucinations, perceptual distortions, and hostility; (2) may have a small role in relieving depression.

▷ **Typical Dosage Range:** (Dosage or schedule must be determined by the doctor for each individual.)

Initially 50 to 75 mg per day in three or four divided doses; dose may be increased gradually in 3 days to 100 mg/day as needed and tolerated. For maintenance: mild psychosis—5 to 15 mg, three or four times per day; moderate psychosis—10 to 25 mg, three or four times per day; severe psychosis—up to 225 mg/day, in three or four divided doses. The total daily dose should not exceed 225 mg.

▷ **Conditions Requiring Dosing Adjustments:**

Liver function: No specific dosage adjustments for patients with liver compromise are defined. Patients with liver compromise should use this drug with caution, as it is a rare cause of liver toxicity.

▷ **How Best to Take This Medicine:** Take with food or milk to reduce stomach irritation. The liquid concentrate may be diluted with water, milk, fruit juice, or carbonated beverages. The tablet may be crushed.

▷ **How Long This Medicine Is Usually Taken:** Continual use on a regular schedule for 3 to 6 weeks is usually necessary to determine the effectiveness of this drug in controlling the features of schizophrenia. Long-term use (months to years) requires supervision and periodic evaluation. See your doctor regularly.

▷ **Tell Your Doctor Before Taking This Medicine If You:**
- ever had an allergic reaction to it.
- have acute alcoholic intoxication or use alcohol excessively.
- are taking any drugs that have sedative effects.
- have any type of seizure disorder.
- have any type of glaucoma.
- have Parkinson's disease or an enlarged prostate gland.
- have impaired liver or kidney function.
- have a history of breast cancer.

▷ **Possible Side Effects:** Drowsiness, dry mouth, nasal congestion, constipation, impaired urination. May lead to abnormally low blood pressure on standing.
Parkinson-like reactions.

▷ **Possible Adverse Effects:**
If any of the following develop, call your doctor promptly for guidance.
Some Mild Problems Drug Can Cause
Allergic reaction: skin rash.
Headache, dizziness, blurred vision, insomnia, depression, euphoria, ringing in ears.
Rapid heartbeat, low blood pressure, fainting.
Loss of appetite, indigestion, nausea.
Some Serious Problems Drug Can Cause
Allergic reactions: liver reaction with jaundice (rare, questionable).
Idiosyncratic reactions: neuroleptic malignant syndrome.
Spasms of face and neck muscles, abnormal involuntary movements of extremities, severe restlessness.
Development of tardive dyskinesias.

Rare muscle damage.

May lower the seizure threshold and make seizures more likely.

▷ **Possible Effects on Sex Life:**   Increased libido; male breast enlargement and tenderness; female breast enlargement with milk formation.

Altered timing and pattern of menstruation.

▷ **Adverse Effects That May Mimic Natural Diseases or Disorders:**
Parkinson-like reactions may be mistaken for naturally occurring Parkinson's disease.

Rare liver reaction may suggest viral hepatitis.

▷ *CAUTION*
1. This drug may alter the pattern of epileptic seizures and require dosage adjustments of anticonvulsants.
2. Obtain prompt evaluation of any change or disturbance of vision.
3. There is a very narrow margin between the effective therapeutic dose and the dose that causes Parkinson-like reactions. Tell your doctor promptly if suggestive symptoms develop.
4. Safety and effectiveness of this drug for those under 12 years old have not been established.
5. Small-dose treatment is indicated for people over 60. This drug can aggravate an existing prostatism. You may be more susceptible to the development of Parkinson-like reactions or tardive dyskinesia. Report any suggestive symptoms promptly.

Advisability of Use During Pregnancy or If Breast-Feeding:
Pregnancy Category: C. Because of its inherent toxicity for brain tissue, avoid use of this drug during pregnancy if possible. Present in breast milk is unknown; avoid taking this drug or refrain from nursing.

▷ **Overdose Symptoms:**   Marked drowsiness, weakness, tremor, agitation, impaired stance and gait, stupor progressing to coma, possible seizures.

▷ **Suggested Periodic Examinations While Taking This Drug:** (at doctor's discretion)
Complete blood cell counts, liver function tests.

▷ **While Taking This Drug the Following Apply:**
Beverages: May be taken with milk.
Alcohol: Avoid completely. Alcohol can increase the sedative action of this drug and enhance its depressant effects on brain function. This drug can also increase the intoxicating effects of alcohol.
Other Drugs:
Molindone may *increase* the effects of
• all drugs containing atropine or having atropinelike effects.
• all drugs with sedative effects, causing excessive sedation.

Molindone *taken concurrently* with

- antiepileptics (anticonvulsants) may require close monitoring for changes in seizure patterns and a need for dosage adjustments.
- monoamine oxidase inhibitors (MAOIs—see Drug Classes) may result in serious increases in temperature or convulsions.

Driving, Hazardous Activities: May cause dizziness and drowsiness. Restrict your activities as necessary.

Exposure to Heat: Use caution and avoid excessive heat as much as possible. This drug may impair the regulation of body temperature and increase the risk of heatstroke.

Discontinuation: Do not stop taking this drug suddenly after long-term use. Ask your doctor for guidance regarding gradual dosage reduction and withdrawal.

▷ **Saving Money When Using This Medicine:**

- Many drugs are available to treat mental disorders. Ask your doctor if this medicine offers the best balance of cost and outcome for you.
- A new medicine called olanzapine appears to avoid some of the side effects of older medicines for schizophrenia. Talk with your doctor about the benefits versus risks of olanzapine.

MORPHINE (MOR feen)

Other Name: MS (morphine sulfate)

Prescription Needed: Yes   **Controlled Drug:** C-II*   **Generic:** Yes

Brand Names: Astramorph, Astramorph/PF, Duramorph, MS Contin, MSIR, Oramorph SR, RMS Uniserts, Roxanol, Roxanol 100, Roxanol SR

Overview of BENEFITS versus RISKS	
Possible Benefits	*Possible Risks*
EFFECTIVE RELIEF OF MODERATE TO SEVERE PAIN	POTENTIAL FOR HABIT FORMATION (DEPENDENCE)
	Respiratory depression
	Weakness, fainting
	Disorientation, hallucinations
	Interference with urination
	Constipation

▷ **Illness This Medication Treats:**

Moderate to severe pain of any cause; also as an adjunct to anesthesia, and in the management of pulmonary edema due to heart failure.

*See Controlled Drug Schedules inside this book's cover.

▷ **Typical Dosage Range:** (Dosage or schedule must be determined by the doctor for each individual.)

Infants and Children: 0.1 to 0.2 mg per kilogram of body weight every 4 hours. Single dose should not exceed 15 mg.

12 to 60 Years of Age: By injection: 5 to 20 mg every 4 hours; may be scheduled (given on a regular basis for severe pain).

By mouth (regular solution, syrup, and tablets): 10 to 30 mg every 4 hours.

By mouth (sustained-release forms [SR]): 30 mg every 8 to 12 hours. For cancer pain this should be combined with a rescue dose (graduated dosing based on pain that breaks through the SR form) of immediate-release morphine liquid.

By suppository: 10 to 30 mg every 4 hours, as needed.

Over 60 Years of Age: Same as for 12 to 60 years of age, using the lower end of the range initially; increase dose cautiously, to achieve effective pain control.

▷ **Conditions Requiring Dosing Adjustments:**

Liver function: The dose and frequency **must** be adjusted for patients with liver compromise. When the drug is being titrated to acceptable pain relief, small incremental doses should be used.

Kidney function: Adjust dose and frequency for patients with renal compromise.

▷ **How Best to Take This Medicine:**   May be taken with or following food to reduce stomach irritation or nausea. The regular tablet may be crushed for administration. The sustained-release tablet should be swallowed whole; do not break it in half, crush it, or chew it. The oral liquid may be mixed with fruit juice to improve its taste.

Scheduled use, such as every hour until the pain is controlled, is not unusual for severe pain and avoids the peaks and valleys of dosing as needed.

▷ **How Long This Medicine Is Usually Taken:**   As required to control pain. For short-term, self-limiting conditions, continual use should not exceed 5 to 7 days without interruption and reassessment of need. For the long-term management of severe chronic pain, an optimal fixed-dosage schedule should be determined.

Cancer pain may require ongoing therapy and be combined with other drugs such as NSAIDs, tricyclic antidepressants, or stimulants.

▷ **Tell Your Doctor Before Taking This Medicine If You:**
- ever had an allergic reaction to it.
- are having an acute attack of asthma.
- are taking, or have taken within the past 14 days, any MAO type A inhibitor.
- have low blood pressure or sickle cell anemia.
- tend to become constipated.

- are taking any atropinelike drugs, antihypertensives, metoclopramide (Reglan), or zidovudine (AZT).
- are taking any other drugs that have a sedative effect.
- have a history of drug abuse or alcoholism.
- have impaired liver or kidney function.
- have prostate gland enlargement.
- have a history of asthma, emphysema, epilepsy, gallbladder disease, or inflammatory bowel disease.
- plan to have surgery under general anesthesia soon.

▷ **Possible Side Effects:**   Drowsiness, light-headedness, weakness, euphoria, dry mouth, urinary retention, constipation.

▷ **Possible Adverse Effects:**
If any of the following develop, call your doctor promptly for guidance.

Some Mild Problems Drug Can Cause
Allergic reactions: skin rash, hives, itching.
Headache, dizziness, sensation of drunkenness, depression, blurred or double vision.
Facial flushing, sweating, heart palpitation.
Nausea, vomiting, constipation.

Some Serious Problems Drug Can Cause
Allergic reactions: swelling of throat or vocal cords, spasm of larynx or bronchial tubes.
Drop in blood pressure, causing severe weakness and fainting.
Disorientation, hallucinations, unstable gait, tremor, muscle twitching.
Rare drug-induced myasthenia gravis.
Rare drug-induced porphyria.
Respiratory depression.

▷ **Possible Effects on Sex Life.**   Reduced libido and/or potency.

▷ **Adverse Effects That May Mimic Natural Diseases or Disorders:**
Paradoxical behavioral disturbances may suggest a psychotic disorder.

▷ *CAUTION*
1. If you have asthma, chronic bronchitis, or emphysema, the excessive use of this drug may cause significant respiratory difficulty, thickening of bronchial secretions, and suppression of coughing.
2. Concurrent use with atropinelike drugs can increase the risk of urinary retention and reduced intestinal function.
3. Do not take this drug following acute head injury.
4. Use this drug very cautiously in infants under 2 years of age, because of their vulnerability to life-threatening respiratory depression. Observe for any indication of paradoxical excitement.

5. Small doses should be given to those over 60 initially, with slow increases in dosage as needed and tolerated. If possible, limit use of this drug to short-term treatment only. Susceptibility to the development of drowsiness, dizziness, unsteadiness, falling, urinary retention, and constipation (often leading to fecal impaction) may be increased.

Advisability of Use During Pregnancy or If Breast-Feeding:

Pregnancy Category: C. Avoid using this drug during the first 3 months. Use sparingly and in small doses during the last 6 months only if clearly needed. Present in breast milk; avoid taking this drug or refrain from nursing.

▷ **Habit-Forming Potential:**   This drug can cause psychological and physical dependence.

▷ **Overdose Symptoms:**   Marked drowsiness, dizziness, confusion, restlessness, depressed breathing, tremors, convulsions, stupor progressing to coma.

▷ **Possible Effects of Long-Term Use:**   Psychological and physical dependence, chronic constipation.

▷ **While Taking This Drug the Following Apply:**

Beverages: May be taken with milk.

Alcohol: Best avoided. Opioid analgesics can intensify the intoxicating effects of alcohol, and alcohol can intensify the depressant effects of opioids on brain function, breathing, and circulation.

Marijuana Smoking: Increase in drowsiness and pain relief; impairment of mental and physical performance.

Other Drugs:

Morphine may *increase* the effects of
* other drugs with sedative effects.
* antihypertensives, causing excessive lowering of blood pressure.
* atropinelike drugs, increasing the risk of constipation and urinary retention.

Morphine may *decrease* the effects of
* metoclopramide (Reglan).

Morphine *taken concurrently* with
* benzodiazepines (see Drug Classes) may result in increased risk of respiratory depression.
* cimetidine (Tagamet) may result in morphine toxicity.
* fluoxetine (Prozac) may lessen pain relief from morphine.
* hydroxyzine (Vistaril) may increase pain relief, but also poses an increased risk of respiratory depression.
* MAO type A inhibitors may cause the equivalent of an acute narcotic overdose: unconsciousness; severe depression of breathing, heart action, and circulation. A variation of this reaction can be excitability, convulsions, high fever, and rapid heart action.

- phenothiazines may cause excessive and prolonged depression of brain functions, breathing, and circulation.
- zidovudine (AZT) may increase the toxicity of both drugs; avoid concurrent use.

Driving, Hazardous Activities: This drug can impair mental alertness, judgment, reaction time, and physical coordination. Avoid hazardous activities.

Discontinuation: It is best to limit this drug to short-term use. If extended use is necessary, discontinuation should be gradual to minimize possible effects of withdrawal: body aches, fever, sweating, nervousness, trembling, weakness, runny nose, sneezing, rapid heart rate, nausea, vomiting, stomach cramps, diarrhea.

▷ **Saving Money When Using This Medicine:**
- Ask your doctor if this medicine offers the best balance of cost and outcome for you, and if it can be combined with other medicines to manage pain more effectively. Also ask who will be assessing your pain (using an algometer) and adjusting your medicines to give the best relief.
- This medicine is treating a symptom that we call pain. Ask your doctor if the CAUSE of the pain can be removed, and the medicine gradually stopped.
- If your liver or kidneys are compromised, ask your doctor if your dosage has been decreased accordingly.
- It is not unusual for this medicine to be slowly decreased over time, once the pain caused by the condition is lessened.
- If higher dose therapy over a longer period of time is used, a stool softener or other medicine to help prevent constipation should be given.
- If an ongoing oral sustained-release form is used, a rescue dose of an immediate-release form of morphine should be provided.
- Effective pain management ALWAYS includes regular assessment of pain and changes in doses in response to that pain.
- Talk with your doctor about prescribing medicine for constipation to be taken WITH this medicine.

NABUMETONE (na BYU me tohn)

Prescription Needed: Yes   **Controlled Drug:** No   **Generic:** No

Brand Name: Relafen

```
Overview of BENEFITS versus RISKS
     Possible Benefits              Possible Risks
EFFECTIVE RELIEF OF MILD     Gastrointestinal ulceration
  TO MODERATE PAIN AND       Drug-induced hepatitis
  INFLAMMATION               Drug-induced kidney damage
  ASSOCIATED WITH            Very rare lung fibrosis.
  OSTEOARTHRITIS AND         Mild fluid retention
  RHEUMATOID ARTHRITIS
```

See the acetic acids (NSAIDs) drug profile for more details.

NADOLOL (nay DOH lohl)

Prescription Needed: Yes   **Controlled Drug:** No   **Generic:** No

Brand Names: Corgard, Corzide [CD], Syn-Nadol

```
Overview of BENEFITS versus RISKS
     Possible Benefits              Possible Risks
EFFECTIVE,                   CONGESTIVE HEART
  WELL-TOLERATED               FAILURE in advanced heart
  ANTIHYPERTENSIVE for         disease
  mild to moderate high blood Provocation of asthma (in
  pressure                     patients with asthma)
EFFECTIVE ANTIANGINAL        Masking of hypoglycemia in
  DRUG FOR CLASSICAL           drug-dependent diabetes
  CORONARY ARTERY            Worsening of angina following
  DISEASE with moderate to     abrupt withdrawal
  severe angina
```

▷ **Illness This Medication Treats:**
  (1) Moderately high blood pressure; (2) helps prevent attacks of effort-induced angina (contraindicated in Prinzmetal's vasospastic angina).
  As Combination Drug Product [CD]: This drug is available in combination with bendroflumethiazide, a mild diuretic. This combination product is more effective and convenient for long-term use.

▷ **Typical Dosage Range:** (Dosage or schedule must be determined by the doctor for each individual.)
  For hypertension: Initially 40 mg daily in one dose; this may be increased gradually as needed and tolerated, up to 640 mg/24 hr. The usual maintenance dose is 80 to 320 mg every 24 hours. The total daily dosage should not exceed 640 mg. For angina: Initially 40 mg

daily in one dose; increase gradually at intervals of 3 to 7 days up to 240 mg/24 hr. The usual maintenance dose is 80 to 240 mg every 24 hours. The total daily dose should not exceed 240 mg.

▷ **Conditions Requiring Dosing Adjustments:**
Kidney function: For patients with moderate kidney compromise, the usual dose should be given every 24 to 36 hours. For patients with severe kidney failure, the drug can be given every 40 to 60 hours.

▷ **How Best to Take This Medicine:**   May be taken without regard to eating. The tablet may be crushed for administration. Do not discontinue this drug abruptly.

▷ **How Long This Medicine Is Usually Taken:**   Use on a regular schedule for 10 to 14 days is usually needed to see the effectiveness of this drug in lowering blood pressure and preventing effort-induced angina. Long-term use of this drug (months to years) is determined by the course of your blood pressure and angina over time and your response to the overall treatment program (weight reduction, salt restriction, smoking cessation, etc.). See your doctor regularly.

▷ **Tell Your Doctor Before Taking This Medicine If You:**
- ever had an allergic reaction to it.
- have congestive heart failure.
- have an abnormally slow heart rate or a serious form of heart block.
- are subject to bronchial asthma.
- are presently experiencing seasonal hay fever or have a history of hay fever (allergic rhinitis), asthma, chronic bronchitis, or emphysema.
- are taking, or have taken within the past 14 days, any MAO type A inhibitor.
- had an adverse reaction to any beta-blocker in the past.
- have a history of serious heart disease, with or without episodes of heart failure.
- have a history of overactive thyroid function.
- have a history of low blood sugar.
- have impaired liver or kidney function.
- have diabetes or myasthenia gravis.
- are currently taking any form of digitalis, quinidine, or reserpine, or any calcium blocker.
- plan to have surgery under general anesthesia soon.

▷ **Possible Side Effects:**   Lethargy and fatigability, cold extremities, rare severe slowing of heart rate, light-headedness in upright position. Increased blood potassium. Rare cramping when walking (intermittent claudication).

▷ **Possible Adverse Effects:**
If any of the following develop, call your doctor promptly for guidance.

Some Mild Problems Drug Can Cause
Allergic reactions: skin rash, itching, drug fever.
Headache, dizziness, insomnia, vivid dreaming, visual disturbances, ringing in ears, slurred speech.
Indigestion, nausea, vomiting, diarrhea, abdominal pain.
Numbness and tingling of extremities.

Some Serious Problems Drug Can Cause
Allergic reaction: facial swelling.
Chest pain, shortness of breath, precipitation of congestive heart failure.
Intensification of heart block.
May cause an acute asthma attack in people with asthma.
Masking of warning indications of acute hypoglycemia in drug-treated diabetes.
Rare carpal tunnel syndrome or spasm of the bronchi.

▷ **Possible Effects on Sex Life:** Decreased libido, impotence, impaired erection.

▷ *CAUTION*

1. ***Do not STOP taking this drug suddenly*** without the knowledge and guidance of your doctor. Carry a notation that states you are taking this drug.
2. Ask your doctor or pharmacist before using nasal decongestants, which are usually present in over-the-counter cold preparations and nose drops. These can cause sudden increases in blood pressure when taken concurrently with beta-blockers.
3. Report the development of any tendency to emotional depression.
4. Safety and effectiveness of this drug for those under 12 years old have not been established. However, if this drug is used, watch for low blood sugar during periods of reduced food intake.
5. Those over 60 should proceed *cautiously* with all antihypertensive drugs. Unacceptably high blood pressure should be reduced without the risks associated with excessively low blood pressure. Start with small doses and monitor the blood pressure response frequently. Sudden, rapid, and excessive blood pressure reduction can predispose to stroke or heart attack. Observe for dizziness, unsteadiness, tendency to fall, confusion, hallucinations, depression, or urinary frequency.

Advisability of Use During Pregnancy or If Breast-Feeding:
Pregnancy Category: C. Avoid use of this drug during the first 3 months if possible. Use only if clearly needed. Ask your doctor for guidance.

Present in breast milk in large amounts. Avoid taking this drug or refrain from nursing.

▷ **Overdose Symptoms:** Weakness, slow pulse, low blood pressure, fainting, cold and sweaty skin, congestive heart failure, possible coma and convulsions.

▷ **Suggested Periodic Examinations While Taking This Drug:** (at doctor's discretion)
Measurements of blood pressure, evaluation of heart function.

▷ **While Taking This Drug the Following Apply:**
Foods: Avoid excessive salt intake.

Beverages: May be taken with milk.

Alcohol: Alcohol may exaggerate this drug's ability to lower blood pressure and increase its mild sedative effect.

Tobacco Smoking: Nicotine may reduce this drug's effectiveness in treating high blood pressure and angina. In addition, high doses may potentiate the constriction of the bronchial tubes caused by regular smoking.

Other Drugs:

Nadolol may *increase* the effects of

- other antihypertensives, causing excessive lowering of blood pressure. Dosage adjustments may be necessary.
- reserpine (Scr-Ap-Es, etc.), causing sedation, depression, slowing of the heart rate, and lowering of blood pressure.
- verapamil (Calan, Isoptin), causing excessive depression of heart function; watch this combination closely.

Nadolol may *decrease* the effects of

- epinephrine.
- ritodrine (Yutopar).
- theophyllines (aminophylline, Theo-Dur, etc.), reducing their effectiveness in treating asthma.

Nadolol *taken concurrently* with

- antacids containing aluminum can block absorption of nadolol and lessen its therapeutic effects.
- amiodarone (Cordarone) can lead to severe slowing of the heart and potentially stop the heart.
- clonidine (Catapres) requires close monitoring for rebound high blood pressure if clonidine is withdrawn while nadolol is still being taken.
- epinephrine can lead to serious increases in blood pressure and slowing of the heart.
- ergot derivatives (see Drug Classes) can worsen blood flow to the extremities (peripheral ischemia).
- insulin requires close monitoring to avoid undetected hypoglycemia.

- lidocaine may lead to lidocaine toxicity.
- oral hypoglycemic agents (see Drug Classes) may cause slowed recovery from any episode of lowered blood sugar.

The following drugs may **decrease** the effects of nadolol

- indomethacin (Indocin), and possibly other NSAID aspirin substitutes; can impair nadolol's antihypertensive effect.

Driving, Hazardous Activities: Use caution until the full extent of drowsiness, lethargy, and blood pressure change has been determined.

Exposure to Heat: Caution is advised. Hot environments can lower the blood pressure and exaggerate this drug's effects.

Exposure to Cold: Caution is advised. Cold environments can enhance the circulatory deficiency in the extremities that may occur. The elderly should take precautions to prevent hypothermia.

Heavy Exercise or Exertion: It is best to avoid exertion that produces light-headedness, excessive fatigue, or muscle cramping. Use of this drug may intensify the hypertensive response to isometric exercise.

Occurrence of Unrelated Illness: The fever that accompanies systemic infections can lower blood pressure and require dosage adjustment. Illnesses that cause nausea or vomiting may interrupt the regular dosage schedule. Ask your doctor for guidance.

Discontinuation: It is advisable to avoid sudden discontinuation of this drug in all situations. If possible, gradual reduction of dose over a period of 2 to 3 weeks is recommended. Ask your doctor for specific guidance.

▷ **Saving Money When Using This Medicine:**

- Many new drugs are available to treat high blood pressure. There are also many different beta-blockers. Ask your doctor if this medicine offers the best balance of cost and outcome for you.
- Ask your doctor how often he or she recommends you to have your blood pressure checked and if taking aspirin every other day makes sense for you.

NAFARELIN (NAF a re lin)

Prescription Needed: Yes **Controlled Drug:** No **Generic:** No

Brand Name: Synarel

Overview of BENEFITS versus RISKS

Possible Benefits	*Possible Risks*
VERY EFFECTIVE TREATMENT OF ENDOMETRIOSIS: relief of symptoms; reduction of lesions	Symptoms of estrogen deficiency (during treatment)
	Masculinizing effects (during treatment)
	Loss of vertebral bone density (at 6 months after treatment)
	Lowered white blood cell counts

▷ **Illness This Medication Treats:**
 (1) Endometriosis: reduction in the size and activity of endometrial implants within the pelvis; relief of pelvic pain associated with menstruation; (2) precocious puberty due to excessive gonadotropic hormone production.

▷ **Typical Dosage Range:** (Dosage or schedule must be determined by the doctor for each individual.)
 Endometriosis (PREGNANCY MUST be negative prior to starting therapy): 400 mcg daily; spray one dose of 200 mcg into one nostril in the morning and one dose of 200 mcg into the other nostril in the evening, 12 hours apart. Begin treatment between days 2 and 4 of the menstrual cycle.
 If regular menstruation persists after 2 months of treatment, the dose may be increased to 800 mcg daily: one spray into each nostril (a total of two sprays, 400 mcg) in the morning and again in the evening.

▷ **How Best to Take This Medicine:** Carefully read and follow the patient instructions provided with this drug. The solution is sprayed directly into the nostrils where it is absorbed into the bloodstream; it should not be swallowed. Time the beginning of treatment and your daily dosage exactly as directed.
 If the use of a nasal decongestant (spray or drops, as for a head cold) is necessary, it should not be used for at least 30 minutes after administration of the nafarelin spray; earlier use could impair absorption of nafarelin.

▷ **How Long This Medicine Is Usually Taken:** Continual use on a regular schedule for 2 to 3 months is usually necessary to determine the effectiveness of this drug in relieving endometriosis. The standard course of treatment is limited to 6 months.
 On completion of 6 months of treatment, 60% of users are free of symptoms, 32% have mild symptoms, 7% have moderate symptoms, and 1% have severe symptoms. Six months after discontinuing this drug, of the 60% who obtain complete relief, 50% will

remain free of symptoms, 33% will have mild symptoms, and 17% will have moderate symptoms.

If symptoms of endometriosis recur following a 6-month course of treatment and a repeat course is considered, bone density should be measured before retreatment.

▷ **Tell Your Doctor Before Taking This Medicine If You:**
- ever had an allergic reaction to it.
- are pregnant, planning pregnancy, or breast-feeding.
- have abnormal vaginal bleeding of unknown cause.
- have used this drug, danazol, or similar drugs previously.
- are taking any type of estrogen, progesterone, or oral contraceptive.
- have a family history of osteoporosis.
- use alcohol or tobacco regularly.
- have a history of low white blood cells.
- are using anticonvulsants or cortisonelike drugs.
- are subject to allergic or infectious rhinitis and use nasal decongestants frequently.

▷ **Possible Side Effects:**   Effects due to reduced estrogen production: hot flashes, headaches, emotional lability, insomnia.

Masculinizing effects: acne, muscle aches, fluid retention, increased skin oil, weight gain, excessive hair growth.

▷ **Possible Adverse Effects:**
If any of the following develop, call your doctor promptly for guidance.
Some Mild Problems Drug Can Cause
   Allergic reactions: skin rash, hives.
   Nasal irritation.
   Depression.
Some Serious Problems Drug Can Cause
   Loss of vertebral bone density: at completion of 6 months of treatment, bone density decreases an average of 8.7%, and bone mass decreases an average of 4.3%; partial recovery during the posttreatment period restores bone density loss to 4.9% and bone mass loss to 3.3%.
   Lowering of white blood cell count.
   Uterine bleeding.

▷ **Possible Effects on Sexual Function:**   Decreased libido, vaginal dryness, reduced breast size. Impotence when used in men for prostate problems.

▷ *CAUTION*
   1. With continual use of this drug at proper dosage, menstruation will cease. If regular menstruation persists, tell your doctor. Dosage adjustment may be necessary.

2. Use this drug consistently on a regular basis. Missed doses can result in breakthrough bleeding and ovulation.
3. It is advisable to avoid pregnancy during the course of treatment. Use a nonhormonal method of birth control, not oral contraceptives. Tell your doctor promptly if you think you may be pregnant.
4. If you find nasal decongestant sprays or drops necessary, delay their use for at least 30 minutes following the intranasal spray of nafarelin.
5. Safety and effectiveness of this drug for those under 18 years old are not established.
6. If this drug is used for prostatism, impotence is a common side effect.

Advisability of Use During Pregnancy or If Breast-Feeding:
Pregnancy Category: X. Avoid using this drug during entire pregnancy. Presence in breast milk is unknown; avoid taking this drug or refrain from nursing.

▷ **Suggested Periodic Examinations While Taking This Drug:** (at doctor's discretion)
Blood cholesterol and triglyceride profiles.
Bone density and mass measurements.

▷ **While Taking This Drug the Following Apply:** *Other Drugs:*
The following drugs will *decrease* the effects of nafarelin
• estrogens.
• oral contraceptives.
Discontinuation: Normal ovarian function (ovulation, menstruation, etc.) is usually restored within 4 to 8 weeks after this drug is discontinued.
Special Storage Instructions: Store in an upright position at room temperature. Protect it from light.

▷ **Saving Money When Using This Medicine:**
• Ask your doctor if this medicine offers the best balance of cost and outcome for you.

NAPROXEN (na PROX en)

Prescription Needed: No (200 mg); Yes (250 mg)   **Controlled Drug:** No   **Generic:** No

Brand Names: Aleve (nonprescription), Anaprox, Anaprox DS, Naprosyn

```
Overview of BENEFITS versus RISKS
     Possible Benefits              Possible Risks
EFFECTIVE RELIEF OF MILD     Gastrointestinal pain,
 TO MODERATE PAIN AND          ulceration, bleeding (rare)
 INFLAMMATION               Drug-induced hepatitis with
                               jaundice (rare)
                            Kidney damage (rare)
                            Mild fluid retention
                            Reduced white blood cell and
                               platelet counts
```

See the propionic acids (NSAID) drug profile for further information.

NEDOCROMIL (na DOK ra mil)

Prescription Needed: Yes   **Controlled Drug:** No   **Generic:** No

Brand Name: Tilade

```
Overview of BENEFITS versus RISKS
     Possible Benefits              Possible Risks
EFFECTIVE PREVENTION OF     Acute bronchospasm (rare)
 RECURRENT ASTHMA           Taste disorder
Prevention of exercise-induced
 asthma
```

▷ **Illness This Medication Treats:**
   (1) Mild to moderate bronchial asthma as a maintenance therapy; (2) has a steroid-sparing effect that can let steroid doses be reduced (avoiding the side effects of those medicines) or even eliminated.

▷ **Typical Dosage Range:** (Dosage or schedule must be determined by the doctor for each individual.)
   Infants and Children: Safety and efficacy of this drug are not established.
   12 to 60 Years of Age: Two (puffs) inhalations four times daily to provide a total of 14 mg/day.
   Over 60 Years of Age: Same as for 12 to 60 years of age.

▷ **How Best to Take This Medicine:** Follow the instructions on the leaflet provided in the medication box carefully. Usage of this drug must be continued, even when you are symptom-free.

▷ **How Long This Medicine Is Usually Taken:** Use on a regular schedule for a week usually determines the effectiveness of this drug in helping prevent acute asthma. Long-term use (months to years) requires periodic physician evaluation.

▷ **Tell Your Doctor Before Taking This Medicine If You:**
- ever had an allergic reaction to it.
- have impaired kidney function.
- have angina or a heart rhythm disorder.
- are uncertain of how or how often to take nedocromil.

▷ **Possible Side Effects:**   Unpleasant taste.
Mild throat irritation or hoarseness; may be lessened by taking a few swallows of water after each inhalation.

▷ **Possible Adverse Effects:**
If any of the following develop, call your doctor promptly for guidance.
Some Mild Problems Drug Can Cause
Allergic reactions: skin rash, hives.
Headache, dizziness.
Unpleasant taste.
Some Serious Problems Drug Can Cause
Allergic reactions: anaphylactic reaction, allergic pneumonitis (allergic reaction of the lung tissue).
Bronchospasm.

▷ **Possible Delayed Adverse Effects:**   Pneumonitis (very rare).

▷ *CAUTION*
1. This drug does NOT act as a bronchodilator and should not be used for immediate relief of acute asthma.
2. If use of this drug has allowed you to stop taking a cortisone-related drug, you may need to resume the cortisone-related drug if you are injured, have an infection, or need surgery.
3. If severe asthma returns, contact your doctor promptly.
4. If you use a bronchodilator drug by inhalation, it is best to take it about 5 minutes before inhaling nedocromil.
5. Safety and effectiveness of this drug for those under 12 years old are not established.
6. This drug does not work for chronic bronchitis or emphysema.

Advisability of Use During Pregnancy or If Breast-Feeding:
Pregnancy Category: B. Ask your doctor for guidance. Presence in breast milk is unknown; avoid using this drug or refrain from nursing.

▷ **Overdose Symptoms:**   Head shaking, tremor, and salivation were seen in dogs given high doses.

▷ **While Taking This Drug the Following Apply:**
Beverages: Avoid all beverages to which you may be allergic.

Other Drugs:
Nedocromil may make it possible to reduce the dose or frequency of use of cortisonelike drugs. Ask your doctor for guidance.
Driving, Hazardous Activities: May cause dizziness. Restrict your activities as necessary.
Heavy Exercise or Exertion: You may be able to exercise without causing an acute asthma attack while taking this drug. Ask your doctor how long before exercising it should be taken.
Discontinuation: If this drug has made it possible for you to reduce or stop usage of cortisonelike drugs and you must stop taking nedocromil, you may have to resume the cortisonelike drug as well as take other measures to control asthma.

▷ **Saving Money When Using This Medicine:**
  • Many new drugs are available to treat asthma. Ask your doctor if this medicine offers the best balance of cost and outcome for you.
  • Ask your doctor if using nebulized lidocaine makes sense for you.

NEOSTIGMINE   (nee oh STIG meen)

Prescription Needed: Yes   **Controlled Drug:** No   **Generic:** Yes

Brand Names: Prostigmin, Viaderm-KC

Overview of BENEFITS versus RISKS	
Possible Benefits	*Possible Risks*
MODERATELY EFFECTIVE TREATMENT OF OCULAR AND MILD FORMS OF MYASTHENIA GRAVIS (symptomatic relief of muscle weakness)	Cholinergic crisis (overdose): excessive salivation, nausea, vomiting, stomach cramps, diarrhea, shortness of breath (asthmalike wheezing), excessive weakness
Eases postoperative bowel slowing or block	

▷ **Illness This Medication Treats:**
  (1) Ocular and milder forms of myasthenia gravis by providing temporary relief of muscle weakness and fatigability; (2) reverses depression of bowel function that can happen after surgery; (3) eases symptoms of bladder instability.

▷ **Typical Dosage Range:** (Dosage or schedule must be determined by the doctor for each individual.)
  Initially: 15 mg every 3 to 4 hours; adjust dosage as needed and toler-

ated. Maintenance: Up to 300 mg/24 hr; the average dose is 75 to 150 mg every 24 hours.

▷ **Conditions Requiring Dosing Adjustments:**

Liver function: Specific guidelines for dosage adjustment are not available. Patients with compromised livers should use this drug with caution.

Kidney function: Specific guidelines for decreasing doses are not available; use of this drug is contraindicated for patients with urine flow obstruction.

▷ **How Best to Take This Medicine:** Take with food or milk to reduce the intensity of side effects. Larger portions of the daily maintenance dose should be timed according to pattern of fatigue and weakness. The tablet may be crushed.

▷ **How Long This Medicine Is Usually Taken:** Use on a regular schedule (with dosage adjustment) for 10 to 14 days is usually necessary to determine the effectiveness of this drug in myasthenia gravis. Long-term use (months to years) requires periodic physician evaluation.

▷ **Tell Your Doctor Before Taking This Medicine If You:**
- ever had an allergic reaction to it.
- are allergic to bromide compounds.
- have any type of seizure disorder.
- are subject to heart rhythm disorders or bronchial asthma.
- have recurrent urinary tract infections.
- have prostatism.
- plan to have surgery under general anesthesia soon.

▷ **Possible Side Effects:** Small pupils, watering of eyes, slow pulse, excessive salivation, nausea, vomiting, stomach cramps, diarrhea, urge to urinate, increased sweating.

▷ **Possible Adverse Effects:**
If any of the following develop, call your doctor promptly for guidance.

Some Mild Problems Drug Can Cause

Allergic reaction: skin rash.

Nervousness, anxiety, unsteadiness, muscle cramps.

Some Serious Problems Drug Can Cause

Confusion, slurred speech, seizures, difficult breathing.

Increased muscle weakness or paralysis.

Excessive vomiting or diarrhea may induce abnormally low blood potassium levels (hypokalemia), accentuating muscle weakness.

Rare porphyria or abnormally slowed heartbeat.

▷ **Adverse Effects That May Mimic Natural Diseases or Disorders:**
Seizures may suggest epilepsy.

▷ *CAUTION*

1. Certain drugs can block the action of this drug and reduce its effectiveness in treating myasthenia gravis. Ask your doctor before starting any new drug.

2. The dosage schedule must be carefully individualized for each patient. Because generalized muscle weakness is a major symptom of both myasthenia crisis (underdosage) and cholinergic crisis (overdosage), it may be difficult to recognize the correct cause. As a rule, weakness that begins within 1 hour after taking this drug probably represents overdosage; weakness that begins 3 or more hours after taking this drug is probably due to underdosage. Observe these time relationships and inform your doctor.

3. During long-term use, observe for the possible development of resistance to this drug's therapeutic action. Ask your doctor about the advisability of discontinuing this drug for a few days to see if responsiveness can be restored.

4. The natural decline of kidney function with aging may require smaller doses for the elderly to prevent accumulation of this drug to toxic levels.

Advisability of Use During Pregnancy or If Breast-Feeding:
Pregnancy Category: C. There are no reports of birth defects due to the use of this drug during pregnancy. However, significant muscular weakness occurred in 20% of newborn infants whose mothers took this drug during pregnancy. Ask your doctor for guidance. Probably not present in breast milk. Monitor the nursing infant closely and discontinue drug or nursing if adverse effects develop.

▷ **Overdose Symptoms:**   Generalized muscular weakness, blurred vision, very small pupils, slow heart rate, difficult breathing (wheezing), excessive salivation, nausea, vomiting, stomach cramps, diarrhea, muscle cramps or twitching. This syndrome constitutes the cholinergic crisis.

▷ **Suggested Periodic Examinations While Taking This Drug:** (at doctor's discretion)
Assessment of drug effectiveness and dosage schedule for optimal therapeutic results.

▷ **While Taking This Drug the Following Apply:**   *Beverages:* May be taken with milk.
Alcohol: Use caution until the combined effects are determined. Weakness and unsteadiness may be accentuated.
Other Drugs:
The following drugs may *decrease* the effects of neostigmine
- atropine (belladonna).
- clindamycin (Cleocin).
- guanadrel (Hylorel).

- guanethidine (Esimil, Ismelin).
- procainamide (Procan SR, Pronestyl).
- quinidine (Cardioquin, Duraquin, etc.).
- quinine (Quinamm).

Neostigmine *taken concurrently* with

- edrophonium may lead to cholinergic crisis in patients with myasthenic weakness.
- hydrocortisone or other corticosteroids (see Drug Classes) may blunt neostigmine's effectiveness.
- physostigmine may give additive adverse effects.

Driving, Hazardous Activities: May cause blurred vision, confusion, or generalized weakness. Restrict your activities as necessary.

Exposure to Heat: Use caution. This drug may cause excessive sweating and increased weakness.

Exposure to Environmental Chemicals: Avoid excessive exposure (inhalation, skin contamination) to the insecticides Baygon, Diazinon, and Sevin; which can accentuate this drug's potential toxicity.

Discontinuation: Do not discontinue this drug abruptly without your doctor's knowledge and guidance.

▷ **Saving Money When Using This Medicine:**
- A generic form can be substituted for the brand name.
- Ask your doctor if this drug offers the best balance of cost and outcome for you.
- If you also take steroids to help your myasthenia gravis, talk with your doctor about calcium supplements, risk factors, and bone mineral density testing.
- Learn as much as possible about your condition. *The Essential Guide to Chronic Illness* is an excellent resource.

NIACIN (NI a sin)

Other Names: Nicotinic acid, vitamin B3

Prescription Needed: Tablets and liquid: No; Capsules: Yes
Controlled Drug: No   **Generic:** Yes

Brand Names: Niac, Nicobid, Nico-400, Nicolar, Nicotinex, SK-Niacin, Slo-Niacin, Span-Niacin-150

Overview of BENEFITS versus RISKS

Possible Benefits	*Possible Risks*
EFFECTIVE REDUCTION OF TOTAL CHOLESTEROL, LOW-DENSITY CHOLESTEROL, AND TRIGLYCERIDES IN TYPES II, III, IV, AND V CHOLESTEROL DISORDERS and elevation of HDL cholesterol (a beneficial effect)	Activation of peptic ulcer Drug-induced hepatitis Aggravation of diabetes or gout
Specific prevention and treatment of pellagra (niacin-deficiency disease)	

▷ **Illness This Medication Treats:**
(1) Helps certain patterns of abnormally high blood levels of cholesterol and triglycerides; (2) pellagra, a niacin (vitamin B3) deficiency disorder characterized by dementia, dermatitis, and diarrhea; and (3) treatment of Hartnup disease.
As Combination Drug Product [CD]: In Canada this drug is combined with meclizine to enhance its effectiveness in treating motion sickness and vertigo.

▷ **Typical Dosage Range:** (Dosage or schedule must be determined by the doctor for each individual.)
For cholesterol disorders: Initially 100 mg three times daily. Dose may be increased in increments of 300 mg daily at intervals of 4 to 7 days as needed and tolerated. The usual maintenance dose is 1 to 2 g three times daily. The total daily dosage should not exceed 6 g.
For prevention of pellagra: 10 to 20 mg daily.
For treatment of pellagra: 50 mg 3 to 10 times daily.

▷ **Conditions Requiring Dosing Adjustments:**
Liver function: This drug is metabolized in the liver and is contraindicated in patients with liver disease.

Kidney function: Elimination of niacin metabolites occurs via the urine; however, no specific guidelines for adjustment of dosing are available.

▷ **How Best to Take This Medicine:** Take with or immediately following meals to prevent stomach irritation. Take one-half of an adult's aspirin tablet or one children's aspirin tablet with each dose of niacin to prevent facial flushing and itching. Dosage should be increased very slowly over 2 to 3 months as needed. The prolonged-action form of niacin is preferable to improve tolerance. The regular tablet may be crushed, but the prolonged-action capsules and tablets should not be altered.

▷ **How Long This Medicine Is Usually Taken:** Use on a regular schedule for 3 to 5 weeks usually determines the effectiveness of this drug in reducing elevated levels of cholesterol and triglycerides. Long-term use (months to years) requires periodic physician evaluation.

▷ **Tell Your Doctor Before Taking This Medicine If You:**
- ever had an allergic reaction to it.
- have active peptic ulcer disease or inflammatory bowel disease.
- have active liver disease.
- are prone to low blood pressure.
- have a heart rhythm disorder of any kind.
- have a history of peptic ulcer disease, inflammatory bowel disease, liver disease, jaundice, or gallbladder disease (with or without gallstones).
- have diabetes or gout.

▷ **Possible Side Effects:** Flushing, itching, tingling, and feeling of warmth usually in the face and neck. Sensitive individuals may experience orthostatic hypotension.

▷ **Possible Adverse Effects:**
If any of the following develop, call your doctor promptly for guidance.
Some Mild Problems Drug Can Cause
Allergic reactions: skin rash, itching, hives.
Headache, dizziness, faintness, impaired vision.
Nausea, vomiting, diarrhea.
Dryness of skin, grayish-black pigmentation of skin folds.
Some Serious Problems Drug Can Cause
Drug-induced hepatitis with jaundice: yellow eyes and skin, dark-colored urine, light-colored stools.
Worsening of diabetes and gout.
Development of heart rhythm disorders.
Rare muscle damage or peptic ulcers.

▷ *CAUTION*

1. Large doses may cause significant increases in blood levels of sugar and uric acid. Those who have diabetes or gout should monitor their status regularly.

2. Periodic measurements of blood cholesterol and triglyceride levels are essential to check your response to treatment and determine the need for changes in dosage or medication.

3. Recent reports indicate that the prolonged-action dosage forms may be more likely to cause liver damage than the rapidly absorbed (crystalline) forms. Ask your doctor about the most appropriate dosage form and schedule for you.

4. Safety and effectiveness of large doses of this drug for those under 12 years old have not been established.

5. Those over 60 should watch for development of low blood pressure (light-headedness, dizziness, faintness) and heart rhythm disorders.

Advisability of Use During Pregnancy or If Breast-Feeding:

Pregnancy Category: C. Use only if clearly needed. Avoid using this drug completely during the first 3 months. Presence in breast milk is unknown; avoid taking this drug or refrain from nursing.

▷ **Overdose Symptoms:** Generalized flushing, nausea, vomiting, stomach cramps, diarrhea, weakness, fainting.

▷ **Suggested Periodic Examinations While Taking This Drug:** (at doctor's discretion)

Measurements of blood levels of total cholesterol, HDL and LDL cholesterol fractions, triglycerides, sugar, and uric acid.

Liver function tests.

▷ **While Taking This Drug the Following Apply:**

Foods: Follow the low-cholesterol diet prescribed by your doctor.

Beverages: May be taken with milk.

Alcohol: Alcohol used with large doses of this drug may cause excessive lowering of blood pressure.

Tobacco Smoking: Can increase flushing or dizziness.

Other Drugs:

Niacin may *increase* the effects of

• some antihypertensives, causing excessive lowering of blood pressure.

Niacin may *decrease* the effects of

• antidiabetics (insulin and sulfonylureas), by raising the level of blood sugar.

• probenecid (Benemid) and sulfinpyrazone (Anturane), by raising the level of blood uric acid.

Niacin *taken concurrently* with
- isoniazid (INH) may decrease niacin levels and require increases in dose to get the same effect.
- lovastatin—and perhaps other cholesterol-lowering drugs—may result in muscle damage.
- nicotine (especially transdermal) can cause increased flushing or dizziness.

Driving, Hazardous Activities: May cause dizziness and faintness. Restrict your activities as necessary.

Discontinuation: Do not discontinue without your doctor's knowledge and guidance. Abrupt withdrawal may be followed by excessive increase in blood cholesterol and triglyceride levels.

▷ **Saving Money When Using This Medicine:**
- Many new drugs are available to treat high cholesterol. Ask your doctor if this medicine offers the best balance of cost and outcome for you. HMG CoA inhibitors have outcome data that demonstrate they can prevent a first heart attack.
- A generic form can be substituted for the brand name.
- Long-term effects can only be avoided by effective lowering of undesirable cholesterol fractions.
- Ask your doctor if taking aspirin every other day makes sense for you.

NICARDIPINE (ni KAR de peen)

Prescription Needed: Yes   **Controlled Drug:** No   **Generic:** No

Brand Name: Cardene

Controversies in Medicine: Results of several studies have indicated that medicines in this chemical family should NOT be used by some patients with extremely compromised hearts. Amlodipine (Norvasc) is the only calcium channel blocker that presently has data to show that it is SAFE, even in the most severely ill congestive heart failure patients. Amlodipine is the only calcium channel blocker to be FDA approved as safe for use in treating hypertension or angina in patients who also have congestive heart failure. There have been several FDA hearings on calcium channel blockers in general.

One retrospective chart review yielded data showing that there was increased risk if nifedipine immediate-release forms were used for treating conditions other than angina in those over 71. There was a caution advised, but the form of nifedipine in question was not approved for uses other than angina. A recent FDA panel found medicines in this class to be safe and effective. A study of nearly 6,000 patients at Tel Aviv Medical Center found that there was no statistically significant risk of death in patients who took calcium-channel blockers versus those who did not take these medicines.

Overview of BENEFITS versus RISKS

Possible Benefits	*Possible Risks*
EFFECTIVE PREVENTION OF CLASSICAL ANGINA-OF-EFFORT	Increase in angina upon starting treatment
EFFECTIVE TREATMENT OF HYPERTENSION	Water retention, ankle swelling

---

▷ **Illness This Medication Treats:**
(1) Classical angina-of-effort (due to atherosclerotic disease of the coronary arteries) or angina caused by artery spasms; (2) mild to moderate hypertension.

▷ **Typical Dosage Range:** (Dosage or schedule must be determined by the doctor for each individual.)
Initially 20 mg three times daily, 6 to 8 hours apart. Dose may be increased gradually at 3-day intervals (as needed and tolerated) up to 40 mg three times daily. The total daily dosage should not exceed 120 mg. The sustained-release form is started at 30 mg twice daily, and increased as needed and tolerated to 60 mg twice daily.

▷ **Conditions Requiring Dosing Adjustments:**
Liver function: For patients with liver compromise, the dose should be started at 20 mg twice a day. If the dose is increased, it should be slowly titrated and the twice-a-day dosing interval retained.
Kidney function: For patients with moderate to severe kidney failure, the starting dose should be 20 mg twice daily. If the dose is increased, it should be titrated slowly, and the twice-daily dosing interval retained. Nicardipine can cause urine retention; a benefit-to-risk decision is necessary for patients with urine outflow problems.

▷ **How Best to Take This Medicine:**   May be taken with or following food to reduce stomach irritation. However, if this drug is taken after a high-fat meal, total absorption may be reduced by 20 to 30%. The capsule should be swallowed whole (not altered).

▷ **How Long This Medicine Is Usually Taken:**   Use on a regular schedule for 2 to 4 weeks is usually necessary to determine the effectiveness of this drug in reducing the frequency and severity of angina or controlling hypertension. For long-term use (months to years) the smallest effective dose should be used. Periodic evaluation is essential.

▷ **Tell Your Doctor Before Taking This Medicine If You:**
- ever had an allergic reaction to it.
- have advanced aortic stenosis.
- had an unfavorable response to any calcium blocker in the past.
- have Duchenne muscular dystrophy.
- are currently taking any form of digitalis or a beta-blocker.
- are taking any drugs that lower blood pressure.
- are taking cimetidine (Tagamet) or cyclosporine (Sandimmune).
- have a history of congestive heart failure, heart attack, or stroke.
- are subject to disturbances of heart rhythm.
- have impaired liver or kidney function.

▷ **Possible Side Effects:**   Rapid heart rate, swelling of the feet and ankles, flushing and sensation of warmth.

▷ **Possible Adverse Effects:**
If any of the following develop, call your doctor promptly for guidance.
Some Mild Problems Drug Can Cause
Allergic reaction: skin rash.
Headache, dizziness, weakness, nervousness, blurred vision, confusion.
Palpitation, shortness of breath.
Indigestion, nausea, vomiting, constipation.
Some Serious Problems Drug Can Cause
Increased frequency or severity of angina on initiation of treatment or following an increase in dose.
Marked drop in blood pressure with fainting.
Rare liver toxicity or problems urinating.
Decreased white blood cell counts have been reported with medicines in the same class.

▷ **Possible Effects on Sex Life:**   Rare impotence.

▷ **Adverse Effects That May Mimic Natural Diseases or Disorders:**
Flushing and warmth may resemble menopausal hot flashes.

▷ *CAUTION*
1. If you are monitoring your own blood pressure, make your measurements just before each dose and 1 to 2 hours after each dose, for an accurate picture of this drug's effect. This will detect excessive fluctuations between high and low readings.
2. Be sure to tell all physicians and dentists you consult that you are taking this drug. Note the use of this drug on your personal identification card.
3. You may use nitroglycerin and other nitrate drugs as needed to relieve acute episodes of angina pain. However, if your angina at-

tacks become more frequent or intense, call your doctor promptly.

4. Safety and effectiveness of this drug for those under 18 years old are not established.

5. Nicardipine is usually well tolerated by those over 60; however, watch for weakness, dizziness, fainting, and falling. Take the necessary precautions to prevent injury. Report promptly any changes in your pattern of thirst and urination.

Advisability of Use During Pregnancy or If Breast-Feeding:

Pregnancy Category: C. Avoid using this drug during the first 3 months. Use during the last 6 months only if clearly needed. Ask your doctor for guidance. Probably present in breast milk; avoid taking this drug or refrain from nursing.

▷ **Overdose Symptoms:** Weakness, light-headedness, fainting, fast pulse, low blood pressure, shortness of breath, flushed and warm skin, tremors.

▷ **Suggested Periodic Examinations While Taking This Drug:** (at doctor's discretion)

Evaluations of heart function, including electrocardiograms; measurements of blood pressure in supine, sitting, and standing positions.

▷ **While Taking This Drug the Following Apply:**

Food: Avoid excessive salt intake.

Beverages: No restrictions. This drug may be taken with milk.

Alcohol: Alcohol may exaggerate the drop in blood pressure experienced by some individuals.

Tobacco Smoking: Nicotine may reduce the effectiveness of this drug.

Marijuana Smoking: Possible reduced effectiveness of this drug; mild to moderate increase in angina; possible changes in electrocardiogram, confusing interpretation.

Other Drugs:

Nicardipine may *increase* the effects of

• cyclosporine (Sandimmune), causing kidney toxicity.

Nicardipine *taken concurrently* with

• amiodarone (Cordarone) may lead to cardiac arrest.

• beta-blockers or digitalis preparations may affect heart rate and rhythm adversely. Careful monitoring by your doctor is necessary if these drugs are taken concurrently.

• magnesium may worsen neuromuscular blockade, and lower blood pressure further.

• nonsteroidal anti-inflammatory drugs (NSAIDs—see Drug Classes) may blunt nicardipine's benefits.

• phenytoin (Dilantin) may lead to phenytoin toxicity as well as blunted benefits of nicardipine.

- rifampin (Rifadin, others) has led to loss of blood pressure control with some other medicines in the same family. Caution is advised.

The following drug may *increase* the effects of nicardipine

- cimetidine (Tagamet).

Driving, Hazardous Activities: Usually no restrictions. This drug may cause drowsiness or dizziness. Restrict your activities as necessary.

Exposure to Heat: Caution is advised. Hot environments can exaggerate the blood pressure–lowering effects of this drug. Observe for light-headedness or weakness.

Heavy Exercise or Exertion: This drug may allow you to be more active without resulting angina pain. Use caution and avoid excessive exercise that could impair heart function without warning pain.

Discontinuation: Do not stop taking this drug abruptly. Ask your doctor about gradual withdrawal. Watch for development of rebound angina.

▷ **Saving Money When Using This Medicine:**

- Many new drugs are available to treat high blood pressure. Ask your doctor if this medicine offers the best balance of cost and outcome for you.
- Ask your doctor how often he or she wants you to have your blood pressure checked.
- Talk with your doctor about taking aspirin every other day in order to help prevent a heart attack.

NICOTINE (NIK oh teen)

Prescription Needed: Yes   **Controlled Drug:** No   **Generic:** No

Brand Names: Habitrol, Nicoderm, Nicorette, Nicorette DS, Nicotrol, Nicotrol NS, Prostep

Author's note: A patient guide to quitting smoking is available from the Agency for Health Care Policy & Research by calling 1-800-358-9295. Two brands of nicotine patches and the nicotine gum are now available without a prescription for those over 18 years old.

Overview of BENEFITS versus RISKS

Possible Benefits	*Possible Risks*
EFFECTIVE REDUCTION OF NICOTINE CRAVING AND WITHDRAWAL EFFECTS when used adjunctively in smoking-cessation treatment programs	Aggravation of existing angina, heart rhythm disorders, hypertension, insulin-dependent diabetes, peptic ulcer, and vascular diseases Increased risk of abortion (if used during pregnancy)

▷ **Illness This Medication Treats:**

Gum, nasal, or transdermal systems used adjunctively with behavior modification programs/support groups to assist cigarette smokers who wish to stop smoking.

▷ **Typical Dosage Range:** (Dosage or schedule must be determined by the doctor for each individual.)

Infants and Children: Avoid use of this drug completely in children. Avoid accidental exposure to patches.

12 to 60 Years of Age: For gum tablets: Initially one piece every hour while awake (10 to 12 pieces daily); supplement with one additional piece if and when needed to control urge to smoke. Total daily dosage should not exceed 30 pieces (60 mg).

For transdermal systems: Dosage depends upon patient characteristics and the product used.

For those weighing 100 lb or more, who smoke 10 or more cigarettes daily, and do *not* have cardiovascular disease: 16-hr system (Nicotrol)—Initially one 15-mg patch applied for 16 hours daily for 4 to 12 weeks. For those who have abstained from smoking, reduce dose to one 10-mg patch applied for 16 hours daily for the next 2 to 4 weeks; then to one 5-mg patch applied for 16 hours daily for the following 2 to 4 weeks.

24-hr system (Habitrol, Nicoderm)—Initially one 21-mg patch applied daily for 4 to 8 weeks. For those who have abstained from smoking, reduce dose to one 14-mg patch daily for the next 2 to 4 weeks; then to one 7-mg patch daily for the following 2 to 4 weeks. Prostep—Initially one 22-mg patch applied daily for 4 to 8 weeks. For those who have abstained from smoking, reduce dose to one 11-mg patch daily for 2 to 4 weeks.

For those weighing less than 100 lb, who smoke less than 10 cigarettes daily, or who *have* cardiovascular disease: 24-hr system (Habitrol, Nicoderm)—Initially one 14-mg patch applied daily for 4 to 8 weeks. For those who have abstained from smoking, reduce dose to one

7-mg patch daily for the next 2 to 4 weeks. Prostep—Initially one 11-mg patch applied daily for 4 to 8 weeks.

For adults using the nasal form: 1–2 doses per hour, up to 5 doses per hour or 40 doses per day. This pattern is continued for 6–8 weeks, followed by a period of gradual reduction of 4–6 weeks using half the usual dose and a decreased number of uses per hour.

Over 60 Years of Age: Same as for 12 to 60 years of age.

▷ **Conditions Requiring Dosing Adjustments:**

Liver function: If the liver is compromised, a decrease of the starting dose must be considered.

Kidney function: Severe renal compromise requires dosing adjustment to avoid accumulation.

▷ **How Best to Take This Medicine:** Carefully follow the manufacturer's directions provided with each product.

For chewing gum: Limit use to one piece of gum at a time. This product is much harder than typical chewing gum. Chew each piece slowly and intermittently for 30 minutes. Tingling gum tissue or peppery taste usually indicates release of a sufficient amount of nicotine. Gradually reduce the number of pieces chewed each day by using it only when there is an urge to smoke. During participation in a smoking-cessation program, always have the gum available as a defense against smoking.

For transdermal systems: Apply a new patch at the same time each day to the upper arm or body where the skin is clean, dry, and free of hair, oil, scars, and irritation of any kind; alternate sites of application. Do not alter the patch in any way. Press the patch firmly in place for 10 seconds; ensure good contact throughout. Wash your hands when you have finished applying the patch. Replace patches that are dislodged by showering, bathing, or swimming.

▷ **How Long This Medicine Is Usually Taken:** Use on a regular schedule for 2 to 3 months usually determines the effectiveness of this drug in achieving lasting cessation of smoking. Nicotine chewing gum should not be used for more than 6 months; transdermal systems should not be used for more than 20 weeks. Best results are realized when these products are part of an organized smoking-cessation program. Long-term use requires periodic evaluation of response and dosage adjustment. See your doctor or pharmacist regularly.

▷ **Tell Your Doctor Before Taking This Medicine If You:**
- ever had an allergic reaction to it.
- have severe, uncontrolled angina, or a pattern of worsening angina.
- have uncontrolled, life-threatening heart rhythm disorders.
- have had a heart attack recently or at any time.
- have any form of angina (coronary heart disease).

- are subject to heart rhythm disorders.
- have insulin-dependent diabetes.
- have hypertension.
- have hyperthyroidism.
- have a pheochromocytoma.
- have a history of esophagitis or peptic ulcer disease.
- have a history of Buerger's disease or Raynaud's disorder.
- have already tried a 3-month course.
- currently have any dental problems or skin disorders.
- have a history of kidney or liver disease.
- think you are pregnant or plan to become pregnant.

▷ **Possible Side Effects:**   For chewing gum: mouth or throat irritation; injury to teeth or dental repairs.

For transdermal systems: redness, itching, or burning at site of application (mild and transient).

▷ **Possible Adverse Effects:**
If any of the following develop, call your doctor promptly for guidance.
Some Mild Problems Drug Can Cause
Allergic reactions: skin rash, itching, local or generalized swellings.
Headache, light-headedness, dizziness, drowsiness, irritability, nervousness, insomnia, joint pain, muscle aches, abnormal dreams.
Rapid heartbeat, palpitation, increased sweating.
Increased or decreased appetite, dry mouth, constipation or diarrhea.
Nasal irritation for the nasal form.
Some Serious Problems Drug Can Cause
Irregular heart rhythms, chest pain, edema.
Rare stroke.

▷ *CAUTION*
1. For these drug products to be safe and effective, IT IS MANDATORY THAT ALL SMOKING BE STOPPED IMMEDIATELY AT THE BEGINNING OF DRUG TREATMENT.
2. Extended use of chewing gum may cause damage to mouth tissues and teeth, loosen fillings, stick to dentures, and initiate or aggravate temporomandibular joint (TMJ) dysfunction.
3. Smoking cessation and the use of these drug products can result in increased blood levels of insulin (in insulin-dependent diabetics); reduced dosage of insulin may be necessary to prevent hypoglycemic reactions.
4. If you are taking any of the following drugs, ask your doctor about the need to reduce their dosage while participating in a smoking-cessation program: aminophylline, oxtriphylline, theophylline,

beta-blockers, propoxyphene, oxazepam, prazosin, pentazocine, imipramine.

5. If you are taking any of the following drugs, ask your doctor about the need to increase their dosage while participating in a smoking-cessation program: isoproterenol, phenylephrine.

6. Used patches should be folded in half with the adhesive sides sealed together, placed in the original pouch or aluminum foil, and disposed of promptly; keep out of reach of children and animals.

7. Use of antacids such as TUMS prior to chewing nicotine gum can increase the amount of nicotine absorbed from the gum.

8. Habitrol patches have been shown to be effective only when they are part of a complete smoking-cessation program that includes counseling.

9. Safety and effectiveness of this drug for those under 12 years old have not been established.

10. Because of the increased possibility of cardiovascular disorders in those over 60, treatment should be initiated with caution and response monitored very closely for adverse effects.

Advisability of Use During Pregnancy or If Breast-Feeding:
Pregnancy Category: For nicotine chewing gum: X; for nicotine transdermal systems: D. Use of this drug is not recommended during pregnancy. Present in breast milk; avoid taking this drug or refrain from nursing.

▷ **Habit-Forming Potential:** Prolonged use (beyond 6 months) may perpetuate physical dependence in nicotine-dependent smokers.

▷ **Overdose Symptoms:** Nausea, vomiting, increased salivation, diarrhea, headache, dizziness, impaired vision and hearing, weakness, confusion, difficult breathing, seizures.

▷ **Suggested Periodic Examinations While Taking This Drug:** (at doctor's discretion)
Evaluation of patient's ability to abstain from smoking.
Evaluation of patient's blood pressure and heart function.

▷ **While Taking This Drug the Following Apply:**
Alcohol: May increase cardiovascular effects.
Tobacco Smoking: Avoid all forms of tobacco completely.
Marijuana Smoking: Avoid completely.
Other Drugs:
Nicotine may *increase* the effects of
• adenosine.
• niacin (flushing and dizziness).
The following drugs may *increase* the effects of nicotine
• antacids such as TUMS used prior to chewing nicotine-containing gum may increase the absorption of nicotine from the gum.

- cimetidine (Tagamet).
- lithium (Lithobid, others).
- ranitidine (Zantac).

Driving, Hazardous Activities: May cause dizziness or drowsiness. Restrict your activities as necessary.

Exposure to Cold: Use caution until tolerance is determined. Cold environments may enhance the vasospastic action of nicotine.

Heavy Exercise or Exertion: Use caution in the presence of angina, known coronary artery disease, or hypertension.

Special Storage Instructions: Store nicotine gum at room temperature and protect it from light. Store nicotine patches at room temperature; avoid exposing to temperatures greater than 86° F (30° C). Do not store unpouched. Once opened, patches should be used promptly.

Discontinuation: As soon as you have been able to stop smoking for a significant time, gradually reduce dosage and then stop using this medicine. Continual use of the chewing gum should not exceed 6 months; continual use of the transdermal systems should not exceed 20 weeks.

▷ **Saving Money When Using This Medicine:**
- Several drugs are available to treat nicotine addiction. All products work best combined with a formal counseling program. Ask your doctor if this medicine offers the best balance of cost and outcome for you.
- Ask your doctor when you will be able to stop taking this drug.

NIFEDIPINE   (ni FED i peen)

Prescription Needed: Yes   **Controlled Drug:** No   **Generic:** Yes

Brand Names: Adalat, Procardia, Procardia XL

Controversies in Medicine: Results of several studies have indicated that medicines in this chemical family should NOT be used by some patients with extremely compromised hearts. Amlodipine (Norvasc) is the only calcium channel blocker that presently has data to show that it is SAFE, even in the most severely ill congestive heart failure patients. Amlodipine is the only calcium channel blocker to be FDA-approved as safe for use in treating hypertension or angina in patients who also have congestive heart failure. There have been several FDA hearings on calcium channel blockers in general.

One retrospective chart review yielded data showing that there was increased risk if nifedipine immediate-release forms were used for treating conditions other than angina in those over 71. There was a caution advised, but the form of nifedipine in question was not approved for uses other than angina. A recent FDA panel found medicines in this class to be safe and effective. A study of nearly 6,000 patients at Tel Aviv Medical Center found that there was no statistically significant risk of death in patients who took calcium channel blockers versus those who did not take these medicines.

Overview of BENEFITS versus RISKS

Possible Benefits	*Possible Risks*
EFFECTIVE PREVENTION OF BOTH MAJOR TYPES OF ANGINA	Rare increase in angina upon starting treatment
EFFECTIVE TREATMENT OF HYPERTENSION	Rare precipitation of congestive heart failure
	Rare drug-induced hepatitis or fainting
	Rare anemia or lowered white blood cell counts

▷ **Illness This Medication Treats:**

(1) Spontaneous angina pectoris due to coronary artery spasm (Prinzmetal's variant angina) and not associated with exertion; and (2) classical angina-of-effort (due to atherosclerotic disease of the coronary arteries) in individuals who have not responded to or cannot tolerate nitrates or beta-blockers. (3) Sustained-release tablets are used to treat mild to moderate hypertension.

▷ **Typical Dosage Range:** (Dosage or schedule must be determined by the doctor for each individual.)

Infants and Children: Dosage not established.

12 to 60 Years of Age: Extended-release form for high blood pressure: Initially 30 mg once daily. Dose may be increased as needed or tolerated at 14-day intervals to 60 mg daily.

For hypertension: Initially a single 30- or 60-mg sustained-release form daily.

Sublingual: Hypertensive crisis: The immediate-release form is NOT recommended for treating hypertension, heart attack, hypertensive crisis, or some forms of unstable angina.

Over 60 Years of Age: Same as for 12 to 60 years of age. The immediate-release form has been associated with an almost fourfold increase in all-cause death when compared to ACE inhibitors, beta-blockers, or other calcium channel blockers.

▷ **Conditions Requiring Dosing Adjustments:**

Liver function: Specific dosage adjustments for patients with liver compromise are not defined, and the dose should be empirically decreased. This drug is also a rare cause of liver toxicity (allergic hepatitis), and should be used with caution by patients with compromised livers. It is also a potential cause of portal hypertension, and should not be used by patients with portal hypertension.

Kidney function: For patients with renal compromise nifedipine requires a benefit-to-risk decision, as it can lead to renal failure.

▷ **How Best to Take This Medicine:**   May be taken with or following food to reduce stomach irritation. The capsule should be swallowed whole (not altered). The sustained-release tablet should be taken whole (not altered). The sustained-release form permits effective once-a-day treatment for both angina and hypertension.

▷ **How Long This Medicine Is Usually Taken:**   Continual use on a regular schedule for 2 to 4 weeks is usually necessary to determine the effectiveness of this drug in reducing the frequency and severity of angina and controlling hypertension. For long-term use (months to years), determine the smallest effective dose. Supervision and periodic evaluation by your doctor are essential. See your doctor regularly.

▷ **Tell Your Doctor Before Taking This Medicine If You:**
- ever had an allergic reaction to it.
- have active liver disease.
- have low blood pressure—systolic pressure below 90.
- had an unfavorable response to any calcium blocker in the past.
- are currently taking any form of digitalis or a beta-blocker.
- are over 71 years old and have been prescribed the immediate-release form of nifedipine.
- are taking any drugs that lower blood pressure.
- have a history of congestive heart failure, heart attack, or stroke.
- are subject to disturbances of heart rhythm.
- have impaired liver or kidney function.
- have diabetes.
- have a history of drug-induced liver damage.

▷ **Possible Side Effects:**   Low blood pressure, rapid heart rate, swelling of the feet and ankles, flushing and sensation of warmth, sweating. Ringing in the ears.

▷ **Possible Adverse Effects:**
If any of the following develop, call your doctor promptly for guidance.
Some Mild Problems Drug Can Cause
  Allergic reactions: skin rash, itching, fever.
  Headache, dizziness, weakness, nervousness, blurred vision.
  Palpitation, shortness of breath, wheezing, cough.
  Heartburn, nausea, diarrhea.
  Tremors, muscle cramps.

Some Serious Problems Drug Can Cause

Allergic reaction: drug-induced hepatitis (very rare).

Idiosyncratic reactions: joint stiffness and inflammation.

Increased frequency or severity of angina when therapy is started or dose is increased.

Rare abnormal muscle movements, kidney toxicity, pulmonary edema, acute psychosis, or lowered white blood cells or hemoglobin.

Marked drop in blood pressure with fainting.

▷ **Possible Effects on Sex Life:**   Altered timing and pattern of menstruation; excessive menstrual bleeding. Tenderness or swelling of male breast tissue.

▷ **Adverse Effects That May Mimic Natural Diseases or Disorders:**
An allergic rash and swelling of the legs may resemble erysipelas. Drug-induced hepatitis may suggest viral hepatitis.

▷ *CAUTION*

1. Tell everyone who prescribes medicines for you that you are taking this drug. Note its use on your personal identification card.

2. You may use nitroglycerin and other nitrate drugs as needed to relieve acute episodes of angina pain. However, if your angina attacks are becoming more frequent or intense, call your doctor promptly.

3. Safety and effectiveness of this drug for those under 12 years old have not been established.

4. Those over 60 may be more susceptible to weakness, dizziness, fainting, and falling. Take the necessary precautions to prevent injury. Report promptly any changes in your pattern of thirst and urination.

5. This drug may cause kidney failure and is NOT ideal for patients with compromised kidneys.

Advisability of Use During Pregnancy or If Breast-Feeding:

Pregnancy Category: C. Avoid this drug during the first 3 months. Use during the last 6 months only if clearly needed. Ask your doctor for guidance. Present in breast milk; avoid taking this drug or refrain from nursing.

▷ **Overdose Symptoms:** Weakness, light-headedness, fainting, fast pulse, low blood pressure, shortness of breath, flushed and warm skin, tremors.

▷ **Suggested Periodic Examinations While Taking This Drug:** (at doctor's discretion)

Evaluations of heart function, including electrocardiograms; measurements of blood pressure in supine, sitting, and standing positions.

▷ **While Taking This Drug the Following Apply:**

Foods: Grapefruit juice may GREATLY increase the amount of medicine that gets into your body. Water is the best liquid to take with this medicine. Avoid excessive salt intake.

Beverages: May be taken with milk.

Alcohol: Alcohol may exaggerate the drop in blood pressure experienced by some people.

Tobacco Smoking: Nicotine may reduce nifedipine's effectiveness.

Marijuana Smoking: Possible reduced effectiveness of this drug; mild to moderate increase in angina; possible changes in electrocardiogram, confusing interpretation.

Other Drugs:

Nifedipine **taken concurrently** with

- amiodarone (Cordarone) may cause the heart to stop beating.
- beta-blockers or digitalis preparations may adversely affect heart rate and rhythm. Careful monitoring by your doctor is necessary if these drugs are taken concurrently.
- cyclosporine (Sandimmune) may lead to nifedipine toxicity.
- digoxin (Lanoxin) can lead to digoxin toxicity.
- diltiazem can lead to nifedipine toxicity.
- oral hypoglycemic agents (see Drug Classes) may result in loss of blood sugar control.
- magnesium may lead to additive lowering of blood pressure.
- phenytoin (Dilantin) can cause phenytoin toxicity.
- rifampin (Rifadin) can blunt nifedipine's benefits.
- theophylline (Theo-Dur, others) can blunt nifedipine's effects and also lead to theophylline toxicity.
- vincristine (Oncovin) can lead to vincristine toxicity.

The following drugs may **increase** the effects of nifedipine

- cimetidine (Tagamet).
- quinidine (Quinaglute, others) may lead to nifedipine toxicity and blunted quinidine benefits as well.
- ranitidine (Zantac).

Driving, Hazardous Activities: Usually no restrictions. This drug may cause drowsiness or dizziness. Restrict your activities as necessary.

Exposure to Heat: Caution is advised. Hot environments can exaggerate the blood pressure–lowering effects. Observe for light-headedness or weakness.

Heavy Exercise or Exertion: This drug may allow you to be more active without resulting angina pain. Use caution and avoid excessive exercise that could impair heart function without warning pain.

Discontinuation: Do not discontinue this drug abruptly. Ask your doctor about gradual withdrawal. Observe for the development of rebound angina.

▷ **Saving Money When Using This Medicine:**
- Many new drugs are available to treat high blood pressure. There are also many calcium channel blockers. Ask your doctor if this medicine offers the best balance of cost and outcome for you.
- Talk with your doctor to see how often he or she recommends you have your blood pressure checked.
- Ask your doctor if taking aspirin every other day to help prevent a heart attack makes sense for you.

NITROFURANTOIN (ni troh fyur AN toin)

Prescription Needed: Yes **Controlled Drug:** No **Generic:** Yes

Brand Names: Furadantin, Furalan, Macrodantin, Macrodantin MACPAC, Parfuran

Overview of BENEFITS versus RISKS	
Possible Benefits	*Possible Risks*
EFFECTIVE TREATMENT OF SOME URINARY TRACT INFECTIONS	Allergic reactions: anaphylaxis; rashes; hives; repetitive asthma; lung inflammation; drug-induced hepatitis
	Peripheral neuropathy
	Blood cell disorders: hemolytic anemia
	Reduced white blood cell count
	Superinfections

▷ **Illness This Medication Treats:**
Infections in the urinary tract.

▷ **Typical Dosage Range:** (Dosage or schedule must be determined by the doctor for each individual.)
For treatment of active infections: 50 to 100 mg every 6 hours. For prevention: 50 to 100 mg once every day at bedtime. The total daily dosage should not exceed 600 mg.

▷ **Conditions Requiring Dosing Adjustments:**
Liver function: Specific dosage adjustments for patients with liver compromise are not defined. This drug is also a rare cause of liver toxicity, and should be used with caution by patients with compromised livers.
Kidney function: This drug should NOT be used by patients with moderate kidney failure. Drink adequate quantities of water.

▷ **How Best to Take This Medicine:**   Preferably taken with or following food to facilitate absorption and reduce stomach irritation. The tablet may be crushed and the capsule opened for administration, but this drug can stain the teeth yellow on contact.

▷ **How Long This Medicine Is Usually Taken:**   Scheduled use for 7 to 10 days usually determines the effectiveness of this drug in curing urinary tract infections. Long-term use for prevention (months to years) requires physician supervision.

NITROGLYCERIN   (ni troh GLIS er in)

Prescription Needed: Yes   **Controlled Drug:** No   **Generic:** Yes

Brand Names: Deponit, Minitran Transdermal Delivery System, Nitro-Bid, Nitrodisc, Nitro-Dur, Nitro-Dur II, Nitrogard, Nitrogard-SR, Nitroglyn, Nitrol, Nitrolingual Spray, Nitrong, Nitrospan, Nitrostat, Nitroglycerin Transdermal System Patch, Transderm-Nitro

Overview of BENEFITS versus RISKS	
Possible Benefits	*Possible Risks*
EFFECTIVE RELIEF AND PREVENTION OF ANGINA	Orthostatic hypotension with and without fainting
EFFECTIVE ADJUNCTIVE TREATMENT IN SELECTED CASES OF CONGESTIVE HEART FAILURE	Skin rash (rare)
	Rare altered hemoglobin with large doses
	Rare lowering of blood platelet counts

▷ **Illness This Medication Treats:**
   (1) Symptomatic coronary artery disease. Rapid-action forms relieve acute attacks of anginal pain. Sustained-action forms prevent development of angina. (2) Helps in improving difficult breathing caused by heart failure or after a heart attack; (3) used intravenously in surgery for controlling blood pressure.

▷ **Typical Dosage Range:** (Dosage or schedule must be determined by the doctor for each individual.)
   According to dosage form:
   Sublingual spray: One metered spray (0.4 mg) under the tongue every 3 to 5 minutes, up to three doses within 15 minutes, to relieve acute angina. To prevent angina, one spray taken 5 to 10 minutes before exertion.
   Sublingual tablets: 0.15 to 0.6 mg dissolved under the tongue at 5-minute intervals to relieve acute angina.

Prolonged-action tablets: 1.3 to 6.5 mg at 8- to 12-hour intervals to prevent angina.

Prolonged-action capsules: 2.5 to 9 mg at 8- to 12-hour intervals to prevent angina.

Ointment: 2.5 to 5 cm (1–2 in, 15–30 mg) applied in a thin, even, uniform layer to hairless skin at 3- to 4-hour intervals to prevent angina.

Buccal tablets: 1 to 2 mg every 4 to 5 hours placed between the cheek and gum.

Transdermal patches: 5-cm^2 to 30-cm^2 patch applied to hairless skin once every 24 hours to prevent angina.

Author's note: In order to preserve its effectiveness, a nitrate-free interval of 12 hours daily is recommended. 24-hour patches are removed after being on for 12 hours. Oral sustained-release forms are dosed to give a 6- to 12-hour nitrate-free interval.

▷ **Conditions Requiring Dosing Adjustments:**
Kidney function: Specific guidelines for dosing changes are not available. This drug can discolor urine.

▷ **How Best to Take This Medicine:**   Dosage forms to be swallowed are best taken when stomach is empty (1 hour before or 2 hours after eating) to obtain maximal blood levels. Tablets should not be crushed for administration. Capsules may be opened, but the contents should not be crushed or chewed before swallowing.

▷ **How Long This Medicine Is Usually Taken:**   Scheduled use for 3 to 5 days usually determines the effectiveness of this drug in preventing and relieving acute anginal attacks. Individual dosage adjustments are necessary for optimal results. Long-term use (months to years) requires physician supervision.

▷ **Tell Your Doctor Before Taking This Medicine If You:**
 • ever had an allergic reaction to it.
 • are severely anemic.
 • have any form of glaucoma, or inadequately treated closed-angle glaucoma.
 • have had an unfavorable response to other nitrate drugs in the past.
 • have abnormal growth of heart muscle (hypertrophy).
 • have low blood pressure.

▷ **Possible Side Effects:**   Flushing of face, headaches, orthostatic hypotension, rapid heart rate, palpitation.

▷ **Possible Adverse Effects**
If any of the following develop, call your doctor promptly for guidance.
Some Mild Problems Drug Can Cause
Allergic reaction: skin rash.

Throbbing headaches (may be severe), dizziness, fainting.
Nausea, vomiting.

Some Serious Problems Drug Can Cause

Allergic reactions: severe skin reactions with peeling.
Idiosyncratic reaction: methemoglobinemia (very rare).
Rare abnormal slowing of the heart.

▷ **Possible Effects on Sex Life:**   Correction of impotence (one report, following sublingual use).

Preventive use prior to sexual activity has been recommended to eliminate or reduce the risk of angina. Consult your doctor for guidance.

▷ **Adverse Effects That May Mimic Natural Diseases or Disorders:**
Hypotensive spells (sudden drops in blood pressure) may be mistaken for late-onset epilepsy.

▷ *CAUTION*

1. This drug can provoke migraine headaches in susceptible individuals.
2. In the presence of impaired brain circulation (cerebral arteriosclerosis), this drug can cause transient ischemic attacks—periods of temporary speech impairment, paralysis, numbness, etc.
3. Development of tolerance to long-acting nitrates renders the sublingual tablets ineffective in relieving acute angina. Sensitivity to the drug's antianginal effect is restored after 1 week of abstinence from the long-acting forms.
4. Many over-the-counter products for allergies, colds, and coughs contain drugs that counteract the desired effects of this drug. Ask your doctor or pharmacist for guidance before using any such medications.
5. Limited usefulness and experience of usage of nitroglycerin in infants and children. Dosage schedules are not established.
6. Small doses with slow increases as needed and tolerated should be given to those over 60. You may be more susceptible to flushing, throbbing headache, dizziness, blackout spells, fainting, and falling.

Advisability of Use During Pregnancy or If Breast-Feeding:
Pregnancy Category: C. Use this drug only if clearly needed. Ask your doctor for guidance. Presence in breast milk is unknown. Monitor the nursing infant closely and discontinue drug or nursing if adverse effects develop.

▷ **Overdose Symptoms:** Throbbing headache, dizziness, marked flushing, nausea, vomiting, abdominal cramps, confusion, delirium, paralysis, seizures, circulatory collapse.

▷ **Suggested Periodic Examinations While Taking This Drug:** (at doctor's discretion)

Measurements of blood pressure and internal eye pressures.
Evaluation of hemoglobin.

▷ **While Taking This Drug the Following Apply:**

Beverages: May be taken with milk.

Alcohol: Avoid alcohol completely in the presence of any side effects or adverse effects. Never use alcohol in the presence of a nitroglycerin headache.

Tobacco Smoking: Nicotine can reduce nitroglycerin's effectiveness.

Marijuana Smoking: Possible reduced effectiveness of this drug; mild to moderate increase in angina; possible changes in the electrocardiogram, confusing interpretation.

Other Drugs:

Nitroglycerin *taken concurrently* with

- acetylcysteine (NAC) may reverse tolerance to the intravenous nitroglycerin form.
- antihypertensives may cause excessive lowering of blood pressure. Careful dosage adjustments may be necessary.
- diltiazem (Cardizem) may result in abnormally low blood pressure if taken with sustained-release nitroglycerine.
- dihydroergotamine or similar ergot derivatives may lead to ergotamine toxicity.
- heparin may blunt heparin's benefits.
- isosorbide dinitrate (Isordil) or mononitrate (Ismo) may result in decreased therapeutic benefits.

The following drug may *increase* the effects of nitroglycerin

- aspirin, in analgesic doses (500 mg or more).

Driving, Hazardous Activities: Usually no restrictions. This drug may cause dizziness or faintness. Restrict your activities as necessary.

Exposure to Heat: Use caution. Hot environments can cause significant lowering of blood pressure.

Exposure to Cold: Cold environments can increase the need for this drug and limit its effectiveness.

Heavy Exercise or Exertion: This drug can increase your tolerance for exercise. Use good judgment regarding excessive exertion in the absence of anginal pain.

Discontinuation: Do not stop taking this drug abruptly after long-term use. It is advisable to reduce the dose (of the prolonged-action dosage forms) gradually over a period of 4 to 6 weeks. Observe for rebound angina.

Special Storage Instructions: For sublingual tablets: To prevent loss of this medicine's strength, keep tablets in the original glass container; do not transfer them to a plastic or metallic container or place absorbent cotton, paper (such as the prescription label), or other material inside the container; do not store other drugs in the same

container. Close the container tightly immediately after each use
and store at room temperature.

▷ **Saving Money When Using This Medicine:**
- Many new nitroglycerine forms are available to treat angina. Ask
  your doctor if this medicine offers the best balance of cost and outcome for you.
- A generic form can be substituted for the brand name.
- Talk with your doctor to see if taking aspirin every other day to help
  prevent a heart attack makes sense for you.
- If you have elevated cholesterol with your angina, talk with your
  doctor about using an HMG CoA inhibitor.

NIZATIDINE (ni ZA te deen)

Prescription Needed: Yes   **Controlled Drug:** No   **Generic:**
No

Brand Names: Axid, Axid AR (nonprescription)

Overview of BENEFITS versus RISKS

Possible Benefits	*Possible Risks*
EFFECTIVE TREATMENT OF PEPTIC ULCER DISEASE: relief of symptoms, acceleration of healing, prevention of recurrence	Drug-induced liver damage (rare) Abnormally low blood platelet count (rare)
CONTROL OF HYPERSECRETORY STOMACH DISORDERS	
Beneficial in treatment of reflux esophagitis	

See the histamine (H2) blocker drug profile for more information.

NORFLOXACIN (nor FLOX a sin)

Prescription Needed: Yes   **Controlled Drug:** No   **Generic:**
No

Brand Names: Noroxin, Noroxin Ophthalmic

▷ **Warning:** (1) Some physicians use the name Norflox to identify the
  generic drug norfloxacin when issuing orders for inpatients or
  writing prescriptions for outpatients. This coinage has resulted in
  serious medication errors: the dispensing of the brand-name drug

Norflex—the generic drug orphenadrine—which is a skeletal muscle relaxant. Ask your pharmacist to verify that you are getting the right drug—an anti-infective, not a muscle relaxant.

(2) Other medicines in this class have caused tendon rupture. If this drug is prescribed for you, ask if you should limit exercise or exertion during therapy. Call your doctor immediately if pain or inflammation appears while you are taking this medicine. A rare idiosyncratic reaction has also been reported, which appears as confusion and disorientation. Call your doctor if you notice a change in thinking or mental status in you or a loved one after this medicine has been started.

Overview of BENEFITS versus RISKS

Possible Benefits	*Possible Risks*
HIGH CURE RATE (95%) IN TREATMENT OF URINARY TRACT INFECTIONS	Infrequent nausea, indigestion
	Impairment of vision (rare)
Effective treatment of bacterial gastroenteritis and gonorrhea	Seizure (rare)

▷ **Illness This Medication Treats:**
(1) Urinary tract infections (in adults) caused by a wide variety of bacteria sensitive to this drug; (2) in ophthalmic solution for treatment of eye infections and conjunctivitis.

▷ **Typical Dosage Range:** Uncomplicated urinary tract infections: 400 mg/12 hr for 3 days. Complicated urinary tract infections: 400 mg/12 hr for 10 to 21 days. Total daily dosage should not exceed 800 mg.
Ophthalmic: One to two drops in the affected eye four times daily.

▷ **Conditions Requiring Dosing Adjustments:**
Liver function: This drug should be used with caution by patients with compromised livers, and blood levels and liver function tests should be obtained.
Kidney function: For patients with moderate kidney compromise, the dose should be decreased to 400 mg daily. Drink adequate quantities of water since norfloxacin is a rare cause of crystalluria.

▷ **How Best to Take This Medicine:** Preferably taken with a full glass of water 1 hour before or 2 hours after eating. Avoid antacids for 2 hours after taking this drug. The tablet may be crushed. Take the full course prescribed.

▷ **How Long This Medicine Is Usually Taken:** Continual use on a regular schedule for 3 to 21 days (depending on the nature of the infection) is usually necessary to determine the effectiveness of this drug in eradicating the infection.

▷ **Tell Your Doctor Before Taking This Medicine If You:**
- ever had an allergic reaction to it.
- are pregnant or breast-feeding.
- are given a prescription for a child under 18 years of age.
- are allergic to cinoxacin (Cinobac) or nalidixic acid (NegGram).
- have a history of psychosis.
- have a seizure disorder.
- have impaired liver or kidney function.

▷ **Possible Adverse Effects:**
If any of the following develop, call your doctor promptly for guidance.

Some Mild Problems Drug Can Cause
> Allergic reactions: skin rash, localized swelling, itching.
> Headache, dizziness, mental depression, seizures.
> Drowsiness, mood alterations, nervousness, insomnia, hallucinations.
> Visual disturbances: blurred or double vision, altered color vision, increased sensitivity to light.
> Dry mouth, decreased appetite, nausea, indigestion, vomiting, diarrhea.
> Swollen or painful tendons and joints.

Some Serious Problems Drug Can Cause
> Allergic reactions: exfoliative dermatitis, anaphylactic reaction.
> Idiosyncratic reaction: confusion, delirium, aphasia reported with another medicine in this same family.
> Seizures.
> Rare kidney toxicity (from crystals formed in the urine).
> Worsening of myasthenia gravis.

▷ **CAUTION**
1. With high doses or prolonged use, crystals can form in the kidney. This can be prevented by drinking copious amounts of water, up to 2 qt/24 hr.
2. This drug may decrease the formation of saliva and predispose to dental cavities or gum disease. See your dentist if mouth dryness persists.
3. The safety of this drug for those who have not attained complete bone growth has not been established. This drug can impair normal bone growth and development in test animals. Avoid using this drug until bone development is complete.
4. The dose must be decreased for patients with reduced kidney function.
5. Talk with your doctor about exercise and any limitations.
6. If you become disoriented or have difficulty thinking after starting this medicine, call your doctor.

Advisability of Use During Pregnancy or If Breast-Feeding:
Pregnancy Category: C. Avoid use of this drug during entire pregnancy. Presence in breast milk is unknown; avoid taking this drug or refrain from nursing.

▷ **Overdose Symptoms:**   Nausea, vomiting, and diarrhea. Confusion and seizures.

▷ **Suggested Periodic Examinations While Taking This Drug:** (at doctor's discretion)
Liver function tests, urine analysis.

▷ **While Taking This Drug the Following Apply:**
Other Drugs:
Norfloxacin *taken concurrently* with
- magnesium will blunt the effectiveness of norfloxacin.
- nitrofurantoin (Macrodantin, etc.) may antagonize the antibacterial action of norfloxacin in the urinary tract. Avoid this combination.
- theophylline may result in SERIOUS toxicity. Ask your doctor for help.
- warfarin poses a threat of SEVERE bleeding. More frequent INR (prothrombin time) testing is needed with adjustment of doses to laboratory results.
- caffeine—caffeine tends to stay in the body longer in higher levels than usual.
- cyclosporine (Sandimmune) may result in a serious increase in cyclosporine levels and toxicity.
The following drug may *increase* the effects of norfloxacin
- probenecid (Benemid).
The following drugs may *decrease* the effects of norfloxacin
- antacids; may reduce its absorption.
- dairy foods; reduces its absorption.
- iron compounds; may reduce its absorption.
- sucralfate; reduces its absorption.
- zinc; reduces its absorption.
Driving, Hazardous Activities: May cause dizziness or impaired vision. Restrict your activities as necessary.
Exposure to Sun: Sunglasses are advised if eyes are overly sensitive to bright light.
Discontinuation: If you experience no adverse effects from this drug, take the full course prescribed for maximal results. See your doctor regarding stopping treatment.

▷ **Saving Money When Using This Medicine:**
- Many new drugs are available to treat infections. Ask your doctor if this medicine offers the best balance of cost and outcome for you.
- Talk with your doctor to make sure that the power of this antibiotic matches the severity of your infection.

- The dose MUST be decreased for people with compromised kidneys. Ask your doctor if your dose has been decreased appropriately.

NORTRIPTYLINE   (nor TRIP ti leen)

Prescription Needed: Yes   **Controlled Drug:** No   **Generic:** No

Brand Names: Aventyl, Pamelor

Overview of BENEFITS versus RISKS	
Possible Benefits	*Possible Risks*
EFFECTIVE RELIEF OF ENDOGENOUS DEPRESSION	ADVERSE BEHAVIORAL EFFECTS: confusion, disorientation, hallucinations, delusions
May help other depressive disorders	CONVERSION OF DEPRESSION TO MANIA in manic-depressive disorders
May help some types of chronic, severe pain	Aggravation of schizophrenia
	Irregular heart rhythms
	Blood cell abnormalities (rare)

▷ **Illness This Medication Treats:**
  (1) Symptoms associated with spontaneous (endogenous) depression. Use only when a true primary depression of significant degree has been diagnosed. This drug should not be used to treat mild or transient (reactive) depression associated with many life situations. (2) Also used in conjunction with other drugs to manage chronic, severe pain associated with such conditions as cancer, migraine headache, severe arthritis, peripheral neuropathy, AIDS, etc.

▷ **Typical Dosage Range:** (Dosage or schedule must be determined by the doctor for each individual.)
  Initially 25 mg three or four times daily. Dose may be increased cautiously as needed and tolerated, by 10 to 25 mg daily at intervals of 1 week. Usual maintenance dose is 50 to 100 mg every 24 hours. Total dose should not exceed 150 mg/24 hr. When the optimal requirement is determined, it may be taken at bedtime as one dose.

▷ **Conditions Requiring Dosing Adjustments:**
  Liver function: This drug is metabolized in the liver, and the metabolites are subsequently eliminated via the urine and bile. Specific dosage adjustments for patients with liver compromise are not defined; however, the patient should be closely followed and levels ob-

tained. A rare cause of hepatoxicity, it should be used with caution by patients with compromised livers.

Kidney function: Specific dosing changes for patients with renal compromise are not usually needed. Nortriptyline can cause decreased urine outflow; its use by patients with urine outflow problems requires a benefit-to-risk decision.

▷ **How Best to Take This Medicine:** May be taken without regard to meals. The capsule may be opened for administration.

▷ **How Long This Medicine Is Usually Taken:** Some benefit may be apparent within 1 to 2 weeks, but adequate response may require continual use for 3 months or longer. Long-term use should not exceed 6 months without evaluation regarding the need for continuation. See your doctor regularly.

▷ **Tell Your Doctor Before Taking This Medicine If You:**
- ever had an allergic reaction to it.
- are taking or have taken within the past 14 days any MAO type A inhibitor.
- are recovering from a recent heart attack.
- have narrow-angle glaucoma.
- are allergic or sensitive to any other tricyclic antidepressant.
- have a history of diabetes, epilepsy, glaucoma, heart disease, prostate gland enlargement, or overactive thyroid function.
- plan to have surgery under general anesthesia soon.

▷ **Possible Side Effects:** Light-headedness, drowsiness, blurred vision, dry mouth, constipation, impaired urination.

▷ **Possible Adverse Effects:**
If any of the following develop, call your doctor promptly for guidance.
Some Mild Problems Drug Can Cause
> Allergic reactions: skin rash, hives, swelling of face or tongue, drug fever.
> Headache, dizziness, weakness, fainting, tremors.
> Peculiar taste, irritation of tongue or mouth, nausea, indigestion.
> Fluctuation of blood sugar levels.

Some Serious Problems Drug Can Cause
> Allergic reactions: hepatitis, with or without jaundice.
> Confusion, disorientation, hallucinations, delusions.
> Aggravation of paranoid psychoses and schizophrenia; seizures.
> Heart palpitation and irregular rhythm.
> Bone marrow depression—fatigue, fever, abnormal bleeding or bruising.
> Rare porphyria.
> Peripheral neuritis—numbness, tingling, pain.

Parkinson-like disorders—usually mild and infrequent; more likely to occur in the elderly.

▷ **Possible Effects on Sex Life:** Decreased libido, increased libido (antidepressant effect), male impotence, inhibited female orgasm, male and female breast enlargement, milk production, swelling of testicles.

▷ *CAUTION*

1. Dosage must be adjusted for each person individually. Report for follow-up evaluation and laboratory tests as directed by your doctor.
2. Withhold this drug if electroconvulsive therapy is to be used for your depression.
3. Safety and effectiveness of this drug for children have not been established.
4. This drug is not indicated for those over 60 years old. The usual dose is 30 to 50 mg daily in divided doses. During the first 2 weeks of treatment, observe for the development of confusion, agitation, forgetfulness, disorientation, delusions, and hallucinations. Reduction of dosage or discontinuation may be necessary. Unsteadiness may predispose to falling and injury. This drug can increase the degree of impaired urination associated with prostate gland enlargement.

Advisability of Use During Pregnancy or If Breast-Feeding:
Pregnancy Category: D. Avoid use of this drug during first 3 months. Use during last 6 months only if clearly needed. Ask your doctor for guidance. Present in breast milk in small amounts. Monitor the nursing infant closely and discontinue this drug or nursing if adverse effects develop: excessive drowsiness and failure to feed.

▷ **Habit-Forming Potential:** Psychological or physical dependence is rare and unexpected.

▷ **Overdose Symptoms:** Confusion, hallucinations, marked drowsiness, heart palpitations, dilated pupils, tremors, stupor, deep sleep, coma, convulsions.

▷ **Suggested Periodic Examinations While Taking This Drug:** (at doctor's discretion)
Complete blood cell counts, liver function tests, serial blood pressure readings and electrocardiograms.

▷ **While Taking This Drug the Following Apply:**
Foods: This drug may increase the appetite and cause excessive weight gain.
Beverages: May be taken with milk.
Alcohol: Avoid completely. This drug can markedly increase the intox-

icating effects of alcohol and accentuate its depressant action on brain function.

Tobacco Smoking: May hasten the elimination of this drug. Higher doses may be necessary.

Other Drugs:

Nortriptyline may *increase* the effects of

- atropinelike drugs.
- dicumarol, increasing the risk of bleeding.
- epinephrine (Adrenalin).
- phenytoin (Dilantin).
- warfarin (Coumadin) and require more frequent INR (prothrombin time) testing with doses adjusted to laboratory results.

Nortriptyline may *decrease* the effects of

- clonidine (Catapres).
- ephedrine (Primatene tablets).
- guanethidine (Ismelin).

Nortriptyline *taken concurrently* with

- activated charcoal will decrease and almost block its absorption.
- benzodiazepines (see Drug Classes) may result in additive sedation.
- disulfiram (Antabuse) may cause acute dementia: confusion, disorientation, hallucinations.
- MAO inhibitor drugs may cause high fever, delirium, and convulsions.
- thyroid preparations may impair heart rhythm and function. Ask your doctor for guidance regarding adjustment of the thyroid dose.
- fluconazole (Diflucan) may result in large increases in nortriptyline levels and cause toxic reactions.
- lithium (Lithobid, others) may pose an increased neurotoxicity risk in elderly patients.
- nifedipine (Adalat, others) may inhibit nortriptyline's antidepressant effects.
- norepinephrine can cause serious increases in blood pressure, abnormal heart rhythm and function. AVOID COMBINING.
- phenothiazines (see Drug Classes) can result in increased phenothiazine levels and toxicity.
- venlafaxine (Effexor) can lead to nortriptyline or venlafaxine toxicity.

The following drugs may *increase* the effects of nortriptyline

- cimetidine (Tagamet)—can cause nortriptyline toxicity.
- fluoxetine (Prozac).
- quinidine (Quinaglute, etc.)—can cause nortriptyline toxicity.
- sertraline (Zoloft).

The following drugs may *decrease* the effects of nortriptyline

- ascorbic acid (Vitamin C) in high doses.
- barbiturates—can reduce its effectiveness.

- carbamazepine (Tegretol).
- conjugated estrogens.
- rifampin (Rifadin).

Driving, Hazardous Activities: May impair mental alertness, judgment, physical coordination, and reaction time. Avoid hazardous activities.

Exposure to Sun: Use caution—this drug may cause photosensitivity.

Exposure to Heat: This drug can inhibit sweating and impair the body's adaptation to hot environments, increasing the risk of heatstroke. Avoid saunas.

Exposure to Cold: The elderly should use caution and avoid conditions conducive to hypothermia.

Discontinuation: It is advisable to discontinue this drug gradually. Abrupt withdrawal after long-term use can cause headache, malaise, and nausea.

▷ **Saving Money When Using This Medicine:**
- Many new drugs are available to treat depression. Ask your doctor if this medicine offers the best balance of cost and outcome for you.
- Once therapy is started and a reasonable time has passed, talk with your doctor if your results are not as good as expected. Sometimes several agents must be tried in helping depression before the best medicine is found.
- Depression has recently been found to be associated with increased risk of osteoporosis. Talk with your doctor about exercise, calcium supplements, and need for bone mineral density testing based on risk factors.

OFLOXACIN (oh FLOX a sin)

Prescription Needed: Yes   **Controlled Drug:** No   **Generic:** No

Brand Names: Floxin, Floxin Uropak, Ocuflox

▷ **Warning:** This drug may rarely cause tendon rupture. If it is prescribed for you, ask if you should limit exercise or exertion during therapy. Call your doctor immediately if pain or inflammation appears while you are taking this medicine. This medicine has also been associated with a very rare idiosyncratic reaction that includes confusion, disorientation, and other changes in mental status. Call your doctor at once if you develop changes in your ability to think while taking this medicine.

Overview of BENEFITS versus RISKS

Possible Benefits	*Possible Risks*
HIGHLY EFFECTIVE TREATMENT FOR INFECTIONS OF THE LOWER RESPIRATORY TRACT, URINARY TRACT, SKIN AND SKIN STRUCTURES, due to susceptible organisms	Rare but serious allergic reactions
	Rare seizures or disorientation or hallucinations
EFFECTIVE TREATMENT FOR SOME SEXUALLY TRANSMITTED DISEASES	Rare tendon rupture
Effective treatment for some infections of the prostate gland	

▷ **Illness This Medication Treats:**

Adult infections in (1) the lower respiratory tract (lungs and bronchial tubes); (2) the urinary tract (kidneys, bladder, urethra, and prostate gland); (3) skin and related tissues. (4) Certain sexually transmitted diseases: gonorrheal and chlamydial infections of the urethra and cervix; (5) eye infections.

▷ **Typical Dosage Range:** (Dosage or schedule must be determined by the doctor for each individual.)

Oral form: 200 to 400 mg every 12 hours, depending upon the nature and severity of the infection. The total daily dosage should not exceed 800 mg.

▷ **Conditions Requiring Dosing Adjustments:**

Liver function: Dosage adjustments do not appear to be needed for patients with liver compromise. A rare cause of hepatoxicity, this drug should be used with caution by patients with compromised livers.

Kidney function. For patients with mild to moderate kidney failure, the usual dose can be given every 12 hours. For patients with moderate to severe kidney failure, the usual dose can be given every 24 hours. For patients with severe kidney failure, half the usual dose should be given every 24 hours.

▷ **How Best to Take This Medicine:** Do not take with food. Best taken 1 hour before or 2 hours after eating. Drink fluids liberally during the entire course of treatment. Avoid antacids containing aluminum or magnesium and supplements containing iron or zinc for 2 hours before and after dosing. The tablet may be crushed for administration.

▷ **How Long This Medicine Is Usually Taken:**   Use on a regular schedule for up to 10 days is usually necessary to determine the effectiveness of this drug in eradicating the infection. The drug should be continued for at least 2 days after all indications of infection have disappeared. Prostate infections may require continual treatment for 6 weeks. Long-term use requires periodic physician evaluation of response and dosage adjustment.

▷ **Tell Your Doctor Before Taking This Medicine If You:**
- ever had an allergic reaction to it.
- are pregnant or breast-feeding.
- have a seizure disorder that is not adequately controlled or a history of a seizure disorder or a circulatory disorder of the brain.
- are given a prescription for a person under 18 years old.
- are allergic to cinoxacin (Cinobac), nalidixic acid (NegGram), ciprofloxacin (Cipro), or norfloxacin (Noroxin).
- have impaired liver or kidney function.
- have a job involving heavy manual labor.
- are taking any form of probenecid or theophylline.

▷ **Possible Side Effects:**   Superinfections: vaginitis.

▷ **Possible Adverse Effects:**
If any of the following develop, call your doctor promptly for guidance.
Some Mild Problems Drug Can Cause
Allergic reactions: rash, itching, fever.
Headache, dizziness, drowsiness, nervousness, insomnia, visual disturbances.
Altered taste, dry mouth, nausea, vomiting, diarrhea.
Some Serious Problems Drug Can Cause
Allergic reactions: anaphylactic reactions.
Idiosyncratic reactions: rare extreme confusion, speech problems (aphasia), and other mental status changes.
Central nervous system stimulation: restlessness, tremor, confusion, hallucinations, seizures (all rare).
Rare tendon rupture with heavy exertion.
Rare drug-induced hepatitis.

▷ **Possible Effects on Sex Life:**   Painful menstruation, excessive menstrual bleeding.

▷ *CAUTION*
1. With high doses or prolonged use of other drugs of this class, crystals may form in the kidney. This can be prevented by drinking copious amounts of water, up to 2 qt/24 hr.
2. Drugs of this class may decrease the formation of saliva and pre-

dispose to dental cavities or gum disease. See your dentist if dry mouth persists.

3. This drug should NOT BE USED by those under 18 years old. This drug may impair normal cartilage and bone development.

4. Impaired kidney function in those over 60 may require dosage reduction. If you are taking theophylline concurrently with this drug, the dose must be decreased. Watch for early signs of possible theophylline accumulation and toxicity.

Advisability of Use During Pregnancy or If Breast-Feeding:

Pregnancy Category: C. The potential for adverse effects on fetal bone development contraindicates the use of this drug during entire pregnancy. Present in breast milk; avoid taking this drug or refrain from nursing.

▷ **Overdose Symptoms:** Nausea, vomiting, and diarrhea. Confusion and seizures.

▷ **Suggested Periodic Examinations While Taking This Drug:** (at doctor's discretion)

Liver function tests, urine analysis.

▷ **While Taking This Drug the Following Apply:**

Beverages: Caffeine from any beverage may stay in the body longer than expected. Take care to limit caffeine intake while using this medicine. This drug may be taken with milk.

Other Drugs:

Ofloxacin may ***increase*** the effects of

• theophylline, causing theophylline toxicity.

• warfarin (Coumadin) may lead to bleeding. More frequent INR (prothrombin time) testing is needed with dosing adjusted to laboratory results.

The following drug may ***increase*** the effects of ofloxacin

• probenecid (Benemid)

The following drugs may ***decrease*** the effects of ofloxacin

• antacids containing aluminum or magnesium—can reduce the absorption of ofloxacin and lessen its effectiveness.

• calcium supplements.

• iron compounds—can decrease the absorption of ofloxacin.

• sucralfate (Carafate)—can decrease ofloxacin absorption.

• zinc salts.

Driving, Hazardous Activities: May cause drowsiness, dizziness, and impaired vision. Restrict your activities as necessary.

Exposure to Sun: This drug may rarely cause photosensitivity. Sunglasses are advised if your eyes are overly sensitive to bright light.

Discontinuation: If you experience no adverse effects from this drug, take the full course prescribed for maximal results. Ask your doctor about stopping treatment.

▷ **Saving Money When Using This Medicine:**
 • Many new drugs as well as several quinolones are available to treat infections. Ask your doctor if this medicine offers the best balance of cost and outcome for you.

OLANZAPINE (oh LAN za peen)

Prescription Needed: Yes   **Controlled Drug:** No   **Generic:** No

Brand Name: Zyprexa

Overview of BENEFITS versus RISKS	
Possible Benefits	*Possible Risks*
BENEFICIAL EFFECTS ON MOOD, THINKING, AND BEHAVIOR IN PSYCHOSIS	Possible increased liver enzymes
DIFFERENT SITES OF ACTION IN THE BRAIN THAN OTHER AGENTS	Very rare orthostatic hypotension
MUCH IMPROVED SIDE-EFFECT PROFILE VERSUS OTHER AGENTS	Very rare neuroleptic malignant syndrome
SIGNIFICANTLY DECREASED RISK OF PARKINSON-LIKE PROBLEMS	
DOES NOT APPEAR TO INCREASE PROLACTIN LEVELS	

▷ **Illness This Medication Treats:**
 Uses currently included in FDA labeling: used to treat sudden schizophrenia or severe worsening of long-standing schizophrenia. Clinical trials lasted 6 weeks. Longer-term use must be reevaluated by the physician on a patient-by-patient basis.

▷ **Typical Dosage Range:** (Dosage or schedule must be determined by the doctor for each individual.)
 18 to 65 Years of Age: Dosing is started with 5 mg with a goal of 10 mg daily, to be achieved in several days. Doses above 10 mg daily have not been demonstrated to be more effective than the 10-mg dose. Safety of doses above 20 mg daily has not been evaluated in clinical trials.
 Over 65 Years of Age: Careful adjustment with lower starting doses and slow increases are recommended, although specific large-scale data

are not available. One small study found the half-life to be 1.5 times longer in those over 65.

▷ **Conditions Requiring Dosing Adjustments:**

Liver function: This medicine is mostly removed from the body by the liver. Caution is advised, and lower doses appear prudent.

Kidney function: Does not appear to be an issue with this medicine, but specific studies have not been done.

▷ **How Best to Take This Medicine:**   Olanzapine may be taken without regard to food.

▷ **How Long This Medicine Is Usually Taken:**   Regular use for at least one week is needed to determine how well this medicine will help psychosis. Clinical trials which lead to approval lasted six weeks. Use for longer than six weeks was not studied in clinical trials and very clearly requires a benefit to risk decision by your doctor.

▷ **Tell Your Doctor Before Taking This Medicine If You:**
- ever had an allergic reaction to it.
- have a severely damaged liver.
- have had neuroleptic malignant syndrome in the past.
- have a history of heart disease, cerebrovascular disease, low blood pressure, or are dehydrated.
- have a history of seizures.
- are pregnant.

▷ **Possible Side Effects:**   Sudden lowering of blood pressure on standing (orthostatic hypotension) has been reported, with a small number of patients passing out (syncope) in early studies. Weight gain

▷ **Possible Adverse Effects:**

If any of the following develop, call your doctor promptly for guidance.

Some Mild Problems This Drug Can Cause
  Allergic reactions: hives, itching, rash.
  Somnolence, dizziness.
  Change in ability to regulate body temperature.
  Increased salivation or nausea.
  Dysphagia, constipation.
Some Serious Problems This Drug Can Cause
  Allergic reactions: not reported as yet.
  Possible tardive dyskinesia.
  Possible increased liver enzymes.
  Rare seizures.
  Movement disorders.
  Very rare neuroleptic malignant syndrome (reported with other antipsychotic medicines).

▷ **Possible Effects on Sex Life:**   Rare priapism.

▷ *CAUTION*

1. Smokers remove this drug 40% faster than nonsmokers, and dosing adjustments may be needed.
2. Safety and effectiveness of this drug in those less than 18 years old have not been established.
3. This drug should be used with caution and started at lower initial doses by those over 65. Dose is slowly increased if needed.
4. Women remove this medicine roughly 30% more slowly than men.
5. Patients who are at risk for aspiration pneumonia may have this risk increased if they take this medicine.
6. This drug may worsen prostate problems.

Advisability of Use During Pregnancy or If Breast-Feeding:

Pregnancy Category: C. Adequate trials of use of this drug in pregnant women have NOT been conducted. Discuss the use of this drug in pregnancy with your doctor as a benefit-to-risk decision. Present in breast milk in animals, unknown in humans; avoid taking this drug or refrain from nursing.

▷ **Overdose Symptoms:**   Supportive treatment for possible: low blood pressure and circulatory collapse, heart arrhythmias, seizures, and obtundation.

▷ **Suggested Periodic Examinations While Taking This Drug:** (at doctor's discretion)

Periodic checks of liver enzymes, complete blood counts.

▷ **While Taking This Drug the Following Apply:**

Alcohol: Alcohol should be avoided while taking this medicine.

Tobacco Smoking: Smoking causes this medicine to be removed from the body 40% faster than in nonsmokers.

Other Drugs:

Olanzapine *taken concurrently* with

- activated charcoal will decrease absorption of olanzapine (may be useful in overdose situations).
- antihypertensives (high blood pressure medicines) may increase their blood pressure–lowering effect.
- carbamazepine (Tegretol) increases the removal of olanzapine from the body by 50%.
- calcium channel blockers (see Drug Classes) may excessively lower blood sugar.
- fluvoxamine (Luvox) may (not yet demonstrated) increase olanzapine blood levels and lead to toxicity.
- levodopa or dopamine agonists may block the therapeutic effects of these agents.

- narcotic analgesics or other medicines (such as benzodiazepines) that have central nervous system effects may be increased.

Driving, Hazardous Activities: Caution: this medicine may cause drowsiness. Use caution until you know the degree of this effect on you.

Exposure to Heat: Caution: this medicine can alter the ability of the body to regulate temperature.

▷ **Saving Money When Using This Medicine:**
- Talk with your doctor to make sure that this medicine offers you the best balance of cost and outcomes.

OLSALAZINE (ohl SAL a zeen)

Prescription Needed: Yes   **Controlled Drug:** No   **Generic:** No

Brand Name: Dipentum

Overview of BENEFITS versus RISKS	
Possible Benefits	*Possible Risks*
EFFECTIVE SUPPRESSION OF INFLAMMATORY BOWEL DISEASE	BONE MARROW DEPRESSION (rare) Drug-induced hepatitis (rare) Occasional aggravation of ulcerative colitis

▷ **Illness This Medication Treats:**
Maintains remission of chronic ulcerative colitis and proctitis.

▷ **Typical Dosage Range:** (Dosage or schedule must be determined by the doctor for each individual.)
Infants and Children. Dosage not established.
12 to 60 Years of Age: 500 mg twice daily, morning and evening.
Over 60 Years of Age: Same as for 12 to 60 years of age.

▷ **Conditions Requiring Dosing Adjustments:**
Liver function: Dosage adjustments do not appear to be needed for patients with liver compromise. This drug is also a rare cause of hepatoxicity (granulomatous hepatitis), and should be used with caution by patients with compromised livers.
Kidney function: With its potential for kidney damage, use of this drug by patients with compromised kidneys requires a benefit-to-risk decision.

▷ **How Best to Take This Medicine:** Take with food, preferably with breakfast and dinner. The capsule may be opened for administration.

▷ **How Long This Medicine Is Usually Taken:** Regularly scheduled use for 1 to 3 weeks usually determines the effectiveness of this drug in controlling the symptoms of ulcerative colitis. Long-term use (months to years) requires physician supervision.

▷ **Tell Your Doctor Before Taking This Medicine If You:**
- ever had an allergic reaction to it.
- have severely impaired kidney function.
- are allergic to aspirin (or other salicylates), mesalamine, or sulfasalazine.
- are allergic by nature: history of hay fever, asthma, hives, eczema.
- have impaired kidney function.
- are currently taking sulfasalazine (Azulfidine).

▷ **Possible Adverse Effects:**
If any of the following develop, call your doctor promptly for guidance.
Some Mild Problems Drug Can Cause
Allergic reactions: skin rash, itching.
Headache, drowsiness, depression, dizziness, rare blurred vision, or paresthesias.
Nausea, vomiting, diarrhea.
Joint aches and pains.
Some Serious Problems Drug Can Cause
Allergic reactions: dermatitis, hair loss (rare).
Rare bone marrow depression: weakness, fever, sore throat, abnormal bleeding or bruising.
Rare drug-induced hepatitis.
Rare pancreatitis or pericarditis.
Rare kidney damage.
Rare spasm of the bronchi.

▷ **Possible Effects on Sex Life:** Rare impotence, excessive menstrual flow.

▷ *CAUTION*
1. Report promptly any early indications of infection or unusual bleeding or bruising.
2. Report promptly any indications of active or intensified ulcerative colitis: abdominal cramping, bloody diarrhea, fever.
3. Safety and effectiveness of this drug for those under 12 years old have not been established.

Advisability of Use During Pregnancy or If Breast-Feeding:
Pregnancy Category: C. Use this drug only if clearly needed. Ask your doctor for guidance. Presence in breast milk is unknown; avoid taking this drug or refrain from nursing.

▷ **Overdose Symptoms:** Headache, dizziness, nausea, vomiting, abdominal cramping.

▷ **Suggested Periodic Examinations While Taking This Drug:** (at doctor's discretion)

Complete blood cell counts.

Liver function tests.

Kidney function tests, urinalysis.

▷ **While Taking This Drug the Following Apply:**

Foods: Follow prescribed diet.

Beverages: May be taken with milk.

Other Drugs:

Olsalazine *taken concurrently* with

- varicella vaccine (Varivax) may increase risk of Reye's syndrome. Olsalazine should be avoided for 6 weeks after the vaccine has been given.

Driving, Hazardous Activities: May cause drowsiness or dizziness. Restrict your activities as necessary.

Exposure to Sun: Use caution until its full effect has been determined. This drug can cause photosensitization.

▷ **Saving Money When Using This Medicine:**

- Several drugs are available to treat inflammatory bowel disease. Ask your doctor if this medicine offers the best balance of cost and outcome for you.

OMEPRAZOLE   (oh ME pra zohl)

Prescription Needed: Yes   **Controlled Drug:**   No   **Generic:** No

Brand Name: Prilosec (formerly Losec)

Overview of BENEFITS versus RISKS

Possible Benefits	*Possible Risks*
VERY EFFECTIVE TREATMENT OF CONDITIONS ASSOCIATED WITH EXCESSIVE PRODUCTION OF GASTRIC ACID: Zollinger-Ellison syndrome, mastocytosis, endocrine adenoma	Rare aplastic anemia Rare liver failure
VERY EFFECTIVE TREATMENT OF REFLUX ESOPHAGITIS	
VERY EFFECTIVE TREATMENT OF GASTRIC AND DUODENAL ULCERS	
TREATMENT OF *HELICOBACTER PYLORI* INFECTIONS	

▷ **Illness This Medication Treats:**
(1) Secretion of stomach acid, inhibiting excessive stomach acid associated with: acute and chronic gastritis, reflux esophagitis, Zollinger-Ellison syndrome, mastocytosis, endocrine adenomas, active gastric and duodenal ulcer; (2) also used in combination with clarithromycin (Biaxin) for refractory duodenal ulcers where the bacteria *Helicobacter pylori* has been cultured.

▷ **Typical Dosage Range:** (Dosage or schedule must be determined by the doctor for each individual.)
Reflux esophagitis: 20 to 40 mg once daily for 4 to 8 weeks.
Excessive stomach acid conditions: 60 mg once daily for as long as necessary.
Gastric and duodenal ulcer: 20 mg once daily for 4 to 8 weeks.
In extreme conditions, doses of 120 mg daily, in divided doses, have been used.

▷ **Conditions Requiring Dosing Adjustments:**
Liver function: Dosage adjustments are not defined; however, patients should be watched carefully for adverse effects. This drug is a rare

cause of liver toxicity, and should be used with caution by patients with compromised livers.

▷ **How Best to Take This Medicine:** Take immediately before eating, preferably the morning meal. The capsule should be swallowed whole without opening; the contents should not be crushed or chewed. This drug may be taken concurrently with antacids if needed to relieve stomach pain.

▷ **How Long This Medicine Is Usually Taken:** Continual use on a regular schedule for 2 to 3 weeks is usually necessary to determine the effectiveness of this drug in suppressing stomach acid production. Long-term use (months) requires periodic physician evaluation.

▷ **Tell Your Doctor Before Taking This Medicine If You:**
- ever had an allergic reaction to it.
- have a currently active bone marrow or blood cell disorder or a history of such disorders, especially one that is drug-induced.
- have a history of liver disease or impaired liver function.
- are currently taking any anticoagulant, diazepam (Valium), or phenytoin (Dilantin, etc.).

▷ **Possible Side Effects:** May increase chances of *Campylobacter* infection. Call your doctor if you start to have frequent mucousy stools and a fever.

▷ **Possible Adverse Effects:**
If any of the following develop, call your doctor promptly for guidance.
Some Mild Problems Drug Can Cause
  Allergic reactions: skin rash, itching.
  Headache, dizziness, drowsiness.
  Indigestion, nausea, vomiting, diarrhea, constipation.
Some Serious Problems Drug Can Cause
  Rare bone marrow depression: weakness, fever, sore throat, infections, abnormal bleeding or bruising.
  Rare liver damage with jaundice.
  Rare urinary tract infection: painful urination, cloudy or bloody urine.
  Rare kidney inflammation (interstitial nephritis).
  Rare half-facial pain.

▷ **Possible Effects on Sex Life:** Drug-induced male breast enlargement and tenderness (gynecomastia) has been rarely reported.

▷ **Adverse Effects That May Mimic Natural Diseases or Disorders:**
Persistent infection or bruising may reflect bone marrow depression; blood counts are advisable.
Liver reactions suggest viral hepatitis.

▷ **CAUTION**

1. Follow your doctor's instructions exactly regarding the length of time you take this drug. Do not extend its use without his or her guidance.
2. Report promptly any indications of infection.
3. Tell your doctor if you plan to take any other medications (prescription or over-the-counter) while taking omeprazole.
4. If acid in the stomach is decreased, the risk that a *Campylobacter* infection may occur is increased. Call your doctor if you start to have frequent loose stools and a fever.
5. Safety and effectiveness of this drug for those under 12 years old have not been established.
6. Slower elimination of this drug by those over 60 makes a satisfactory response possible with smaller doses; this reduces the risk of adverse effects. Limit the daily dose to 20 mg if possible.

Advisability of Use During Pregnancy or If Breast-Feeding:

Pregnancy Category: C. Avoid using this drug if possible. Use only if clearly necessary and for the shortest possible time. Presence in breast milk is unknown; avoid taking this drug or refrain from nursing.

▷ **Overdose Symptoms:**   Possible drowsiness, dizziness, lethargy, abdominal pain, nausea.

▷ **While Taking This Drug the Following Apply:**

Beverages: May be taken with milk.

Alcohol: Alcohol is best avoided as it stimulates the secretion of stomach acid.

Tobacco Smoking: No interactions expected. However, smoking is best avoided; it may stimulate the secretion of stomach acid.

Other Drugs:

Omeprazole may *increase* the effects of

- anticoagulants (warfarin, etc.), increasing the risk of bleeding.
- clonazepam (Klonopin) and perhaps some other benzodiazepines (see Drug Classes), leading to benzodiazepine toxicity.
- cyclosporine (Sandimmune) by increasing blood levels; however, decreased levels have also been reported.
- diazepam (Valium), causing excessive sedation.
- digoxin (Lanoxin) and lead to toxicity.
- phenytoin (Dilantin, etc.), causing phenytoin toxicity.
- warfarin (Coumadin), requiring more frequent INR (prothrombin time) testing and adjustment of dosing to laboratory results.

Omeprazole may *decrease* the effects of

- ampicillin.
- amoxacillin.

- iron preparations.
- ketoconazole (Nizoral).

Driving, Hazardous Activities: May cause drowsiness and dizziness. Restrict your activities as necessary.

Discontinuation: Follow your doctor's instructions. The duration of use varies according to the condition under treatment and individual patient response. Premature discontinuation could result in incomplete healing or prompt recurrence of symptoms.

▷ **Saving Money When Using This Medicine:**
- Many new drugs are available to treat ulcer disease. Ask your doctor if this medicine offers the best balance of cost and outcome for you.
- Some recent data show that the use of omeprazole in combination with clarithromycin offers better outcomes than traditional therapy in patients with *Helicobacter-pylori*–associated ulcers.

ONDANSETRON (on DAN sa tron)

Prescription Needed: Yes   **Controlled Drug:** No   **Generic:** No

Brand Name: Zofran

Overview of BENEFITS versus RISKS	
Possible Benefits	*Possible Risks*
EFFECTIVE ORAL TREATMENT AND RELIEF OR PREVENTION OF SEVERE VOMITING AFTER CHEMOTHERAPY OR RADIATION TREATMENTS	EXTRAPYRAMIDAL REACTIONS (RARE) BRONCHOSPASM (RARE) GRAND MAL SEIZURES (RARE) Rare liver failure Rare heart rate or rhythm changes

▷ **Illness This Medication Treats:**

(1) Prevents nausea and vomiting associated with chemotherapy that can cause vomiting; (2) prevents postoperative nausea or vomiting; (3) prevents nausea or vomiting after radiation therapy.

▷ **Typical Dosage Range:** (Dosage or schedule must be determined by the doctor for each individual.)

Infants and Children: Little information is available regarding the use of this drug in those less than 4 years old.

4 to 11 Years of Age: Vomiting from chemotherapy: One 4-mg tablet given three times by mouth daily. The method and frequency is the same as for adults.

12 to 60 Years of Age: One 8-mg tablet given three times a day. The first dose should be given 30 minutes before the start of the emetogenic chemotherapy. Subsequent doses should be given 4 hours and 8 hours after the first dose.

Over 60 Years of Age: Same as for 12 to 60 years of age.

▷ **Conditions Requiring Dosing Adjustments:**

Liver function: Patients with severe decreases in liver function should not take more than 8 mg/day.

▷ **How Best to Take This Medicine:**   May be taken on an empty stomach.

▷ **How Long This Medicine Is Usually Taken:**   Because chemotherapy can cause vomiting long after it has been given, continual use on a regular schedule for 3 days is usually necessary.

▷ **Tell Your Doctor Before Taking This Medicine If You:**
- ever had an allergic reaction to it.
- have chronic renal failure.
- have a history of liver disease.
- have a history of alcoholism.

▷ **Possible Side Effects:**   Constipation, sedation.

▷ **Possible Adverse Effects:**
If any of the following develop, call your doctor promptly for guidance.

Some Mild Problems Drug Can Cause
   Allergic reactions: skin rash.
   Headache, sedation, dizziness and light-headedness, constipation, diarrhea, dry mouth.

Some Serious Problems Drug Can Cause
   Allergic reactions: anaphylaxis (rare).
   Rare: extrapyramidal reactions (abnormal body movements), seizures, angina, tachycardia, bronchospasm, liver failure, hypokalemia (low potassium).

▷ **Adverse Effects That May Mimic Natural Diseases or Disorders:**
Changes in liver enzymes may mimic hepatitis; however, specific antibodies will not be present. Bronchospasm may mimic asthma.

▷ *CAUTION*
Safety and effectiveness of this drug for those under 3 years old have not been established.

Advisability of Use During Pregnancy or If Breast-Feeding:

Pregnancy Category: B. Ask your doctor for help. This drug is present in breast milk in rats, but its presence in humans is unknown. Caution should be used by nursing mothers.

▷ **Overdose Symptoms:**   Doses 10 times greater than the recommended amounts have not resulted in illness.

▷ **Suggested Periodic Examinations While Taking This Drug:** (at doctor's discretion)

Observe for vomiting occurrence and frequency.

▷ **While Taking This Drug the Following Apply:**

Alcohol: Additive sedation and potential additive urge to vomit if alcohol is taken in large quantities. Liver problems from alcohol abuse may limit the total dose which can be taken.

Marijuana Smoking: May cause additive sedation and provide additive antiemetic effects.

Other Drugs:

The following drugs may *increase* the effects of ondansetron

- allopurinol (Zyloprim).
- cimetidine (Tagamet).
- ranitidine (Zantac).
- disulfiram (Antabuse).
- fluconazole (Diflucan).
- isoniazid (Nydrazid).
- macrolide antibiotics (erythromycin, azithromycin, and clarithromycin).
- metronidazole (Flagyl).
- monoamine oxidase inhibitor (MAOI) antidepressants (Nardil).

The following drugs may *decrease* the effects of ondansetron

- barbiturates.
- carbamazepine (Tegretol).
- phenylbutazone (Butazolidin, Azolid).
- phenytoin (Dilantin).
- rifampin (Rifadin) and rifabutin (Mycobutin).
- tolbutamide (Orinase).

Driving, Hazardous Activities: May cause drowsiness and dizziness. Restrict your activities as necessary.

Storage Instructions: Keep at room temperature. Avoid exposing this drug to extreme humidity.

Discontinuation: Take this medication exactly as your doctor has instructed. Ondansetron may be stopped after you've completed the prescribed course (usually 3 days) of therapy.

▷ **Saving Money When Using This Medicine:**

- Many new drugs are available to stop vomiting. Ask your doctor if this medicine offers the best balance of cost and outcome for you. Know when it is acceptable to stop this drug. It is very expensive, and the exact amount should be purchased.

ORAL CONTRACEPTIVES   (or al kon tra SEP tivs)

Other Names: Estrogens/progestins, BCPs, OCs

Prescription Needed: Yes   **Controlled Drug:** No   **Generic:**
No

Brand Names: Brevicon, Demulen, Enovid, Levlen, Loestrin, Lo/
Ovral, Micronor (progestin-only mini-pill), Modicon, Nelova,
Nelova 1/50M, Nelova 10/11, Norcept-E 1/35, Nordette, Norethin
1/35E, Norethin 1/50M, Norinyl, Norlestrin, Nor-QD (progestin-
only mini-pill), Ortho-Cyclen, Ortho-Novum, Ovcon, Ovral, Ovrette
(progestin-only mini-pill), Tri-Levlon, Tri-Norinyl, Triphasil

Overview of BENEFITS versus RISKS	
Possible Benefits	*Possible Risks*
HIGHLY EFFECTIVE FOR CONTRACEPTIVE PROTECTION	SERIOUS, LIFE-THREATENING THROMBOEMBOLIC DISORDERS in susceptible individuals
Moderately effective as adjunctive treatment in managing excessive menses and endometriosis	Hypertension
	Fluid retention
	Intensification of migrainelike headaches
	Intensification of fibrocystic breast changes
	Accelerated growth of uterine fibroid tumors
	Drug-induced hepatitis with jaundice
	Benign liver tumors (rare)

▷ **Illness This Medication Treats:**

(1) Prevention of unwanted pregnancy; (2) the mini-pill contains only
one component—a progestin—which is slightly less effective than
the combination of estrogen and progestin in preventing pregnancy;
(3) used in women who do not make enough hormones (female hy-
pogonadism); (4) eases excessive blood flow of menstruation;
(5) one combination (mestranol and norethynodrel) may be useful
in endometriosis.

As Combination Drug Product [CD]: Most oral contraceptives consist
of a combination of estrogen and progestin. These are the most effective form of contraception available. Used primarily to prevent
pregnancy, they are sometimes used to treat menstrual irregularity,
excessively heavy menstrual flow, and endometriosis.

▷ **Typical Dosage Range:** (Dosage or schedule must be determined by the doctor for each individual.)

Start with the first tablet on the fifth day after the onset of menstruation. Follow with one tablet daily (taken at the same time each day) for 21 consecutive days. Resume treatment on the eighth day following the last tablet taken during the preceding cycle. The schedule is to take the drug daily for 3 weeks and omit it for 1 week. For the mini-pill (progestin only): Initiate treatment on the first day of menstruation and take one tablet daily, throughout the year (no interruption).

▷ **Conditions Requiring Dosing Adjustments:**

Liver function: This drug should NOT be taken if you have liver disease.

▷ **How Best to Take This Medicine:** May be taken with or after food to reduce stomach irritation. To ensure regular (daily) use and uniform blood levels, it is advisable to take the tablet at the same time daily. The tablets may be crushed.

▷ **How Long This Medicine Is Usually Taken:** Varies according to individual needs and circumstances. Long-term use (months to years) requires supervision and periodic evaluation by your doctor every 6 months.

▷ **Tell Your Doctor Before Taking This Medicine If You:**
- ever had an allergic reaction to it or any other oral contraceptive.
- have a history of thrombophlebitis, embolism, heart attack, or stroke.
- have breast cancer or a history of it or cancer of the reproductive organs.
- have active liver disease, seriously impaired liver function, or a history of liver tumor.
- have abnormal and unexplained vaginal bleeding.
- have sickle cell disease.
- are pregnant.
- have fibrocystic breast changes, fibroid tumors of the uterus, endometriosis, migrainelike headaches, epilepsy, asthma, heart disease, high blood pressure, gallbladder disease, diabetes, or porphyria.
- smoke tobacco on a regular basis.
- plan to have surgery soon.

▷ **Possible Side Effects:** Fluid retention, weight gain, breakthrough bleeding (spotting in middle of menstrual cycle), altered menstrual pattern, lack of menstruation (during and following cessation of drug), increased susceptibility to yeast infection of the genital tissues.

▷ **Possible Adverse Effects:**

If any of the following develop, call your doctor promptly for guidance.

Some Mild Problems Drug Can Cause

Allergic reactions: skin rash, itching.

Headache, irritability, accentuation of migraine headaches.

Nausea, vomiting, bloating, diarrhea.

Tannish pigmentation of the face.

Reduced tolerance to contact lenses.

Impaired color vision: blue tinge to objects, blue halo around lights.

Some Serious Problems Drug Can Cause

Allergic reactions: erythema multiforme and nodosum (skin reactions), loss of scalp hair.

Idiosyncratic reactions: joint and muscle pains.

Emotional depression, rise in blood pressure.

Eye changes: optic neuritis, retinal thrombosis, altered curvature of the cornea, cataracts.

Gallbladder disease, benign liver tumors, jaundice, rise in blood sugar.

Erosion of uterine cervix, enlargement of uterine fibroid tumors, cystitislike syndrome.

Thrombophlebitis—pain or tenderness in thigh or leg.

Pulmonary embolism—sudden shortness of breath, pain in chest, coughing, bloody sputum.

Stroke—headaches, blackout, sudden weakness or paralysis, severe dizziness, altered vision, slurred speech, inability to speak.

Heart attack (blood clot in coronary artery)—sudden pain in chest, neck, jaw or arm; weakness; sweating; nausea.

Mesenteric thrombosis—blood clot in abdominal artery.

▷ **Possible Effects on Sex Life:**   Decreased libido.

Altered character of menstruation; midcycle spotting.

Breast enlargement and tenderness with milk production.

Absent menstruation and infertility (temporary) after discontinuation of drug.

▷ **Possible Delayed Adverse Effects:**   Estrogens taken during pregnancy can predispose the female child to later development of cancer of the vagina or cervix following puberty. Nonpregnant use DOES NOT increase breast cancer risk.

▷ **Adverse Effects That May Mimic Natural Diseases or Disorders:** Liver reactions may suggest viral hepatitis.

▷ *CAUTION*

1. The incidence of serious adverse effects of these drugs is very low. However, any unusual development should be reported and evaluated promptly.

2. Studies indicate that women over 30 years old who smoke and use

oral contraceptives are at significantly greater risk of having a serious cardiovascular event than nonusers.

3. The risk of thromboembolism increases with the amount of estrogen in the product and the age of the user. Low-estrogen combinations are advised.

4. It is best to stop these drugs 1 month prior to elective surgery, to reduce the risk of postsurgical thromboembolism.

5. Investigate promptly any alteration or disturbance of vision during the use of these drugs.

6. Investigate promptly the nature of recurrent, persistent, or severe headaches that develop while taking these drugs.

7. Observe for significant change of mood. Discontinue this drug if depression develops.

8. Certain commonly used drugs may reduce the effectiveness of oral contraceptives (some are listed under "Other Drugs," below).

9. Diarrhea lasting more than a few hours (and occurring during the days the drug is taken) can prevent adequate absorption of these drugs and impair their effectiveness.

10. If two consecutive menstrual periods are missed, ask your doctor about the advisability of performing a pregnancy test. Do not continue to use these drugs until your pregnancy status is determined.

Advisability of Use During Pregnancy or If Breast-Feeding:

Pregnancy Category: X. Estrogens taken during pregnancy can predispose the female child to the development of cancer of the vagina or cervix following puberty. ***Avoid these drugs completely during entire pregnancy.*** Present in breast milk in minute amounts. These drugs may suppress milk formation if started early following delivery. Breast-feeding is considered to be safe during the use of oral contraceptives.

▷ **Overdose Symptoms:** Headache, drowsiness, nausea, vomiting, fluid retention, abnormal vaginal bleeding, breast enlargement and discomfort.

▷ **Suggested Periodic Examinations While Taking This Drug:** (at doctor's discretion)

Regular (every 6 months) evaluation of the breasts and pelvic organs, including Pap smears. Liver function tests as indicated.

▷ **While Taking This Drug the Following Apply:**

Foods: Avoid excessive use of salt if fluid retention occurs. Ascorbic acid (vitamin C) may result in increased ethinyl estradiol levels and breakthrough bleeding if vitamin C is stopped.

Beverages: May be taken with milk.

Tobacco Smoking: Recent studies indicate that heavy smoking (15 or more cigarettes daily) in association with the use of oral contraceptives significantly increases the risk of heart attack (coronary thrombosis). Heavy smoking should be considered a contraindication.

Other Drugs:
Oral contraceptives may ***increase*** the effects of

- some benzodiazepines, causing excessive sedation.
- cyclosporine (Sandimmune) and cause toxicity.
- metoprolol (Lopressor), causing excessive beta-blocker effects.
- prednisolone and prednisone, causing excessive cortisonelike effects.
- theophyllines (Theo-Dur, others), increasing the risk of toxic effects.

Oral contraceptives ***taken concurrently*** with

- antibiotics (such as amoxicillin or ampicillin) may blunt the contraceptive's effectiveness, **and result in unwanted pregnancy**.
- antidiabetics may cause unpredictable fluctuations of blood sugar.
- tricyclic antidepressants (Elavil, Sinequan, etc.) may enhance their adverse effects and reduce their antidepressant effectiveness.
- troleandomycin (Tao) may increase the incidence of liver toxicity and jaundice.
- warfarin (Coumadin) may unpredictably alter prothrombin activity. More frequent INR (prothrombin time) testing is needed.

The following drugs may ***decrease*** the effects of oral contraceptives (and impair their effectiveness)

- barbiturates (phenobarbital, etc.).
- carbamazepine (Tegretol).
- griseofulvin (Fulvicin, etc.).
- penicillins (ampicillin, penicillin V).
- phenytoin (Dilantin).
- primidone (Mysoline).
- rifampin (Rifadin, Rimactane).
- tetracyclines.

Driving, Hazardous Activities: Ask your doctor for assessment of individual risk and guidance regarding specific restrictions.

Exposure to Sun: Use caution until full effect is known. These drugs can cause photosensitivity.

Discontinuation: If spotting or bleeding occurs, call your doctor; a pill with a higher estrogen content may be required. Remember: omitting this drug for only 1 day may allow pregnancy to occur. After discontinuing this drug, it is best to avoid pregnancy for 3 to 6 months, because of a significant likelihood of chromosome abnormalities in a fetus conceived during this time.

▷ **Saving Money When Using This Medicine:**
- Many kinds of birth control pills are available as well as an injectable form. Ask your doctor if this medicine offers the best balance of cost and outcome for you.

- If you are prescribed an antibiotic, talk with your doctor to see if it will blunt the benefits of this form of birth control and ask if you should use another method.

OXICAMS

(Nonsteroidal Anti-Inflammatory Drugs)
Piroxicam (peer OX i kam)

Prescription Needed: Yes **Controlled Drug:** No **Generic:** Yes

Brand Names: Feldene

Overview of BENEFITS versus RISKS	
Possible Benefits	*Possible Risks*
EFFECTIVE RELIEF OF MILD TO MODERATE PAIN AND INFLAMMATION	Gastrointestinal pain, ulceration, bleeding.
	Drug-induced hepatitis (rare)
	Kidney damage (rare)
	Mild fluid retention -
	Reduced white blood cell and platelet counts

▷ **Illness This Medication Treats:**

Mild to moderate pain and inflammation associated with (1) rheumatoid arthritis, (2) osteoarthritis.

Also treats terminal cancer pain in combination with doxepin.

▷ **Typical Dosage Range:** (Dosage or schedule must be determined by the doctor for each individual.)

As antiarthritic: 10 mg twice daily, 12 hours apart; or 20 mg once daily. The total daily dosage should not exceed 40 mg, and then for no more than 5 days.

▷ **Conditions Requiring Dosing Adjustments:**

Liver function: This drug should be used with caution by patients with liver compromise, and the dose should be empirically decreased.

Kidney function: This drug should be used with caution by patients with renal compromise, and kidney function should be followed closely.

▷ **How Best to Take This Medicine:** Take with or following food to prevent stomach irritation. Take with a full glass of water and remain upright (do not lie down) for 30 minutes. The capsule may be opened for administration.

▷ **How Long This Medicine Is Usually Taken:** Use on a regular schedule for 2 weeks usually determines the effectiveness of this drug in relieving the discomfort of arthritis. Long-term use (months to years) requires your doctor's supervision and periodic evaluation.

▷ **Tell Your Doctor Before Taking This Medicine If You:**
- ever had an allergic reaction to it or aspirin or aspirin substitutes.
- are subject to asthma or nasal polyps caused by aspirin.
- have active peptic ulcer disease or any form of gastrointestinal bleeding, or a history of peptic ulcer disease, regional enteritis, or ulcerative colitis.
- have a bleeding disorder, a blood cell disorder, or a history of any type of bleeding disorder.
- have active liver disease or impaired liver or kidney function.
- have high blood pressure or a history of heart failure.
- are taking acetaminophen, aspirin or aspirin substitutes, anticoagulants, or oral antidiabetic drugs.
- plan to have surgery of any type soon.

▷ **Possible Side Effects:**   Fluid retention (weight gain), prolongation of bleeding time.

▷ **Possible Adverse Effects:**
If any of the following develop, call your doctor promptly for guidance.
Some Mild Problems Drug Can Cause
Allergic reactions: skin rash, itching, spontaneous bruising.
Headache, dizziness, altered or blurred vision, ringing in the ears, drowsiness, inability to concentrate.
Nausea, vomiting, abdominal pain, diarrhea.
Some Serious Problems Drug Can Cause
Active peptic ulcer, stomach or intestinal bleeding.
Drug-induced liver damage.
Kidney damage with painful urination, bloody urine, reduced urine formation.
Rare pancreatitis.
Rare serious skin damage (toxic epidermal necrolysis or TEN).
Rare bone marrow depression: weakness, fever, sore throat, abnormal bleeding or bruising.

▷ **Possible Delayed Adverse Effects:**   Mild anemia due to "silent" blood loss from the stomach (less than that caused by aspirin).

▷ **Adverse Effects That May Mimic Natural Diseases or Disorders:**
Liver reaction may suggest viral hepatitis.

▷ *CAUTION*
1. The smallest effective dose should always be used.
2. This drug may hide early signs of infection. Tell your doctor if you think you are developing an infection.
3. Safety and effectiveness of this drug for those under 12 years old have not been established.

4. Those over 60 should take small doses until their tolerance is determined. Watch for any indications of liver or kidney toxicity, fluid retention, dizziness, confusion, impaired memory, stomach bleeding, or constipation.

Advisability of Use During Pregnancy or If Breast-Feeding:

Pregnancy Category: B. Category D in the last 3 months. The manufacturer does not recommend use of this drug during pregnancy. Present in breast milk; avoid taking this drug or refrain from nursing.

▷ **Overdose Symptoms:**   Possible drowsiness, dizziness, ringing in the ears, nausea, vomiting, indigestion.

▷ **Suggested Periodic Examinations While Taking This Drug:** (at doctor's discretion)

Complete blood cell counts, liver and kidney function tests.

Complete eye examinations if vision is altered in any way.

Hearing examinations if ringing in the ears or hearing loss develops.

▷ **While Taking This Drug the Following Apply:**

Beverages: May be taken with milk.

Alcohol: Use with caution. Both alcohol and piroxicam can irritate the stomach lining, and increase the risk of stomach ulceration and/or bleeding.

Other Drugs:

Piroxicam may ***increase*** the effects of

- acetaminophen (Tylenol, etc.), increasing the risk of kidney damage; avoid prolonged use of this combination.
- anticoagulants (Coumadin, etc.), increasing the risk of bleeding; monitor prothrombin time and adjust dose accordingly.
- lithium (Lithobid, others) may lead to lithium toxicity.
- methotrexate (Mexate) may lead to methotrexate toxicity.

Piroxicam ***taken concurrently*** with the following drugs may increase the risk of bleeding; avoid these combinations:

- aspirin.
- dipyridamole (Persantine).
- indomethacin (Indocin).
- sulfinpyrazone (Anturane).
- valproic acid (Depakene).

Driving, Hazardous Activities: May cause drowsiness or dizziness. Restrict your activities as necessary.

▷ **Saving Money When Using This Medicine:**

- Many NSAID medications are available. Ask your doctor if this medicine offers the best combination of cost and outcome for you.
- If you are at risk for ulcers, talk with your doctor about using misoprostol to help prevent them while you take this medicine.
- A generic form may be substituted for the brand name.
- Ask your doctor how long this medicine is usually taken to treat

your condition, and how soon it should be changed to another drug if it is ineffective.

- If your pain persists, talk to your doctor about visiting a chronic pain center.

OXAPROZIN (OX a proh zin)

Prescription Needed: Yes   **Controlled Drug:** No   **Generic:** No

Brand Name: Daypro

Overview of BENEFITS versus RISKS	
Possible Benefits	*Possible Risks*
EFFECTIVE RELIEF OF MILD TO MODERATE PAIN AND INFLAMMATION	Gastrointestinal pain, ulceration, and bleeding (rare)
ONCE-DAILY DOSING	Palpitations
	Sleep disturbances
	Confusion
	Kidney toxicity (rare)
	Fluid retention (rare)

See the propionic acids (NSAIDs) drug profile for further information.

OXTRIPHYLLINE (ox TRY fi lin)

Other Names: Choline theophyllinate, theophylline cholinate

Prescription Needed: Yes   **Controlled Drug:** No   **Generic:** Yes

Brand Names: Choledyl, Choledyl Delayed-Release, Choledyl SA, Choledyl Expectorant [CD]

Overview of BENEFITS versus RISKS

Possible Benefits	*Possible Risks*
EFFECTIVE PREVENTION AND RELIEF OF ACUTE BRONCHIAL ASTHMA	NARROW TREATMENT RANGE
MODERATELY EFFECTIVE CONTROL OF CHRONIC, RECURRENT BRONCHIAL ASTHMA	FREQUENT STOMACH DISTRESS
Moderately effective symptomatic relief in chronic bronchitis and emphysema	Gastrointestinal bleeding
	Central nervous system toxicity, seizures
	Heart rhythm disturbances

▷ **Illness This Medication Treats:**
(1) Shortness of breath and wheezing characteristic of acute bronchial asthma, and prevention of the recurrent asthmatic episodes; (2) also useful in relieving the asthmaticlike symptoms associated with some types of chronic bronchitis and emphysema.

As Combination Drug Product [CD]: In combination with guaifenesin this drug provides an expectorant effect that thins the mucus secretions in the bronchial tubes.

Author's note: This medicine yields 64% free theophylline, the active medicine. See the theophylline drug profile for further information.

OXYCODONE (ox ee KOH dohn)

Prescription Needed: Yes   **Controlled Drug:** C-II*   **Generic:** Yes

Brand Names: Percocet [CD], Percodan [CD], Percodan-Demi [CD], Roxicet, Roxicodone, Roxiprin [CD], SK-Oxycodone, Tylox [CD]

*See Controlled Drug Schedules inside this book's cover.

```
┌─────────────────────────────────────────────────────┐
│           Overview of BENEFITS versus RISKS          │
│   Possible Benefits            Possible Risks        │
│  EFFECTIVE RELIEF OF      POTENTIAL FOR HABIT         │
│   MODERATE TO SEVERE       FORMATION                  │
│   PAIN                     (DEPENDENCE)               │
│                           Sedative effects            │
│                           Body movement disorders if  │
│                            abruptly stopped (rare)    │
│                           Mild allergic reactions     │
│                            (infrequent)               │
│                           Nausea                      │
│                           Constipation                │
└─────────────────────────────────────────────────────┘
```

▷ **Illness This Medication Treats:**
Used to relieve moderate to severe pain.
As Combination Drug Product [CD]: Oxycodone is available in combinations with acetaminophen and aspirin. These milder pain relievers enhance the analgesic effect and reduce fever when present.

▷ **Typical Dosage Range:** (Dosage or schedule must be determined by the doctor for each individual.)
Percodan is given as one tablet (5 mg) every 6 hours. Current pain theory supports scheduled, rather than as-needed, use. The dose may be increased to 10 mg/4 hr if needed for severe pain. The total daily dosage should not exceed 60 mg.

▷ **Conditions Requiring Dosing Adjustments:**
Liver function: The liver plays a significant role in eliminating this drug. Dose should be decreased.

▷ **How Best to Take This Medicine:**   May be taken with or following food to reduce stomach irritation or nausea. The tablet may be crushed.

▷ **How Long This Medicine Is Usually Taken:**   As required to control pain. Continual use should not exceed 5 to 7 days without interruption and reassessment of need.

▷ **Tell Your Doctor Before Taking This Medicine If You:**
- ever had an allergic reaction it.
- are having an acute attack of asthma.
- had an unfavorable reaction to any narcotic drug in the past.
- have a history of drug abuse or alcoholism.
- have chronic lung disease with impaired breathing.
- have impaired liver or kidney function or have difficulty emptying the urinary bladder.
- have gallbladder disease, a seizure disorder, or an underactive thyroid gland.

- are taking any other drugs that have a sedative effect.
- plan to have surgery under general anesthesia soon.

▷ **Possible Side Effects:**   Drowsiness, light-headedness, dry mouth, urinary retention, constipation.

▷ **Possible Adverse Effects:**
If any of the following develop, call your doctor promptly for guidance.
Some Mild Problems Drug Can Cause
Allergic reactions: skin rash, itching.
Idiosyncratic reactions: skin rash and itching when combined with dairy products (milk or cheese).
Dizziness, sensation of drunkenness, confusion, depression, blurred or double vision.
Nausea, vomiting.
Some Serious Problems Drug Can Cause
Impaired breathing: patients with chronic lung disease should use this drug with caution.

▷ **Possible Effects on Sex Life:**   Blunted sexual responses.

▷ *CAUTION*
1. If you have asthma, chronic bronchitis, or emphysema, excessive use of this drug may cause significant respiratory difficulty, thickening of bronchial secretions, and suppression of coughing.
2. Concurrent use of this drug with atropinelike drugs can increase the risk of urinary retention and reduced intestinal function.
3. Do not take this drug following acute head injury.
4. This drug should not be used in those under 2 years old because of the potential for life-threatening respiratory depression.
5. Those over 60 should take small doses initially, and increase dosage as needed and tolerated. Limit the use of this drug to short-term treatment only. Increased susceptibility to drowsiness, dizziness, unsteadiness, falling, urinary retention, and constipation (often leading to fecal impaction) may occur.

Advisability of Use During Pregnancy or If Breast-Feeding:
Pregnancy Category: C. Use this drug only if clearly needed and in small, infrequent doses. Presence in breast milk is unknown; avoid taking this drug or refrain from nursing.

▷ **Habit-Forming Potential:**   Psychological and/or physical dependence can develop with use of large doses for an extended period of time.

▷ **Overdose Symptoms:**   Drowsiness, restlessness, agitation, nausea, vomiting, dry mouth, vertigo, weakness, lethargy, stupor, coma, seizures.

▷ **Possible Effects of Long-Term Use:** Psychological and physical dependence, chronic constipation.

▷ **While Taking This Drug the Following Apply:**

Beverages: May be taken with milk.

Alcohol: Oxycodone can intensify the intoxicating effects of alcohol, and alcohol can intensify the depressant effects of oxycodone on brain function, breathing, and circulation. Avoid alcohol.

Marijuana Smoking: Increase in drowsiness and pain relief; impairment of mental and physical performance.

Other Drugs:

Oxycodone may ***increase*** the effects of

• other drugs with sedative effects.

• atropinelike drugs, increasing the risk of constipation and urinary retention.

Driving, Hazardous Activities: This drug can impair mental alertness, judgment, reaction time, and physical coordination. Avoid hazardous activities accordingly.

Discontinuation: It is best to limit this drug to short-term use. If its use is necessary for longer periods, discontinuation should be gradual to minimize possible effects of withdrawal.

▷ **Saving Money When Using This Medicine:**

• Current pain management theory advocates scheduled use rather than as-needed use. Ask your doctor if this is appropriate for you.

• Many medications are available to treat pain. Ask your doctor if this drug provides the best combination of cost and outcome for you, and who will regularly assess your pain and adjust medicines.

• If you are prone to constipation, ask your doctor if stool softener should be started WITH this medicine.

• Ask your doctor how the pain being treated typically behaves, and how long this medicine is usually used to treat it.

• A generic form can be substituted for the brand name.

• Ask your doctor if you should visit a chronic pain center.

PENBUTOLOL   (pen BYU toh lohl)

Prescription Needed: Yes   **Controlled Drug:** No   **Generic:** No

Brand Names: Levatol

```
┌─────────────────────────────────────────────────────────┐
│              Overview of BENEFITS versus RISKS          │
│    Possible Benefits              Possible Risks        │
│ EFFECTIVE,                    CONGESTIVE HEART          │
│   WELL-TOLERATED                FAILURE in advanced     │
│   ANTIHYPERTENSIVE for          heart disease          │
│   mild to moderate high blood Worsening of angina in   │
│   pressure                      coronary heart disease │
│                                 (abrupt withdrawal)    │
│                               Masking of low blood     │
│                                 sugar in drug-treated  │
│                                 diabetes               │
│                               Provocation of asthma    │
│                                 (in asthmatics)        │
└─────────────────────────────────────────────────────────┘
```

▷ **Illness This Medication Treats:**
Mild to moderate high blood pressure. This drug may be used alone or concurrently with other antihypertensives, such as diuretics. Penbutolol may reduce the number deaths following a heart attack.

▷ **Typical Dosage Range:** (Dosage or schedule must be determined by the doctor for each individual.)
Initially 20 mg once daily. The dose may be increased gradually by 10 mg/day at intervals of 2 weeks, as needed and tolerated, up to 80 mg/day. For maintenance, 20 to 40 mg once daily is usually adequate. The total daily dose should not exceed 80 mg.

▷ **Conditions Requiring Dosing Adjustments:**
Liver function: Penbutolol is contraindicated for patients with severe liver compromise. Dosage adjustments should be considered for patients with mild to moderate liver disease; however, no specific guidelines are available.

▷ **How Best to Take This Medicine:**   May be taken without regard to eating. The tablet may be crushed for administration. Do not stop taking this drug abruptly.

▷ **How Long This Medicine Is Usually Taken:**   Continual use on a regular schedule for up to 2 weeks usually determines the effectiveness of this drug in lowering blood pressure. Long-term use (months to years) is determined by the course of your blood pressure over time and your response to the overall treatment program (weight reduction, salt restriction, smoking cessation, etc.). Consult your doctor regularly.

▷ **Tell Your Doctor Before Taking This Medicine If You:**
• ever had an allergic reaction to it.
• have congestive heart failure.
• have an abnormally slow heart rate or a serious form of heart block.

- are subject to bronchial asthma.
- had an adverse reaction to any beta-blocker in the past.
- have a history of serious heart disease, with or without episodes of heart failure.
- have a history of hay fever (allergic rhinitis), chronic bronchitis, or emphysema.
- have a history of overactive thyroid function.
- have a history of low blood sugar.
- have impaired liver or kidney function.
- have diabetes or myasthenia gravis.
- have impaired circulation in the extremities (Raynaud's disorder, claudication pains in legs).
- are currently taking any form of digitalis, quinidine, or reserpine, or any calcium blocker.
- plan to have surgery under general anesthesia soon.

▷ **Possible Side Effects:**   Lethargy and fatigability. Worsening of circulatory problems in those with preexisting conditions. Slow heart rate, light-headedness in upright position.

▷ **Possible Adverse Effects:**
If any of the following develop, call your doctor promptly for guidance.
Some Mild Problems Drug Can Cause
Allergic reactions: skin rash, itching, reversible hair loss.
Headache, dizziness, blurred vision, insomnia, abnormal dreams.
Nausea, vomiting, constipation, diarrhea.
Joint and muscle discomfort.
Some Serious Problems Drug Can Cause
Allergic reactions: anaphylactic reaction.
Mental depression, anxiety, disorientation, short-term memory loss, hallucinations.
Chest pain, shortness of breath, congestive heart failure.
Induction of bronchial asthma (in asthmatic individuals).
Aggravation of myasthenia gravis.
Abnormally low white blood cell and platelet counts: fever, sore throat, abnormal bleeding or bruising.

▷ **Possible Effects on Sex Life:**   Decreased libido and impotence, rare but more common with higher doses; Peyronie's disease.

▷ *CAUTION*
1. *Do not stop taking this drug suddenly* without the knowledge and guidance of your doctor. Carry a note stating that you are taking penbutolol.
2. Consult your doctor or pharmacist before using nasal decongestants, usually present in over-the-counter cold preparations and

nose drops. These can cause sudden increases in blood pressure when taken concurrently with beta-blockers.

3. Report the development of any tendency to emotional depression.

4. Safety and effectiveness of this drug for those under 12 years old have not been established. However, if this drug is used, observe for the development of low blood sugar during periods of reduced food intake.

5. Those over 60 should proceed *cautiously* with all antihypertensives. Unacceptably high blood pressure should be reduced without the risks associated with excessively low blood pressure. Small starting doses are advisable, with frequent blood pressure checks. Sudden, rapid, and excessive reduction of blood pressure can predispose to stroke or heart attack. Observe for dizziness, unsteadiness, tendency to fall, confusion, hallucinations, depression, or urinary frequency.

Advisability of Use During Pregnancy or If Breast-Feeding:

Pregnancy Category: C. Use this drug only if clearly needed. Ask your doctor for guidance. Presence in breast milk is unknown; avoid taking this drug or refrain from nursing.

▷ **Overdose Symptoms:** Weakness, slow pulse, low blood pressure, fainting, cold and sweaty skin, congestive heart failure, possible coma and convulsions.

▷ **Suggested Periodic Examinations While Taking This Drug:** (at doctor's discretion)
Measurements of blood pressure, evaluation of heart function. Complete blood cell counts.

▷ **While Taking This Drug the Following Apply:**

Foods: Avoid excessive salt intake.

Beverages: May be taken with milk.

Alcohol: Alcohol may exaggerate this drug's ability to lower the blood pressure and increase its mild sedative effect.

Tobacco Smoking: Nicotine may reduce this drug's effectiveness in treating high blood pressure. In addition, high doses may potentiate the constriction of the bronchial tubes caused by regular smoking.

Other Drugs:

Penbutolol may *increase* the effects of

- other antihypertensives, causing excessive lowering of the blood pressure. Dosage adjustments may be necessary.
- reserpine (Ser-Ap-Es, etc.), causing sedation, depression, slowing of the heart rate, and lowering of the blood pressure. This combination is best avoided.
- verapamil (Calan, Isoptin), causing excessive depression of heart function; monitor this combination closely.

Penbutolol *taken concurrently* with

- clonidine (Catapres) requires close monitoring for rebound high blood pressure if clonidine is withdrawn while penbutolol is still being taken.
- fluvoxamine (Luvox) may lead to excessive slowing of the heart rate or blood pressure.
- insulin requires close monitoring to avoid undetected hypoglycemia.
- amiodarone (Cordarone) may cause a dangerously slow heart rate and arrest; AVOID this combination.
- venlafaxine (Effexor) may result in increased risk of toxicity.

The following drugs may *increase* the effects of penbutolol

- methimazole (Tapazole).
- oral contraceptives (birth control pills).
- propylthiouracil (Propacil).

The following drugs may *decrease* the effects of penbutolol

- barbiturates (phenobarbital, etc.).
- indomethacin (Indocin), and possibly other aspirin substitutes or NSAIDs; these may impair penbutolol's antihypertensive effect.
- rifampin (Rifadin, Rimactane).

Driving, Hazardous Activities: Use caution until the full extent of fatigue, dizziness, and blood pressure change have been determined.

Exposure to Heat: Caution is advised. Hot environments can lower the blood pressure and exaggerate the effects of this drug.

Exposure to Cold: Caution is advised. Cold environments can enhance the circulatory deficiency in the extremities that may occur with this drug. The elderly should take precautions to prevent hypothermia.

Heavy Exercise or Exertion: It is advisable to avoid exertion that produces light-headedness, excessive fatigue, or muscle cramping. The use of penbutolol may intensify the hypertensive response to isometric exercise.

Occurrence of Unrelated Illness: The fever that accompanies systemic infections can lower blood pressure and require dosage adjustment. Illnesses that cause nausea or vomiting may interrupt the regular dosage schedule. Ask your doctor for guidance.

Discontinuation: Avoid sudden discontinuation of this drug in all situations. If possible, gradual reduction of dose over a period of 2 to 3 weeks is recommended. Ask your doctor for specific guidance.

▷ **Saving Money When Using This Medicine:**

- Many new drugs as well as many beta-blockers are available to treat high blood pressure. Ask your doctor if this medicine offers the best balance of cost and outcome for you.

- Ask your doctor how often your blood pressure should be checked. Also ask if taking aspirin every other day makes sense for you.
- Once-a-day dosing may offer a considerable advantage if it is hard to remember to take your medicine.

PENICILLAMINE (pen i SIL a meen)

Prescription Needed: Yes **Controlled Drug:** No **Generic:** No

Brand Names: Cuprimine, Depen

Overview of BENEFITS versus RISKS	
Possible Benefits	*Possible Risks*
EFFECTIVE TREATMENT OF WILSON'S DISEASE (COPPER TOXICITY)	SEVERE ALLERGIC REACTIONS
Partially effective treatment of rheumatoid arthritis	BONE MARROW DEPRESSION
Effective treatment of cystinuria and cystine kidney stones	Drug-induced damage of lungs, liver, pancreas, kidneys
Partially effective treatment of heavy metal poisoning: iron, lead, mercury, and zinc	

▷ **Illness This Medication Treats:**
   (1) Wilson's disease (copper toxicity of brain, cornea, liver, and kidneys); (2) severe rheumatoid arthritis that has failed to respond to less hazardous conventional treatment; (3) cystinuria and cystine stone formation.

▷ **Typical Dosage Range:** (Dosage or schedule must be determined by the doctor for each individual.)

Infants and Children: For Wilson's disease: From 6 months to 12 years old—20 mg/kg of body weight daily, in four divided doses.

For rheumatoid arthritis: Initially 3 mg per kilogram of body weight (up to 250 mg) daily, in two divided doses for 3 months; then 6 mg per kilogram of body weight (up to 500 mg) daily, in two divided doses for 3 months; gradually increase dose, as needed and tolerated, to a maximum of 10 mg per kilogram of body weight daily, in three to four divided doses.

For cystinuria: 30 mg per kilogram of body weight daily, in four divided doses.

For lead poisoning: 25 to 40 mg per kilogram of body weight daily, in two to three divided doses.

12 to 60 Years of Age: For Wilson's disease: 250 mg four times daily.

For rheumatoid arthritis: Initially 125 or 250 mg once daily as a single dose; increase dose gradually, as needed and tolerated, by 125 or 250 mg daily at intervals of 2 to 3 months. The total daily dose should not exceed 1000 mg for small individuals, 1500 mg for large individuals.

For cystinuria and cystine stones: 500 mg four times daily.

For heavy metal poisoning: 500 to 1500 mg daily for 1 to 2 months.

Over 60 Years of Age: Initially 125 mg daily; gradually increase dose, as needed and tolerated, by 125 mg daily at intervals of 2 to 3 months. The total daily dose should not exceed 750 mg.

▷ **Conditions Requiring Dosing Adjustments:**

Liver function: Dosing adjustments do not appear to be needed; however, this drug is a rare cause of hepatoxicity and should be used with caution by patients with compromised livers.

Kidney function: This drug should NOT be taken by patients with moderate kidney failure. Penicillamine is a cause of nephropathy and kidney failure, and for patients with compromised kidneys its use should be based on a benefit-to-risk decision.

▷ **How Best to Take This Medicine:**   Take this drug on an empty stomach, 1 hour before or 2 hours after eating. The capsule may be opened and the tablet may be crushed for administration.

▷ **How Long This Medicine Is Usually Taken:**   Use on a regular schedule for 2 to 3 months is usually needed to see the effectiveness of this drug in relieving the symptoms of Wilson's disease or rheumatoid arthritis. Long-term use (months to years) requires periodic physician evaluation.

PENICILLIN V   (pen i SIL in VEE)

Prescription Needed: Yes   **Controlled Drug:** No   **Generic:** Yes

Brand Names: Beepen VK, Betapen-VK, Ledercillin VK, Penapar VK, Pen-Vee K, Robicillin VK, SK-Penicillin VK, Uticillin VK, V-Cillin K, Veetids

Overview of BENEFITS versus RISKS	
Possible Benefits	*Possible Risks*
EFFECTIVE TREATMENT OF INFECTIONS due to susceptible microorganisms	ALLERGIC REACTIONS, mild to severe
	Superinfections (yeast)
	Drug-induced colitis

▷ **Illness This Medication Treats:**
(1) Infections of the respiratory tract, middle ear, and skin; (2) helps prevent rheumatic fever and bacterial endocarditis in people with valvular heart disease.

▷ **Typical Dosage Range:** (Dosage or schedule must be determined by the doctor for each individual.)
Dosage is based on the results of sensitivity testing of the causative organism, the severity of the infection, and the patient's response. Depending on the specific infection, the dosage range is 125 to 500 mg every 6 to 8 hours. For the prevention of bacterial endocarditis: 2 g (2000 mg) taken 1 hour before the procedure, followed by 1 g 6 hours later. The total daily dosage should not exceed 7 g (7000 mg).

▷ **Conditions Requiring Dosing Adjustments:**
Kidney function: Patients with renal compromise should take no more than 250 mg every 6 hours. This drug can cause interstitial nephritis, and its use should be based on a benefit-to-risk decision for patients with compromised kidneys.

▷ **How Best to Take This Medicine:**   May be taken on an empty stomach or with food or milk. Absorption may be slightly faster if this drug is taken when the stomach is empty. The tablet may be crushed.

▷ **How Long This Medicine Is Usually Taken:**   For all streptococcal infections: not less than 10 consecutive days (without interruption) to reduce the possibility of developing rheumatic fever or glomerulonephritis. For all other infections: as long as necessary to eradicate the infection.

▷ **Tell Your Doctor Before Taking This Medicine If You:**
• ever had an allergic reaction to it or are allergic by nature (hay fever, asthma, hives, eczema).
• suspect you are allergic to *any* form of penicillin.
• are allergic to any cephalosporin antibiotic (Ancef, Anspor, Ceclor, Ceporan, Ceporex, Kafocin, Keflex, Keflin, Kefzol, Loridine, Ultracef, Velosef).

▷ **Possible Side Effects:**   Superinfections, often due to yeast organisms.

▷ **Possible Adverse Effects:**
If any of the following develop, call your doctor promptly for guidance.
Some Mild Problems Drug Can Cause
Allergic reactions: skin rashes, hives, itching.
Irritations of mouth and tongue, black tongue, nausea, vomiting, mild diarrhea, dizziness (rare).

Some Serious Problems Drug Can Cause
Allergic reactions: anaphylactic reaction, severe skin reactions, drug fever, swollen painful joints, sore throat, abnormal bleeding or bruising.
Drug-induced colitis.
Rare hemolytic anemia, porphyria, or abnormal liver function.

▷ **CAUTION**
1. Take the exact dose and the full course prescribed.
2. This drug should not be used at the same time as antibiotics such as erythromycin or tetracycline.
3. Watch children closely for evidence of a developing allergy to penicillin. This drug may cause diarrhea, which sometimes necessitates discontinuation.
4. Those over 60 typically have natural changes in the skin that may predispose them to prolonged itching reactions in the genital and anal regions. Report such reactions promptly.

Advisability of Use During Pregnancy or If Breast-Feeding:
Pregnancy Category: B. Considered safe for use during any period of pregnancy. Present in breast milk; avoid taking this drug if possible or refrain from nursing.

▷ **Overdose Symptoms:** Possible nausea, vomiting, and/or diarrhea.

▷ **Suggested Periodic Examinations While Taking This Drug:** (at doctor's discretion)
Complete blood cell counts, kidney function tests.

▷ **While Taking This Drug the Following Apply:**
Beverages: May be taken with milk.
Other Drugs:
Penicillin V *decrease* the effects of
• oral contraceptives (birth control pills) in some women, impairing their effectiveness in preventing pregnancy.
Penicillin V *taken concurrently* with
• aminoglycoside antibiotics (see Drug Classes) may blunt the aminoglycoside benefits.
• probenecid (Benemid) will increase and sustain penicillin blood levels—this is often used to benefit therapy.
The following drugs may *decrease* the effects of penicillin V
• antacids; may reduce the absorption of penicillin V.
• chloramphenicol (Chloromycetin).
• erythromycin (Erythrocin, E-Mycin, etc.).
• tetracyclines (Achromycin, Declomycin, doxycycline, etc.).
Driving, Hazardous Activities: Be alert to the rare occurrence of dizziness and/or nausea, and restrict your activities accordingly.
Special Storage Instructions: Oral solutions should be refrigerated.

Observe the Following Expiration Times: Do not take oral solution older than 7 days (kept at room temperature) or 14 days (refrigerated).

▷ **Saving Money When Using This Medicine:**
- Ask your doctor if this medicine offers the best balance of cost and outcome for you.
- The dose must be adjusted for people with kidney compromise. Ask your doctor whether the dose has been decreased for you.
- A generic form can be substituted for the brand name.
- Ask your doctor how long this medicine is usually used to treat your infection, and if the power of this drug matches the severity of your infection.

PENTAMIDINE (pen TAM i deen)

Prescription Needed: Yes   **Controlled Drug:** No   **Generic:** No

Brand Names: NebuPent

Overview of BENEFITS versus RISKS	
Possible Benefits	*Possible Risks*
PREVENTION AND TREATMENT OF *PNEUMOCYSTIS CARINII* PNEUMONIA (AIDS-RELATED)	Pancreatitis (rare) Hypoglycemia (rare) Cough and bronchospasm Kidney damage Liver damage

▷ **Saving Money When Using This Medicine:**
- Many drugs are available to treat or prevent *Pneumocystis carinii* pneumonia (PCP), and this medicine is not the drug of first choice. Ask your doctor if this medicine offers the best balance of cost and outcome for you.

PENTAZOCINE (pen TAZ oh seen)

Prescription Needed: Yes   **Controlled Drug:** C-IV*   **Generic:** No

Brand Names: Talacen [CD], Talwin, Talwin Compound [CD], Talwin Nx [CD]

*See Controlled Drug Schedules inside this book's cover.

```
┌─────────────────────────────────────────────────────────┐
│              Overview of BENEFITS versus RISKS           │
│      Possible Benefits           Possible Risks          │
│   EFFECTIVE RELIEF OF         POTENTIAL FOR HABIT         │
│     MODERATE TO SEVERE          FORMATION                │
│     PAIN                        (DEPENDENCE)             │
│                               Sedative effects           │
│                               Mental and behavioral      │
│                                 disturbances             │
│                               Low blood pressure, fainting│
│                               Nausea                     │
│                               Constipation               │
└─────────────────────────────────────────────────────────┘
```

▷ **Illness This Medication Treats:**

Moderate to severe acute or chronic pain from any cause.

As Combination Drug Product [CD]: Pentazocine is used in combinations with milder pain relievers such as acetaminophen and aspirin, which enhance the analgesic effect and reduce fever. In the United States the tablet form also contains naloxone (Talwin Nx), a narcotic antagonist that renders the drug ineffective if injected.

▷ **Typical Dosage Range:** (Dosage or schedule must be determined by the doctor for each individual.)

50 mg every 3 to 4 hours. Dose may be increased to 100 mg/4 hr if needed for severe pain. The total daily dosage should not exceed 600 mg. Current pain theory calls for scheduled use of pain medicines, seeking to prevent rather than treat pain.

▷ **Conditions Requiring Dosing Adjustments:**

Liver function: Dose should be decreased for patients with liver compromise.

Kidney function: For patients with moderate to severe kidney failure, the dose should be decreased by 25 to 50%.

▷ **How Best to Take This Medicine:**   May be taken with or following food to reduce stomach irritation or nausea. The tablet may be crushed.

▷ **How Long This Medicine Is Usually Taken:**   As required to control pain. Continual use should not exceed 5 to 7 days without interruption and reassessment of need.

▷ **Tell Your Doctor Before Taking This Medicine If You:**
- ever had an allergic reaction to it.
- are having an acute attack of asthma.
- have had an unfavorable reaction to any narcotic in the past.
- have a history of drug abuse or alcoholism.
- have chronic lung disease with impaired breathing.
- have impaired liver or kidney function.

- have gallbladder disease, a seizure disorder, or an underactive thyroid gland.
- have difficulty emptying your urinary bladder.
- are taking any other drugs that have a sedative effect.
- plan to have surgery under general anesthesia soon.

▷ **Possible Side Effects:** Drowsiness, light-headedness, weakness, urinary retention, constipation.

▷ **Possible Adverse Effects:**

If any of the following develop, call your doctor promptly for guidance.

Some Mild Problems Drug Can Cause

Allergic reactions: skin rash, itching, swelling of face.

Headache, dizziness, impaired concentration, sensation of drunkenness, blurred or double vision, flushing, sweating.

Nausea, vomiting, indigestion, diarrhea.

Some Serious Problems Drug Can Cause

Marked drop in blood pressure, possible fainting.

Impaired breathing: patients with chronic lung disease should use this drug with caution.

Mental and behavioral disturbances, hallucinations, tremor.

Bone marrow depression of a mild and reversible nature (rare).

Aggravation of prostatism.

Rare drug-induced seizures, porphyria, fixed positioning of the eyes, or bone marrow depression (mild and reversible).

▷ *CAUTION*

1. Use of this drug with atropinelike drugs may increase the risk of urinary retention and reduced intestinal function.
2. Do not take this drug following acute head injury.
3. Safety and effectiveness of this drug for those under 12 years old have not been established.
4. Those over 60 should proceed *cautiously* with small doses and small increases, as needed and tolerated. Limit use of this drug to short-term treatment only. Pentazocine may increase susceptibility to drowsiness, dizziness, unsteadiness, falling, urinary retention, and constipation.

Advisability of Use During Pregnancy or If Breast-Feeding:

Pregnancy Category: C. (may be B or D in high-dose or extended use at term). Avoid use of this drug during the first 3 months. Use only if clearly needed and in small, infrequent doses during the last 6 months. Presence in breast milk is expected. Avoid taking this drug or refrain from nursing.

▷ **Habit-Forming Potential:** Psychological and/or physical dependence can develop with large doses used for an extended period.

▷ **Overdose Symptoms:**   Anxiety, disturbed thoughts, hallucinations, progressive drowsiness, stupor, depressed breathing.

▷ **Suggested Periodic Examinations While Taking This Drug:** (at doctor's discretion)
Complete blood cell counts if this drug is used for an extended period.

▷ **While Taking This Drug the Following Apply:**

Beverages: May be taken with milk.

Alcohol: Pentazocine can intensify the intoxicating effects of alcohol, and alcohol can intensify the depressant effects of pentazocine on brain function, breathing, and circulation. NOT ADVISED.

Tobacco Smoking: Heavy smoking may reduce this drug's effectiveness and make larger doses necessary.

Marijuana Smoking: Increase in drowsiness and pain relief; impairment of mental and physical performance.

Other Drugs:

Pentazocine may *increase* the effects of

- other drugs with sedative effects.
- atropinelike drugs, increasing the risk of constipation and urinary retention.
- cyclosporine (Sandimmune) and lead to toxicity.
- MAO inhibitors (see Drug Classes), and may result in muscle rigidity.

Driving, Hazardous Activities: This drug can impair mental alertness, judgment, reaction time, and physical coordination. Avoid hazardous activities accordingly.

Discontinuation: It is advisable to limit this drug to short-term use. If extended use is necessary, discontinuation should be gradual to minimize possible effects of withdrawal.

▷ **Saving Money When Using This Medicine:**

- A large number of available drugs provide similar effectiveness. Ask your doctor to prescribe the drug that offers the best combination of cost and outcome. Also ask who will be regularly assessing your pain and adjusting your medicines.
- If you have a problem with constipation, ask your doctor to add a stool softener.
- If your pain continues, talk with your doctor about visiting a chronic pain center.

PENTOXIFYLLINE (pen tox I fi leen)

Other Name: Oxpentifylline

Prescription Needed: Yes   **Controlled Drug:** No   **Generic:** No

Brand Names: Trental

Overview of BENEFITS versus RISKS

Possible Benefits	*Possible Risks*
IMPROVED BLOOD FLOW IN PERIPHERAL ARTERIAL DISEASE	Reduced blood pressure, angina, abnormal heart rhythms
REDUCTION OF INTERMITTENT CLAUDICATION PAIN	Indigestion, nausea, vomiting
	Rare lowering of blood counts or aplastic anemia
	Dizziness, flushing

▷ **Illness This Medication Treats:**
  Peripheral obstructive arterial disease; used to improve arterial blood flow and reduce the frequency and severity of muscle pain due to intermittent claudication.

▷ **Typical Dosage Range:** (Dosage or schedule must be determined by the doctor for each individual.)
  400 mg three times per day. If adverse nervous system or gastrointestinal effects occur, reduce the dose to 400 mg twice per day.

▷ **Conditions Requiring Dosing Adjustments:**
  Kidney function: The dose should be empirically decreased for patients with compromised kidneys.

▷ **How Best to Take This Medicine:** Take with or following food to reduce stomach irritation. Swallow the tablet whole without breaking, crushing, or chewing.

▷ **How Long This Medicine Is Usually Taken:** Continual use on a regular schedule for 2 to 4 weeks is usually necessary to determine the effectiveness of this drug in preventing or delaying the pains of intermittent claudication associated with walking. Treatment for a minimum of 3 months is recommended to determine full effectiveness. Long-term use (months to years) requires physician supervision.

▷ **Tell Your Doctor Before Taking This Medicine If You:**
  • ever had an allergic reaction to it.
  • are allergic to other xanthine drugs: caffeine, theophylline, theobromine.
  • have impaired kidney function.

- have low blood pressure, impaired brain circulation, or coronary artery disease.
- smoke tobacco.
- are taking any antihypertensives.

▷ **Possible Adverse Effects:**
If any of the following develop, call your doctor promptly for guidance.
Some Mild Problems Drug Can Cause
Allergic reaction: skin rash.
Headache dizziness, tremor.
Rare: nosebleeds or flu-like syndrome.
Indigestion, nausea, vomiting.
Some Serious Problems Drug Can Cause
Development of angina or heart rhythm disorders in the presence of coronary artery disease.
Rare: liver toxicity; retinal bleeding; decreased blood platelets or all cells; or auditory hallucinations.

▷ *CAUTION*
1. Use with caution in the presence of impaired brain circulation (cerebral arteriosclerosis) or coronary artery disease. If any related symptoms develop, see your doctor for prompt evaluation.
2. Safety and effectiveness of this drug for those under 18 years old have not been established. The use of pentoxifylline in this age group is not anticipated.
3. Those over 60 may be more susceptible to adverse effects. Report any indications of dizziness or chest pain promptly.

Advisability of Use During Pregnancy or If Breast-Feeding:
Pregnancy Category: C. Avoid use during the first 3 months. Otherwise, this drug should be used only if clearly needed. Present in breast milk; avoid taking this drug or refrain from nursing.

▷ **Overdose Symptoms:**   Drowsiness, flushing, faintness, excitement, seizures.

▷ **Suggested Periodic Examinations While Taking This Drug:** (at doctor's discretion)
Blood pressure measurements, evaluation of heart status.

▷ **While Taking This Drug the Following Apply:**
Beverages: May be taken with milk.
Alcohol: Use caution until the combined effects have been determined. Alcohol may increase the blood pressure–lowering effect.
Tobacco Smoking: Nicotine constricts arteries and impairs pentoxifylline's effectiveness significantly. Avoid all use of tobacco.

Other Drugs:

Pentoxifylline may *increase* the effects of

- antihypertensives, causing excessive lowering of blood pressure.
- warfarin (Coumadin, etc.), increasing the possibility of unwanted bleeding; have INR (prothrombin times) checked more frequently and medicine doses adjusted to lab results.
- cimetidine (Tagamet), nizatidine (Axid), famotidine (Pepcid), or ranitidine (Zantac); may lead to pentoxifylline toxicity due to increased drug absorption. Pentoxifylline doses may need to be decreased.
- theophylline (Theo-Dur, others), which may lead to theophylline toxicity.

Driving, Hazardous Activities: May cause drowsiness or dizziness. Restrict your activities as necessary.

▷ **Saving Money When Using This Medicine:**

- Ask your doctor if this drug offers the best combination of cost and outcome.
- If there is an elevated cholesterol component to your problem, talk with your doctor about using an HMG CoA inhibitor.
- Talk with your doctor about the benefits of taking aspirin every other day to help prevent a heart attack.

PERGOLIDE (PER go lide)

Prescription Needed: Yes   **Controlled Drug:** No   **Generic:** No

Brand Names: Permax

Overview of BENEFITS versus RISKS	
Possible Benefits	*Possible Risks*
ADDITIVE RELIEF OF PARKINSON'S DISEASE SYMPTOMS when used concurrently with levodopa/carbidopa (Sinemet) PERMITS A REDUCTION IN SINEMET DOSAGE	ABNORMAL INVOLUNTARY MOVEMENTS HALLUCINATIONS INITIAL FALL IN BLOOD PRESSURE/ORTHOSTATIC HYPOTENSION Possible premature heart contractions

▷ **Illness This Medication Treats:**

Parkinson's disease; used as an adjunct treatment to levodopa/carbidopa for those who experience intolerable abnormal movements (dyskinesia) and/or increasing on-off episodes due to levodopa. The addition of pergolide (1) permits reduction of the daily dose of levodopa, with consequent lessening of dyskinesia and erratic drug response, and (2) provides additional relief of parkinsonian symptoms.

▷ **Typical Dosage Range:** (Dosage or schedule must be determined by the doctor for each individual.)

Initially 0.05 mg daily for the first 2 days; gradually increase the daily dose by 0.1 or 0.15 mg every third day over the next 12 days. If needed and tolerated, the daily dose may be increased further by 0.25 mg every third day until an optimal response is achieved. The total daily dosage should be divided into three equal portions and given at 6- to 8-hour intervals. The usual maintenance dose is 3 mg/24 hr; do not exceed 5 mg/24 hr.

During gradual introduction, the concurrent dose of levodopa/carbidopa (Sinemet) may be cautiously decreased in accord with your doctor's instructions.

▷ **Conditions Requiring Dosing Adjustments:**

Liver function: No specific guidelines for dosing adjustments for patients with liver compromise are available. This drug should be used with caution by patients with compromised livers.

Kidney function: The dose should be decreased for patients with kidney compromise; however, specific guidelines are not available.

▷ **How Best to Take This Medicine:** Take with food or milk to reduce stomach irritation. The tablet may be crushed.

▷ **How Long This Medicine Is Usually Taken:** Continual use on a regular schedule for 4 to 6 weeks is usually necessary to determine the effectiveness of this drug in controlling the symptoms of Parkinson's disease and permitting reduced levodopa/carbidopa dosage. Long-term use (months to years) requires periodic evaluation of response and dosage adjustment. See your doctor regularly.

▷ **Tell Your Doctor Before Taking This Medicine If You:**
- ever had an allergic reaction to it.
- had a serious adverse effect from any ergot preparation in the past.
- have severe coronary artery disease or peripheral vascular disease; or any degree of coronary artery disease, especially angina; or a history of heart attack.
- have constitutionally low blood pressure.
- are pregnant or breast-feeding.
- are taking any antihypertensives or antipsychotics.
- have any type of heart rhythm disorder.
- have impaired liver or kidney function.
- have a seizure disorder.

▷ **Possible Side Effects:** Weakness, chest pain—possibly anginal, peripheral edema, orthostatic hypotension.

▷ **Possible Adverse Effects:**

If any of the following develop, call your doctor promptly for guidance.

Some Mild Problems Drug Can Cause

Allergic reactions: skin rash, facial swelling.

Headache, dizziness, confusion, drowsiness, insomnia, double vision.

Nasal congestion, shortness of breath, palpitation, fainting.

Altered taste, loss of appetite, dry mouth, nausea, vomiting, constipation, diarrhea.

Some Serious Problems Drug Can Cause

Idiosyncratic reactions: flu-like symptoms.

Abnormal involuntary movements (dyskinesia), psychotic behavior.

Hallucinations.

Rare anemia.

Paranoid delusions.

▷ **Possible Effects on Sex Life:** Infrequent reports of altered libido (both increased and decreased), impotence, breast pain, priapism.

▷ **Adverse Effects That May Mimic Natural Diseases or Disorders:** Effects on mental function and behavior may resemble psychotic disorders.

▷ *CAUTION*

1. This drug can initiate dyskinesias and worsen existing dyskinesias. Watch carefully for tremors, twitching, or abnormal involuntary movements of any kind. Report these promptly.

2. Begin treatment with low doses to prevent the possibility of excessive blood pressure drop (see "Typical Dosage Range," above).

3. Tell your doctor promptly if you become pregnant or plan pregnancy. This drug has been reported (rarely) to cause abortion and birth defects.

4. For those over 60, small initial doses are mandatory. Watch closely for any tendency to light-headedness or faintness, especially on arising from a lying or sitting position. You may be more susceptible to impaired thinking, confusion, agitation, nightmares, or hallucinations.

Advisability of Use During Pregnancy or If Breast-Feeding:

Pregnancy Category: B. Prudence advises against the use of this drug during pregnancy. Ask your doctor for guidance. Presence in breast milk is unknown; avoid taking this drug or refrain from nursing.

▷ **Overdose Symptoms:** Nausea, vomiting, palpitations, low blood pressure, agitation, severe involuntary movements, hallucinations, seizures.

▷ **Possible Effects of Long-Term Use:** Increased risk of developing dyskinesias.

▷ **Suggested Periodic Examinations While Taking This Drug:** (at
  doctor's discretion)
  Regular evaluation of drug response, heart function, and blood pressure status.

▷ **While Taking This Drug the Following Apply:**
  Beverages: May be taken with milk.
  Alcohol: Use caution until the combined effects have been determined.
    Alcohol can exaggerate blood pressure–lowering and sedative ef-
    fects.
  Other Drugs:
  Pergolide *taken concurrently* with
  • antihypertensives (and other drugs that can lower blood pressure)
    requires careful monitoring for excessive drops in pressure. Dosage
    adjustments may be necessary.
  The following drugs may *decrease* the effects of pergolide and dimin-
  ish its effectiveness:
  • chlorprothixene (Taractan).
  • haloperidol (Haldol).
  • metoclopramide (Reglan).
  • phenothiazines (see Drug Classes).
  • thiothixene (Navane).
  Driving, Hazardous Activities: May cause dizziness, drowsiness, im-
    paired coordination, or fainting. Restrict your activities as neces-
    sary.
  Exposure to Heat: Use caution until the combined effects have been
    determined. Hot environments can lower blood pressure.
  Discontinuation: Do not stop taking this drug abruptly. Sudden with-
    drawal can cause confusion, paranoid thinking, and severe halluci-
    nations. Ask your doctor about a schedule for gradual withdrawal.

▷ **Saving Money When Using This Medicine:**
  • Ask your doctor if this drug offers the best combination of cost and
    outcome.
  • A new medicine currently in trials takes a different approach to Par-
    kinson's and may offer better outcomes. Discuss new treatments
    and treatment trials with your doctor.

PERPHENAZINE (per FEN a zeen)

Prescription Needed: Yes   **Controlled Drug:** No   **Generic:**
No

Brand Names: Etrafon [CD], Etrafon-A [CD], Etrafon Forte [CD],
  Triavil [CD], Trilafon

```
┌─────────────────────────────────────────────────────────┐
│              Overview of BENEFITS versus RISKS           │
│      Possible Benefits              Possible Risks       │
│   EFFECTIVE CONTROL OF        SERIOUS TOXIC EFFECTS ON    │
│     ACUTE MENTAL                BRAIN with long-term use  │
│     DISORDERS (in most        Infrequent liver damage with│
│     patients)                   jaundice                 │
│   Beneficial effects on thinking, Rare blood cell disorders:│
│     mood, and behavior          hemolytic anemia,        │
│   Relief of anxiety and tension   abnormally low white blood│
│   Moderately effective control of cell and platelet counts│
│     nausea and vomiting                                  │
└─────────────────────────────────────────────────────────┘
```

▷ **Illness This Medication Treats:**
(1) Acute and chronic psychotic disorders such as agitated depression, schizophrenia; (2) may be used as a tranquilizer in the management of agitated and disruptive behavior in the absence of true psychosis; (3) may be used to relieve severe nausea or vomiting.

▷ **Typical Dosage Range:** (Dosage or schedule must be determined by the doctor for each individual.)
For psychotic symptoms: Initially 4 to 8 mg three times daily. Dose may be increased by 4 mg at 3- to 4-day intervals, as needed and tolerated. Usual dosage range is 8 to 24 mg daily. Total daily dosage should not exceed 64 mg.

▷ **Conditions Requiring Dosing Adjustments:**
Liver function: The dose should be decreased for patients with liver compromise; this drug is contraindicated for patients with moderate to severe liver compromise.
Kidney function: This drug should be used with caution by patients with urine outflow problems; perphenazine can cause urine retention.

▷ **How Best to Take This Medicine:** May be taken with or following meals to reduce stomach irritation. The regular tablets may be crushed for administration; the prolonged-action tablets should be taken whole, not broken, crushed, or chewed.

▷ **How Long This Medicine Is Usually Taken:** Continual use on a regular schedule for several weeks is usually necessary to determine the effectiveness of this drug in controlling psychotic disorders. Stop using perphenazine if it is not significantly beneficial within 6 weeks. Long-term use (months to years) requires periodic physician evaluation of response.

▷ **Tell Your Doctor Before Taking This Medicine If You:**
• ever had an allergic reaction to it.
• have active liver disease.

- have cancer of the breast.
- have a current blood cell or bone marrow disorder.
- are allergic or abnormally sensitive to any phenothiazine.
- are pregnant or breast-feeding your child.
- have impaired liver or kidney function.
- have any type of seizure disorder.
- have diabetes, glaucoma, or heart disease.
- have a history of lupus erythematosus.
- are taking any drug with sedative effects.
- plan to have surgery under general or spinal anesthesia soon.

▷ **Possible Side Effects:** Drowsiness (usually during the first 2 weeks), orthostatic hypotension, blurred vision, dry mouth, nasal congestion, constipation, impaired urination.

Pink or purple coloration of urine, of no significance.

▷ **Possible Adverse Effects:**

If any of the following develop, call your doctor promptly for guidance.

Some Mild Problems Drug Can Cause

Allergic reactions: skin rash, hives, low-grade fever.

Lowering of body temperature, especially in the elderly.

Increased appetite and weight gain.

Dizziness, weakness, agitation, insomnia, impaired day and night vision.

Chronic constipation, fecal impaction.

Some Serious Problems Drug Can Cause

Allergic reactions: hepatitis with jaundice, severe skin reactions, anaphylactic reaction.

Idiosyncratic reactions: neuroleptic malignant syndrome.

Depression; seizures; deposits in cornea, lens, and retina.

Rapid heart rate, heart rhythm disorders.

Blood cell disorders: hemolytic anemia, reduced white blood cell and blood platelet counts.

Drug-induced porphyria.

Nervous system reactions: Parkinson-like disorders, severe restlessness, muscle spasms involving the face and neck, tardive dyskinesia.

▷ **Possible Effects on Sex Life:** Altered timing and pattern of menstruation.

Female breast enlargement with milk production.

Male breast enlargement and tenderness.

Inhibited ejaculation.

False-positive pregnancy test results.

▷ **Adverse Effects That May Mimic Natural Diseases or Disorders:**
Nervous system reactions may suggest true Parkinson's disease.
Liver reactions may suggest viral hepatitis.
Reactions resembling systemic lupus erythematosus can occur.

▷ *CAUTION*

1. Many over-the-counter medications for allergies, colds, and coughs contain drugs that can interact unfavorably with this drug. Ask your doctor or pharmacist for guidance before using any such medications.
2. Antacids that contain aluminum and/or magnesium can prevent absorption and reduce perphenazine's effectiveness.
3. Get prompt evaluation of any change or disturbance of vision.
4. Use of this drug is not recommended in children under 12 years old. Do not use this drug in the presence of symptoms suggestive of Reye's syndrome. Children with acute infectious diseases (flu-like infections, chickenpox, measles, etc.) are more prone to muscular spasms of the face, back, and extremities when this drug is given to control nausea or vomiting.
5. For people over 60, small doses of this drug are advisable until individual response has been determined. You may be more susceptible to drowsiness, lethargy, constipation, lowered body temperature, and orthostatic hypotension. This drug can enhance existing prostatism. You may also be more susceptible to Parkinson-like reactions and/or tardive dyskinesia. These reactions must be recognized early since they may become unresponsive to treatment and irreversible.

Advisability of Use During Pregnancy or If Breast-Feeding:

Pregnancy Category: C. Avoid using this drug during the first 3 months; avoid during the last month because of possible effects on the newborn infant. Present in breast milk in minute amounts. Monitor nursing infant closely and discontinue drug or nursing if adverse effects develop.

▷ **Overdose Symptoms:**   Marked drowsiness, weakness, tremor, agitation, unsteadiness, deep sleep, coma, convulsions.

▷ **Suggested Periodic Examinations While Taking This Drug:** (at doctor's discretion)

Complete blood cell counts, especially between the 4th and 10th weeks of treatment.
Liver function tests, electrocardiograms.
Complete eye examinations—eye structure and vision.
Careful inspection of the tongue for early evidence of fine, involuntary, wavelike movements that could indicate the beginning of tardive dyskinesia.

▷ **While Taking This Drug the Following Apply:**

Nutritional Support: A riboflavin (vitamin B2) supplement should be taken with long-term use.

Beverages: May be taken with milk.

Alcohol: Avoid completely. Alcohol can increase the sedative action of phenothiazines and accentuate their depressant effects on brain function and blood pressure. Phenothiazines can increase the intoxicating effects of alcohol.

Tobacco Smoking: Possible reduction of drowsiness.

Marijuana Smoking: Moderate increase in drowsiness; accentuation of orthostatic hypotension; increased risk of precipitating latent psychoses, confusing the interpretation of mental status and drug responses.

Other Drugs:

Perphenazine may *increase* the effects of

- all sedatives, especially meperidine (Demerol), causing excessive sedation.
- all atropinelike drugs, causing nervous system toxicity.

Perphenazine may *decrease* the effects of

- guanethidine (Ismelin, Esimil), reducing its effectiveness in lowering blood pressure.

Perphenazine *taken concurrently* with

- ascorbic acid (vitamin C) may blunt perphenazine's benefits.
- lithium (Lithobid, Lithotabs) may impair the effectiveness of lithium and cause nervous system toxicity.
- monoamine oxidase inhibitors (MAOIs—see Drug Classes) may increase risk of abnormal movements.

The following drugs may *decrease* the effects of perphenazine

- antacids containing aluminum and/or magnesium.
- barbiturates.
- benztropine (Cogentin).
- disulfiram (Antabuse).
- trihexyphenidyl (Artane).

Driving, Hazardous Activities: This drug can impair mental alertness, judgment, and physical coordination. Avoid hazardous activities.

Exposure to Sun: Use caution until your sensitivity has been determined. Some phenothiazines can cause photosensitivity.

Exposure to Heat: Use caution and avoid excessive heat as much as possible. This drug may impair the regulation of body temperature and increase the risk of heatstroke.

Exposure to Cold: Use caution and dress warmly. This drug can increase the risk of hypothermia in the elderly.

Discontinuation: After a period of long-term use, do not discontinue this drug suddenly. Gradual withdrawal over 2 to 3 weeks under your doctor's supervision is recommended. Do not discontinue this drug without your doctor's knowledge and approval. The relapse rate of schizophrenia after discontinuation is 50 to 60%.

▷ **Saving Money When Using This Medicine:**
- A large number of drugs are available to treat depression and schizophrenia. Ask your doctor if this drug offers the best combination of cost and outcome.
- A new medicine called olanzapine may offer fewer side effects than previously available medicines.

PHENELZINE (FEN el zeen)

Prescription Needed: Yes   **Controlled Drug:** No   **Generic:** No

Brand Names: Nardil

Overview of BENEFITS versus RISKS

Possible Benefits	*Possible Risks*
EFFECTIVE RELIEF OF REACTIVE, NEUROTIC, ATYPICAL DEPRESSIONS with associated anxiety or phobia	DANGEROUS INTERACTIONS WITH MANY DRUGS AND FOODS
Beneficial in some depressions that are unresponsive to other treatments	CONDUCIVE TO HYPERTENSIVE CRISIS
	DISORDERED HEART RATE AND RHYTHM
	Drug-induced hepatitis (rare)
	Mental changes: agitation, confusion, impaired memory, hypomania

---

▷ **Illness This Medication Treats:**
Severe situational (reactive or neurotic) depression, atypical depression, and (though less effective) severe endogenous depression. Because of the supervision required during its use and its potential for serious adverse effects, this monoamine oxidase (MAO) type A inhibitor is usually reserved for depressions that have not responded satisfactorily to other antidepressants.

▷ **Typical Dosage Range.** (Dosage or schedule must be determined by the doctor for each individual.)
Initially 15 mg three times per day (or 1 mg per kilogram of body weight divided into three equal doses, given three times a day); increase rapidly up to 60 mg/day, as needed and tolerated, until improvement is apparent. For maintenance, dose is slowly decreased over several weeks to the smallest dose that maintains improve-

ment, which may be as low as 15 mg daily or every other day. Total daily dosage should not exceed 90 mg.

▷ **Conditions Requiring Dosing Adjustments:**
Liver function: This drug should not be used by patients with increased liver function tests or a history of liver compromise.
Kidney function: No specific dosing changes are indicated for patients with renal compromise. This drug should be used with caution by patients with urine outflow problems, as phenelzine can cause urine retention.

▷ **How Best to Take This Medicine:**   May be taken on an empty stomach or with food. Do not take in late evening; it can interfere with sleep. The tablet may be crushed for administration.

▷ **How Long This Medicine Is Usually Taken:**   Continual use on a regular schedule for 3 to 4 weeks is usually necessary to determine the effectiveness of this drug in relieving depression. Once the optimal maintenance dose has been determined, it may be continued indefinitely. Long-term use (months to years) requires physician supervision.

▷ **Tell Your Doctor Before Taking This Medicine If You:**
- ever had an allergic reaction to it.
- have advanced heart disease.
- have active liver disease or impaired liver function.
- have an adrenaline-producing tumor.
- are taking any another MAO type A inhibitor, a tricyclic antidepressant, or carbamazepine.
- have high blood pressure.
- have had a stroke, or have impaired circulation to the brain.
- have coronary heart disease.
- have frequent or severe headaches.
- have diabetes, epilepsy, schizophrenia, or an overactive thyroid gland.
- have impaired kidney function.
- plan to have surgery under general or spinal anesthesia soon.

▷ **Possible Side Effects:**   Insomnia if taken in the evening.
Orthostatic hypotension.
Fluid retention (swelling of feet and ankles).

▷ **Possible Adverse Effects:**
If any of the following develop, call your doctor promptly for guidance.
Some Mild Problems Drug Can Cause
Allergic reaction: skin rash.
Headache, dizziness, drowsiness, agitation, confusion, impaired

memory, tremors, muscle twitching, blurred vision, impaired red-green color vision.

Dry mouth, increased appetite, indigestion, constipation.

Some Serious Problems Drug Can Cause

Drug-induced hepatitis with jaundice.

Hypertensive crisis: rapid and extreme rise in blood pressure, severe throbbing headache, palpitation, nausea, vomiting, sweating, risk of brain hemorrhage.

Unusual excitement or nervousness.

Rare Parkinson-like syndrome, porphyria, eye toxicity, lowered white blood cell count, seizures, neuroleptic malignant syndrome.

Disturbances of heart rate and rhythm.

▷ **Possible Effects on Sex Life:** Decreased libido, impaired erection, inhibited ejaculation.

Inhibited orgasm.

▷ **Adverse Effects That May Mimic Natural Diseases or Disorders:**

Drug-induced hepatitis may suggest viral hepatitis.

▷ *CAUTION*

1. Careful dosage adjustment is mandatory. Do not exceed the lowest effective dose.

2. A severe headache or palpitations may indicate a dangerous elevation of blood pressure. Discontinue this drug immediately and call your doctor.

3. This drug may suppress anginal pain that would normally warn of excessive demand on the heart.

4. This drug may increase the possibility of hypoglycemic reactions if used concurrently with insulin or oral antidiabetic drugs (sulfonylureas). It may also delay recovery from hypoglycemia.

5. This drug can alter the threshold for convulsions with epilepsy or seizure disorder. Dosages of anticonvulsants may require adjustment.

6. Discontinue 2 weeks before elective surgery under general or spinal anesthesia. Consult your surgeon or anesthesiologist

7. Many over-the-counter drug products contain ingredients that can cause serious interactions if taken concurrently. Avoid use of the following: cold and sinus medications, nasal decongestants, hay fever preparations, asthma inhalants, appetite and weight control products, pep pills. Consult your doctor or pharmacist regarding their safe use with this drug.

8. It is best to carry a personal identification card that states you are taking this drug. Tell all medical personnel who provide care that you are taking this drug.

9. Safety and effectiveness of this drug for those under 16 years old have not been established.

10. This drug is not recommended for use by anyone over 60. However, if poor response to other treatment justifies consideration of a trial, it is inadvisable to use it in the presence of high blood pressure, hardening of the arteries, impaired circulation within the brain, or coronary artery disease. This drug intensifies existing prostatism. Fluid retention is more prominent in this age group.

Advisability of Use During Pregnancy or If Breast-Feeding:

Pregnancy Category: C. Avoid using this drug completely if possible. Ask your doctor for guidance. Probably present in breast milk; avoid taking this drug or refrain from nursing.

▷ **Overdose Symptoms:**   Overstimulation, agitation, anxiety, restlessness, insomnia, confusion, delirium, hallucinations, seizures, high fever, circulatory collapse, coma.

▷ **Suggested Periodic Examinations While Taking This Drug:** (at doctor's discretion)

Blood pressure measurements in lying, sitting, and standing positions.

Complete blood cell counts, liver function tests.

▷ **While Taking This Drug the Following Apply:**

*Foods: **All tyramine-rich foods should be avoided completely**.*

Beverages: Limit coffee, tea, and cola beverages to one serving daily.

Alcohol: Use extreme caution until the combined effects have been determined. Alcohol can increase the depressant effects on brain function.

Other Drugs:

Phenelzine may *increase* the effects of

• amphetamines and related drugs.

• appetite suppressants.

• all drugs with stimulant effects on the nervous system, causing excessive rise in blood pressure.

• all drugs with sedative effects, causing excessive sedation.

• insulin.

• sulfonylureas (see Drug Classes) and perhaps other oral hypoglycemic agents.

Phenelzine *taken concurrently* with

• antihistamines (see Drug Classes) may worsen anticholinergic side effects of antihistamines.

• buspirone (BuSpar) may lead to undesirable increases in blood pressure.

• carbamazepine (Tegretol) may cause severe toxic reactions.

- dextromethorphan (as in many nonprescription cough medicines with a "DM" on the label) may cause severe toxic reactions. DO NOT COMBINE.
- fluoxetine (Prozac)—phenelzine combined with another medicine in this same class has resulted in fatal reactions. Avoid this combination.
- fluvoxamine (Luvox) and perhaps other serotonin reuptake inhibitors may result in serious reactions. DO NOT COMBINE.
- levodopa (Dopar, Sinemet) may cause a dangerous rise in blood pressure.
- meperidine (Demerol) may cause high fever, seizures, and coma.
- methyldopa (Aldomet) may cause a dangerous rise in blood pressure.
- methylphenidate (Ritalin) may cause severe headache, weakness, and numbness in the extremities.
- nadolol and perhaps other beta-blockers (see Drug Classes) may lead to serious decreases in heart rate.
- nefazodone (Serzone) may lead to serious adverse effects. DO NOT combine these medicines.
- paroxetine (Paxil) can lead to serious adverse effects. DO NOT combine these medicines.
- phenothiazines (see Drug Classes) may lead to exaggerated central nervous system effects.
- phenylpropanolamine (various) can lead to serious increases in blood pressure. DO NOT combine.
- tricyclic antidepressants may cause severe toxic reactions including high fever, delirium, tremor, seizures, and coma.
- venlafaxine (Effexor) may result in serious adverse reactions. DO NOT combine.

Note: Ask your doctor before taking *any other drugs* while taking phenelzine.

Driving, Hazardous Activities: May cause dizziness, drowsiness, and blurred vision. Restrict your activities as necessary.

Occurrence of Unrelated Illness: Because of the very serious and life-threatening interactions that can occur between this drug and many others, it is mandatory that you tell each doctor and dentist you visit that you are taking this drug.

Discontinuation: If this drug is not effective after 4 weeks of continual use, it should be discontinued. If it is effective, continue taking it in proper dosage until advised to stop. Do not discontinue it abruptly. If another antidepressant is tried, allow a drug-free waiting period of 14 days between the discontinuation of this drug and initiation of the new one. All precautions regarding the avoidance of tyramine-rich foods and other drugs must be observed during this 14-day period.

▷ **Saving Money When Using This Medicine:**
- A large number of drugs as well as several monoamine oxidase (MAO) inhibitors are available to treat depression. Ask your doctor to prescribe the drug that offers the best combination of cost and outcome.

PHENOBARBITAL   (fee noh BAR bi tawl)

Other Name: Phenobarbitone

Prescription Needed: Yes   **Controlled Drug:**   C-IV*   **Generic:**   Yes

Brand Names: Barbidonna [CD], Barbidonna Elixir [CD], Barbita, Belladenal [CD], Belladenal-S [CD], Bellergal-S [CD], Bronkotabs [CD], Bronkolixir [CD], Chardonna—2 [CD], Dilantin w/Phenobarbital [CD], Donnatal [CD], Kinesed [CD], Luminal, Mudrane GG Elixir & Tablets [CD], Mudrane Tablets [CD], Phenergan w/Codeine [CD], Quadrinal [CD], Solfoton, Tedral Preparations [CD]

Overview of BENEFITS versus RISKS

Possible Benefits	*Possible Risks*
EFFECTIVE CONTROL OF TONIC-CLONIC SEIZURES AND ALL TYPES OF PARTIAL SEIZURES	POTENTIAL FOR DEPENDENCE LIFE-THREATENING TOXICITY WITH OVERDOSAGE
EFFECTIVE CONTROL OF FEBRILE SEIZURES OF CHILDHOOD	Drug-induced hepatitis
Effective relief of anxiety and nervous tension	Rare blood cell disorders: abnormally low red cell, white cell, and platelet counts

---

▷ **Illness This Medication Treats:**
(1) Mild sedative in relief of anxiety, nervous tension, and insomnia—however, newer agents have fewer drug interactions or effects on sleep cycles; (2) anticonvulsant in control of grand mal epilepsy and all types of partial seizures. Also used to control febrile seizures of childhood.

As Combination Drug Product [CD]: This drug is available in many combinations with derivatives of belladonna, an antispasmodic commonly used to treat functional disorders of the gastrointestinal tract. It is also available in combination with bronchodilators for asthma, and with ergotamine for headaches.

▷ **Typical Dosage Range:** (Dosage or schedule must be determined by the doctor for each individual.)

*See Controlled Drug Schedules inside this book's cover.

As sedative: 15 to 30 mg two to four times a day. As hypnotic: 100 to 200 mg at bedtime. As anticonvulsant: 100 to 200 mg given as a single dose at bedtime. The total daily dosage should not exceed 600 mg. Some clinicians dose phenobarbital as 2–3 mg per kilogram of body weight in order to maintain a blood level of 15–40 mcg/ml.

▷ **Conditions Requiring Dosing Adjustments:**

Liver function: This drug should be used with caution and in decreased doses by patients with liver compromise. Blood levels should be obtained more frequently than for patients with normal liver function. Phenobarbital is a rare cause of toxicity.

Kidney function: This drug should be used with caution and in decreased doses by patients with compromised kidneys. Blood levels should be obtained at prudent intervals. Patients with alkaline urine will have more rapid elimination of this drug in the urine.

▷ **How Best to Take This Medicine:** May be taken with or after food to reduce stomach irritation. Regular tablets may be crushed and capsules opened for administration. Prolonged-action dosage forms should be swallowed whole without alteration.

▷ **How Long This Medicine Is Usually Taken:** Continual use on a regular schedule for 3 to 5 days is usually necessary to determine the effectiveness of this drug in relieving anxiety and tension, and for 4 to 6 weeks to determine its ability to control seizures. To treat anxiety-tension states, use should not exceed 4 weeks without reappraisal of continued need. Long-term use for seizure control (months to years) requires your doctor's supervision.

▷ **Tell Your Doctor Before Taking This Medicine If You:**
- ever had an allergic reaction to it.
- are subject to acute intermittent porphyria.
- are allergic or overly sensitive to any barbiturate.
- are pregnant or planning pregnancy.
- have a history of alcohol or drug abuse.
- are taking any drugs with sedative effects.
- have any type of seizure disorder or breathing problem.
- have myasthenia gravis or porphyria.
- have impaired liver, kidney, or thyroid gland function.
- plan to have surgery under general anesthesia soon.

▷ **Possible Side Effects:** Drowsiness, impaired concentration, mental and physical sluggishness.

▷ **Possible Adverse Effects:**

If any of the following develop, call your doctor promptly for guidance.

Some Mild Problems Drug Can Cause

Allergic reactions: skin rashes, localized swellings of face, drug fever.

Dizziness, unsteadiness, impaired vision, double vision.

Nausea, vomiting, diarrhea.

Shoulder-hand syndrome: pain and stiffness in the shoulder, pain and swelling in the hand.

Some Serious Problems Drug Can Cause

Allergic reactions: drug-induced hepatitis with jaundice.

Idiosyncratic reactions: paradoxical excitement and delirium (instead of sedation).

Mental depression, abnormal involuntary movements.

Blood cell disorders: deficiencies of all blood cell types causing fatigue, weakness, fever, sore throat, abnormal bleeding or bruising.

Dose-related breathing depression.

Rare kidney disease or vision problems.

▷ **Possible Effects on Sex Life:** Decreased libido and/or impotence. Decreased effectiveness of oral contraceptives taken concurrently.

▷ **Adverse Effects That May Mimic Natural Diseases or Disorders:** Liver reactions may suggest viral hepatitis.

▷ *CAUTION*

1. Anticonvulsant therapy must be carefully individualized. Accurate diagnosis and seizure pattern typing are critical for prescription of the best medications.

2. Emotional stress or physical trauma (including surgery) may require increased anticonvulsant dosage to control seizures.

3. Prolonged-action dosage forms are not appropriate for the treatment of seizures and should not be used.

4. This drug should not be given to the hyperkinetic child. Observe for possible paradoxical stimulation and hyperactivity; this can occur in 10 to 40% of children. Changes associated with puberty characteristically slow the metabolism of this drug and permit its gradual accumulation. Blood levels in young adolescents should be monitored every 3 months to detect rising concentrations and early toxicity. Adjust dosage as necessary.

5. The elderly should avoid usage of all barbiturates. If use of this drug is attempted, start with small doses until tolerance has been determined. Watch for confusion, delirium, agitation, and excitement. Do not use this drug concurrently with other drugs for mental disorders. This drug is conducive to the development of hypothermia.

Advisability of Use During Pregnancy or If Breast-Feeding:

Pregnancy Category: D. Avoid use of this drug during entire pregnancy if possible. If it is clearly needed to control seizures, the mother should receive vitamin K prior to delivery and the infant should receive it at birth. Present in breast milk in small amounts. Monitor the nursing infant closely and discontinue drug or nursing if adverse effects develop.

▷ **Habit-Forming Potential:** Psychological and physical dependence can occur with prolonged use of excessive doses—300 to 700 mg per day for 1 to 2 months. Dependence is not likely to occur with the usual sedative or anticonvulsant doses.

▷ **Overdose Symptoms:** Behavior similar to alcoholic intoxication: confusion, slurred speech, physical incoordination, staggering gait, drowsiness, stupor progressing to coma.

▷ **Suggested Periodic Examinations While Taking This Drug:** (at doctor's discretion)

For control of seizures, monitoring of blood phenobarbital levels to guide dosage. Time to sample blood for phenobarbital level: just before next dose. Recommended therapeutic ranges: For adults, 20–40 mcg/ml; for children, 15–30 mcg/ml.

Complete blood cell counts, liver function tests.

During long-term use: blood levels of folic acid, vitamin B12, calcium, and phosphorus; skeletal X-ray studies for bone demineralization.

▷ **While Taking This Drug the Following Apply:**

Foods: Eat liberally of foods rich in folic acid: fortified breakfast cereals, liver, legumes, green leafy vegetables.

Beverages: May be taken with milk or fruit juices.

Alcohol: Avoid completely. Alcohol can greatly increase the sedative and depressant actions of this drug on brain functions.

Tobacco Smoking: May enhance the sedative effects of this drug and increase drowsiness.

Marijuana Smoking: Increased drowsiness, unsteadiness; significantly impaired mental and physical performance.

Other Drugs:

Phenobarbital may *increase* the effects of

• all other drugs with sedative effects, causing excessive sedation.

Phenobarbital may *decrease* the effects of

• anticoagulants (Coumadin, etc.), requiring dosage adjustments.
• certain beta-blockers (Inderal, Lopressor), reducing their effectiveness.
• cortisonelike drugs.
• cyclosporine (Sandimmune).
• diltiazem (Cardizem)
• doxycycline (Vibramycin), reducing its effectiveness.
• griseofulvin (Fulvicin, etc.), reducing its effectiveness.
• metoprolol (Lopressor).
• oral contraceptives, reducing their effectiveness in preventing pregnancy.
• quinidine (Quinaglute, etc.), reducing its effectiveness.
• propranolol (Inderal).

- theophyllines (aminophylline, Theo-Dur, etc.), reducing their antiasthmatic effectiveness.
- verapamil (Calan), reducing its effectiveness.
- warfarin (Coumdin), requiring increased INR (prothrombin time) testing.

Phenobarbital *taken concurrently* with

- chloramphenicol (Chloromycetin) may blunt chloramphenicol's benefits.
- colestipol (Colestid) and other cholesterol-lowering resins may blunt phenobarbital's benefits.
- influenza (flu) vaccine may lead to phenobarbital toxicity.
- itraconazole (and perhaps other antifungals) may blunt the antifungal's therapeutic effect.
- phenytoin (Dilantin) may alter phenytoin blood levels: a high phenobarbital level will increase the phenytoin level; a low phenobarbital level will decrease the phenytoin level. Periodic determination of blood levels of both drugs is advised.
- primidone (Mysoline) may lead to phenobarbital toxicity.

The following drugs may *increase* the effects of phenobarbital

- ascorbic acid (vitamin C).
- felbamate (Felbatol).
- valproic acid (Depakene).

Driving, Hazardous Activities: May cause drowsiness and impair mental alertness, judgment, physical coordination, and reaction time. Restrict your activities as necessary.

Exposure to Sun: Use caution until your sensitivity has been determined; this drug may cause photosensitivity.

Exposure to Cold: Observe the elderly for possible hypothermia while taking this drug.

Discontinuation: If used as an anticonvulsant, this drug must not be discontinued abruptly. Sudden withdrawal can precipitate status epilepticus (repetitive seizures). Dosage should be reduced gradually over a period of 3 months. Total drug withdrawal may be attempted after a period of 3 to 5 years without a seizure. However, seizures are likely to recur in 40% of adults and in 20 to 30% of children.

▷ **Saving Money When Using This Medicine:**

- A large number of drugs are available that provide similar effectiveness. Ask your doctor to prescribe the drug that offers the best combination of cost and outcome.
- It may be possible (after a significant seizure-free period) to stop taking this medicine. Ask your doctor for help.
- Drug levels are expensive. Make sure they are drawn with prudent, not excessive, frequency.
- Generic forms may be substituted for the brand name.

PHENYTOIN (FEN i toh in)

Other Name: Diphenylhydantoin

Prescription Needed: Yes   **Controlled Drug:** No   **Generic:** Yes

Brand Names: Dilantin, Dilantin w/Phenobarbital [CD], Ekko-JR, Diphenylan

Overview of BENEFITS versus RISKS	
Possible Benefits	*Possible Risks*
EFFECTIVE CONTROL OF TONIC-CLONIC (GRAND MAL), PSYCHOMOTOR (TEMPORAL LOBE), MYOCLONIC, AND FOCAL SEIZURES	VERY NARROW TREATMENT MARGIN
	POSSIBLE BIRTH DEFECTS
	Overgrowth of gums
	Excessive hair growth
	Rare blood cell disorders: impaired production of all blood cells
	Drug-induced hepatitis
	Drug-induced nephritis

▷ **Illness This Medication Treats:**

Grand mal, psychomotor, myoclonic, and focal seizures.

Though not officially approved, this drug is also used to treat trigeminal neuralgia, relieving pain.

As Combination Drug Product [CD]: Available in combination with phenobarbital. Some seizure disorders require the combined actions of these two drugs for effective control.

▷ **Typical Dosage Range:** (Dosage or schedule must be determined by the doctor for each individual.)

Initially 100 mg three times a day. Dose may be increased cautiously by 100 mg/week as needed and tolerated. After the optimal maintenance dose has been determined, the total daily dose may be taken as a single dose every 24 hours if Dilantin capsules are used. No other formulation is approved for once-a-day use. The total daily dosage should not exceed 600 mg. Blood levels are needed.

▷ **Conditions Requiring Dosing Adjustments:**

Liver function: The maintenance dose should be decreased based on blood levels.

Kidney function: The dose or dosing interval must be adjusted for patients with moderate kidney compromise.

Obesity: Dose MUST be calculated on ideal (NOT actual) body weight. The product of 1.33 times the actual weight divided by the ideal weight is then added to the final loading dose.

▷ **How Best to Take This Medicine:**   May be taken with or after food to reduce stomach irritation. The capsule may be opened and the tablet may be crushed.

▷ **How Long This Medicine Is Usually Taken:**   Continual use on a regular schedule for 2 to 3 weeks is usually necessary to determine the effectiveness of this drug in reducing the frequency and severity of seizures. Optimal control requires careful dosage adjustments over a period of several months. Long-term use (months to years) requires ongoing physician supervision.

▷ **Tell Your Doctor Before Taking This Medicine If You:**
  • ever had an allergic reaction to this or other hydantoin drugs.
  • are taking any other drugs at this time.
  • have a history of liver disease or impaired liver function.
  • have low blood pressure, diabetes, or any type of heart disease.
  • plan to have surgery under general anesthesia soon.

▷ **Possible Side Effects:**   Mild fatigue, sluggishness, and drowsiness. Pink-red to brown coloration of urine (of no significance).

▷ **Possible Adverse Effects:**
If any of the following develop, call your doctor promptly for guidance.
Some Mild Problems Drug Can Cause
  Allergic reactions: skin rashes, drug fever.
  Headache, dizziness, nervousness, insomnia, muscle twitching.
  Nausea, vomiting, constipation.
  Joint pain or swelling.
  Overgrowth of gum tissues (most common in children).
  Excessive growth of body hair (most common in young girls).
Some Serious Problems Drug Can Cause
  Allergic reactions: drug-induced hepatitis, with or without jaundice.
    Drug-induced nephritis, with acute kidney failure. Severe skin reactions. Generalized enlargement of lymph glands.
  Idiosyncratic reaction: hemolytic anemia.
  Bone marrow depression: fatigue, fever, sore throat, abnormal bleeding or bruising.
  Mental confusion, unsteadiness, double vision, jerky eye movements, slurred speech.
  Rare drug-induced seizure, acute psychosis, low thyroid, myasthenia gravis, heart rhythm problems, porphyria, or myopathy.
  Elevated blood sugar, due to inhibition of insulin release.

▷ **Possible Effects on Sex Life:**   Decreased libido and/or impotence. Peyronie's disease.

Decreased effectiveness of oral contraceptives taken concurrently **and possible unwanted pregnancy.**

Rare swelling or tenderness of male breast tissue.

▷ **Adverse Effects That May Mimic Natural Diseases or Disorders:**
Drug-induced hepatitis may suggest viral hepatitis.

Skin reactions may resemble lupus erythematosus.

▷ *CAUTION*

1. Some brand-name capsules have a significantly longer duration of action than generic capsules of the same strength. To ensure a correct dosing schedule, it is necessary to distinguish between "prompt-" and "extended-action" capsules. Do not substitute one for the other without your doctor's knowledge and guidance.

2. When used for the treatment of epilepsy, *this drug must not be stopped abruptly.*

3. The wide variation of action from person to person requires careful individualization of dosage schedules. Periodic measurements of blood levels can be helpful in determining the appropriate dosage.

4. Regularity of drug use is essential for successful management of seizure disorders. Take this drug at the same time each day.

5. Shake the suspension form thoroughly before measuring the dose. Use a standard measuring device to ensure the dose is based on a 5-ml teaspoon.

6. Side effects and mild adverse effects are usually most apparent during the first several days of treatment, and often subside with continued use.

7. It may be necessary to take folic acid to prevent anemia while taking this drug. Talk with your doctor about this.

8. It is advisable to carry a personal identification card that states you are taking this drug.

9. Careful monitoring by periodic measurement of blood levels is essential for all ages. Some children require more than one daily dose for good control. Watch for early indications of toxicity: jerky eye movements, unsteadiness in stance and gait, slurred speech, abnormal involuntary movements of the extremities, and odd behavior.

10. This medicine is removed by the liver in a way that can only remove so much of the drug at a given time. If this pathway fills up, a small change in dose may result in a huge increase in level.

11. Those over 60 may be more sensitive to all of this drug's actions and require smaller doses. Look for signs of early toxicity: drowsiness, fatigue, confusion, unsteadiness, disturbances of vision, slurred speech, muscle twitching.

Advisability of Use During Pregnancy or If Breast-Feeding:
Pregnancy Category: D. Talk with your doctor about the advantages and possible disadvantages of use of this drug during pregnancy. It is advisable to use the smallest maintenance dose that will control seizures. In addition, take vitamin K during the last month of pregnancy to prevent a deficiency of blood clotting factors in the fetus. Present in breast milk in trace amounts. Monitor the nursing infant closely and discontinue the drug or nursing if adverse effects develop.

▷ **Overdose Symptoms:** Drowsiness, jerky eye movements, hand tremor, unsteadiness, slurred speech, hallucinations, delusions, nausea, vomiting, stupor progressing to coma.

▷ **Possible Effects of Long-Term Use:** Low blood calcium resulting in rickets or osteomalacia; megaloblastic anemia; peripheral neuropathy; schizophreniclike psychosis. Lymphosarcoma, malignant lymphoma, and leukemia have been associated with long-term use; no cause-and-effect relationship has been established.

▷ **Suggested Periodic Examinations While Taking This Drug:** (at doctor's discretion)
Monitoring of blood phenytoin levels to guide dosage. Time to sample blood for phenytoin level: just before the next dose. Recommended therapeutic range: 10–20 ng/ml.
Complete blood cell counts, liver function tests.
Measurements of the following blood levels: glucose, calcium, phosphorus, folic acid, vitamin B12.
Skeletal X-ray studies for bone demineralization.

▷ **While Taking This Drug the Following Apply:**
Nutritional Support: Supplements of folic acid, calcium, vitamin D, and vitamin K may be necessary.
Beverages: May be taken with milk.
Alcohol: Alcohol (in large quantities or with continual use) may reduce this drug's effectiveness in preventing seizures.

Other Drugs:
Phenytoin may *decrease* the effects of
- acetaminophen.
- conjugated estrogens (Premarin).
- cortisonelike drugs.
- cyclosporine (Sandimmune).
- doxycycline (Vibramycin, etc.).
- itraconazole (Sporanox).
- levodopa (Larodopa, Sinemet).
- levothyroxine.
- meperidine (Demerol).
- methadone (Dolophine).

- mexiletine (Mexitil).
- miconazole (Monistat, others).
- oral contraceptives (birth control pills).
- oral hypoglycemics (see Drug Classes).
- paroxetine (Paxil).
- quinidine (Quinaglute, etc.).

Phenytoin *taken concurrently* with

- oral anticoagulants (Coumadin, etc.) can either increase or decrease the anticoagulant effect; this combination should be closely checked with INR (prothrombin time) testing.
- carbamazepine (Tegretol) may increase or decrease blood levels of phenytoin.
- chlordiazepoxide (Librium) and perhaps other benzodiazepines (see Drug Classes) may change phenytoin blood levels. More frequent testing of blood levels is needed.
- ciprofloxacin (Cipro) may change phenytoin blood levels.
- dopamine can result in very low blood pressure.
- ketorolac (Toradol) may lead to seizures. DO NOT combine these medicines.
- primidone (Mysoline) may alter primidone's actions and enhance its toxicity.
- theophyllines (aminophylline, Theo-Dur, etc.) may decrease the effectiveness of both drugs.
- valproic acid (Depakene) may change levels of either medicines. More frequent checks of blood levels of both medicines are needed if the medicines are to be combined.
- warfarin (Coumadin) may change warfarin's effects. More frequent INR (prothrombin time) testing is needed.

The following drugs may *increase* the effects of phenytoin

- amiodarone (Cordarone).
- chloramphenicol (Chloromycetin).
- chlorpheniramine.
- cimetidine (Tagamet).
- co-trimoxazole (Bactrim).
- diltiazem (Cardizem).
- disulfiram (Antabuse).
- felbamate (Felbatol).
- fluconazole (Diflucan).
- fluoxetine (Prozac).
- fluvoxamine (Luvox).
- ibuprofen and perhaps other NSAIDs (see Drug Classes).
- isoniazid (INH, Niconyl, etc.).
- nifedipine (Adalat).
- omeprazole (Prilosec).
- phenacemide (Phenurone).

- phenylbutazone (Butazolidin).
- sulfonamides (see Drug Classes).
- tricyclic antidepressants (see Drug Classes).
- trimethoprim (Proloprim, Trimpex).
- valproic acid (Depakene).

The following drugs may *decrease* the effects of phenytoin

- bleomycin.
- carmustine.
- cisplatin.
- diazoxide.
- folic acid.
- methotrexate (Mexate).
- rifampin (Rifadin).
- vinblastine.

Driving, Hazardous Activities: May impair mental alertness, vision, and coordination. Restrict your activities as necessary.

Exposure to Sun: Use caution. This drug may cause photosensitivity.

Occurrence of Unrelated Illness: Intercurrent infections may slow elimination of this drug and increase the risk of toxicity due to higher blood levels.

Discontinuation: **This drug must not be stopped abruptly.** Sudden withdrawal can lead to severe and repeated seizures. If this drug is to be discontinued, gradual reduction in dosage should be made over a period of 3 months. Total drug withdrawal may be attempted after a period of 3 to 4 years without a seizure. However, seizures are likely to recur in 40% of adults and in 20 to 30% of children.

▷ **Saving Money When Using This Medicine:**

- A large number of drugs are available to treat seizures and pain syndromes. Ask your doctor to prescribe the drug that offers the best combination of cost and outcome.
- It may be possible (after a significant seizure-free period) to stop taking this medicine. Ask your doctor for help.
- Generic forms may be substituted for the brand name. If you change to a generic, tell your doctor. The amount absorbed may vary from form to form.
- Blood levels are expensive. Make sure levels are checked at prudent, not excessive, intervals.
- A new medicine called gabapentin has been useful in treating some chronic pain syndromes as well as add-on therapy for seizures. Talk to your doctor about this.

PILOCARPINE   (pi loh KAR peen)

Prescription Needed: Yes   **Controlled Drug:** No   **Generic:** Yes

Brand Names: Adsorbocarpine, Almocarpine, E-Pilo Preparations [CD], Isopto Carpine, Ocusert Pilo-20, -40, PE Preparations [CD], Pilagan, Pilocar, Salagen

---

Overview of BENEFITS versus RISKS

Possible Benefits	*Possible Risks*
EFFECTIVE REDUCTION OF INTERNAL EYE PRESSURE FOR CONTROL OF ACUTE AND CHRONIC GLAUCOMA	Mild side effects with systemic absorption Minor eye discomfort Altered vision

---

▷ **Illness This Medication Treats:**
  (1) Management of all types of glaucoma. Selection of the appropriate dosage form and strength must be carefully individualized. (2) Can be of help for dry mouth (xerostomia).
  As Combination Drug Product [CD]: This drug is combined with epinephrine (in eyedrop solutions) to utilize the actions of both drugs for lowering internal eye pressure. The opposite effects of these two drugs on the size of the pupil (pilocarpine constricts, epinephrine dilates) prevents excessive constriction or dilation.

▷ **Typical Dosage Range:** (Dosage or schedule must be determined by the doctor for each individual.)
  For chronic glaucoma: Eyedrop solutions —One drop of a 1 to 2% solution three to four times a day. Eye gel—Apply a 0.5-inch strip of gel into the eye once daily at bedtime; Ocusert—Insert one into the affected eye and replace every 7 days with a new one.

▷ **Conditions Requiring Dosing Adjustments:**
  Liver function: The specific elimination of this drug is unclear.
  Kidney function: The elimination of this drug has yet to be defined.

▷ **How Best to Take This Medicine:** To avoid excessive absorption into the body, press finger against inner corner of the eye (to close off the tear duct) during and for 2 minutes following instillation of the eyedrop. Place the gel and the Ocusert in the eye at bedtime.

▷ **How Long This Medicine Is Usually Taken:** Continual use on a regular schedule for 1 to 2 weeks is usually necessary to determine the effectiveness of this drug in controlling internal eye pressure. Long-term use (months to years) requires supervision and periodic evaluation by your doctor. See your doctor regularly.

▷ **Tell Your Doctor Before Taking This Medicine If You:**
- ever had an allergic reaction to it.
- have active bronchial asthma or a history of bronchial asthma.
- have a history of acute iritis.
- have gallstones, heart disease, or chronic obstructive pulmonary (lung) disease.

▷ **Possible Side Effects:** Temporary impairment of vision, usually lasting 2 to 3 hours following instillation of eyedrops.

▷ **Possible Adverse Effects:**
If any of the following develop, call your doctor promptly for guidance.
Some Mild Problems Drug Can Cause
Allergic reactions: itching of the eyes, itching and/or swelling of the eyelids.
Headache, heart palpitation, tremors.
Some Serious Problems Drug Can Cause
Provocation of acute asthma in susceptible individuals.
Rare retinal detachment or mental status changes.
Atrioventricular block (abnormal heart conduction).

▷ **Possible Effects on Laboratory Tests:** Red blood cell and white blood cell counts: increased.

▷ *CAUTION*
Maintaining personal cleanliness to prevent eye infections is especially important for those over 60 years of age. Report promptly any indication of possible infection involving the eyes.
Advisability of Use During Pregnancy or If Breast-Feeding:
Pregnancy Category: C. Limit use of this drug to the smallest effective dose. Minimize systemic absorption of this drug. This drug may be present in breast milk in small amounts. Monitor the nursing infant closely and discontinue taking this drug or nursing if adverse effects develop.

▷ **Overdose Symptoms:** Flushing of face, increased flow of saliva, sweating. If solution is swallowed: nausea, vomiting, diarrhea, profuse sweating, rapid pulse, difficult breathing, loss of consciousness.

▷ **Suggested Periodic Examinations While Taking This Drug:** (at doctor's discretion)
Measurement of internal eye pressure on a regular basis.
Examination of eyes for development of cataracts.

▷ **While Taking This Drug the Following Apply:**
Alcohol: Use caution until the combined effect has been determined. If this drug is absorbed, it may prolong the effect of alcohol on the brain.

Marijuana Smoking: Sustained additional decrease in internal eye pressure.

Other Drugs:

The following drugs may *decrease* the effects of pilocarpine
• atropine and drugs with atropinelike actions (see Drug Classes).

Pilocarpine *taken concurrently* with
• epinephrine will result in increased myopia.
• timolol can produce additive effects in treating glaucoma.

Driving, Hazardous Activities: May impair your ability to focus vision properly. Restrict your activities as necessary.

Discontinuation: Do not discontinue regular use of this drug without consulting your doctor. Periodic discontinuation and temporary substitution of another drug may be necessary to preserve this drug's effectiveness in treating glaucoma.

▷ **Saving Money When Using This Medicine:**
• Several drugs are available to treat glaucoma. Ask your doctor if this medicine offers the best balance of cost and outcome for you.
• A generic form can be substituted for the brand name.

PINDOLOL   (PIN doh lohl)

Prescription Needed: Yes   **Controlled Drug:** No   **Generic:** No

Brand Names: Visken

Overview of BENEFITS versus RISKS	
Possible Benefits	*Possible Risks*
EFFECTIVE, WELL-TOLERATED ANTIHYPERTENSIVE for mild to moderate high blood pressure	CONGESTIVE HEART FAILURE in advanced heart disease
	Worsening of angina in coronary heart disease (abrupt withdrawal)
	Masking of low blood sugar in drug-treated diabetes
	Provocation of asthma (with high doses)

▷ **Illness This Medication Treats:**
Mild to moderate high blood pressure, alone or with other medicines such as diuretics.

As Combination Drug Product [CD]: In Canada this drug is available in combination with hydrochlorothiazide. The addition of a thiazide diuretic to this beta-blocker enhances its antihypertensive effectiveness.

▷ **Typical Dosage Range:** (Dosage or schedule must be determined by the doctor for each individual.)

Initially 5 mg twice daily (12 hours apart). The dose may be increased gradually by 10 mg/day at intervals of 2 to 3 weeks, as needed and tolerated, up to 60 mg/day. For maintenance: 5 to 10 mg two or three times a day. The total daily dose should not exceed 60 mg.

▷ **Conditions Requiring Dosing Adjustments:**

Liver function: The dose should be decreased for patients with severe liver compromise and combined liver and kidney compromise.

Kidney function: Decrease dose if urine output is significantly decreased.

▷ **How Best to Take This Medicine:**   May be taken without regard to eating. The tablet may be crushed. Do not stop taking this medicine abruptly.

▷ **How Long This Medicine Is Usually Taken:**   Continual use on a regular schedule for 2 to 3 weeks is usually necessary to determine the effectiveness of this drug in lowering blood pressure. Long-term use (months to years) is determined by the course of your blood pressure over time and your response to the overall treatment program (weight reduction, salt restriction, smoking cessation, etc.). See your doctor regularly.

▷ **Tell Your Doctor Before Taking This Medicine If You:**

- ever had an allergic reaction to it.
- have congestive heart failure.
- have an abnormally slow heart rate or a serious form of heart block.
- are taking, or have taken within the past 14 days, any MAO type A inhibitor.
- have had an adverse reaction to any beta-blocker in the past.
- have a history of serious heart disease, with or without episodes of heart failure.
- have a history of hay fever (allergic rhinitis), asthma, chronic bronchitis, or emphysema.
- have a history of overactive thyroid function (hyperthyroidism).
- have a history of low blood sugar.
- have impaired liver or kidney function.
- have diabetes or myasthenia gravis.
- are currently taking any form of digitalis, quinidine, or reserpine, or any calcium blocker.
- plan to have surgery under general anesthesia soon.

▷ **Possible Side Effects:**   Lethargy and fatigability, cold extremities, slow heart rate, light-headedness in upright position.

▷ **Possible Adverse Effects:**

If any of the following develop, call your doctor promptly for guidance.

Some Mild Problems Drug Can Cause

Allergic reactions: skin rash, itching.

Headache, dizziness, insomnia, abnormal dreams.

Nausea, vomiting, constipation, diarrhea.

Joint and muscle discomfort, fluid retention (edema).

Some Serious Problems Drug Can Cause

Mental depression, anxiety.

Chest pain, shortness of breath, precipitation of congestive heart failure.

Induction of bronchial asthma (in asthmatic individuals).

Rare drug-induced lupus erythematosus.

Very rare carpal tunnel syndrome (reported with other medicines in the same class).

▷ **Possible Effects on Sex Life:** Decreased libido or impaired erection.

▷ *CAUTION*

1. ***Do not stop taking this drug suddenly*** without the knowledge and guidance of your doctor. Carry a personal identification card that states you are taking this drug.
2. Talk with your doctor or pharmacist before using nasal decongestants (usually present in over-the-counter cold preparations and nose drops). These can cause sudden increases in blood pressure when taken concurrently with beta-blockers.
3. Report the development of any tendency to emotional depression.
4. Safety and effectiveness of this drug for those under 12 years old have not been established. However, if this drug is used, observe for the development of low blood sugar during periods of reduced food intake.
5. Those over 60 should proceed *cautiously* with all antihypertensives. Unacceptably high blood pressure should be reduced without creating the risks associated with excessively low blood pressure. Start treatment with small doses, and monitor the blood pressure response frequently. Sudden, rapid, and excessive reduction of blood pressure can predispose to stroke or heart attack. Observe for dizziness, unsteadiness, tendency to fall, confusion, hallucinations, depression, or urinary frequency.

Advisability of Use During Pregnancy or If Breast-Feeding:

Pregnancy Category: B. Use this drug only if clearly needed. Ask your doctor for guidance. Present in breast milk; avoid taking this drug or refrain from nursing.

▷ **Overdose Symptoms:** Weakness, slow pulse, low blood pressure, fainting, cold and sweaty skin, congestive heart failure, possible coma, and convulsions.

▷ **Suggested Periodic Examinations While Taking This Drug:** (at doctor's discretion)
Measurements of blood pressure, evaluation of heart function.

▷ **While Taking This Drug the Following Apply:**
Foods: Avoid excessive salt intake.
Beverages: May be taken with milk.
Alcohol: Use with caution until the combined effect has been determined. Alcohol may exaggerate pindolol's ability to lower the blood pressure and increase its mild sedative effect.
Tobacco Smoking: Nicotine may reduce this drug's effectiveness in treating high blood pressure. In addition, high doses may potentiate the constriction of the bronchial tubes caused by regular smoking.
Other Drugs:
Pindolol may *increase* the effects of
- other antihypertensives, causing excessive lowering of the blood pressure. Dosage adjustments may be necessary.
- reserpine (Ser-Ap-Es, etc.), causing sedation, depression, slowing of the heart rate, and lowering of the blood pressure.
- verapamil (Calan, Isoptin), causing excessive depression of heart function; monitor this combination closely.

Pindolol *taken concurrently* with
- amiodarone (Cordarone) may cause extremely slow heartbeats and risk of cardiac arrest.
- clonidine (Catapres) requires close monitoring for rebound high blood pressure if clonidine is withdrawn while pindolol is still being taken.
- epinephrine may result in a large increase in blood pressure and change in heart rate.
- fluoxetine (Prozac) can lead to increased risk of pindolol toxicity.
- fluvoxamine (Luvox) may lead to pindolol toxicity.
- insulin requires close monitoring to avoid undetected hypoglycemia.
- oral hypoglycemic agents (see Drug Classes) may slow recovery from any lowered blood sugar that occurs.
- phenylpropanolamine may lead to serious increases in blood pressure. Avoid this combination.
- venlafaxine (Effexor) may lead to beta-blocker or venlafaxine toxicity. It is best to avoid this combination, or reduce doses of both medicines if they are combined.

The following drugs may *increase* the effects of pindolol

- cimetidine (Tagamet).
- methimazole (Tapazole).
- oral contraceptives (birth control pills).
- propylthiouracil (Propacil).

The following drugs may *decrease* the effects of pindolol

- barbiturates (phenobarbital, etc.).
- indomethacin (Indocin), and possibly other aspirin substitutes (NSAIDs); these may impair pindolol's antihypertensive effect.
- rifampin (Rifadin, Rimactane).
- theophylline (Theo-Dur, others).

Driving, Hazardous Activities: Use caution until the full extent of fatigue, dizziness, and blood pressure change have been determined.

Exposure to Heat: Caution is advised. Hot environments can lower the blood pressure and exaggerate the effects of this drug.

Exposure to Cold: Caution is advised. Cold environments can enhance circulatory deficiency in the extremities. The elderly should take precautions to prevent hypothermia.

Heavy Exercise or Exertion: Avoid exertion that produces light-headedness, excessive fatigue, or muscle cramping. This drug may intensify the hypertensive response to isometric exercise.

Occurrence of Unrelated Illness: The fever that accompanies systemic infections can lower the blood pressure and require an adjustment of dosage. Illnesses that cause nausea or vomiting may interrupt the regular dosage schedule. Ask your doctor for guidance.

Discontinuation: Avoid sudden discontinuation of this drug in all situations. If possible, gradual reduction of dose over a period of 2 to 3 weeks is recommended. Ask your doctor for specific guidance.

▷ **Saving Money When Using This Medicine:**

- Many drugs are available to treat high blood pressure. Ask your doctor if this medicine offers the best balance of cost and outcome for you. Ask how often your blood pressure should be checked.
- Talk with your doctor about the benefits and risks of taking aspirin every other day to help prevent heart attacks.
- Ask your doctor about available stress management and exercise programs in your community.

PIRBUTEROL (peer BYU ter ohl)

Prescription Needed: Yes   **Controlled Drug:** No   **Generic:** No

Brand Name: Maxair

```
┌─────────────────────────────────────────────────────────┐
│           Overview of BENEFITS versus RISKS              │
│      Possible Benefits              Possible Risks       │
│   VERY EFFECTIVE RELIEF OF    Increased blood pressure   │
│      BRONCHOSPASM             Nervousness                │
│                               Fine hand tremor           │
│                               Irregular heart rhythm (with│
│                                  excessive use)          │
└─────────────────────────────────────────────────────────┘
```

▷ **Illness This Medication Treats:**
   (1) Eases acute attacks of bronchial asthma; (2) reduces the frequency
   and severity of chronic, recurrent asthmatic attacks (prevention);
   (3) relieves reversible bronchospasm seen in chronic bronchitis,
   bronchiectasis, and emphysema.

▷ **Typical Dosage Range:** (Dosage or schedule must be determined by
   the doctor for each individual.)
   Inhaler: One to two inhalations (200–400 mcg) every 4 to 6 hours. **Do
   not exceed** 12 inhalations (2400 mcg) every 24 hours. Oral: 10 to 15
   mg three to four times daily. Maximum dose is 60 mg daily.

▷ **Conditions Requiring Dosing Adjustments:**
   Liver function: This drug should be used with caution by patients with
   liver compromise who use it frequently. Guidelines for dosage adjustments are not available.

▷ **How Best to Take This Medicine:**   Carefully follow the instructions
   for use provided with the inhaler. Do not overuse.

▷ **How Long This Medicine Is Usually Taken:**   According to individual requirements. Do not use beyond the time necessary to terminate episodes of asthma.

▷ **Tell Your Doctor Before Taking This Medicine If You:**
   • ever had an allergic reaction to it.
   • currently have an irregular heart rhythm.
   • are taking, or have taken within the past 2 weeks, any MAO type A
     inhibitor.
   • have any type of heart or circulatory disorder, especially high blood
     pressure, coronary heart disease, or heart rhythm abnormality.
   • have diabetes or hyperthyroidism.
   • have any type of seizure disorder.
   • are taking any form of digitalis or stimulant.

▷ **Possible Side Effects:**   Aerosol—dryness or irritation of mouth or
   throat, altered taste.

▷ **Possible Adverse Effects:**
   If any of the following develop, call your doctor promptly for guidance.

Some Mild Problems Drug Can Cause
Allergic reactions: skin rash, itching.
Headache, dizziness, fine hand tremor.
Palpitations, rapid heart rate, chest pain, cough.
Nausea, diarrhea.

Some Serious Problems Drug Can Cause
Irregular heart rhythm, increased blood pressure.

▷ **CAUTION**

1. Concurrent use by inhalation with beclomethasone aerosol (Beclovent, Vanceril) may increase the risk of toxicity due to fluorocarbon propellants. It is advisable to use pirbuterol aerosol 20 to 30 minutes *before* beclomethasone aerosol, to reduce the risk of toxicity and enhance the penetration of beclomethasone.

2. Excessive or prolonged use by inhalation can reduce this drug's effectiveness and cause serious heart rhythm disturbances, including cardiac arrest.

3. Safety and effectiveness of this drug in children under 12 years old have not been established.

4. Those over 60 should avoid excessive and continual use. If acute asthma is not relieved promptly, other drugs will have to be tried. Watch for nervousness, palpitations, irregular heart rhythm, and muscle tremors.

Advisability of Use During Pregnancy or If Breast-Feeding:
Pregnancy Category: C. Avoid use of this drug during the first 3 months if possible. Presence in breast milk is unknown; avoid taking this drug or refrain from nursing.

▷ **Overdose Symptoms:** Nervousness, palpitation, rapid heart rate, sweating, headache, tremor, vomiting, chest pain.

▷ **While Taking This Drug the Following Apply:**
Beverages: Avoid excessive use of caffeine-containing beverages—coffee, tea, cola, chocolate.

Other Drugs:
Pirbuterol *taken concurrently* with

• albuterol (Proventil, Ventolin) may increase the risk of adverse heart effects.

• MAO type A inhibitors may cause an excessive increase in blood pressure and undesirable heart stimulation.

• phenothiazines (see Drug Classes) may lessen the therapeutic benefits of pirbuterol.

Driving, Hazardous Activities: Use caution if excessive nervousness or dizziness occurs.

Heavy Exercise or Exertion: Use caution. Excessive exercise can induce asthma in sensitive individuals.

▷ **Saving Money When Using This Medicine:**
• A large number of drugs are available to treat asthma. Ask your doc-

tor to prescribe the drug that offers the best combination of cost and outcome.

- It may be possible (after a significant asthma-free period) to stop taking this medicine. Ask your doctor for help.
- Talk with your doctor about the usage of nebulized lidocaine for asthma.

PIROXICAM (peer OX i kam)

Prescription Needed: Yes   **Controlled Drug:** No   **Generic:** Yes

Brand Names: Feldene

Overview of BENEFITS versus RISKS	
Possible Benefits	*Possible Risks*
EFFECTIVE RELIEF OF MILD TO MODERATE PAIN AND INFLAMMATION	Gastrointestinal pain, ulceration, bleeding Drug-induced hepatitis (rare) Kidney damage (rare) Mild fluid retention Reduced white blood cell and platelet counts

See the oxicams (NSAIDs) drug profile for further information.

PRAVASTATIN (pra vah STA tin)

Prescription Needed: Yes   **Controlled Drug:** No   **Generic:** No

Brand Name: Pravachol

Overview of BENEFITS versus RISKS	
Possible Benefits	*Possible Risks*
EFFECTIVE REDUCTION OF TOTAL BLOOD CHOLESTEROL AND LDL CHOLESTEROL DECREASES THE NUMBER OF FIRST-TIME HEART ATTACKS DECREASES THE NUMBER OF PATIENT DEATHS	Drug-induced hepatitis, without jaundice Drug-induced myositis

▷ **Illness This Medication Treats:**

(1) High total blood cholesterol levels (in people with Types IIa and IIb hypercholesterolemia) due to increased fractions of low-density lipoprotein (LDL) cholesterol, in conjunction with a cholesterol-lowering diet. Pravastatin should not be used until an adequate trial of nondrug cholesterol-lowering methods has proved to be ineffective. (2) USED TO PREVENT A FIRST HEART ATTACK and reduce deaths from cardiovascular disease in people with increased blood cholesterol who are at risk of a first heart attack.

▷ **Typical Dosage Range:** (Dosage or schedule must be determined by the doctor for each individual.)

Infants and Children: Under 2 years: Do not use this drug.

2 to 18 years: Dosage not established.

18 to 60 Years of Age: Initially 10 to 40 mg daily (depending on cholesterol level), taken at bedtime. Maintenance dosage is 10 to 20 mg daily; adjust as needed and tolerated, at intervals of 4 weeks.

Over 60 Years of Age: Same as for 18 to 60 years of age.

▷ **Conditions Requiring Dosing Adjustments:**

Liver function: This drug should be used with caution by patients with liver compromise, and the starting dose should be decreased to 10 mg/day. Pravastatin is contraindicated for patients with acute liver disease.

Kidney function: Patients with significant renal compromise can take a starting dose of 10 mg/day. This drug should be used with caution by patients with renal compromise.

▷ **How Best to Take This Medicine:** Can be taken without regard to eating, preferably at bedtime (the highest rates of cholesterol production occur between midnight and 5 A.M.). The tablet may be crushed for administration.

▷ **How Long This Medicine Is Usually Taken:** Continual use on a regular schedule for 4 to 6 weeks is usually necessary to determine the effectiveness of this drug in reducing blood levels of total and LDL cholesterol. Long-term use (months to years) requires periodic evaluation of response and dosage adjustment. See your doctor regularly.

▷ **Tell Your Doctor Before Taking This Medicine If You:**

- ever had an allergic reaction to it.
- have active liver disease.
- are pregnant or breast-feeding, are not using any method of birth control, or are planning pregnancy.
- previously took any other drugs in this class: lovastatin (Mevacor), simvastatin (Zocor).
- have a history of liver disease or impaired liver function.

- have unexplained muscle weakness or tenderness.
- regularly consume substantial amounts of alcohol.
- have cataracts or impaired vision.
- have any type of chronic muscular disorder.
- plan to have major surgery in the near future.

▷ **Possible Side Effects:**   Development of abnormal liver function tests without associated symptoms.

▷ **Possible Adverse Effects:**
If any of the following develop, call your doctor promptly for guidance.
Some Mild Problems Drug Can Cause
Allergic reactions: skin rash, itching.
Headache, dizziness.
Indigestion, stomach pain, nausea, excessive gas, constipation, diarrhea.
Muscle cramps and/or pain.
Some Serious Problems Drug Can Cause
Marked and persistent abnormal liver function tests with focal hepatitis.
Acute myositis (muscle pain and tenderness).
Rare lowering of white blood cells or nerve damage.

▷ *CAUTION*
1. If pregnancy occurs while taking this drug, discontinue it immediately and call your doctor.
2. Report promptly any development of muscle pain or tenderness, especially if accompanied by fever or malaise.
3. Report promptly altered or impaired vision so that an appropriate evaluation can be made.
4. Safety and effectiveness of this drug for those under 18 years old have not been established.
5. Those over 60 should tell their doctor about any personal or family history of cataracts. Comply with all recommendations regarding periodic eye examinations. Report promptly any alterations in vision.
6. This drug dose must be decreased for patients with liver compromise and should NOT be used by people with acute liver disease.

Advisability of Use During Pregnancy or If Breast-Feeding:
Pregnancy Category: X. This drug should be avoided during entire pregnancy. Present in breast milk in small amounts; avoid taking this drug or refrain from nursing.

▷ **Overdose Symptoms:**   Increased indigestion, stomach distress, nausea, diarrhea.

▷ **Suggested Periodic Examinations While Taking This Drug:** (at doctor's discretion)

Blood cholesterol studies: total cholesterol, HDL and LDL fractions.

Liver function tests before treatment, every 6 weeks during the first 3 months of use, every 8 weeks for the rest of the first year, and at 6-month intervals thereafter.

Complete eye examination at beginning of treatment and any time a significant change in vision occurs. Ask your doctor for guidance.

▷ **While Taking This Drug the Following Apply:**

Foods: Follow a standard low-cholesterol diet.

Beverages: May be taken with milk.

Alcohol: No interactions expected. Use sparingly.

Other Drugs:

Pravastatin *taken concurrently* with

- clofibrate (Atromid-S) has been associated with muscle damage.
- cyclosporine (Sandimmune) increases the risk of muscle damage.
- gemfibrozil (Lopid) may alter the absorption and excretion of pravastatin; these should not be taken concurrently.
- warfarin (Coumadin) increases the risk of bleeding. More frequent INR (prothrombin time) testing is needed.

The following drug may *decrease* the effects of pravastatin

- cholestyramine (Questran) may reduce absorption of pravastatin; take pravastatin 1 hour before or 4 hours after cholestyramine.

Driving, Hazardous Activities: May cause dizziness. Restrict your activities as necessary.

Discontinuation: Do not discontinue this drug without your doctor's knowledge and guidance. Blood cholesterol levels may increase significantly following discontinuation.

▷ **Saving Money When Using This Medicine:**

- A large number of available drugs lower cholesterol. Ask your doctor to prescribe the drug that offers the best combination of cost and outcome.
- Talk with your doctor about taking aspirin every other day to help prevent a heart attack.

PRAZOSIN (PRA zoh sin)

Prescription Needed: Yes   **Controlled Drug:** No   **Generic:** Yes

Brand Names: Minipress, Minizide [CD]

Overview of BENEFITS versus RISKS

Possible Benefits	*Possible Risks*
EFFECTIVE INITIAL THERAPY FOR MILD TO MODERATE HYPERTENSION	First-dose drop in blood pressure, with fainting
EFFECTIVE IN COMBINATION THERAPY OF MODERATE TO SEVERE HYPERTENSION	Induction of paroxysmal tachycardia
EFFECTIVE CONTROL OF HYPERTENSION IN PHEOCHROMOCYTOMA	
Effective in presence of impaired kidney function	
REDUCES BENIGN PROSTATIC HYPERPLASIA	

▷ **Illness This Medication Treats:**

(1) Mild to moderate hypertension; (2) also used in conjunction with other drugs to treat moderate to severe hypertension; (3) benign prostatic hyperplasia.

▷ **Typical Dosage Range:** (Dosage or schedule must be determined by the doctor for each individual.)

Hypertension: Usually a test dose of 1 mg is taken to determine the patient's response within the first 2 hours. If this is tolerated satisfactorily, the dose is cautiously increased up to 15 mg/24 hr in two or three divided doses. The total daily dosage should not exceed 20 mg.

Benign prostatic hyperplasia: Starting dose is 0.5 mg to 1 mg twice daily. The dose is increased as needed or tolerated up to 2 mg twice daily.

▷ **Conditions Requiring Dosing Adjustments:**

Liver function: This drug should be used with caution and in lower doses by patients with liver compromise.

Kidney function: Small starting doses may achieve the same effect as larger doses for patients with compromised kidneys.

▷ **How Best to Take This Medicine:** May be taken without regard to food. The capsule may be opened.

▷ **How Long This Medicine Is Usually Taken:** Continual use on a regular schedule for 4 to 6 weeks is usually necessary to determine the effectiveness of this drug in controlling hypertension. Long-term use (months to years) requires physician supervision.

▷ **Tell Your Doctor Before Taking This Medicine If You:**
- ever had an allergic reaction to it.
- are experiencing mental depression, or have a history of mental depression.
- have angina (active coronary artery disease) and are not taking a beta-blocker.
- have experienced orthostatic hypotension when using other antihypertensives.
- have impaired circulation to the brain, or a history of stroke.
- have coronary artery disease.
- have active liver disease or impaired liver function.
- plan to have surgery under general anesthesia soon.

▷ **Possible Side Effects:** Orthostatic hypotension, drowsiness, salt and water retention, dry mouth, nasal congestion, constipation.

▷ **Possible Adverse Effects:**
If any of the following develop, call your doctor promptly for guidance.
Some Mild Problems Drug Can Cause
Allergic reactions: skin rash, itching.
Headache, dizziness, fatigue, nervousness, sweating, numbness and tingling, blurred vision, reddened eyes, ringing in the ears. Sleep disturbance.
Palpitation, rapid heart rate, shortness of breath.
Nausea, vomiting, diarrhea, abdominal pain.
Urinary frequency and incontinence.
Some Serious Problems Drug Can Cause
Mental depression.
Paroxysmal tachycardia (heart rates of 120–160 beats/min).

▷ **Possible Effects on Sex Life:** Decreased libido; impotence. Retrograde ejaculation. Priapism.

▷ *CAUTION*
1. Watch for a possible first-dose response of a precipitous drop in blood pressure, with or without fainting, usually within 30 to 90 minutes. Limit initial doses to 1 mg taken at bedtime for the first 3 days; remain supine after taking these trial doses.
2. Impaired kidney function may increase your sensitivity to this drug and require smaller than usual doses.
3. Safety and effectiveness of this drug for those under 12 years old have not been established
4. Those over 60 should start therapy with no more than 1 mg/day for the first 3 days. Subsequent dose increases must be very gradual and carefully supervised. The occurrence of orthostatic hypotension can cause unexpected falls and injury; sit or lie down

promptly if you feel light-headed or dizzy. Report any indications of dizziness or chest pain promptly.

Advisability of Use During Pregnancy or If Breast-Feeding:

Pregnancy Category: C. Use this drug only if clearly needed. Ask your doctor for guidance. Present in breast milk in small amounts. Monitor the nursing infant closely and discontinue taking this drug or nursing if adverse effects develop.

▷ **Overdose Symptoms:** Orthostatic hypotension, headache, generalized flushing, rapid heart rate, extreme weakness, irregular heart rhythm, circulatory collapse.

▷ **While Taking This Drug the Following Apply:**

Foods: Avoid excessive salt intake.

Beverages: May be taken with milk.

Alcohol: Use with extreme caution until the combined effects have been determined. Alcohol can cause excessive reduction in blood pressure.

Tobacco Smoking: Nicotine can significantly worsen this drug's ability to intensify coronary insufficiency in susceptible individuals. All forms of tobacco should be avoided.

Other Drugs:

The following drugs may *increase* the effects of prazosin

• other medicines for high blood pressure (often used to help).

• beta-adrenergic—blockers; the severity and duration of the first-dose hypotensive response may be increased.

• verapamil (Calan) may increase blood levels of prazosin and require decreased doses.

Prazosin *taken concurrently* with

• NSAIDs (see Drug Classes) may blunt the blood pressure–lowering effect of prazosin.

Driving, Hazardous Activities: May cause dizziness or drowsiness. Restrict your activities as necessary.

Exposure to Cold: Use caution until combined effect has been determined. Cold environments may increase prazosin's ability to cause coronary insufficiency (angina) in susceptible individuals.

Heavy Exercise or Exertion: Excessive exertion can augment this drug's ability to induce angina.

Discontinuation: If this drug is part of your treatment program for congestive heart failure, do not discontinue it abruptly. Ask your doctor for guidance.

▷ **Saving Money When Using These Medicines:**

• Many medicines are available to treat high blood pressure. Ask your doctor to start you on the least expensive drug in the class that is most appropriate for you. Ask how often your blood pressure should be checked.

- A generic form can be substituted for the brand name.
- Talk with your doctor about stress management and exercise programs available in your community.
- Ask if taking aspirin every other day could help prevent a heart attack for you.

PREDNISOLONE (pred NIS oh lohn)

Prescription Needed: Yes   **Controlled Drug:** No   **Generic:** Yes

Brand Names: Blephamide, Cortalone, Econopred Ophthalmic, Pred-G [CD], Prelone

Overview of BENEFITS versus RISKS	
Possible Benefits	*Possible Risks*
EFFECTIVE RELIEF OF SYMPTOMS IN A WIDE VARIETY OF INFLAMMATORY AND ALLERGIC DISORDERS	Short-term use (up to 10 days) is usually well tolerated
EFFECTIVE IMMUNOSUPPRESSION in selected benign and malignant disorders	Long-term use (exceeding 2 weeks) is associated with many possible adverse effects: ALTERED MOOD AND PERSONALITY; CATARACTS; GLAUCOMA; HYPERTENSION;
Prevention of rejection in organ transplantation	OSTEOPOROSIS; ASEPTIC BONE NECROSIS; INCREASED SUSCEPTIBILITY TO INFECTIONS

▷ **Illness This Medication Treats:**
(1) A wide variety of allergic and inflammatory conditions; most commonly used in management of serious skin disorders, asthma, regional enteritis, ulcerative colitis, and all types of major rheumatic disorders including bursitis, tendonitis, most forms of arthritis, and inflammatory eye conditions; (2) part of combination therapy of lymphoma; (3) symptoms of ulcerative colitis.

▷ **Typical Dosage Range:** (Dosage or schedule must be determined by the doctor for each individual.)
Oral form: 5 to 60 mg daily as a single dose or in divided doses. The total daily dosage should not exceed 250 mg. Dose should be lowered to the lowest effective dose.
Ophthalmic form: One to two drops placed (instilled) into the eye sac every 3 to 12 hours. Rarely increased to once every hour.

▷ **Conditions Requiring Dosing Adjustments:**

Kidney function: Dosing adjustments for patients with renal compromise do not appear to be needed. This drug can cause proteinuria, and the use of prednisolone by patients with protein-losing renal compromise (nephropathy) may require a benefit-to-risk decision.

▷ **How Best to Take This Medicine:**   Take with or following food to prevent stomach irritation, preferably in the morning. The tablet may be crushed.

▷ **How Long This Medicine Is Usually Taken:**   For acute disorders: 4 to 10 days. For chronic disorders: according to individual requirements. The duration of use should not exceed the time necessary to obtain adequate symptomatic relief in acute self-limiting conditions, or the time required to stabilize a chronic condition and permit gradual withdrawal. Its intermediate duration of action makes this drug appropriate for alternate-day administration. See your doctor regularly.

▷ **While Taking This Drug the Following Apply:**

Other Drugs:

Prednisolone may *decrease* the effects of
- isoniazid (INH, Niconyl, etc.).
- salicylates (aspirin, sodium salicylate, etc.).

Prednisolone *taken concurrently* with
- oral anticoagulants may either increase or decrease their effectiveness; consult your doctor regarding the need for prothrombin time testing and dosage adjustment.

The following drugs may *decrease* the effects of prednisolone
- antacids; may reduce its absorption.
- barbiturates (Amytal, Butisol, phenobarbital, etc.).
- phenytoin (Dilantin, etc.).
- rifampin (Rifadin, Rimactane, etc.).

▷ **Author's Note:**   The information categories provided in this profile are appropriate for prednisolone. Refer to the following profile of prednisone for information that has been omitted. A derivative of prednisone, prednisolone shares its significant actions and effects.

PREDNISONE   (PRED ni sohn)

Prescription Needed: Yes   **Controlled Drug:** No   **Generic:** Yes

Brand Names: Deltasone, Meticorten, Orasone

Overview of BENEFITS versus RISKS

Possible Benefits	*Possible Risks*
EFFECTIVE RELIEF OF SYMPTOMS IN A WIDE VARIETY OF INFLAMMATORY AND ALLERGIC DISORDERS	Short-term use (up to 10 days) is usually well tolerated
EFFECTIVE IMMUNOSUPPRESSION in selected benign and malignant disorders	Long-term use (exceeding 2 weeks) is associated with many possible adverse effects: ALTERED MOOD AND PERSONALITY; CATARACTS; GLAUCOMA; HYPERTENSION; OSTEOPOROSIS; ASEPTIC BONE NECROSIS; INCREASED SUSCEPTIBILITY TO INFECTIONS
Prevention of organ transplantation rejection	

▷ **Illness This Medicine Treats:**   (1) A wide variety of allergic and inflammatory conditions; serious skin disorders, asthma, regional enteritis, ulcerative colitis, gout, lupus erythematosus, and all types of major rheumatic disorders including bursitis, tendonitis, and most forms of arthritis; (2) combination therapy of lymphoma; (3) insufficient function of the adrenal gland; (4) combination therapy of several kinds of leukemia; (5) helps kidney transplant patients; (6) multiple sclerosis.

▷ **Typical Dosage Range:** (Dosage or schedule must be determined by the doctor for each individual.)
5 to 60 mg daily as a single dose or in divided doses. The total daily dosage should not exceed 250 mg.

▷ **Conditions Requiring Dosing Adjustments:**
Kidney function: Dosing adjustments for patients with kidney compromise do not appear to be needed. This drug is a possible cause of proteinuria and its use by patients with protein-losing renal compromise (nephropathy) may require a benefit-to-risk decision.

▷ **How Best to Take This Medicine:**   Take with or following food to prevent stomach irritation, preferably in the morning. The tablet may be crushed for administration.

▷ **How Long This Medicine Is Usually Taken:**   For acute disorders: 4 to 10 days. For chronic disorders: according to individual requirements. The duration of use should not exceed the time necessary to obtain adequate symptomatic relief in acute self-limiting conditions or to stabilize a chronic condition and permit gradual withdrawal. Its intermediate duration of action makes this drug appropriate for alternate-day administration. See your doctor regularly.

▷ **Tell Your Doctor Before Taking This Medicine If You:**
- ever had an allergic reaction to it.
- have active peptic ulcer disease.
- have an active infection of the eye caused by the herpes simplex virus.
- have active tuberculosis.
- had an unfavorable reaction to any cortisonelike drug in the past.
- have osteoporosis.
- have a history of peptic ulcer disease, thrombophlebitis, or tuberculosis.
- have diabetes, glaucoma, high blood pressure, diverticulitis, deficient thyroid function, or myasthenia gravis.
- plan to have surgery of any kind soon.

▷ **Possible Side Effects:**   Increased appetite, weight gain, retention of salt and water, excretion of potassium, increased susceptibility to infection.

▷ **Possible Adverse Effects:**
If any of the following develop, call your doctor promptly for guidance.
Some Mild Problems Drug Can Cause
Allergic reaction: skin rash.
Headache, dizziness, insomnia.
Acid indigestion, abdominal distention.
Muscle cramping and weakness.
Acne, excessive growth of facial hair.
Some Serious Problems Drug Can Cause
Mental and emotional disturbances of serious magnitude.
Reactivation of latent tuberculosis.
Development of peptic ulcer.
Increased blood pressure or blood sugar.
Development of inflammation of pancreas.
Thrombophlebitis—pain or tenderness in thigh or leg.
Pulmonary embolism—sudden shortness of breath, chest pain, coughing, bloody sputum.
Bone necrosis.
Rare Kaposi's sarcoma or low blood platelets.

▷ **Possible Effects on Sex Life:**   Altered timing and pattern of menstruation.
Correction of male infertility when due to autoantibodies that suppress sperm activity.

▷ **Adverse Effects That May Mimic Natural Diseases or Disorders:**
Pattern of symptoms and signs resembling Cushing's syndrome.

▷ *CAUTION*

1. It is prudent to carry a personal identification card that states you are taking this drug, if your course of treatment is to exceed 1 week.

2. Do not stop taking this drug abruptly if you are using it for long-term treatment.

3. If vaccination against measles, rabies, smallpox, or yellow fever is required, discontinue this drug 72 hours before vaccination, and do not resume it for at least 14 days after vaccination.

4. Avoid prolonged use of prednisone in infants and children if possible. During long-term use, observe for suppression of normal growth and the possibility of increased intracranial pressure. Following long-term use, the child may be at risk for adrenal gland deficiency during stress for as long as 18 months after cessation.

5. Cortisonelike drugs should be used very sparingly by those over 60, and only when the disorder is unresponsive to adequate trials of unrelated drugs. Avoid prolonged use. Continual use (even in small doses) can increase the severity of diabetes, enhance fluid retention, raise blood pressure, weaken resistance to infection, induce stomach ulcer, and accelerate development of cataracts and osteoporosis.

Advisability of Use During Pregnancy or If Breast-Feeding:

Pregnancy Category: B or C. Avoid using this drug completely during the first 3 months. Limit use during the last 6 months as much as possible. If this drug is used, examine the infant for possible deficiency of adrenal gland function. Present in breast milk; avoid taking this drug or refrain from nursing.

▷ **Habit-Forming Potential:** Use of this drug to suppress symptoms over an extended period may produce a state of functional dependence. In the treatment of conditions such as asthma and rheumatoid arthritis, keep the dose as small as possible and attempt withdrawal after periods of reasonable improvement. Such procedures may reduce the degree of steroid rebound—the return of symptoms as the drug is withdrawn.

▷ **Overdose Symptoms:** Fatigue, muscle weakness, stomach irritation, acid indigestion, excessive sweating, facial flushing, fluid retention, swelling of extremities, increased blood pressure.

▷ **Suggested Periodic Examinations While Taking This Drug:** (at doctor's discretion)

Measurements of blood pressure, blood sugar, and potassium levels.

Complete eye examinations at regular intervals.

Chest X ray if you have a history of tuberculosis.

Determination of child's rate of development to detect growth retardation.

Bone mineral density testing (to assess osteoporosis or fracture risk).

▷ **While Taking This Drug the Following Apply:**

Foods: No interactions expected. Ask your doctor about the need to restrict your salt intake or eat potassium-rich foods. During long-term use, a high-protein diet is advisable.

Nutritional Support: During long-term use, take a vitamin D supplement. During wound repair, take a zinc supplement.

Beverages: Drink all forms of milk liberally.

Alcohol: Use caution if you are prone to peptic ulcer disease.

Tobacco Smoking: Nicotine increases the blood levels of naturally produced cortisone and related hormones. Heavy smoking may add to the expected drug actions and requires close observation for excessive effects.

Marijuana Smoking: May cause additional impairment of immunity.

Other Drugs:

Prednisone may **decrease** the effects of

- isoniazid (INH, Niconyl, etc.).
- salicylates (aspirin, sodium salicylate, etc.).

Prednisone **taken concurrently** with

- amphotericin B may lead to additive potassium loss.
- oral anticoagulants may either increase or decrease their effectiveness; consult your doctor regarding the need for INR (prothrombin time) testing and dosage adjustment.
- oral contraceptives (birth control pills) may prolong prednisone's effects.
- cyclosporine (Sandimmune) can cause increased cyclosporine levels and increased prednisone levels. Decreased doses are needed for both medications.
- foscarnet (Foscavir) can lead to additive potassium loss.
- ketoconazole (Nizoral) will blunt ketoconazole's effects.
- loop or thiazide diuretics (see Drug Classes) may blunt the diuretic's benefits.
- NSAIDs can lead to increased intestinal and stomach irritation.
- oral hypoglycemic agents (see Drug Classes) can result in loss of blood sugar control.
- theophylline (Theo-Dur, others) may result in variable theophylline responses. Blood levels are needed more often.
- vaccines such as smallpox or pneumococcal vaccine may not give the expected protection or immunity.

The following drugs may **decrease** the effects of prednisone

- antacids; may reduce its absorption.
- barbiturates (Amytal, Butisol, phenobarbital, etc.).
- carbamazepine (Tegretol).
- phenytoin (Dilantin, etc.).
- primidone (Mysoline).
- rifampin (Rifadin, Rimactane, etc.).

Driving, Hazardous Activities: Be alert to the rare occurrence of dizziness.

Occurrence of Unrelated Illness: This drug may decrease your natural resistance to infection. Tell your doctor if you develop an infection of any kind. It may also reduce your body's ability to respond to the stress of acute illness, injury, or surgery.

Discontinuation: If you have been taking this drug for an extended period of time, do not discontinue it abruptly. Ask your doctor about gradual withdrawal. For a period of 2 years after discontinuation, it is essential in the event of illness, injury, or surgery to inform attending medical personnel of your past use of this drug. The period of impaired response to stress following the use of cortisonelike drugs may last for 1 to 2 years.

▷ **Saving Money When Using These Medicines:**
- Many medications are available to help inflammation. Ask your doctor if this drug offers the best combination of cost and outcome for you.
- Generics may be substituted for the brand name.
- Ask your doctor exactly how long you will need to take this medicine to treat your condition.
- If this medicine will be used long-term, talk with your doctor about calcium supplements, exercise, and osteoporosis risk factors. Also ask whether bone mineral density testing is needed, based on your history.

PRIMAQUINE (PRIM a kween)

Prescription Needed: Yes   **Controlled Drug:** No   **Generic:** Yes

Brand Names: None in U.S. or Canada, available only as generic.

Overview of BENEFITS versus RISKS	
Possible Benefits	*Possible Risks*
EFFECTIVE PREVENTION AND TREATMENT OF CERTAIN TYPES OF MALARIA	HEMOLYTIC ANEMIA Methemoglobinemia Decreased white blood cell counts (rare)
EFFECTIVE ADJUNCTIVE TREATMENT OF *PNEUMOCYSTIS CARINII* PNEUMONIA	

▷ **Illness This Medication Treats:**

Prevention and treatment of malaria caused by *Plasmodium vivax* and *Plasmodium falciparum*.

May also be used (in combination with clindamycin) for AIDS-related *Pneumocystis carinii* pneumonia. Combined therapy is used in patients who are unresponsive or intolerant to standard treatment.

▷ **Typical Dosage Range:** (Dosage or schedule must be determined by the doctor for each individual.)

Infants and Children: 0.3 mg of the base per kilogram of body weight. This dose is taken once daily for 14 days during the last two weeks of chloroquine therapy. Some clinicians give 0.9 mg per kilogram of body weight of the base weekly for 8 weeks in conjunction with the chloroquine therapy.

12 to 60 Years of Age: For malaria: 26.3 mg (15 mg of base), once daily for 14 days.

For *Pneumocystis carinii* pneumonia: 15 to 30 mg of the base, once daily for 21 days.

Over 60 Years of Age: Same as for 12 to 60 years of age.

PRIMIDONE (PRI mi dohn)

Prescription Needed: Yes   **Controlled Drug:** No   **Generic:** Yes

Brand Names: Myidone, Mysoline

Overview of BENEFITS versus RISKS	
Possible Benefits	*Possible Risks*

EFFECTIVE CONTROL OF TONIC-CLONIC (GRAND MAL) AND ALL TYPES OF PARTIAL SEIZURES	Allergic skin reactions
	Blood cell disorders:
	    megaloblastic anemia,
	    deficient white blood cells
	    and platelets (rare)

▷ **Illness This Medication Treats:**

Generalized grand mal seizures and all types of partial seizures; supplements the anticonvulsant action of phenytoin.

▷ **Typical Dosage Range:** (Dosage or schedule must be determined by the doctor for each individual.)

Initially 100 mg/24 hr as a single dose at bedtime for 3 days; 100 to 125 mg twice a day for days 4 through 6; 100 to 125 mg three times a day for days 7 through 9; and an ongoing (maintenance) dose of 250 mg three or four times a day, 6 to 8 hours apart. Total daily dosage should not exceed 2000 mg.

▷ **Conditions Requiring Dosing Adjustments:**

Liver function: The dose **must** be decreased and blood levels obtained more frequently for patients with liver compromise.

Kidney function: Patients with mild to moderate kidney failure can take the usual dose every 8 hours. Patients with moderate to severe kidney failure can take the usual dose every 8 to 12 hours. Patients with severe kidney failure should take the usual dose every 12 to 24 hours. This drug should be used with caution by patients with renal compromise, as it can cause urine crystals.

▷ **How Best to Take This Medicine:** May be taken with or following food to reduce stomach irritation. The tablet may be crushed. Shake the suspension well before measuring the dose.

▷ **How Long This Medicine Is Usually Taken:** Continual use on a regular schedule for 2 to 4 weeks usually determines the effectiveness of this drug in reducing the frequency and severity of seizures. Long-term use (months to years) requires supervision and periodic evaluation. See your doctor regularly.

▷ **Tell Your Doctor Before Taking This Medicine If You:**
- ever had an allergic reaction to it.
- are allergic to phenobarbital.
- have a history of porphyria.
- had an allergic or idiosyncratic reaction to any barbiturate in the past.
- have impaired liver, kidney, or thyroid gland function.
- have asthma, emphysema, or myasthenia gravis.
- are pregnant or planning pregnancy.
- plan to have surgery under general anesthesia soon.

▷ **Possible Side Effects:** Drowsiness, impaired concentration, mental and physical sluggishness.

▷ **Possible Adverse Effects:**

If any of the following develop, call your doctor promptly for guidance.

Some Mild Problems Drug Can Cause

Allergic reactions: skin rashes, localized swellings.

"Hangover" effect, dizziness, impaired vision, double vision, fatigue, emotional disturbances.

Low blood pressure, faintness.

Nausea, vomiting, thirst, increased urine volume.

Some Serious Problems Drug Can Cause

Allergic reaction: swelling of lymph glands.

Idiosyncratic reactions: paradoxical anxiety, rage.

Rare visual or auditory hallucinations.
Blood cell disorders: megaloblastic anemia due to folic acid deple-
tion; deficient production of white blood cells and blood platelets.
Rare systemic lupus erythematosus or porphyria.

▷ **Possible Effects on Sex Life:** Decreased libido and/or impotence.
Decreased effectiveness of oral contraceptives taken concurrently.

▷ **Adverse Effects That May Mimic Natural Diseases or Disorders:**
Allergic swelling of lymph glands may suggest a naturally occurring lymphoma.

▷ *CAUTION*
1. This drug must not be discontinued abruptly.
2. The wide variation of this drug's action from person to person
requires careful individualization of dosage schedules.
3. Regularity of use of this drug is essential for the successful management of seizure disorders. Take your medication at the same
time each day.
4. Side effects and mild adverse effects are usually most apparent
during the first several weeks of treatment and often subside with
continued use.
5. Folic acid may be necessary to prevent anemia while taking this
drug. Ask your doctor.
6. Carry a personal identification card that states you are taking this
drug.
7. Use this drug with caution in the hyperkinetic (overactive) child.
Observe for possible paradoxical hyperactivity. Changes associated with puberty characteristically slow the metabolism of
phenobarbital and permit its gradual accumulation. Blood level
measurements in young adolescents can detect rising concentrations of this drug, which could lead to toxicity.
8. The elderly should avoid the usage of all barbiturates. If use is
attempted, start with small doses until tolerance has been determined. Watch for confusion, delirium, agitation, or paradoxical
excitement. This drug may be conducive to hypothermia.

Advisability of Use During Pregnancy or If Breast-Feeding:
Pregnancy Category: D. Talk with your doctor about the advantages
and disadvantages of primidone use during pregnancy. Determine
the smallest maintenance dose that will prevent seizures.
The newborn infants of mothers who take this drug during pregnancy
may develop abnormal bleeding or bruising due to the deficiency of
certain blood clotting factors. Ask your doctor about taking vitamin
K during the last month of pregnancy. Present in breast milk. Watch
the nursing infant closely and discontinue taking this drug or nursing if adverse effects develop.

▷ **Overdose Symptoms:** Drowsiness, jerky eye movements, blurred vision, staggering gait, incoordination, slurred speech, stupor progressing to coma.

▷ **Suggested Periodic Examinations While Taking This Drug:** (at doctor's discretion)

Complete blood cell counts. Measurements of blood levels of calcium and phosphorus. Evaluation of lymph and thyroid glands. Bone mineral density testing during long-term use.

▷ **While Taking This Drug the Following Apply:**

Nutritional Support: Ask your doctor about the need for supplements of calcium, vitamin D, folic acid, and vitamin K.

Beverages: May be taken with milk or fruit juice.

Alcohol: Avoid completely. Alcohol can greatly increase sedative and depressant effects on brain function.

Tobacco Smoking: May enhance the sedative effects and increase drowsiness.

Other Drugs:

Note: 15% of primidone is converted to phenobarbital in the body. See the phenobarbital drug profile for possible drug interactions.

Driving, Hazardous Activities: May cause drowsiness and dizziness; primidone can also impair mental alertness, vision, and physical coordination. Restrict your activities as necessary.

Occurrence of Unrelated Illness: Notify your doctor of any illness or injury that prevents use of this drug according to your regular dosage schedule.

Discontinuation: Do not stop taking this medicine without your doctor's knowledge and approval. Sudden withdrawal of any anticonvulsant can cause severe and repeated seizures.

▷ **Saving Money When Using These Medicines:**

• Many types of medicines are available to treat seizures. The effectiveness varies with the seizure type. Ask your doctor to start you on the least expensive drug in the most appropriate class.

• Generics are available.

• Ask your doctor exactly how long you will need to take this medicine to treat your condition.

• Drug levels are expensive; make sure levels are drawn at prudent, not excessive, intervals.

• A new medicine called gabapentin is available for add on therapy. Talk to your doctor about this if your seizures continue to be poorly controlled.

PROBENECID (proh BEN e sid)

Prescription Needed: Yes   **Controlled Drug:** No   **Generic:** Yes

Brand Names: Benemid, Colabid [CD], ColBenemid [CD], Polycillin-PRB [CD], Probalan, Probampacin [CD], Proben-C [CD], SK-Probenecid

---

Overview of BENEFITS versus RISKS

Possible Benefits	*Possible Risks*
EFFECTIVE LONG-TERM PREVENTION OF ACUTE ATTACKS OF GOUT	Formation of uric acid kidney stones
Useful adjunct to penicillin therapy (to achieve high blood and tissue levels of penicillin)	Bone marrow depression (aplastic anemia) (rare)
	Drug-induced liver and kidney damage (both rare)

▷ **Illness This Medication Treats:**
(1) Long-term management of gout to prevent acute attacks; (2) helps keep blood levels of penicillin effective; (3) reduces increased uric acid levels caused by thiazide diuretics.

As Combination Drug Product [CD]: Combination with colchicine, a drug often used for acute gout. These drugs have different mechanisms of action; both drugs relieve the acute manifestations of gout and offer some protection from recurrence.

▷ **Typical Dosage Range:** (Dosage or schedule must be determined by the doctor for each individual.)
Antigout: Initially 250 mg twice a day for 1 week; then 500 mg twice a day. Adjunct to penicillin therapy: 500 mg four times a day.

▷ **Conditions Requiring Dosing Adjustments:**
Liver function: No specific guidelines for dosage adjustment for patients with liver compromise are available. This drug should be used with caution by patients with liver compromise.
Kidney function: Patients with moderate kidney failure should **not** take this drug as its effectiveness is questionable. This drug should be used with caution by patients with renal compromise, as it can cause kidney problems.

▷ **How Best to Take This Medicine:** Take with or following food to reduce stomach irritation. Drink 2.5 to 3 qt of liquids daily. The tablet may be crushed for administration.

▷ **How Long This Medicine Is Usually Taken:** Continual use on a regular schedule for several months is usually necessary to determine the effectiveness of this drug in preventing acute attacks of gout. Long-term use (months to years) requires supervision and periodic evaluation. See your doctor regularly.

▷ **Tell Your Doctor Before Taking This Medicine If You:**
  • ever had an allergic reaction to it.
  • have active liver disease.
  • have an active blood cell or bone marrow disorder, or a history of a blood cell or bone marrow disorder.
  • are experiencing an attack of acute gout.
  • have a history of kidney disease or kidney stones.
  • have a history of liver disease or impaired liver function.
  • have a history of peptic ulcer disease.
  • are taking any drugs that contain aspirin or aspirinlike drugs.

▷ **Possible Side Effects:** Development of kidney stones (composed of uric acid); this is preventable. Consult your doctor regarding the use of sodium bicarbonate (or other urine alkalizer) to prevent stone formation.

▷ **Possible Adverse Effects:**
  If any of the following develop, call your doctor promptly for guidance.
  Some Mild Problems Drug Can Cause
  Allergic reactions: skin rash, itching, drug fever.
  Headache, dizziness, flushing of face.
  Reduced appetite, sore gums, nausea, vomiting.
  Some Serious Problems Drug Can Cause
  Allergic reaction: anaphylactic reaction.
  Idiosyncratic reaction: hemolytic anemia.
  Bone marrow depression: fatigue, weakness, fever, sore throat, abnormal bleeding or bruising.
  Drug-induced liver damage with jaundice.
  Drug-induced kidney damage: marked fluid retention, reduced urine formation.
  Rare porphyria or fluid in the retina.

▷ **Adverse Effects That May Mimic Natural Diseases or Disorders:**
  Liver reactions may suggest viral hepatitis.
  Kidney reactions may suggest nephrosis.

▷ *CAUTION*
  1. Dosage of this drug should not be started until 2 to 3 weeks after an acute attack of gout has subsided.

2. This drug may increase the frequency of acute attacks of gout during the first few months of treatment. Concurrent use of colchicine is advised to prevent acute attacks.

3. Aspirin (and aspirin-containing drug products) can reduce this drug's effectiveness. Use acetaminophen or a nonaspirin analgesic for pain relief as needed.

4. Safety and effectiveness of this drug for those under 2 years old have not been established.

5. Those over 60 should proceed *cautiously*. The natural decline in kidney function may require dosage decreases. Susceptibility to serious adverse effects may increase. Call your doctor promptly if any adverse effects occur.

6. Gout can be associated with lead poisoning, and is considered by some clinicians to be a risk factor for coronary heart disease. Your doctor may want to check your lead level and how healthy your heart is.

Advisability of Use During Pregnancy or If Breast-Feeding:
Pregnancy Category: B. This drug has been used during pregnancy with no reports of birth defects or adverse effects on the fetus. Ask your doctor for guidance. Presence in breast milk is unknown; avoid taking this drug or refrain from nursing.

▷ **Overdose Symptoms:** Stomach irritation, nausea, vomiting, nervous agitation, delirium, seizures, coma.

▷ **Suggested Periodic Examinations While Taking This Drug:** (at doctor's discretion)
Complete blood cell counts, measurements of blood uric acid, liver and kidney function tests.

▷ **While Taking This Drug the Following Apply:**
Foods: Follow your doctor's advice regarding the need for a low-purine diet.
Beverages: A large intake of coffee, tea, or cola beverages may reduce this drug's effectiveness.
Alcohol: No interactions are expected. However, large amounts of alcohol can raise the blood uric acid level and reduce the effectiveness of treatment.
Other Drugs:
Probenecid may *increase* the effects of
• acyclovir (Zovirax), resulting in toxicity unless doses are reduced.
• clofibrate (Atromid-S).
• dyphylline (Neothylline).
• ketoprofen and perhaps other NSAIDs (see Drug Classes).
• methotrexate (Mexate), increasing its toxicity.

- midazolam (Versed), increasing CNS depression.
- oral hypoglycemic agents (see Drug Classes).
- thiopental (Pentothal), prolonging its anesthetic effect.
- zalcitabine (Hivid).
- zidovudine (Retrovir), increasing the toxicity risk.

Probenecid *taken concurrently* with

- allopurinol (Zyloprim) may increase the time allopurinol stays in the body (half-life). Dose decreases may be needed.
- penicillins may cause a three- to fivefold increase in penicillin blood levels, greatly increasing the effectiveness of each penicillin dose.
- cephalosporins may cause a doubling of antibiotic levels.
- dapsone may cause up to a 50% increase in dapsone level.
- rifampin (Rifadin, others) may increase rifampin blood levels.

The following drugs may *decrease* the effects of probenecid

- aspirin and other salicylates; reduces its effectiveness in promoting uric acid excretion.
- bismuth subsalicylate (Pepto-Bismol, others).

Driving, Hazardous Activities: May cause dizziness. Restrict your activities as necessary.

Discontinuation: Do not discontinue this drug without consulting your doctor.

▷ **Saving Money When Using These Medicines:**
- Generic forms may be substituted for the brand name.

PROBUCOL (PROH byu kohl)

Prescription Needed: Yes **Controlled Drug:** No **Generic:** No

Brand Name: Lorelco

Author's note: Hoechst Marion Roussel has stopped distribution of this drug in the United States. It will only be available until current supplies are used up.

PROCAINAMIDE (proh kayn A mide)

Prescription Needed: Yes **Controlled Drug:** No **Generic:** Yes

Brand Names: Procamide SR, Procan SR, Pronestyl, Pronestyl-SR, Rhythmin

```
┌─────────────────────────────────────────────────────────┐
│           Overview of BENEFITS versus RISKS              │
│   Possible Benefits              Possible Risks          │
│   EFFECTIVE TREATMENT OF      NARROW TREATMENT           │
│     SELECTED HEART              RANGE                     │
│     RHYTHM DISORDERS          MAY CAUSE SYSTEMIC         │
│                                 LUPUS ERYTHEMATOSUS       │
│                                 SYNDROME                  │
│                               Provocation of abnormal heart│
│                                 rhythms                   │
│                               Blood cell disorders:       │
│                                 insufficient white blood cells│
│                                 and platelets             │
└─────────────────────────────────────────────────────────┘
```

▷ **Illness This Medication Treats:**
Stops and helps prevent recurrent premature beats arising in the heart atria and the ventricles.

▷ **Typical Dosage Range:** (Dosage or schedule must be determined by the doctor for each individual.)
Dose varies according to indication for use. Starting dose is usually 50 mg per kilogram of body weight per day (immediate-release form). This dose is then divided into equal doses and given every 3, 4, or 6 hours. The ongoing dose is adjusted to individual patient response and blood levels. The sustained-release form is usually started in younger patients without kidney problems at 50 mg per kilogram of body weight per day. This dose is divided into equal doses and is given every 6 to 12 hours, depending on patient response and blood levels.

▷ **Conditions Requiring Dosing Adjustments:**
Liver function: This drug should be used with caution by patients with liver compromise, and blood levels obtained. This drug is also a cause of systemic lupus erythematosus (SLE); patients should have periodic SLE testing. The use of this drug by patients with compromised livers requires a benefit-to-risk decision.
Kidney function: Patients with moderate to severe kidney failure can take the usual doses every 6 to 12 hours. Patients with creatinine clearances of less than 10 ml/min can take the usual dose every 8 to 24 hours. This drug should be used with caution by patients with renal compromise, and appropriate blood levels obtained.

▷ **How Best to Take This Medicine:**   Preferably taken on an empty stomach, 1 hour before or 2 hours after eating. However, this drug may be taken with or following food to reduce stomach irritation. The regular capsules may be opened and the regular tablets crushed; however, the prolonged-action tablets should be swallowed whole without alteration.

▷ **How Long This Medicine Is Usually Taken:**   Continual use on a regular schedule for 24 to 48 hours is usually necessary to determine the effectiveness of this drug in correcting or preventing responsive rhythm disorders. Long-term use requires supervision and periodic evaluation. See your doctor regularly.

▷ **Tell Your Doctor Before Taking This Medicine If You:**
- ever had an allergic reaction to it or had any unfavorable reactions to other antiarrhythmic drugs.
- have second- or third-degree heart block as determined by electrocardiogram.
- are allergic to procaine (Novocain) or other local anesthetics of the "-caine" drug class, such as those commonly used for glaucoma testing and dental procedures.
- have a history of heart disease of any kind, especially heart block.
- have a history of low blood pressure.
- have a history of lupus erythematosus.
- have a history of abnormally low blood platelet counts from any cause.
- have impaired liver or kidney function.
- have myasthenia gravis.
- have an enlarged prostate gland.
- are taking any form of digitalis or a diuretic that can cause excessive potassium loss.
- plan to have surgery under general anesthesia soon.

▷ **Possible Side Effects:**   Drop in blood pressure in susceptible individuals.

▷ **Possible Adverse Effects:**
If any of the following develop, call your doctor promptly for guidance.
Some Mild Problems Drug Can Cause
Allergic reactions: skin rash, hives, itching, drug fever.
Weakness, light-headedness.
Loss of appetite, bitter taste, indigestion, nausea, vomiting, diarrhea.
Some Serious Problems Drug Can Cause
Allergic reactions: systemic lupus erythematosus–like syndrome: fever, skin eruptions, joint and muscle pains, pleurisy.
Idiosyncratic reactions: mental depression, hallucinations, psychotic behavior, hemolytic anemia.
Severe drop in blood pressure, fainting.

Asthmalike breathing difficulties.

Induction of new heart rhythm disturbances.

Inability to empty urinary bladder, prostatism.

Blood cell disorders: abnormally low white blood cell count, causing fever, sore throat, infections; abnormally low blood platelet count, causing abnormal bleeding or bruising.

Rare pericardial effusions, anticholinergic syndrome, or peripheral neuropathy.

▷ **Adverse Effects That May Mimic Natural Diseases or Disorders:**
Rare liver reaction may suggest viral hepatitis.

▷ *CAUTION*

1. Thorough evaluation of heart function (including electrocardiograms) is necessary before use.
2. Periodic evaluation of heart function is necessary to determine your response to this drug. Some individuals experience worsening of their heart rhythm disorder and/or deterioration of heart function. Close monitoring of heart rate, rhythm, and overall performance is essential.
3. Dosage must be adjusted carefully for each individual. Do not change your dosage without the knowledge and supervision of your doctor.
4. Do not take any other antiarrhythmic while taking this drug unless directed to do so by your doctor.
5. Infants and children's blood cell counts should be monitored for loss of white blood cells.
6. Those over 60 may require reduction in dosage. Observe carefully for light-headedness, dizziness, unsteadiness, and tendency to fall.

Advisability of Use During Pregnancy or If Breast-Feeding:
Pregnancy Category: C. Use this drug only if clearly needed. Present in breast milk; avoid taking this drug or refrain from nursing.

▷ **Overdose Symptoms:** Loss of appetite, nausea, vomiting, weakness, faintness, irregular heart rhythm, stupor, circulatory collapse, heart arrest.

▷ **Suggested Periodic Examinations While Taking This Drug:** (at doctor's discretion)

Complete blood cell counts.

Blood tests for the development of lupus erythematosus (LE) cells and antinuclear antibodies.

Electrocardiograms to monitor the full effect of this drug on the mechanisms that influence heart rate and rhythm.

▷ **While Taking This Drug the Following Apply:**

Beverages: Avoid excessive intake of coffee, tea, and cola beverages. Avoid iced drinks. This drug may be taken with milk.

Alcohol: Use caution until the combined effects have been determined. Alcohol can increase the blood pressure–lowering effects of this drug.

Tobacco Smoking: Nicotine can cause irritability of the heart and reduce the effectiveness of this drug.

Other Drugs:

Procainamide may *increase* the effects of

• antihypertensives, causing excessive lowering of blood pressure.

The following drugs may *increase* the effects of procainamide

• amiodarone (Cordarone).
• cimetidine (Tagamet).
• propranolol (Inderal).
• quinidine (Quinaglute).
• ranitidine (Zantac).
• trimethoprim (Bactrim, Proloprim)

Driving, Hazardous Activities: May cause dizziness or weakness. Restrict your activities as necessary.

Exposure to Heat: Use caution. Hot environments are conducive to lower blood pressure.

Occurrence of Unrelated Illness: Disorders that cause vomiting, diarrhea, or dehydration can affect this drug's action adversely. Report such developments promptly.

Discontinuation: This drug should not be discontinued abruptly following long-term use. Ask your doctor about gradual dose reduction.

▷ **Saving Money When Using These Medicines:**

• Many drugs are available to treat abnormal heart rhythms. Ask your doctor to start you on the least expensive drug in the class that offers the best combination of cost and outcome for you.
• A generic form may be substituted for the brand name.
• Talk with your doctor to see if taking aspirin every other day to help prevent a heart attack makes sense for you.

PROCHLORPERAZINE (proh klor PER a zeen)

Prescription Needed: Yes   **Controlled Drug:** No   **Generic:** Yes

Brand Name: Compazine, Eskatrol, Ultrazine [CD]

```
┌─────────────────────────────────────────────────────────────┐
│            Overview of BENEFITS versus RISKS                 │
│      Possible Benefits              Possible Risks           │
│  EFFECTIVE CONTROL OF         SERIOUS TOXIC EFFECTS ON       │
│    ACUTE MENTAL                 BRAIN with long-term use     │
│    DISORDERS in the majority  Liver damage with jaundice     │
│    of patients: beneficial effects  (infrequent)            │
│    on thinking, mood, and     Blood cell disorders:          │
│    behavior                     abnormally low white cell and│
│  EFFECTIVE CONTROL OF           platelet counts (rare)       │
│    NAUSEA AND VOMITING                                       │
│  Relief of anxiety and nervous                               │
│    tension                                                   │
└─────────────────────────────────────────────────────────────┘
```

▷ **Illness This Medication Treats:**
   (1) Severe nausea and vomiting; (2) schizophrenia, though rarely; (3) motion sickness.

▷ **Typical Dosage Range:** (Dosage or schedule must be determined by the doctor for each individual.)
   Initially 5 mg of the immediate-release form every 6 to 8 hours. If needed and tolerated, dose may be increased by 5 mg at intervals of 3 to 4 days. Usual range is 35 to 60 mg every 24 hours. The total daily dosage should not exceed 150 mg.
   Nausea or vomiting: 5 to 10 mg three or four times daily. The sustained-release form can be used as 15 mg when you wake up in the morning or 10 mg every 12 hours.

▷ **Conditions Requiring Dosing Adjustments:**
   Liver function: This drug should be used with caution by patients with liver compromise.

▷ **How Best to Take This Medicine:**   May be taken with or following food to reduce stomach irritation. The tablets may be crushed. Prolonged-action capsules should be swallowed whole without alteration.

▷ **How Long This Medicine Is Usually Taken:**   Continual use on a regular schedule for 12 to 24 hours determines the effectiveness of this drug in controlling nausea and vomiting. If this drug is used for severe anxiety-tension states or acute psychotic behavior, a trial of several weeks is usually necessary to determine its effectiveness. Discontinue this drug if no significant benefit occurs within 6 weeks. See your doctor regularly.

▷ **Tell Your Doctor Before Taking This Medicine If You:**
   • ever had an allergic reaction to it.
   • have active liver disease or impaired liver or kidney function.
   • have cancer of the breast.

- have a current blood cell or bone marrow disorder.
- are allergic or abnormally sensitive to any phenothiazine drug.
- have any type of seizure disorder.
- have diabetes, glaucoma, or heart disease.
- have a history of lupus erythematosus.
- have prostate problems or are taking any drug with sedative effects.
- plan to have surgery under general or spinal anesthesia soon.

▷ **Possible Side Effects:** Drowsiness (usually during the first 2 weeks), orthostatic hypotension, blurred vision, dry mouth, nasal congestion, constipation, impaired urination.

Pink or purple coloration of urine, of no significance.

▷ **Possible Adverse Effects:**

If any of the following develop, call your doctor promptly for guidance.

Some Mild Problems Drug Can Cause

Allergic reactions: skin rash, low-grade fever.

Lowering of body temperature, especially in the elderly.

Increased appetite and weight gain.

Dizziness, weakness, agitation, insomnia, impaired day and night vision.

Chronic constipation, fecal impaction.

Some Serious Problems Drug Can Cause

Allergic reactions: hepatitis with jaundice, usually between second and fourth week; high fever; asthma; anaphylactic reaction.

Idiosyncratic reactions: toxic dermatitis, neuroleptic malignant syndrome.

Depression, disorientation, seizures.

Rare disturbances of heart rhythm or porphyria.

Bone marrow depression: fever, sore throat, abnormal bleeding or bruising.

Parkinson-like disorders; muscle spasms of face, jaw, neck, back, extremities; extreme restlessness; slowed movements; muscle rigidity; tremors; tardive dyskinesias.

▷ **Possible Effects on Sex Life:** Altered timing and pattern of menstruation; female breast enlargement with milk production; male breast enlargement and tenderness; inhibited ejaculation; priapism; false-positive pregnancy test result.

▷ **Adverse Effects That May Mimic Natural Diseases or Disorders:**

Nervous system reactions may suggest Parkinson's disease.

Liver reactions may suggest viral hepatitis.

Systemic lupus erythematosus–like reactions can occur.

▷ *CAUTION*

1. Many over-the-counter medications for allergies, colds, and coughs contain drugs that can interact unfavorably with pro-

chlorperazine. Ask your doctor or pharmacist for guidance before using any such medications.

2. Antacids that contain aluminum and/or magnesium can prevent the absorption of this drug and reduce its effectiveness.

3. Obtain prompt evaluation of any change or disturbance of vision.

4. Do not use this drug in infants under 2 years old or children of any age with symptoms suggestive of Reye's syndrome. Children with acute illnesses (flu-like infections, measles, chickenpox, etc.) are very susceptible to adverse effects when prochlorperazine is given to control nausea and vomiting.

5. Small doses are advisable for those over 60 until individual response has been determined. You may be more susceptible to drowsiness, lethargy, constipation, lowered body temperature, and orthostatic hypotension. This drug can enhance existing prostatism. You may also be more susceptible to Parkinson-like reactions and/or tardive dyskinesia. These reactions must be recognized early since they may become unresponsive to treatment and irreversible.

Advisability of Use During Pregnancy or If Breast-Feeding:

Pregnancy Category: C. Limit use of this drug to small and infrequent doses. Avoid during the last month because of possible effects on the newborn infant. Present in breast milk in small amounts. Watch the nursing infant closely and stop taking this drug or nursing if adverse effects develop.

▷ **Overdose Symptoms:**   Marked drowsiness, weakness, tremor, agitation, unsteadiness, deep sleep, coma, convulsions.

▷ **Suggested Periodic Examinations While Taking This Drug:** (at doctor's discretion)

Complete blood cell counts, especially between the fourth and tenth weeks of treatment.

Liver function tests, electrocardiograms.

Complete eye examinations—eye structures and vision.

Careful inspection of the tongue for early evidence of fine, involuntary, wavelike movements that could indicate the beginning of tardive dyskinesia.

▷ **While Taking This Drug the Following Apply:**

Nutritional Support: A riboflavin (vitamin B2) supplement should be taken with long-term use.

Beverages: May be taken with milk.

Alcohol: Avoid completely. Alcohol can increase the sedative action of phenothiazines and accentuate their depressant effects on brain function and blood pressure. Phenothiazines can increase the intoxicating effects of alcohol.

Tobacco Smoking: Possible reduction of drowsiness.

Marijuana Smoking: Moderate increase in drowsiness; accentuation of orthostatic hypotension; increased risk of precipitating latent psychoses, confusing the interpretation of mental status and drug responses.

Other Drugs:

Prochlorperazine may ***increase*** the effects of

- all sedative drugs, especially meperidine (Demerol), causing excessive sedation.
- all atropinelike drugs, causing nervous system toxicity.

Prochlorperazine may ***decrease*** the effects of

- guanethidine (Ismelin, Esimil), reducing its effectiveness in lowering blood pressure.

Prochlorperazine ***taken concurrently*** with

- oral hypoglycemic agents (see Drug Classes) may blunt their therapeutic benefit.
- propranolol (Inderal) may cause increased effects of both drugs; monitor effects closely and adjust dosages as necessary.

The following drugs may ***decrease*** the effects of prochlorperazine

- antacids containing aluminum and/or magnesium.
- benztropine (Cogentin).
- trihexyphenidyl (Artane).

Driving, Hazardous Activities: This drug can impair mental alertness, judgment, and physical coordination. Avoid hazardous activities.

Exposure to Sun: Use caution until your sensitivity has been determined. Some phenothiazines can cause photosensitivity.

Exposure to Heat: Use caution and avoid excessive heat as much as possible. This drug may impair the regulation of body temperature and increase the risk of heatstroke.

Exposure to Cold: Use caution and dress warmly. This drug can increase the risk of hypothermia in the elderly.

Discontinuation: After a period of long-term use, do not suddenly stop taking this drug. Gradual withdrawal over 2 to 3 weeks under your doctor's supervision is recommended.

▷ **Saving Money When Using This Medicine:**

- A large number of available drugs provide similar effectiveness. Ask your doctor to prescribe the drug that offers the best combination of cost and outcome.
- It may be possible (after a significant symptom-free period) to stop taking this medicine. Ask your doctor for help.
- A generic form may be substituted for the brand name.

PROPIONIC ACIDS

(Nonsteroidal Anti-Inflammatory Drugs)
Ibuprofen (i byu PROH fen)
Fenoprofen (FEN oh proh fen)
Flurbiprofen (FLUR bi proh fen)
Ketoprofen (KEY toh proh fen)
Naproxen (na PROX in)
Oxaprozin (ox A proh zin)

Prescription Needed: Varies   **Controlled Drug:** No   **Generic:** Yes (all but oxaprozin)

Brand Names:
Ibuprofen: Advil, Aches-N-Pain, Arthritis Foundation Pain Reliever, Bayer Select, Children's Advil, CoAdvil [CD], Haltran, Ibuprohm, IBU-TAB, Junior Strength Motrin (nonprescription), Medipren, Motrin, Motrin IB, Nuprin, PediaProfen, Rufen
Fenoprofen: Nalfon
Flurbiprofen: Ansaid
Ketoprofen: Actron (12.5 mg nonprescription), Orudis, Oruvail
Naproxen: Naprosyn, Aleve, Anaprox, Anaprox DS, Naprelan (once-daily formulation)
Oxaprozin: Daypro

Overview of BENEFITS versus RISKS

Possible Benefits	*Possible Risks*
EFFECTIVE RELIEF OF MILD TO MODERATE PAIN AND INFLAMMATION	Gastrointestinal pain, ulceration, bleeding (rare)
	Rare kidney damage
	Fluid retention
	Rare bone marrow depression (except oxaprozin)
	Rare liver toxicity (naproxen, ketoprofen, and flurbiprofen)

▷ **Illness This Medication Treats:**

(1) All six agents—treatment of rheumatoid and osteoarthritis; (2) naproxen is useful for: bursitis, gout, dysmenorrhea (ketoprofen and ibuprofen also), pain, juvenile rheumatoid arthritis, and tendonitis; (3) fenoprofen is the only agent approved for treatment of tennis elbow.

Other (unlabeled) generally accepted uses: (1) naproxen has been used to treat migraine and colds caused by rhinoviruses; (2) oxaprozin is useful for gout and tendonitis; (3) ketoprofen may have a role in treating temporal arteritis; (4) flurbiprofen has some support for therapy of periodontal disease and miosis inhibition; (5) fenoprofen has been used successfully in migraine; (6) ibuprofen treats inter-leukin-2 toxicity, chronic urticaria, and decreases IUD-associated bleeding. All agents have been used for a variety of pains and fever.

▷ **Typical Dosage Range:** (Dosage or schedule must be determined by the doctor for each individual.)

Ibuprofen: 200 to 800 mg three or four times daily. Total daily dosage should not exceed 3200 mg.

Fenoprofen: 300 to 600 mg three or four times daily. Daily maximum is 3200 mg.

Flurbiprofen: 100 to 200 mg daily in two to four divided doses. The lowest effective dose should be used. Daily maximum is 300 mg.

Ketoprofen: 75 mg three times daily or 50 mg four times daily. Usual daily dose is 150 to 300 mg divided into three or four doses. Daily maximum is 300 mg.

Naproxen: For gout: 750 mg initially, then 250 mg every 8 hours until attack is relieved. For arthritis: 250, 375, or 500 mg twice daily 12 hours apart.

The new sustained-release form (Naprelan) offers an intestinal protective drug absorption system (IPDAS) and once-daily (two tablets) dosing.

Menstrual pain: 500 mg initially, then 250 mg every 6 to 8 hours as needed.

Oxaprozin: 1200 mg as a single daily dose in the morning. Daily maximum is 1800 mg.

Author's note: When medicines in this class are available in non-prescription forms—usually with smaller dose sizes and shorter usage period—fewer adverse effects occur. Talk with your doctor or pharmacist for more information.

▷ **Conditions Requiring Dosing Adjustments:**

Liver function. All drugs are metabolized in the liver; patients with liver compromise should use these drugs with caution and consider lower doses.

Kidney function: These drugs share the risks common to most NSAIDs. Some patients with kidney compromise depend on prosta-glandins for kidney function. These patients must make a benefit-to-risk decision regarding the use of NSAIDs.

▷ **How Best to Take This Medicine:** Take either on an empty stomach or with food or milk to prevent stomach irritation. Take with a full glass of water and remain upright (do not lie down) for 30 minutes. The tablets may be crushed and the capsules opened except for Naprelan or ketoprofen tablets, which should not be crushed or altered.

▷ **How Long This Medicine Is Usually Taken:** Use on a regular schedule for 1 to 2 weeks usually determines the effectiveness of these drugs. Peak effect may take 6 weeks. Long-term use requires supervision and periodic evaluation by your doctor.

▷ **Tell Your Doctor Before Taking This Medicine If You:**
- ever had an allergic reaction to it.
- are subject to asthma or nasal polyps caused by aspirin, or are allergic to aspirin or other aspirin substitutes.
- have active peptic ulcer disease or any form of gastrointestinal bleeding, or a history of such disorders.
- have active liver disease (naproxen, ketoprofen, and flurbiprofen).
- have a bleeding disorder or a blood cell disorder.
- have impaired liver or kidney function.
- have high blood pressure or a history of heart failure.
- are taking any of the following: acetaminophen, aspirin or aspirin substitutes, or anticoagulants.

▷ **Possible Side Effects:** Fluid retention (weight gain); pink, red, purple, or rust coloration of urine (ibuprofen only). Ringing in the ears.

▷ **Possible Adverse Effects:**
If any of the following develop, call your doctor promptly for guidance.
Some Mild Problems Drug Can Cause
  Allergic reactions: skin rash, hives, itching.
  Headache, dizziness, altered vision, ringing in the ears, depression.
  Sleep disturbances (oxaprozin).
  Palpitations (fenoprofen).
  Mouth sores, nausea, vomiting, constipation, diarrhea.
Some Serious Problems Drug Can Cause
  Allergic reactions: anaphylaxis, severe skin reactions.
  Idiosyncratic reactions: ibuprofen- or naproxen-induced meningitis with fever and coma.
  Active peptic ulcer, with or without bleeding.
  Liver damage with jaundice.
  Kidney damage with painful urination, bloody urine, reduced urine formation.
  Rare bone marrow depression—fatigue, weakness, fever, sore throat, abnormal bleeding or bruising.

▷ **Possible Effects on Sex Life:** Altered timing and pattern of menstruation (ibuprofen, ketoprofen, and naproxen), and excessive menstrual bleeding (ibuprofen and ketoprofen); rare male breast enlargement and tenderness (ibuprofen). Naproxen may rarely inhibit ejaculation; ketoprofen may rarely decrease libido.

▷ **Possible Delayed Adverse Effects:** Mild anemia due to silent blood loss from the stomach.

▷ **Adverse Effects That May Mimic Natural Diseases or Disorders:** Liver reaction may suggest viral hepatitis.

▷ *CAUTION*
1. Dosage should always be limited to the smallest amount that produces reasonable improvement.
2. These drugs may mask early indications of infection. Tell your doctor if you are developing an infection of any kind.
3. Safety and effectiveness of these drugs for those under 12 years old are not established.
4. Those over 60 should take small doses until tolerance is determined. Watch for signs of liver or kidney toxicity, fluid retention, dizziness, confusion, impaired memory, stomach bleeding, or constipation.

Advisability of Use During Pregnancy or If Breast-Feeding:
Pregnancy Category: B for ibuprofen, fenoprofen, flurbiprofen, ketoprofen, and naproxen; C for oxaprozin. Ibuprofen and fenoprofen are D if used in the last 3 months (trimester) of pregnancy. Avoid use of these drugs during the last 3 months. Use during the first 6 months only if clearly needed. The makers of ketoprofen and flurbiprofen say that both medicines should be avoided in late pregnancy. Ask your doctor for guidance. Present in breast milk; avoid taking these drugs or refrain from nursing.

▷ **Overdose Symptoms:** Drowsiness, dizziness, ringing in the ears, nausea, vomiting, diarrhea, confusion, unsteadiness, stupor progressing to coma.

▷ **Suggested Periodic Examinations While Taking This Drug:** (at doctor's discretion)
Complete blood cell counts, liver and kidney function tests, complete eye examinations if vision is altered in any way.

▷ **While Taking This Drug the Following Apply:**
Beverages: May be taken with milk.
Alcohol: Use with caution. The irritant action of alcohol on the stomach lining, added to that of these drugs, increases the risk of stomach ulceration and/or bleeding.
Other Drugs:
These medicines may *increase* the effects of propionic acids
• acetaminophen (Tylenol, etc.), increasing the risk of kidney damage; avoid prolonged use of this combination.

- anticoagulants (Coumadin, etc.), increasing the risk of bleeding; monitor prothrombin time and adjust dose accordingly.
- enoxaparin (Lovenox), if NSAIDs have been used before hip replacement surgery and enoxaparin is used after surgery.
- lithium (Lithobid, others), causing toxic lithium levels.
- methotrexate (Mexate, others), resulting in major methotrexate toxicity with possible anemia, hemorrhage, and blood infections.

These medicines may *decrease* the effects of proprionic acids

- diuretics such as hydrochlorothiazide (Esidrix) and furosemide (Lasix).
- beta-blockers such as carteolol (Cartrol).

Proprionic acids *taken concurrently* with the following drugs may increase the risk of bleeding; avoid these combinations:

- aspirin.
- dipyridamole (Persantine).
- enoxaparin (Lovenox).
- indomethacin (Indocin).
- sulfinpyrazone (Anturane).
- valproic acid (Depakene).
- warfarin (Coumadin).

Driving, Hazardous Activities: These drugs may cause drowsiness or dizziness. Restrict your activities as necessary.

Exposure to Sun: Use caution. Ibuprofen, ketoprofen, flurbiprofen, and naproxen have caused photosensitivity.

▷ **Saving Money When Using These Medicines:**
- The effectiveness of all these medicines is about equal. Ask your doctor to start you on the least expensive drug in the class most appropriate for you.
- Generics are available for several propionic acid NSAIDs.
- Ask your doctor exactly how long you will need to take this medicine to treat your condition.
- If your liver is compromised, ask your doctor if the dose has been decreased appropriately.
- If your pain continues, ask your doctor if visiting a chronic pain center would be appropriate for you.

PROPRANOLOL (proh PRAN oh lohl)

Prescription Needed: Yes   **Controlled Drug:** No   **Generic:** Yes

Brand Names: Inderal, Inderal-LA, Inderide [CD], Inderide LA [CD], Ipran

Overview of BENEFITS versus RISKS	
Possible Benefits	**Possible Risks**
EFFECTIVE, WELL-TOLERATED AS ANTIANGINAL for effort-induced angina; ANTIARRHYTHMIC for certain heart rhythm disorders; antihypertensive for mild to moderate hypertension	CONGESTIVE HEART FAILURE in advanced heart disease
	Worsening of angina in coronary heart disease (if abruptly withdrawn)
	Masking of low blood sugar in diabetics
EFFECTIVE PREVENTION OF MIGRAINE HEADACHES	Provocation of asthma
	Rare depression
Effective adjunct for preventing recurrent heart attack (myocardial infarction)	Rare blood cell disorders: low white cell or platelet counts
Effective adjunct for the management of pheochromocytoma	

▷ **Illness This Medication Treats:**

(1) Several serious cardiovascular disorders: classical effort-induced angina, some heart rhythm disturbances, and high blood pressure. Also beneficial in preventing the recurrence of heart attacks (myocardial infarction). (2) Reduces frequency and severity of migraine headaches.

Other (unlabeled) generally accepted uses: (1) may help control physical symptoms of anxiety and nervous tension (as in stage fright), familial tremors, symptoms associated with markedly overactive thyroid gland function (thyrotoxicosis); (2) amputation pain.

As Combination Drug Product [CP]: In combination with hydrochlorothiazide, treats hypertension. This combination has two drugs with different mechanisms of action, and provide greater long-term effectiveness and convenience.

▷ **Typical Dosage Range:** (Dosage or schedule must be determined by the doctor for each individual.)

Varies with indication.

Antianginal: Initially 10 mg three or four times daily; increase dose gradually every 3 to 7 days, as needed and tolerated. The total daily dosage should not exceed 400 mg.

Antiarrhythmic: 10 to 30 mg three or four times daily, as needed and tolerated.

Antihypertensive: Initially 40 mg twice daily; increase dose gradually as needed and tolerated. The total daily dosage should not exceed 640 mg.

Migraine headache prevention: Initially 20 mg four times daily; increase dose gradually as needed and tolerated. The total daily dosage should not exceed 480 mg.

Author's note: Extended-release or long-acting formulations offer the advantage of once-daily dosing for many patients. Discuss these with your doctor.

▷ **Conditions Requiring Dosing Adjustments:**

Liver function: in patients with liver compromise should use this drug with caution; however, no specific guidelines for adjustment of dosages are available.

Kidney function: Patients with combined renal and hepatic compromise should use this drug with caution.

▷ **How Best to Take This Medicine:**   Preferably taken 1 hour before eating to maximize absorption. The tablet may be crushed for administration; to prevent harmless possible numbing effect, mix with soft food and swallow promptly. The prolonged-action capsules should be swallowed whole without alteration. Do not discontinue abruptly.

▷ **How Long This Medicine Is Usually Taken:**   Continual use on a regular schedule for 10 to 14 days determines the effectiveness of this drug in preventing angina, controlling heart rhythm disorders, and lowering blood pressure. Peak benefits may require continual use for 6 to 8 weeks. Long-term use (months to years) is determined by the course of your symptoms over time and your response to the overall treatment program (weight reduction, salt restriction, smoking cessation, etc.). See your doctor regularly.

▷ **Tell Your Doctor Before Taking This Medicine If You:**

- ever had an allergic reaction to it.
- have bronchial asthma.
- have Prinzmetal's variant angina (coronary artery spasm).
- have congestive heart failure.
- have an abnormally slow heart rate or a serious form of heart block.
- are allergic to insect stings (the epinephrine kits used to ease allergic reactions to stings may be blunted by a beta-blocker).
- are taking, or have taken within the past 14 days, any MAO type A inhibitor.
- had an adverse reaction to any beta-blocker in the past.
- have a history of serious heart disease, with or without episodes of heart failure.
- have a history of hay fever (allergic rhinitis), asthma, chronic bronchitis, or emphysema.
- have a history of overactive thyroid function.

- have a history of low blood sugar.
- have impaired liver or kidney function.
- have diabetes or myasthenia gravis.
- are currently taking any form of digitalis, quinidine, or reserpine, or any calcium blocker.
- plan to have surgery under general anesthesia soon.

▷ **Possible Side Effects:**   Lethargy and fatigability, cold extremities, slow heart rate, light-headedness in upright position.

▷ **Possible Adverse Effects:**

If any of the following develop, call your doctor promptly for guidance.

Some Mild Problems Drug Can Cause

Allergic reactions: skin rash, temporary loss of hair, drug fever.
Headache, dizziness, insomnia, vivid dreams.
Nausea, vomiting, diarrhea.

Some Serious Problems Drug Can Cause

Idiosyncratic reaction: acute behavioral disturbances such as disorientation, confusion, hallucinations, amnesia.
Mental depression, anxiety.
Chest pain, shortness of breath, precipitation of congestive heart failure.
Rare peripheral neuropathy, drug-induced myasthenia gravis, porphyria, interstitial nephritis, hyperthyroidism, carpal tunnel syndrome, or systemic lupus erythematosus.
Induction of bronchial asthma (in asthmatic people).
Rare blood cell disorders: abnormally low white blood cell count, causing fever and sore throat; abnormally low blood platelet count, causing abnormal bleeding or bruising.

▷ **Possible Effects on Sex Life:**   Decreased libido; impaired erection; impotence.

This drug has the highest incidence of libido reduction and erectile impairment of all beta-blockers.
Male infertility (inhibited sperm motility); Peyronie's disease.

▷ **Adverse Effects That May Mimic Natural Diseases or Disorders:**
Reduced blood flow to extremities may resemble Raynaud's phenomenon.

▷ **CAUTION**

1. ***Do not stop taking this drug suddenly*** without knowledge and guidance of your doctor. Carry a personal identification card that states you are taking this drug.
2. Ask your doctor or pharmacist before using nasal decongestants, usually present in over-the-counter cold preparations and nose

drops. These can cause sudden increases in blood pressure when taken concurrently with beta-blockers.

3. Report any tendency to emotional depression.

4. Safety and effectiveness of this drug for those under 12 years old have not been established. However, if used, observe for the development of low blood sugar during periods of reduced food intake.

5. Those over 60 should proceed *cautiously* with all antihypertensives. High blood pressure should be reduced without the risks associated with excessively low blood pressure. Start treatment with small doses, and monitor the blood pressure response frequently. Sudden, rapid, and excessive reduction of blood pressure can predispose to stroke or heart attack. Watch for dizziness, unsteadiness, tendency to fall, confusion, hallucinations, depression, or urinary frequency.

Advisability of Use During Pregnancy or If Breast-Feeding:
Pregnancy Category: C. Avoid use of this drug during the first 3 months if possible. Use only if clearly needed; ask your doctor for guidance. Present in breast milk. Watch the nursing infant closely and taper off this drug or stop nursing if adverse effects develop.

▷ **Overdose Symptoms:** Weakness, slow pulse, low blood pressure, fainting, cold and sweaty skin, congestive heart failure, possible coma and convulsions.

▷ **Possible Effects of Long-Term Use:** Reduced heart reserve and eventual heart failure in susceptible individuals with advanced heart disease.

▷ **Suggested Periodic Examinations While Taking This Drug:** (at doctor's discretion)
Complete blood cell counts.
Measurements of blood pressure, evaluation of heart function.

▷ **While Taking This Drug the Following Apply:**
Foods: Avoid excessive salt intake.
Beverages: May be taken with milk.
Alcohol: Use with caution until combined effect has been determined. Alcohol may exaggerate propranolol's ability to lower the blood pressure and increase its mild sedative effect.
Tobacco Smoking: Nicotine may reduce propranolol's effectiveness in treating angina, heart rhythm disorders, and high blood pressure. Smoking increases the rate of elimination of this drug and decreases its blood levels, especially in younger patients. In addition, high doses may potentiate constriction of bronchial tubes caused by regular smoking.

Other Drugs:

Propranolol may *increase* the effects of

- other antihypertensives, causing excessive lowering of blood pressure. Dosage adjustments may be necessary.
- lidocaine (Xylocaine, etc.).
- reserpine (Ser-Ap-Es, etc.), causing sedation, depression, slowing of the heart rate, and lowering of the blood pressure.
- verapamil (Calan, Isoptin), causing excessive depression of heart function; monitor this combination closely.
- warfarin (Coumadin) and increase bleeding risk. More frequent INR (prothrombin time) testing is needed, with dosing adjusted to test results.

Propranolol may *decrease* the effects of

- albuterol (Proventil).
- theophyllines (aminophylline, Theo-Dur, etc.), reducing their antiasthmatic effectiveness.

Propranolol *taken concurrently* with

- amiodarone (Cordarone) may result in abnormal heart rhythms and low pulse.
- clonidine (Catapres) requires close monitoring for rebound high blood pressure if clonidine is withdrawn while propranolol is still being taken.
- digoxin (Lanoxin) can lead to severe slowing of the heart.
- epinephrine (Adrenalin, etc.) may cause a marked rise in blood pressure and slowing of the heart rate.
- fluoxetine (Prozac) or fluvoxamine (Luvox) may increase the risk of slow heartbeat and sedation.
- insulin requires close monitoring to avoid undetected hypoglycemia.
- oral hypoglycemic agents (see Drug Classes) may slow recovery from any excessively lowered blood sugar that may occur.
- quinidine (Quinaglute) can increase adverse effects without increasing benefits.
- venlafaxine (Effexor) can increase risk of propranolol toxicity.
- X-ray contrast media such as diatrizoate may result in up to an eightfold increased risk of severe allergic reactions.

The following drugs may *increase* the effects of propranolol

- chlorpromazine (Thorazine, etc.).
- cimetidine (Tagamet).
- diltiazem (Cardizem).
- disopyramide (Norpace).
- furosemide and other diuretics.
- methimazole (Tapazole).
- nicardipine (Cardene).
- propylthiouracil (Propacil).

The following drugs may *decrease* the effects of propranolol
- antacids.
- barbiturates (phenobarbital, etc.).
- indomethacin (Indocin) and possibly other aspirin substitutes or NSAIDs; may impair propranolol's antihypertensive effect.
- rifampin (Rifadin, Rimactane).

Driving, Hazardous Activities: Use caution until the full extent of drowsiness, lethargy, and blood pressure change has been determined.

Exposure to Heat: Caution is advised. Hot environments can lower blood pressure and exaggerate the effects of this drug.

Exposure to Cold: Caution is advised. Cold environments can enhance circulatory deficiency in the extremities. The elderly should take precautions to prevent hypothermia.

Heavy Exercise or Exertion: It is advisable to avoid exertion that produces light-headedness, excessive fatigue, or muscle cramping. Use of this drug may intensify the hypertensive response to isometric exercise.

Occurrence of Unrelated Illness: The fever that accompanies systemic infections can lower blood pressure and require adjustment of dosage. Illnesses that cause nausea or vomiting may interrupt the regular dosage schedule. Ask your doctor for guidance.

Discontinuation: Avoid sudden discontinuation of this drug in all situations; this is especially true in the presence of coronary artery disease. If possible, gradual reduction of dose over a period of 2 to 3 weeks is recommended. Ask your doctor for specific guidance.

▷ **Saving Money When Using This Medicine:**
- A large number of available drugs provide similar effectiveness. Ask your doctor to prescribe the drug that offers the best combination of cost and outcome.
- A generic form may be substituted for the brand name.
- Talk with your doctor about stress management and exercise programs available in your area.
- Ask your doctor if taking aspirin every other day to help prevent a heart attack makes sense for you.

PROTRIPTYLINE (proh TRIP ti leen)

Prescription Needed: Yes   **Controlled Drug:** No   **Generic:** No

Brand Name: Vivactil

Overview of BENEFITS versus RISKS

Possible Benefits	*Possible Risks*
EFFECTIVE RELIEF OF MAJOR ENDOGENOUS DEPRESSIONS	ADVERSE BEHAVIORAL EFFECTS: confusion, disorientation, hallucinations, delusions
Possibly beneficial for other depressive disorders	CONVERSION OF DEPRESSION TO MANIA in manic-depressive disorders
Possibly beneficial for managing of attention deficit disorder	Aggravation of schizophrenia
Possibly beneficial for managing narcolepsy/cataplexy syndrome	Irregular heart rhythms
	Rare blood cell abnormalities

▷ **Illness This Medication Treats:**

Relief of symptoms associated with major spontaneous (endogenous) depression, depressed bipolar disorder, and mixed bipolar disorder.

▷ **Typical Dosage Range:** (Dosage or schedule must be determined by the doctor for each individual.)

Infants and Children: Dosage not established.

12 to 60 Years of Age: Initially 5 to 10 mg, three or four times daily. Increase dose cautiously as needed and tolerated by 5 mg daily at intervals of 1 week. The usual maintenance dose is 15 to 40 mg every 24 hours, divided into three or four doses. The total daily dose should not exceed 60 mg.

Over 60 Years of Age: Initially 5 mg two or three times daily to evaluate tolerance. Increase dose cautiously, as needed and tolerated, by 5 mg daily at intervals of 1 week. Doses above 20 mg daily require careful monitoring of heart function and blood pressure. The total daily dose should not exceed 40 mg.

▷ **Conditions Requiring Dosing Adjustments:**

Liver function. People with liver compromise should use this drug with caution. The dose should be decreased, and blood levels obtained at appropriate intervals. Protriptyline is a rare cause of liver toxicity.

Kidney function: Patients with urine outflow problems should use this drug with caution, as it can delay urination.

▷ **How Best to Take This Medicine:**   May be taken without regard to meals. The tablet may be crushed

For those who experience a stimulating effect: (1) necessary dosage increases should be made in the morning; (2) the last daily dose should be taken in the afternoon (3 to 4 P.M.) to avoid insomnia and disturbed dreaming.

▷ **How Long This Medicine Is Usually Taken:**   Some benefit may be apparent within 1 to 2 weeks, but adequate response may require continual use for 3 months or longer. Long-term use should not exceed 6 months without evaluation of the need for continuation. See your doctor regularly.

▷ **Tell Your Doctor Before Taking This Medicine If You:**
- ever had an allergic reaction to it.
- are taking, or have taken within the past 14 days, any MAO type A inhibitor.
- are recovering from a recent heart attack.
- have narrow-angle glaucoma.
- are allergic or sensitive to any other tricyclic antidepressant.
- have a history of diabetes, epilepsy, psychosis, glaucoma, heart disease, prostate gland enlargement, or overactive thyroid function.
- plan to have surgery under general anesthesia soon.

▷ **Possible Side Effects:**   Light-headedness, blurred vision, dry mouth, constipation, impaired urination.

▷ **Possible Adverse Effects:**
If any of the following develop, call your doctor promptly for guidance.
Some Mild Problems Drug Can Cause
   Allergic reactions: skin rash, swelling of face or tongue, drug fever.
   Headache, dizziness, weakness, fainting, unsteady gait, tremors.
   Peculiar taste, irritation of tongue or mouth, nausea, indigestion.
   Fluctuation of blood sugar levels.
Some Serious Problems Drug Can Cause
   Allergic reactions: hepatitis, with or without jaundice.
   Confusion, hallucinations, delusions.
   Aggravation of paranoid psychoses and schizophrenia; seizures.
   Heart palpitation and irregular rhythm.
   Bone marrow depression—fatigue, fever, sore throat, abnormal bleeding or bruising.
   Peripheral neuritis—numbness, tingling, pain.
   Parkinson-like disorders—usually mild and infrequent; more likely to occur in the elderly.

▷ **Possible Effects on Sex Life:**   Decreased libido, increased libido (antidepressant effect), male impotence, inhibited female orgasm, male and female breast enlargement, milk production, swelling of testicles.

▷ **Adverse Effects That May Mimic Natural Diseases or Disorders:**
   Liver toxicity may suggest viral hepatitis.

▷ *CAUTION*

1. Dosage must be adjusted for each person individually. Report for follow-up evaluation and laboratory tests as directed by your doctor.
2. It is advisable to withhold this drug if electroconvulsive therapy is to be used to treat your depression.
3. Safety and effectiveness of this drug for those under 6 years old are not established. This drug may be used to relieve symptoms of attention deficit disorder, with or without hyperactivity, in selected children over 6 years old.
4. Usual dosage for those over 60 is 15 to 30 mg daily in divided doses. During the first 2 weeks of treatment, watch for confusion, agitation, forgetfulness, disorientation, delusions, and hallucinations. Reduction of dosage or discontinuation may be necessary. Unsteadiness may predispose to falling and injury. This drug can increase the degree of impaired urination associated with prostate gland enlargement.

Advisability of Use During Pregnancy or If Breast-Feeding:

Pregnancy Category: C. Avoid use of this drug during the first 3 months. Use during the last 6 months only if clearly needed. Ask your doctor for guidance. Presence in breast milk in small amounts. Monitor the nursing infant closely and discontinue taking this drug or nursing if adverse effects develop: excessive drowsiness and failure to feed.

▷ **Habit-Forming Potential.**   Psychological or physical dependence is rare and unexpected.

▷ **Overdose Symptoms:**

Confusion, hallucinations, marked drowsiness, heart palpitations, dilated pupils, tremors, stupor, deep sleep, coma, convulsions.

▷ **Suggested Periodic Examinations While Taking This Drug:** (at doctor's discretion)

Complete blood cell counts, liver function tests, and electrocardiograms.

▷ **While Taking This Drug the Following Apply:**

Foods: May increase the appetite and cause excessive weight gain.

Beverages: May be taken with milk.

Alcohol: Avoid completely. This drug can markedly increase the intoxicating effects of alcohol and accentuate its depressant action on brain function.

Tobacco Smoking: May hasten the drug's elimination. Higher doses of this drug may be necessary.

Other Drugs:

Protriptyline may *increase* the effects of

• atropinelike drugs.
• dicumarol, increasing the risk of bleeding.

- epinephrine (Adrenalin).
- norepinephrine.
- phenytoin (Dilantin) and lead to toxicity.
- pseudoephedrine and may cause high blood pressure and arrhythmias.

Protriptyline may **decrease** the effects of

- clonidine (Catapres), causing loss of blood pressure control; do not use these drugs concurrently.
- guanethidine (Ismelin).

Protriptyline **taken concurrently** with

- carbamazepine (Tegretol) may lead to increased blood levels and risk of carbamazepine toxicity as well as blunted protriptyline benefits.
- disulfiram (Antabuse) may cause acute dementia: confusion, disorientation, hallucinations.
- MAO inhibitors (see Drug Classes) may cause high fever, delirium, and convulsions.
- thyroid preparations may impair heart rhythm and function. Ask your doctor for guidance regarding adjustment of thyroid dose.
- venlafaxine (Effexor) may lead to increased protriptyline levels and toxicity.
- warfarin (Coumadin) may lead to prolonged anticoagulation. Increased frequency of INR (prothrombin time) testing should be done, and dose adjustment of warfarin to laboratory test results.

The following drugs may **increase** the effects of protriptyline

- cimetidine (Tagamet).
- estrogens (Premarin).
- fluoxetine (Prozac).
- lithium (Lithobid, etc.).
- oral contraceptives (birth control pills).
- ranitidine (Zantac).
- sertraline (Zoloft).

The following drugs may **decrease** the effects of protriptyline

- barbiturates—may reduce protriptyline's effectiveness.

Driving, Hazardous Activities: May impair mental alertness, judgment, physical coordination, and reaction time. Avoid hazardous activities.

Exposure to Sun: May cause photosensitivity.

Exposure to Heat: This drug can inhibit sweating and impair the body's adaptation to hot environments, increasing the risk of heatstroke. Avoid saunas.

Exposure to Cold: The elderly should use caution and avoid conditions conducive to hypothermia.

Discontinuation: Discontinue this drug gradually. Abrupt withdrawal after long-term use can cause headache, malaise, and nausea.

▷ **Saving Money When Using This Medicine:**
- A large number of available drugs provide similar effectiveness. Ask your doctor to prescribe the drug that offers the best combination of cost and outcome.
- It may be possible (after a significant symptom-free period) to stop this medicine. Ask your doctor for help.
- Ask your doctor if stress management and exercise programs available in your area make sense for you.
- Recently depression has been found to be associated with an increased risk of osteoporosis. Talk with your doctor about calcium supplements, risk factors, exercise, and bone mineral density testing.

PYRAZINAMIDE (peer a ZIN a mide)

Prescription Needed: Yes   **Controlled Drug:** No   **Generic:** Yes

Brand Name: Rifater

Overview of BENEFITS versus RISKS	
Possible Benefits	*Possible Risks*
EFFECTIVE ADJUNCTIVE TREATMENT OF TUBERCULOSIS	DRUG-INDUCED HEPATITIS
	Activation of gouty arthritis
	Activation of porphyria
	Rare decreased platelets or hemoglobin

▷ **Illness This Medication Treats:**
Combination treatment of active tuberculosis.

▷ **Typical Dosage Range:** (Dosage or schedule must be determined by the doctor for each individual.)
Infants and Children: 7.5 to 15 mg per kilogram of body weight, twice daily; or 15 to 30 mg per kilogram of body weight, once daily.
Total daily dosage should not exceed 1.5 g.
12 to 60 Years of Age: For tuberculosis: 15 to 30 mg per kilogram of body weight (up to a maximum of 2000 mg) daily. Some patients do better with twice-weekly dosing: 50–75 mg per kilogram of body weight, up to 4000 mg.
Author's note: Because of the current resistant tuberculosis problem, most clinicians start all patients on a four-drug regimen until laboratory culture results are available.
Over 60 Years of Age: Same as for 12 to 60 years of age.

▷ **Conditions Requiring Dosing Adjustments:**

Liver function: Patients with liver compromise should use this drug with caution, in empirically decreased dosages. This drug is a hepatotoxin, and is contraindicated in patients with severe liver dysfunction.

Kidney function: For patients with endstage renal failure, the dose **must** be adjusted to 12 to 20 mg per kilogram of body weight daily. Patients should be closely monitored.

▷ **How Best to Take This Medicine:**   May be taken with or following food to reduce stomach irritation. The tablet may be crushed for administration. Take the full course prescribed. Pyrazinamide should be taken concurrently with other antitubercular drugs to prevent the development of drug-resistant strains of tuberculosis bacteria.

▷ **How Long This Medicine Is Usually Taken:**   Continual use on a regular schedule for 2 months is usually necessary to determine the effectiveness of this drug in controlling active tuberculosis. Long-term use of antitubercular drugs (6 months or more) requires periodic evaluation of response and dosage adjustment. See your doctor regularly.

▷ **Tell Your Doctor Before Taking This Medicine If You:**
- ever had an allergic reaction to it or ethionamide, isoniazid, or niacin (nicotinic acid).
- have permanent liver damage with impaired function.
- have active gout or diabetes.
- have active peptic ulcer disease or a history of peptic ulcer or porphyria.
- have a history of liver disease or impaired kidney function.

▷ **Possible Side Effects:**   Increased blood uric acid levels.

▷ **Possible Adverse Effects:**

If any of the following develop, call your doctor promptly for guidance.

Some Mild Problems Drug Can Cause
Allergic reactions: skin rash, itching, fever.
Loss of appetite, nausea, vomiting.
Joint pain.

Some Serious Problems Drug Can Cause
Idiosyncratic reactions: rare sideroblastic anemia.
Drug-induced hepatitis, with and without jaundice.
Rare seizures, porphyria, decreased blood platelets, or interstitial nephritis.
Gouty arthritis, due to increased blood uric acid levels.

▷ **Adverse Effects That May Mimic Natural Diseases or Disorders:**
Drug-induced hepatitis may suggest viral hepatitis.

▷ *CAUTION*
1. When this drug is used alone, tuberculosis bacteria rapidly develop resistance. To be effective, this drug must be used in combination with other effective antitubercular drugs.
2. This drug may interfere with control of diabetes.
3. Safety and effectiveness of this drug for those under 12 years old have not been established. The rare occurrence of a drug-related seizure has been reported in a 2-year-old child.

Advisability of Use During Pregnancy or If Breast-Feeding:
Pregnancy Category: C. Use this drug only if clearly needed. Ask your doctor for guidance. Present in breast milk; avoid taking this drug or refrain from nursing.

▷ **Overdose Symptoms:** Nausea, vomiting, malaise.

▷ **Possible Effects of Long-Term Use:** Liver damage.

▷ **Suggested Periodic Examinations While Taking This Drug:** (at doctor's discretion)
Complete blood cell counts.
Liver function tests.
Uric acid blood levels.

▷ **While Taking This Drug the Following Apply:**
Beverages: May be taken with milk.
Alcohol: Use sparingly to minimize liver toxicity.
Other Drugs:
Pyrazinamide may *decrease* the effects of
• allopurinol (Zyloprim).
• BCG vaccine.
• colchicine (ColBenemid).
• probenecid (Benemid).
• sulfinpyrazone (Anturane).
Exposure to Sun: Use caution until full effect is known. This drug may cause photosensitivity.
Discontinuation: This drug is usually taken for a minimum of 2 months if tolerated. Do not stop taking it without your doctor's knowledge and guidance.

▷ **Saving Money When Using This Medicine:**
• There is a severe problem with resistant tuberculosis in this country as this book went to press. The best outcomes are achieved with combination therapy of several drugs. Ask your doctor if this medicine offers the best balance of cost and outcome for you.
• A generic form may be substituted for the brand name.

PYRIDOSTIGMINE   (peer id oh STIG meen)

Prescription Needed: Yes   **Controlled Drug:** No   **Generic:**
No

Brand Names: Mestinon, Mestinon Timespan, Regonol

Overview of BENEFITS versus RISKS

Possible Benefits	*Possible Risks*
MODERATELY EFFECTIVE TREATMENT OF OCULAR AND MILD FORMS OF MYASTHENIA GRAVIS (symptomatic relief of muscle weakness)	Cholinergic crisis (overdose): excessive salivation, nausea, vomiting, stomach cramps, diarrhea, shortness of breath (asthmalike wheezing), excessive weakness

---

▷ **Illness This Medication Treats:**
  (1) Ocular and milder forms of myasthenia gravis—gives temporary relief of muscle weakness and fatigability; most useful in long-term treatment when there is little or no difficulty in swallowing; (2) of limited use in reversing effects of muscle relaxants.

▷ **Typical Dosage Range:** (Dosage or schedule must be determined by the doctor for each individual.)
  Myasthenia gravis: Initially one to six normal-release tablets spaced throughout the day when maximum strength is needed. Ongoing dose varies: one to three extended-release tablets every 6 hours. Some patients supplement the extended-release tablets with the 30 mg immediate-release tablets or the syrup in order to best control of symptoms.

▷ **How Best to Take This Medicine:**   Take with food or milk to reduce the intensity of side effects. Larger portions of the daily maintenance dosage should be timed according to the pattern of fatigue and weakness. The syrup will permit a finer adjustment of dosage. The regular tablet may be crushed. The prolonged-action tablet should be taken whole (not altered).

▷ **How Long This Medicine Is Usually Taken:**   Continual use on a regular schedule (with dosage adjustment) for 10 to 14 days usually determines the effectiveness of this drug in relieving the symptoms of myasthenia gravis. Long-term use (months to years) requires periodic evaluation of response and dosage adjustment.

▷ **Tell Your Doctor Before Taking This Medicine If You:**
  • are allergic to bromide compounds.
  • are subject to heart rhythm disorders or bronchial asthma.

- have recurrent urinary tract infections.
- have prostatism.
- plan to have surgery under general anesthesia soon.

▷ **Possible Side Effects:**   Small pupils, watering of eyes, slow pulse, excessive salivation, nausea, vomiting, stomach cramps, diarrhea, urge to urinate, increased sweating.

▷ **Possible Adverse Effects:**
If any of the following develop, call your doctor promptly for guidance.

Some Mild Problems Drug Can Cause
Allergic reaction: skin rash.
Nervousness, anxiety, unsteadiness, muscle cramps, or twitching.
Loss of scalp hair.

Some Serious Problems Drug Can Cause
Confusion, slurred speech, seizures, difficult breathing (asthmatic wheezing).
Increased muscle weakness or paralysis.
Rare psychosis.
Excessive vomiting or diarrhea may induce abnormally low blood potassium levels, accentuating muscle weakness.

▷ **Adverse Effects That May Mimic Natural Diseases or Disorders:**
Seizures may suggest the possibility of epilepsy.

▷ *CAUTION*
1. Certain drugs can block the action of this drug and reduce its effectiveness in treating myasthenia gravis. Talk to your doctor before starting any new drug, prescription or over-the-counter.
2. Dosage schedule must be carefully individualized. Variations in response may occur from time to time. Because generalized muscle weakness is a major symptom of both myasthenia crisis (underdosage) and cholinergic crisis (overdosage), it may be difficult to recognize the correct cause. As a rule, weakness that begins within 1 hour after taking this drug probably represents overdosage; weakness that begins after 3 or more hours is probably due to underdosage. Observe these time relationships and tell your doctor.
3. During long-term use, observe for resistance to the drug's therapeutic action (loss of effectiveness). Ask your doctor about the advisability of discontinuing this drug for a few days to see if responsiveness can be restored.
4. The syrup form permits greater precision of dosage adjustment and ease of administration in children.
5. The natural decline of kidney function with aging may require smaller doses to prevent accumulation to toxic levels.

Advisability of Use During Pregnancy or If Breast-Feeding:

Pregnancy Category: C. There are no reports of birth defects during pregnancy. However, there are reports of significant muscular weakness in newborn infants whose mothers took this drug during pregnancy. Ask your doctor for guidance. Present in breast milk. Watch the nursing infant closely and discontinue taking this drug or nursing if adverse effects develop.

▷ **Overdose Symptoms:** Generalized muscular weakness, blurred vision, very small pupils, slow heart rate, difficult breathing (wheezing), excessive salivation, nausea, vomiting, stomach cramps, diarrhea, muscle cramps, or twitching. This syndrome constitutes the cholinergic crisis.

▷ **While Taking This Drug the Following Apply:**

Beverages: May be taken with milk.

Alcohol: Use caution until the combined effects are determined. Weakness and unsteadiness may be accentuated.

Other Drugs:

The following drugs may *decrease* the effects of pyridostigmine

- atropine (belladonna).
- clindamycin (Cleocin).
- guanadrel (Hylorel).
- guanethidine (Esimil, Ismelin).
- procainamide (Procan SR, Pronestyl).
- quinidine (Cardioquin, Duraquin, etc.).
- quinine (Quinamm).
- steroids (see Drug Classes).

Pyridostigmine *taken concurrently* with

- disopyramide (Norpace) may ease the sweating, problems with urinating, and other *anticholinergic* effects of pyridostigmine.

Driving, Hazardous Activities: May cause blurred vision, confusion, or generalized weakness. Restrict your activities as necessary.

Exposure to Heat: Use caution. This drug may cause excessive sweating and increased weakness.

Exposure to Environmental Chemicals: Avoid excessive exposure (inhalation, skin contamination) to the insecticides Baygon, Diazinon, and Sevin, which can accentuate this drug's potential toxicity.

Discontinuation: Do not stop taking this drug abruptly without your doctor's knowledge and guidance.

▷ **Saving Money When Using This Medicine:**

- Ask your doctor if this medicine offers the best balance of cost and outcome for you.

- People with compromised kidneys should use this drug with caution and in decreased doses.
- Find out as much as possible about your condition. *The Essential Guide to Chronic Illness* is an excellent resource.

PYRIMETHAMINE (peer i METH a meen)

Prescription Needed: Yes   **Controlled Drug:** No   **Generic:** No

Brand Names: Daraprim, Fansidar [CD]

```
                Overview of BENEFITS versus RISKS
      Possible Benefits                 Possible Risks
 EFFECTIVE PREVENTION          BONE MARROW
    AND TREATMENT OF              DEPRESSION, APLASTIC
    CERTAIN TYPES OF              ANEMIA
    MALARIA                     Serious skin reactions
 Effective treatment of
    AIDS-related isosporiasis
    diarrhea
 Effective adjunctive treatment
    of AIDS-related toxoplasmosis
```

▷ **Illness This Medication Treats:**
  (1) Prevents chloroquine-resistant *Plasmodium falciparum* malaria, when taken with sulfadoxine; (2) treats chloroquine-resistant *Plasmodium falciparum* malaria, when taken together with sulfadoxine and quinine; (3) helps toxoplasmosis.
  Other (unlabeled) generally accepted uses: (1) treatment of isosporiasis diarrhea in those with AIDS or AIDS-related complex (ARC); (2) treatment of toxoplasmosis in those with AIDS or ARC; (3) prevention of *Pneumocystis carinii* pneumonia (PCP) in HIV-positive patients.

QUAZEPAM (KWAH zee pam)

Prescription Needed: Yes   **Controlled Drug:** C-IV*   **Generic:** No

Brand Name: Doral, Dormalin

*See Controlled Drug Schedules inside this book's cover.

```
┌─────────────────────────────────────────────────────┐
│          Overview of BENEFITS versus RISKS          │
│   Possible Benefits           Possible Risks        │
│  EFFECTIVE HYPNOTIC during   Habit-forming potential with │
│    4 weeks of continual use    long-term use         │
│  NO SUPPRESSION OF REM       Minor impairment of mental │
│    (RAPID EYE MOVEMENT)        functions ("hangover" effect) │
│    SLEEP                                             │
│  NO REM SLEEP REBOUND                               │
│    after discontinuation                            │
│  Wide margin of safety with                         │
│    therapeutic doses                                │
└─────────────────────────────────────────────────────┘
```

▷ **Illness This Medication Treats:**
(1) Short-term treatment of insomnia (difficulty falling asleep, frequent nighttime awakenings, and/or early morning awakenings); (2) preoperative use as a hypnotic.

▷ **Typical Dosage Range:** (Dosage or schedule must be determined by the doctor for each individual.)
Infants and Children: Up to 18 years of age—use of this drug is not recommended.
18 to 60 Years of Age: Initially 15 mg at bedtime; on the third night, decrease to 7.5 mg and evaluate effectiveness; adjust further dosage as needed and tolerated.
Over 60 Years of Age: Same as for 18 to 60 years of age. The usual maintenance dose is 7.5 mg, once daily at bedtime; use higher doses with caution.

▷ **Conditions Requiring Dosing Adjustments:**
Liver function: The dose **must** be decreased for patients with liver compromise.
Kidney function: Quazepam should be used with caution and in decreased doses by patients with renal compromise.

▷ **How Best to Take This Medicine:** May be taken on an empty stomach or with food or milk. The tablet may be crushed. Do not stop it abruptly if taken for more than 4 weeks.

▷ **How Long This Medicine Is Usually Taken:** Continual use for 3 nights is needed to evaluate benefits in relieving insomnia. If possible, use this drug for periods of 3 to 5 nights intermittently, repeating as needed with appropriate dosage adjustment. Avoid uninterrupted and prolonged use. The duration of use should not exceed 2 weeks without reappraisal of continued need.

▷ **Tell Your Doctor Before Taking This Medicine If You:**
• ever had an allergic reaction to it.
• are pregnant or planning pregnancy.

- have acute narrow-angle glaucoma.
- are allergic to any benzodiazepine drug.
- are told you suffer sleep apnea (periods of momentary cessation of breathing while asleep).
- have a history of alcoholism or drug abuse.
- have impaired liver or kidney function.
- have a history of serious depression or a mental disorder.
- are taking other drugs with sedative effects.
- have asthma, emphysema, epilepsy, or myasthenia gravis.

▷ **Possible Side Effects:** Mild "hangover" effects on arising: drowsiness, lethargy.

▷ **Possible Adverse Effects:**
If any of the following develop, call your doctor promptly for guidance.

Some Mild Problems Drug Can Cause
Allergic reactions: skin rash, itching.
Headache, dizziness, fatigue, blurred vision.
Dry mouth, nausea, vomiting, indigestion, constipation, diarrhea.

Some Serious Problems Drug Can Cause
Idiosyncratic reactions: nervousness, irritability, euphoria, hallucinations (rare paradoxical reactions that may occur with any benzodiazepine).

▷ **Possible Effects on Sex Life:** Decreased libido, impotence (rare and questionable).

▷ *CAUTION*
1. This drug should not be stopped abruptly if it has been taken continually for more than 4 weeks.
2. The concurrent use of some over-the-counter drug products that contain antihistamines (allergy and cold preparations, sleep aids) can cause excessive sedation in sensitive individuals.
3. Regular nightly use of any hypnotic drug should be avoided.
4. The liver transforms this drug into long-acting forms that persist in the body for 24 hours or more. With continual daily use of this drug, these active forms may accumulate and produce increasing sedation. If you experience a "hangover" effect, avoid hazardous activities (driving, etc.) and the use of alcohol.
5. Safety and effectiveness of this drug for those under 18 years old have not been established.
6. Those over 60 should use smaller doses at longer intervals to avoid overdosage. Observe for the possible development of lethargy, indifference, fatigue, weakness, unsteadiness, disturbing dreams, nightmares, and paradoxical reactions of excitement, agitation, anger, hostility, and rage. This long-acting benzodiazepine may cause residual sluggishness and unsteadiness, with increased risk

of falling during the day following bedtime use. This drug may also increase the number of periods of sleep apnea in this age group.

Advisability of Use During Pregnancy or If Breast-Feeding:

Pregnancy Category: X. Several studies indicate an increased risk of birth defects if benzodiazepines are used during the first 3 months. Frequent use in late pregnancy can cause floppy infant syndrome in the newborn: weakness, lethargy, unresponsiveness, depressed breathing, low body temperature. Avoid use of this drug during entire pregnancy. Present in breast milk; avoid taking this drug or refrain from nursing.

▷ **Habit-Forming Potential:** Can produce psychological and/or physical dependence in large doses for an extended period. Avoid continual use.

▷ **Overdose Symptoms:** Marked drowsiness, weakness, feeling of drunkenness, staggering gait, tremor, stupor progressing to deep sleep or coma.

▷ **While Taking This Drug the Following Apply:**

Beverages: Avoid excessive intake of caffeine-containing beverages (coffee, tea, cola, chocolate) within 4 hours of taking this drug. This drug may be taken with milk.

Alcohol: Use with extreme caution until the combined effect is determined. Alcohol may increase the absorption of this drug and add to its depressant effects on the brain. Avoid alcohol completely, throughout the day and night, if you need to drive or engage in any hazardous activity.

Tobacco Smoking: Heavy smoking may reduce the hypnotic action of this drug.

Marijuana Smoking: Increased sedation and significant impairment of intellectual and physical performance.

Other Drugs:

Quazepam may *increase* the effects of
- digoxin (Lanoxin), causing digoxin toxicity.
- phenytoin (Dilantin), causing phenytoin toxicity.

Quazepam may *decrease* the effects of
- levodopa (Sinemet, etc.), reducing its effectiveness in treating Parkinson's disease.

The following drugs may *increase* the effects of quazepam
- cimetidine (Tagamet).
- clindamycin (Cleocin).
- disulfiram (Antabuse).
- isoniazid (INH, Rifamate, etc.).
- omeprazole (Prilosec).

- oral contraceptives (birth control pills).
- valproic acid (Depakene).

The following drugs may **decrease** the effects of quazepam

- rifampin (Rimactane, etc.).
- theophylline (aminophylline, Theo-Dur, etc.).

Driving, Hazardous Activities: May impair mental alertness, judgment, physical coordination, and reaction time. Avoid hazardous activities accordingly.

Exposure to Heat: Use caution until the effect of excessive perspiration is determined. Because of reduced urine volume, this drug may accumulate in the body and produce overdosage effects.

Discontinuation: Avoid sudden discontinuation if this drug has been taken for more than 4 weeks without interruption. Dosage should be tapered gradually to prevent a withdrawal syndrome that could include depression, confusion, hallucinations, tremor, seizures, muscle cramping, sweating, and vomiting.

▷ **Saving Money When Using This Medicine:**

- Ask your doctor if this medicine offers the best balance of cost and outcome for you.
- Talk with your doctor about modifying caffeine (from coffee, tea, sodas, etc.). Also ask if any of your prescription, nonprescription, or herbal medicines could contribute to your sleep problems.
- Dose MUST be decreased for people with compromised livers.
- If your response has been good, ask your doctor if your dose can be decreased, and then discontinued.

QUINAPRIL (KWIN a pril)

Prescription Needed: Yes   **Controlled Drug:** No   **Generic:** No

Brand Name: Accupril

Overview of BENEFITS versus RISKS	
Possible Benefits	*Possible Risks*
EFFECTIVE CONTROL OF MILD TO MODERATE HIGH BLOOD PRESSURE	Rare low blood pressure
	Very rare allergic swelling of face, tongue, vocal cords
	Lowering of white blood cell count (reported with other medicines in this class)

▷ **Illness This Medication Treats:**
(1) Mild to moderate high blood pressure, either alone or concurrently with a thiazide diuretic; (2) treats congestive heart failure.

▷ **Typical Dosage Range:** (Dosage or schedule must be determined by the doctor for each individual.)

Infants and Children: Dosage not established.

12 to 60 Years of Age: Initially 10 mg once daily for those who are not taking a diuretic; 5 mg once daily for those taking a diuretic. The usual maintenance dose is 20 to 40 mg daily, taken in a single dose. If once-a-day dosing does not give stable control of blood pressure over a 24-hour period, divide the dose equally into morning and evening doses. The total daily dosage should not exceed 80 mg.

Over 60 Years of Age: Same as for 12 to 60 years of age, if kidney function is normal. If kidney function is significantly impaired, reduce dose by 50%. The total daily dose should not exceed 40 mg.

▷ **Conditions Requiring Dosing Adjustments:**

Kidney function: Patients with mild kidney failure can take 10 mg daily. Those with moderate kidney failure may take 5 mg daily. Patients with severe kidney failure may take 2.5 mg daily.

▷ **How Best to Take This Medicine:**   Take on an empty stomach or with food at same time each day. The tablet may be crushed.

▷ **How Long This Medicine Is Usually Taken:**   Continual use on a regular schedule for 2 to 3 weeks is usually necessary to determine the effectiveness of this drug in controlling high blood pressure. The proper treatment of high blood pressure usually requires the long-term use of effective medications. See your doctor regularly.

▷ **Tell Your Doctor Before Taking This Medicine If You:**

- ever had an allergic reaction to it or to other ACE inhibitors.
- are in last 6 months of pregnancy or planning pregnancy.
- currently have a blood cell or bone marrow disorder.
- have an abnormally high level of blood potassium.
- have a history of kidney disease or impaired kidney function.
- are taking an immunosuppressant or have a low white blood cell count.
- have scleroderma or systemic lupus erythematosus.
- have cerebral artery disease.
- have any form of heart disease.
- are taking any other antihypertensives, diuretics, nitrates, or potassium supplements.
- plan to have surgery under general anesthesia soon.

▷ **Possible Side Effects:**   Dizziness, orthostatic hypotension, fainting, increased blood potassium level.

▷ **Possible Adverse Effects:**

If any of the following develop, call your doctor promptly for guidance.

Some Mild Problems Drug Can Cause
> Allergic reactions: skin rash, itching.
> Headache, fatigue, drowsiness, numbness and tingling, weakness.
> Cough, chest pain, palpitation.
> Nausea/vomiting, constipation.

Some Serious Problems Drug Can Cause
> Allergic reactions: swelling (angioedema) of face, tongue, and/or vocal cords; can be life-threatening.
> Blood cell problems have been reported with other ACE inhibitors, and caution should be used.
> Impairment of kidney function.

▷ **Possible Effects on Sex Life:**   Swelling or tenderness of male breast tissue (gynecomastia).

▷ *CAUTION*

1. Ask your doctor about the advisability of discontinuing other antihypertensives (especially diuretics) for 1 week before starting this drug.
2. **Tell your doctor immediately if you become pregnant.** This drug should not be taken beyond the first 3 months of pregnancy.
3. **Report promptly** any indications of infection (fever, sore throat) and water retention (weight gain, puffiness, swollen feet or ankles).
4. Do not use a salt substitute without your doctor's knowledge and approval (many contain potassium).
5. Obtain blood cell counts and urine analyses **before** starting this drug.
6. Safety and effectiveness of this drug for infants and children have not been established.
7. For those over 60, small doses are advisable until tolerance has been determined. Sudden and excessive lowering of blood pressure can predispose to stroke or heart attack in those with impaired brain circulation or coronary artery heart disease.

Advisability of Use During Pregnancy or If Breast-Feeding:
Pregnancy Category: C in the first 3 months of pregnancy; D in the last 6 months. Avoid using this drug completely during the last 6 months. During the first 3 months of pregnancy, use only if clearly needed. Ask your doctor for guidance. Presence in breast milk is unknown; avoid taking this drug or refrain from nursing.

▷ **Overdose Symptoms:**   Excessive drop in blood pressure, light-headedness, dizziness, fainting.

▷ **Suggested Periodic Examinations While Taking This Drug:** (at doctor's discretion)
Before starting drug: complete blood cell counts, urine analysis with measurement of protein content, blood potassium level.

During use of drug: blood cell counts, measurements of blood potassium.

▷ **While Taking This Drug the Following Apply:**

Foods: Talk with your doctor about salt intake.

Nutritional Support: **Do not take** potassium supplements unless directed by your doctor.

Beverages: May be taken with milk.

Alcohol: Use caution until the combined effect has been determined. Alcohol may enhance the blood pressure–lowering effect of this drug.

Other Drugs:

Quinapril **taken concurrently** with

- aspirin or other NSAIDs (see Drug Classes) may blunt quinapril's benefits.
- cyclosporine (Sandimmune) may cause increased kidney toxicity.
- furosemide (Lasix) may cause decreased blood pressure on standing (postural hypotension).
- lithium can cause increased lithium blood levels and toxicity; monitor lithium blood levels and adjust dosage as necessary.
- potassium preparations (K-Lyte, Slow-K, etc.) may cause increased blood levels of potassium, with risk of serious heart rhythm disturbances.
- potassium-sparing diuretics—amiloride (Moduretic), spironolactone (Aldactazide), triamterene (Dyazide)—may cause increased blood levels of potassium, with risk of serious heart rhythm disturbances.
- tetracycline can reduce the absorption of tetracycline.

Driving, Hazardous Activities: Be aware of possible drops in blood pressure with resultant dizziness or faintness.

Exposure to Sun: Caution is advised. A similar drug from this class can cause photosensitivity.

Exposure to Heat: Caution is advised. Avoid excessive perspiring with resultant loss of body water and drop in blood pressure.

Occurrence of Unrelated Illness: Report promptly any disorder that causes nausea, vomiting, or diarrhea. Fluid and chemical imbalances must be corrected as soon as possible.

Discontinuation: This drug may be stopped abruptly without causing a sudden increase in blood pressure. However, you should talk with your doctor about withdrawal for any reason.

▷ **Saving Money When Using This Medicine:**

- Many drugs are available to treat high blood pressure. Ask your doctor if this medicine offers the best balance of cost and outcome for you. Ask how often your blood pressure should be checked.

- Ask your doctor if stress management and exercise programs available in your community make sense for you.
- Talk with your doctor about the advisability of taking aspirin every other day to help prevent a heart attack.

QUINIDINE (KWIN i deen)

Prescription Needed: Yes **Controlled Drug:** No **Generic:** Yes

Brand Names: Cardioquin, Cin-Quin, Duraquin, Quinaglute Dura-Tabs, Quinidex Extentabs, Quinora, SK-Quinidine Sulfate

Overview of BENEFITS versus RISKS	
Possible Benefits	*Possible Risks*
EFFECTIVE TREATMENT OF SELECTED HEART RHYTHM DISORDERS	NARROW TREATMENT RANGE
	FREQUENT ADVERSE EFFECTS
	NUMEROUS ALLERGIC AND IDIOSYNCRATIC REACTIONS
	Dose-related toxicity
	Provocation of abnormal heart rhythms
	Rare: abnormally low blood platelet count, hemolytic anemia, kidney or liver toxicity

▷ **Illness This Medication Treats:**
(1) Used to control abnormal heart rhythms: atrial fibrillation and flutter, paroxysmal atrial tachycardia, paroxysmal ventricular tachycardia, premature atrial and ventricular contractions; (2) used intravenously for malaria in people unable to take medicines by mouth.
As Combination Drug Product [CD]: This drug is available in Canada in combination with a barbiturate, a mild sedative added to allay the anxiety and nervous tension that often accompany heart rhythm disorders.

▷ **Typical Dosage Range:** (Dosage or schedule must be determined by the doctor for each individual.)
For premature atrial or ventricular contractions: 200 to 300 mg three or four times each day.
For paroxysmal atrial tachycardia: 400 to 600 mg every 2 to 3 hours until paroxysm is terminated.

For atrial flutter: digitalize first; then individualize dosage schedule as appropriate.

For atrial fibrillation: digitalize first; then try 200 mg every 2 to 3 hours for five to eight doses; increase dose daily until normal rhythm is restored or toxic effects develop.

Maintenance schedule: 200 to 300 mg three or four times each day. The total daily dosage should not exceed 4000 mg.

▷ **Conditions Requiring Dosing Adjustments:**

Liver function: This drug is extensively metabolized in the liver. Blood levels should be obtained to guide dosing. Ongoing doses may need to be lowered by 50%. Quinidine is a rare cause of liver damage, and patients should be followed closely.

Kidney function: Obtain blood levels as a guide to dosing. Increased elimination may be seen in patients with acid urine. Quinidine should be used with caution by patients with renal compromise.

▷ **How Best to Take This Medicine:**   Best taken on an empty stomach to achieve high blood levels rapidly. However, it may be taken with or following food to reduce stomach irritation. The regular tablets may be crushed and the capsules opened. The prolonged-action forms should be swallowed whole without alteration.

▷ **How Long This Medicine Is Usually Taken:**   Continual use on a regular schedule for 2 to 4 days is usually necessary to determine the effectiveness of this drug in correcting or preventing responsive abnormal rhythms. Long-term use (months to years) requires supervision and periodic evaluation. See your doctor regularly.

▷ **Tell Your Doctor Before Taking This Medicine If You:**
- ever had an allergic reaction it.
- currently have an acute infection of any kind.
- have coronary artery disease or myasthenia gravis.
- have a history of hyperthyroidism.
- had a deficiency of blood platelets in the past from any cause.
- have acute rheumatic fever or subacute bacterial endocarditis (SBE).
- are now taking, or have taken recently, any digitalis preparation (digitoxin, digoxin, etc.).
- plan to have surgery under general anesthesia soon.

▷ **Possible Side Effects:**   Drop in blood pressure, which may be marked in some people.

▷ **Possible Adverse Effects:**

If any of the following develop, call your doctor promptly for guidance.

Some Mild Problems Drug Can Cause

   Allergic reactions: skin rash, itching, drug fever (rare).

Dose-related toxicity (cinchonism): blurred vision, ringing in the ears, loss of hearing, dizziness.

Irritation of the esophagus.

Nausea, vomiting, diarrhea.

Some Serious Problems Drug Can Cause

Allergic reactions: severe skin reactions, hemolytic anemia, joint and muscle pains, anaphylactic reaction, reduced blood platelet count, drug-induced hepatitis.

Idiosyncratic reactions: skin rash, rapid heart rate, acute delirium and combative behavior, difficult breathing.

Heart conduction abnormalities.

Rare drug-induced myasthenia gravis, mental changes, kidney toxicity, systemic lupus erythematosus, or carpal tunnel syndrome.

Optic neuritis, impaired vision.

Abnormally low white blood cell count: fever, sore throat, infections.

▷ **Adverse Effects That May Mimic Natural Diseases or Disorders:**
Drug-induced hepatitis may suggest viral hepatitis.

▷ *CAUTION*

1. The effects of this drug are very unpredictable because of the wide variation in individual response. Dosage adjustments must be based upon individual reaction. Tell your doctor about any events you suspect are drug-related.

2. Carry a personal identification card that states you are taking this drug.

3. A test for drug idiosyncrasy should be made before this drug is started. Discontinue quinidine use if there is no beneficial response after 3 days of adequate dosage.

4. Small doses are mandatory for those over 60 until your individual response has been determined. Observe for the development of light-headedness, dizziness, weakness, or sense of impending faint. Use caution to prevent falls.

Advisability of Use During Pregnancy or If Breast-Feeding:
Pregnancy Category: C. Use this drug only if clearly needed. Present in breast milk; avoid taking this drug or refrain from nursing.

▷ **Overdose Symptoms:** Nausea, vomiting, ringing in the ears, headache, jerky eye movements, double vision, altered color vision, confusion, delirium, hot skin, seizures, coma.

▷ **Suggested Periodic Examinations While Taking This Drug:** (at doctor's discretion)
Complete blood cell counts, electrocardiograms.

▷ **While Taking This Drug the Following Apply:**
Beverages: May be taken with milk.

Alcohol: Alcohol may enhance the blood pressure–lowering effects of this drug.

Tobacco Smoking: Nicotine can increase irritability of the heart and aggravate rhythm disorders. Avoid all forms of tobacco.

Other Drugs:

Quinidine may ***increase*** the effects of
- anticoagulants (Coumadin, etc.), increasing the risk of bleeding.
- digitoxin and digoxin (Lanoxin), causing digitalis toxicity.
- disopyramide (Norpace).
- tricyclic antidepressants (see Drug Classes).
- warfarin (Coumadin) and lead to bleeding. More frequent INR (prothrombin times) are needed.

The following drugs may ***increase*** the effects of quinidine
- amiodarone (Cordarone).
- cimetidine (Tagamet).
- ketoconazole (Nizoral).
- verapamil (Verelan, others).

Quinapril ***taken concurrently*** with
- aspirin may prolong the bleeding time.
- beta-blockers (see Drug Classes) may lead to undesirable heart changes.
- codeine may blunt codeine's effectiveness.
- tricyclic antidepressants (see Drug Classes) may result in antidepressant toxicity.
- venlafaxine (Effexor) can lead to venlafaxine toxicity.

The following drugs may ***decrease*** the effects of quinidine
- barbiturates (phenobarbital, etc.).
- phenytoin (Dilantin).
- rifampin (Rifadin, Rimactane).
- sucralfate (Carafate).

Driving, Hazardous Activities: May cause dizziness and alter vision. Restrict your activities as necessary.

▷ **Saving Money When Using This Medicine:**
- Many new drugs are available to treat abnormal heart rhythms. Ask your doctor if this medicine offers the best balance of cost and outcome for you.
- Patients with liver or kidney compromise should obtain blood levels to guide dosing.
- Talk with your doctor about whether you should take aspirin every other day in order to help prevent a heart attack.
- A generic form can be substituted for the brand name.

RAMIPRIL   (ra MI pril)

Prescription Needed: Yes   **Controlled Drug:** No   **Generic:** No

Brand Name: Altace

Overview of BENEFITS versus RISKS

Possible Benefits	*Possible Risks*
EFFECTIVE CONTROL OF MILD TO SEVERE HIGH BLOOD PRESSURE	Rare excessive lowering of blood pressure Rare allergic swelling of face, tongue, or vocal cords (angioedema)

▷ **Illness This Medication Treats:**
(1) High blood pressure, alone or concurrently with thiazide-type diuretics. Mild to moderate high blood pressure usually responds to low doses; severe high blood pressure may require higher doses, with greater risk of serious adverse effects. (2) Decrease in the size of the left ventricle and control of blood pressure in people with abnormally enlarged left ventricles; (3) control of blood pressure caused by kidney artery abnormalities; (4) used for people with atherosclerosis to help prevent heart attacks; (5) used after heart attacks to help prevent death, a second heart attack, and undesirable heart weakness from a first heart attack.

▷ **Typical Dosage Range:** (Dosage or schedule must be determined by the doctor for each individual.)
Initially 2.5 mg once daily for 2 to 4 weeks. The usual maintenance dose is 2.5 to 20 mg each day in a single dose or in two divided doses.
If taking diuretics: either discontinue the diuretic for 3 days before starting this drug or begin treatment with 1.25 mg of this drug.
Total daily dose should not exceed 5 mg if kidney function is significantly impaired.

▷ **Conditions Requiring Dosing Adjustments:**
Liver function: This drug is extensively metabolized in the liver to ramiprilat, with subsequent elimination via the urine. Patients with compromised livers should be followed closely.
Kidney function: For patients with moderate kidney failure or creatinine values of greater than 2.5 mg/dl, use 1.25 mg of ramipril daily. Patients with renal compromise should use this drug with caution.

▷ **How Best to Take This Medicine:** Take on an empty stomach or with food at same time each day. The capsule may be opened.

▷ **How Long This Medicine Is Usually Taken:** Use on a regular schedule for 2 to 4 weeks determines the effectiveness of this drug in controlling high blood pressure. The proper treatment of high blood pressure usually requires the long-term use of effective medications. See your doctor regularly.

▷ **Tell Your Doctor Before Taking This Medicine If You:**
- ever had an allergic reaction to it or to any other ACE inhibitors.
- have a history of angioedema (a serious allergic reaction) from any cause.
- have active liver disease or impaired liver or kidney function.
- have an abnormally high level of blood potassium.
- are pregnant, planning pregnancy, or breast-feeding.
- have scleroderma or systemic lupus erythematosus.
- have any form of heart disease.
- have diabetes.
- have low white blood cell counts.
- are taking any other antihypertensives, diuretics, nitrates, or potassium supplements.
- plan to have surgery under general anesthesia soon.

▷ **Possible Side Effects:**   Dizziness, light-headedness.

▷ **Possible Adverse Effects:**
If any of the following develop, call your doctor promptly for guidance.
Some Mild Problems Drug Can Cause
  Allergic reactions: skin rash, itching.
  Headache, fatigue, nervousness, numbness and tingling, insomnia.
  Chest pain, palpitation, drug-induced cough.
  Stomach pain, nausea, vomiting, diarrhea.
  Excessive sweating, joint and muscle aches.
Some Serious Problems Drug Can Cause
  Allergic reactions: swelling (angioedema) of face, tongue, and/or vocal cords: can be life-threatening.
  Rare liver toxicity.
  Rare pancreatitis reported with some other ACE inhibitors.

▷ **Possible Effects on Sex Life:**   Rare reports of impotence. Swelling or tenderness of male breast tissue (gynecomastia).

▷ *CAUTION*
  1. Talk with your doctor about discontinuing other antihypertensives (especially diuretics) for 1 week before starting this drug.
  2. **Report promptly** any indications of infection (fever, sore throat) and water retention (weight gain, puffiness, swollen feet or ankles).
  3. Do not use a salt substitute without your doctor's knowledge and approval (many contain potassium).

4. Obtain blood cell counts and urine analyses **before** starting this drug.
5. **Tell your doctor immediately if pregnancy occurs.** This drug should not be taken beyond the first 3 months of pregnancy.
6. Safety and effectiveness of this drug for infants and children have not been established.
7. Small doses are advisable for those over 60, until tolerance has been determined. Sudden and excessive lowering of blood pressure can predispose to stroke or heart attack in those with impaired brain circulation or coronary artery heart disease.
8. Dosing MUST be adjusted for patients with compromised kidneys with a creatinine clearance less than 40 ml/min.

Advisability of Use During Pregnancy or If Breast-Feeding:

Pregnancy Category: D. Avoid using this drug completely during the last 6 months. During the first 3 months of pregnancy, use only if clearly needed (C). Ask your doctor for guidance. Present in breast milk; avoid taking this drug or refrain from nursing.

▷ **Overdose Symptoms:** Excessive drop in blood pressure: light-headedness, dizziness, fainting.

▷ **Suggested Periodic Examinations While Taking This Drug:** (at doctor's discretion)

Before starting drug: complete blood cell counts; urine analysis with measurement of protein content; blood potassium level.

During use of drug: blood cell counts; measurements of blood potassium.

▷ **While Taking This Drug the Following Apply:**

Foods: Ask your doctor about salt intake.

Nutritional Support: **Do not take** potassium supplements unless directed by your doctor.

Beverages: May be taken with milk.

Alcohol: Use caution until the combined effect has been determined. Alcohol may enhance this drug's blood pressure–lowering effect.

Other Drugs:

Ramipril *taken concurrently* with

- aspirin or other NSAIDs (see Drug Classes) may blunt the benefits of ramipril.
- cyclosporine (Sandimmune) may increase the risk of kidney toxicity.
- lithium (Lithane, Lithotab, etc.) may cause increased blood lithium levels and symptoms of lithium toxicity. Monitor lithium levels closely.
- loop diuretics (see Drug Classes) may cause excessive lowering of blood pressure on standing.

- phenothiazines (see Drug Classes) has caused excessive lowering of blood pressure with other ACE inhibitors.
- potassium preparations (K-Lyte, Slow-K, etc.) may cause increased blood levels of potassium with risk of serious heart rhythm disturbances.
- potassium-sparing diuretics—amiloride (Moduretic), spironolactone (Aldactazide), triamterene (Dyazide)—may cause increased blood levels of potassium with the risk of serious heart rhythm disturbances.

Driving, Hazardous Activities: Be aware of possible drops in blood pressure with resultant dizziness or faintness.

Exposure to Sun: Caution is advised. A similar drug of this class can cause photosensitivity.

Exposure to Heat: Caution is advised. Avoid excessive perspiring with resultant loss of body water and drop in blood pressure.

Occurrence of Unrelated Illness: Report promptly any disorder that causes nausea, vomiting, or diarrhea. Fluid and chemical imbalances must be corrected as soon as possible.

▷ **Saving Money When Using This Medicine:**
- Many new drugs are available to treat high blood pressure. Ask your doctor if this medicine offers the best balance of cost and outcome for you. Ask how often you should have your blood pressure checked.
- Ask your doctor if stress management and exercise programs available in your community make sense for you.
- Talk with your doctor about taking aspirin every other day in order to prevent heart attacks.

RANITIDINE (ra NI te deen)

Prescription Needed: Yes   **Controlled Drug:** No   **Generic:** No

Brand Name: Zantac, Zantac 75 (nonprescription form)

▷ **Warning:** The brand names Zantac and Xanax can be mistaken for each other, leading to serious medication errors. Zantac (a yellow or peach tablet), the generic drug ranitidine, is used to treat peptic ulcer disease. Xanax (white, yellow, blue oval tablets), the generic drug alprazolam, is a mild tranquilizer. Verify that you are taking the correct drug.

Overview of BENEFITS versus RISKS

Possible Benefits	Possible Risks
EFFECTIVE TREATMENT OF PEPTIC ULCER DISEASE: relief of symptoms, acceleration of healing, prevention of recurrence	Drug-induced hepatitis (rare) Confusion (in severely ill elderly patients) Blood cell disorders (rare)
CONTROL OF HYPERSECRETORY STOMACH DISORDERS	
Beneficial in treatment of reflux esophagitis	

Author's note: All four of the available H2-receptor blocking drugs are now available without prescription. See the histamine (H2) blocking drugs profile for further information.

RIFABUTIN (RIF a byou tin)

Prescription Needed: Yes   **Controlled Drug:** No   **Generic:** No

Brand Name: Mycobutin

▷ **Warning:** Rifabutin prophylaxis must not be given to people with active tuberculosis.

Overview of BENEFITS versus RISKS

Possible Benefits	Possible Risks
PREVENTION OF DISSEMINATED *MYCOBACTERIUM AVIUM-INTRACELLULARE* COMPLEX (MAC) (WITH ADVANCED HIV INFECTION)	NEUTROPENIA, RARE CHEST PAIN WITH DYSPNEA, LEUKOPENIA, ANEMIA, THROMBOCYTOPENIA, HEPATITIS

▷ **Illness This Medication Treats:**

(1) Prevents disseminated *Mycobacterium avium-intracellulare* complex (MAC) in patients with advanced HIV infection; (2) treats *Mycobacterium avium-intracellulare* infections. Typically combined with a number of other medications such as (with or without amikacin) clofazimine, streptomycin, ethambutol, and ciprofloxacin.

▷ **Typical Dosage Range:** (Dosage or schedule must be determined by the doctor for each individual.)

Infants and Children: Safety and effectiveness of this drug in MAC prophylaxis has not clearly been established for this age group. Safety data from a trial of 22 children who were HIV-positive:

Infants 1 year of age—18.5 mg per kilogram of body weight daily

Children 2–10 years—8.6 mg per kilogram of body weight daily

Adolescents 14 years—4.0 mg per kilogram of body weight daily.

14 to 60 Years of Age: 300 mg once a day. People who are prone to nausea and vomiting may take 150 mg two times a day with food.

Over 60 Years of Age: Same as for 12 to 60 years of age.

▷ **Conditions Requiring Dosing Adjustments:**

Liver function: At present, clear adjustments of dose for patients with hepatic compromise are not defined, but the drug should be used with caution.

Kidney function: Elimination of this drug may actually be increased in people with compromised kidneys, yet the clinical effect is unknown. Changes in dose or interval are not currently recommended for patients with kidney compromise.

▷ **How Best to Take This Medicine:**   May be taken with food if you are prone to nausea and vomiting. For children, this drug can be mixed with foods such as applesauce.

▷ **How Long This Medicine Is Usually Taken:**   Continual use on a regular schedule indefinitely is usually necessary to ensure the effectiveness of this drug in prophylaxis of disseminated MAC. Long-term use (months to years) requires periodic evaluation of response. See your doctor regularly.

As a part of combination therapy of a *Mycobacterium avium-intracellulare* infection, the ideal duration of treatment has not been identified, but treatment is usually ongoing.

▷ **Tell Your Doctor Before Taking This Medicine If You:**

- had an allergic reaction to it.
- have active tuberculosis.
- are pregnant or planning pregnancy.
- are taking an oral contraceptive.
- are taking an anticoagulant such as Coumadin.
- take other medicines that were not discussed with your doctor when this medicine was prescribed.

▷ **Possible Side Effects:**   This medication may color saliva, urine, feces, sputum, perspiration, tears, and skin a brown-orange color. Soft contact lenses may become permanently stained by rifabutin or its metabolites.

Emergence of resistant *Mycobacterium* tuberculosis.

▷ **Possible Adverse Effects:**

If any of the following develop, call your doctor promptly for guidance.

Some Mild Problems Drug Can Cause
  Allergic reactions: skin rash, fever.
  Change in taste perceptions, headache, loss of appetite, nausea, vomiting, and diarrhea, muscle aches, joint pains, and a flu-like syndrome.
Some Serious Problems Drug Can Cause
  Very rare confusion, aphasia and seizures, chest pain with dyspnea (trouble breathing), nonspecific T wave changes (change in heartbeat), neutropenia.
  Rare leukopenia, anemia, thrombocytopenia, and hepatitis.

▷ **Possible Effects on Sex Life:**   Potential alteration of pattern and timing of menstruation.
  Decreased effectiveness of oral contraceptives taken together with this drug.

▷ **Adverse Effects That May Mimic Natural Diseases or Disorders:**
  Liver reactions similar to viral hepatitis.

▷ *CAUTION*
  1. The effectiveness of oral contraceptives may be decreased by this drug.
  2. This drug may hasten the development of resistant *Mycobacterium* tuberculosis if used as monotherapy.
  3. Urine, feces, saliva, sputum, sweat, tears, and skin may be colored brown-orange. Soft contact lenses may be permanently stained.
  4. Safety and effectiveness of this drug for children have not been established.
  5. Specific precautions have not yet been developed for those over 60; however, since the drug is similar to rifampin, those over 60 may be more sensitive to its adverse effects.

  Advisability of Use During Pregnancy or If Breast-Feeding:
  Pregnancy Category: B. Ask your doctor for guidance. Presence in breast milk is unknown; avoid taking this drug or refrain from nursing.

▷ **Suggested Periodic Examinations While Taking This Drug:** (at doctor's discretion)
  May cause neutropenia and thrombocytopenia, therefore white blood cell counts and platelet counts should be checked. Liver function tests should also be obtained periodically.

▷ **While Taking This Drug the Following Apply:**
  Alcohol: Potential for additive liver toxicity. It is best to avoid alcohol.
  Marijuana Smoking: May be an additive cause of rashes and seizures in people with existing seizure disorders. Avoid marijuana completely.

Other Drugs:

Rifabutin may **decrease** the effects of

- antianxiety agents such as diazepam.
- anticoagulants such as Coumadin.
- anticonvulsant drugs such as phenytoin.
- barbiturates.
- BCG live attenuated vaccine.
- beta-blockers such as metoprolol, propranolol.
- chloramphenicol (Chloromycetin).
- clofibrate (Atromid-S).
- cortisonelike drugs (see Drug Classes).
- cyclosporine (Sandimmune).
- dapsone.
- digitalis preparations (Lanoxin, others).
- disopyramide (Norpace).
- ketoconazole (Nizoral).
- mexilitine (Mexitil).
- narcotics such as methadone.
- oral contraceptives (birth control pills).
- oral hypoglycemic agents (see Drug Classes).
- quinidine (Quinaglute, others).
- theophylline (Theo-Dur, others).
- verapamil (Verelan, others).
- zidovudine (the effect is decreased by a decreased drug level).

Rifabutin **taken concurrently** with

- anticoagulants such as Coumadin results in a decreased anticoagulant effect INR (the prothrombin time decreases). Doses should be adjusted to laboratory test levels.
- fluconazole (Diflucan) may result in increased rifabutin concentrations.
- trimetrexate (Neutrexin) may blunt benefits of trimetrexate.

Driving, Hazardous Activities: May rarely be associated with confusion and seizures. Restrict your activities as necessary.

Discontinuation: Do not discontinue or interrupt use of this drug without discussing it with your doctor.

▷ **Saving Money When Using This Medicine:**
- Many drugs are available to treat MAC. Combination therapy is often used. Ask your doctor to prescribe the best medicines offering the most desirable balance of cost and outcome for you.
- Ask your doctor about using a viral load to check the continued success of your AIDS therapy.

RIFAMPIN (RIF am pin)

Other Name: Rifampicin

Prescription Needed: Yes

Brand Names: Rifadin, Rifamate [CD], Rifater [CD], Rimactane, Rimactane/INH Dual Pack [CD]

Overview of BENEFITS versus RISKS

Possible Benefits	*Possible Risks*
EFFECTIVE TREATMENT OF TUBERCULOSIS in combination with other drugs	DRUG-INDUCED HEPATITIS DRUG-INDUCED NEPHRITIS Rare coagulation defects or
EFFECTIVE PREVENTION OF MENINGITIS by eliminating meningococcus from the throat of carriers	pseudomembranous colitis Rare blood cell disorder: abnormally low blood platelet count

---

▷ **Illness This Medication Treats:**
(1) Active tuberculosis; usually given concurrently with other antitubercular drugs to enhance its effectiveness; (2) helps eliminate meningitis germ (meningococcus) from the throats of healthy carriers, to prevent its spread. Not effective for active meningitis.

As Combination Drug Product [CD]: Available in combination with isoniazid, another antitubercular drug that delays the development of drug-resistant strains of tuberculosis.

▷ **Typical Dosage Range:** (Dosage or schedule must be determined by the doctor for each individual.)
For tuberculosis: 10 mg per kilogram of body weight daily, up to 600 mg/day. For meningococcus carriers: 600 mg/day for 4 days. The total daily dosage should not exceed 600 mg.

▷ **Conditions Requiring Dosing Adjustments:**
Liver function: This drug is extensively metabolized in the liver and excreted in the feces. For patients with severe failure, 6–8 mg per kilogram of body weight per week is used.
Kidney function: Up to 30% of this drug is eliminated unchanged by the kidneys. One researcher uses 50–100% of the usual dose for people with creatinine clearances of 10–50 ml/min. Talk with your doctor.

▷ **How Best to Take This Medicine:** Preferably taken with 8 oz of water on an empty stomach (1 hour before or 2 hours after eating). However, this drug may be taken with food if necessary to reduce stomach irritation. The capsule may be opened and the contents mixed with applesauce or jelly for administration.

▷ **How Long This Medicine Is Usually Taken:** Use on a regular schedule for several months determines the effectiveness of this drug in promoting recovery from tuberculosis. Long-term use requires ongoing physician supervision.

▷ **Tell Your Doctor Before Taking This Medicine If You:**
- ever had an allergic reaction to it.
- have active liver disease or a history of liver disease, or impaired liver function.
- are pregnant or are taking an oral contraceptive.
- consume alcohol daily.
- are taking an anticoagulant.

▷ **Possible Side Effects:** Red, orange, or brown discoloration of tears, sweat, saliva, sputum, urine, or stool. Yellow discoloration of the skin (not jaundice). Note: In the absence of symptoms indicating illness, any discoloration is harmless and does not indicate toxicity. Possible fungal superinfections.

▷ **Possible Adverse Effects:**
If any of the following develop, call your doctor promptly for guidance.
Some Mild Problems Drug Can Cause
  Allergic reactions: skin rash, itching, drug fever.
  Headache, drowsiness, dizziness, blurred vision, impaired hearing, vague numbness and tingling.
  Heartburn, nausea, vomiting, abdominal cramps, diarrhea.
Some Serious Problems Drug Can Cause
  Serious skin problems (Stevens-Johnson syndrome or toxic epidermal necrolysis).
  Flu-like syndrome: fever, chills, headache, dizziness, musculoskeletal pain, difficult breathing.
  Drug-induced liver damage, with or without jaundice.
  Drug-induced kidney damage: impaired urine production, bloody or cloudy urine.
  Excessively low blood platelet count: abnormal bleeding or bruising.
  Rare porphyria, hemolytic anemia, colitis, gallstones, or pancreatitis.

▷ **Possible Effects on Sex Life:** Altered timing and pattern of menstruation.
Decreased effectiveness of oral contraceptives.

▷ **Adverse Effects That May Mimic Natural Diseases or Disorders:**
  Liver reactions may suggest viral hepatitis.
  Kidney reactions may suggest an infectious nephritis.

▷ *CAUTION*
1. May permanently discolor soft contact lenses.
2. May reduce the effectiveness of oral contraceptives; unplanned pregnancy could occur. An alternate method of contraception is advised.
3. When rifampin is used alone in the treatment of tuberculosis, resistant bacterial strains can develop rapidly. This drug should be used only in conjunction with other antitubercular drugs.
4. To ensure the best possible response to treatment, take the full course of medication prescribed; this may be for several months or years.
5. Monitor infants or children closely for possible liver toxicity or deficiency of blood platelets.
6. Those over 60 have natural changes in body composition and function, which may increase susceptibility to the adverse effects of this drug. Report promptly any indications of possible drug toxicity.

Advisability of Use During Pregnancy or If Breast-Feeding:
Pregnancy Category: C. If possible, avoid use of this drug during the first 3 months. Present in breast milk; avoid taking this drug or refrain from nursing.

▷ **Overdose Symptoms:** Nausea, vomiting, drowsiness, unconsciousness, severe liver damage, jaundice.

▷ **Suggested Periodic Examinations While Taking This Drug:** (at doctor's discretion)
Complete blood cell counts, liver and kidney function tests.
Hearing acuity tests if hearing loss is suspected.

▷ **While Taking This Drug the Following Apply:**
Alcohol: It is best to avoid alcohol completely to reduce the risk of potential liver toxicity
Other Drugs:
Rifampin *taken concurrently* with
• halothane anesthesia may result in serious liver damage.
Rifampin may *decrease* the effects of
• antianxiety drugs (see Drug Classes or benzodiazepines)
• anticoagulants (Coumadin, etc.), reducing their effectiveness. Increased INR (prothrombin time) testing is needed.
• some anticonvulsant drugs (see Drug Classes).
• some antifungals: fluconazole (Diflucan), itraconazole (Sporanox), or ketoconazole (Nizoral).
• barbiturates (see Drug Classes).
• BCG live vaccine.

- beta-blockers: metoprolol, propranolol.
- some calcium channel blockers (see Drug Classes).
- chloramphenicol (Chloromycetin).
- clofibrate (Atromid-S).
- cortisonelike drugs (see Drug Classes).
- cyclosporine (Sandimmune).
- digitoxin.
- methadone (Dolophine).
- mexiletine (Mexitil).
- oral contraceptives (birth control pills).
- oral hypoglycemics (see Drug Classes).
- phenytoin (Dilantin).
- progestins.
- quinidine.
- sulfonylureas: chlorpropamide, tolbutamide.
- theophyllines (aminophylline, Theo-Dur, etc.).
- tricyclic antidepressants (see Drug Classes).
- verapamil (Verelan).
- zidovudine (AZT).

The following drug may *decrease* the effects of rifampin

- p-aminosalicylic acid (PAS); reduces its antitubercular effectiveness.

Driving, Hazardous Activities: May cause dizziness, drowsiness, impaired vision, and hearing. Restrict your activities as necessary.

Discontinuation: It is advisable not to interrupt or discontinue usage of this drug without talking with your doctor. Intermittent administration can increase the possibility of developing allergic reactions.

▷ **Saving Money When Using This Medicine:**

- There is an epidemic of resistant tuberculosis in large cities. Often several drugs must be used at once to treat this infection. Ask your doctor if this medicine offers the best balance of cost and outcome for you.
- It is critical to use this medicine for an extended period of time to cure the infection.

RISPERIDONE (ris PEER i dohn)

Prescription Needed: Yes   **Controlled Drug:** No   **Generic:** No

Brand Names: Risperdal

```
+-------------------------------------------------------------+
|               Overview of BENEFITS versus RISKS             |
|       Possible Benefits              Possible Risks         |
|   TREATMENT OF                   Rare change in heart       |
|     SCHIZOPHRENIA                  function (prolonged QT    |
|     REFRACTORY TO OTHER            interval)                |
|     AGENTS                       Rare involuntary movement  |
|   DECREASED SIDE EFFECTS           disorder                 |
|     COMPARED TO SOME             Rare neuroleptic malignant |
|     OTHER AVAILABLE DRUGS          syndrome                 |
+-------------------------------------------------------------+
```

▷ **Illness This Medication Treats:**

Management of chronic schizophrenia.

Other (unlabeled) generally accepted uses: treatment of (1) acute schizophrenia; (2) aggression; (3) Tourette's syndrome.

▷ **Typical Dosage Range:** (Dosage or schedule must be determined by the doctor for each individual.)

Infants and Children: Safety and efficacy of this drug for those less than 18 years old have not been established.

18 to 60 Years of Age: Usual starting dose is 1 mg taken twice daily. Dosage may be increased as needed and tolerated by 1 mg on the second and third day, for a total of 3 mg twice daily by the third day. Further dose changes, if needed, should be made at 1-week intervals. Doses greater than 6 mg/day are not recommended.

Over 60 Years of Age: Therapy is started with 0.5 mg twice daily. The dose is increased if needed and tolerated by 0.5 mg twice daily. Doses greater than 1.5 mg daily are achieved by small increases made at 1-week intervals. Pay careful attention to blood pressure and development of adverse effects.

▷ **Conditions Requiring Dosing Adjustments:**

Liver function: The starting dose must be decreased and adjusted as for those over 60 years old.

Kidney function: The starting dose must be decreased and adjusted as for those over 60 years old.

▷ **How Best to Take This Medicine:** The tablet may be crushed; its effect is not changed by food.

▷ **How Long This Medicine Is Usually Taken:** Use on a regular schedule for 1 to 2 weeks usually determines the effectiveness of this drug in helping control chronic schizophrenia. If long-term use is attempted, the lowest effective dose should be used. Periodic evaluation of response and dosage adjustment by your doctor is required.

▷ **Tell Your Doctor Before Taking This Medicine If You:**
- ever had an allergic reaction to it.
- have had neuroleptic malignant syndrome (ask your doctor).

- have a history of breast cancer.
- have liver or kidney compromise.
- are pregnant or planning pregnancy.
- have a history of Parkinson's disease or seizures.
- ever had tardive dyskinesia.
- have a history of heart rhythm disturbances.

▷ **Possible Side Effects:** Increased prolactin levels may result in male and female breast tenderness and swelling.

▷ **Possible Adverse Effects:**
If any of the following develop, call your doctor promptly for guidance.
Some Mild Problems Drug Can Cause
Allergic reactions: skin rash.
Somnolence.
Difficulty in concentrating/fatigue.
Increased dreaming.
Weight gain.
Orthostatic hypotension.
Increased urination.
Some Serious Problems Drug Can Cause
Allergic reactions: anaphylactic reactions.
Abnormal heart function.
Tardive dyskinesia.
Neuroleptic malignant syndrome.
Low sodium.
Rare seizures.
Low platelets.
Abnormal liver function.

▷ **Possible Effects on Sex Life:** Diminished sexual desire. Delayed or absent orgasm. Erectile dysfunction including priapism, male or female breast tenderness or swelling. Dry vagina or menstrual changes. Ejaculation failure.

▷ **Possible Delayed Adverse Effects:** Swelling and tenderness of male and female breast tissue.

▷ *CAUTION*
1. This drug should be used with great caution, if at all, by patients with cancer.
2. Call your doctor promptly if you have an increased tendency to infection or abnormal bleeding or bruising while taking this drug.
3. This drug should be used with great caution, if at all, by patients with a history of seizures.
4. Safety and effectiveness of this drug for those under 18 years old have not been established.

5. Those over 60 should take a lower starting dose and slowly increase the dose as needed or tolerated. The elderly may be at increased risk for postural hypotension and problems with motor skills. People with prostate problems may have an increased risk of urine retention.

Advisability of Use During Pregnancy or If Breast-Feeding:
Pregnancy Category: C. Ask your doctor for guidance. Present in breast milk; avoid taking this drug or refrain from nursing.

▷ **Overdose Symptoms:** Drowsiness, hypotension, tachycardia, low sodium and potassium, ECG changes (prolonged QT interval), and seizure.

▷ **Suggested Periodic Examinations While Taking This Drug:** (at doctor's discretion)
Liver function tests.
Electrolytes (sodium and potassium).
ECG.
Prolactin.

▷ **While Taking This Drug the Following Apply:**
Alcohol: Avoid alcohol while taking risperidone.
Marijuana Smoking: Increased somnolence.
Other Drugs:
Risperidone may *decrease* the effects of
• levodopa (Sinemet, others).
Risperidone *taken concurrently* with
• carbamazepine (Tegretol) decreases the drug level and perhaps the therapeutic effect of risperidone.
• other medicines that act on the brain (centrally acting) will increase the effects of these medicines on the brain.
The following drug may *increase* the effects of risperidone
• clozapine (Clozaril).
Driving, Hazardous Activities: May cause drowsiness and difficulty concentrating. Restrict your activities as necessary.
Exposure to Sun: Use caution. This drug may cause photosensitivity.
Discontinuation: Talk with your doctor before discontinuing use of this medication.

▷ **Saving Money When Using This Medicine:**
• Many new drugs are available to treat schizophrenia. Ask your doctor if this medicine offers the best balance of cost and outcome for you.
• Dose must be decreased for those over 60 or those with liver or kidney compromise.

SALMETEROL   (sal ME ter all)

Prescription Needed: Yes   **Controlled Drug:** No   **Generic:** No

Brand Name: Serevent, Aeromax

Overview of BENEFITS versus RISKS

Possible Benefits	*Possible Risks*
LONG-ACTING RELIEF OF BRONCHIAL ASTHMA PREVENTION OF NOCTURNAL ASTHMA SYMPTOMS	Rapid heart rate (tachycardia)

▷ **Illness This Medication Treats:**
(1) Prevention of bronchospasm in asthma; (2) prevention of nocturnal asthma; (3) prevention of exercise-induced bronchospasm.

▷ **Typical Dosage Range:** (Dosage or schedule must be determined by the doctor for each individual.)
Infants and Children: Safety and efficacy of this drug in those less than 12 years old are not established.
12 to 60 Years of Age: For prevention of asthma: Two inhalations (42 mcg) twice daily, in the morning and evening. Doses should be given 12 hours apart.
For prevention of exercise-induced asthma: Two inhalations at least 30 to 60 minutes BEFORE exercise. Additional doses of salmeterol should NOT be given for 12 hours.
Over 60 Years of Age: Same as for 12 to 60 years of age.

▷ **Conditions Requiring Dosing Adjustments:**
Liver function: Use this drug with caution, as it may accumulate in liver failure.
Kidney function: The use of salmeterol in kidney failure patients has not been studied.

▷ **How Best to Take This Medicine:** Follow written instructions on the inhaler closely. The use of salmeterol with a spacer or similar device has not been studied. Shake well before using.

▷ **How Long This Medicine Is Usually Taken:** Use on a regular schedule for 4 to 6 weeks is usually necessary to determine the effectiveness of this drug in preventing asthma attacks. Long-term use (months to years) requires periodic physician evaluation.

▷ **Tell Your Doctor Before Taking This Medicine If You:**
- ever had an allergic reaction to it.
- currently have an irregular heart rhythm.
- are taking, or have taken within the past 2 weeks, any MAO type A inhibitor.
- have an overactive thyroid.
- have diabetes.
- have abnormally high blood pressure.

▷ **Possible Side Effects:** Dryness or irritation of the mouth or throat, altered taste. Nervousness or palpitations.

▷ **Possible Adverse Effects:**
If any of the following develop, call your doctor promptly for guidance.
Some Mild Problems Drug Can Cause
  Allergic reactions: skin rash and urticaria.
  Rhinitis and laryngitis.
  Nervousness and fatigue.
  Headache, tremor, and nervousness.
Some Serious Problems Drug Can Cause
  Rare respiratory arrest.
  Rapid heart rate (tachycardia) and palpitations.
  Paradoxical bronchospasm.

▷ **Possible Effects on Sex Life:** Painful or difficult menstruation.

▷ **Possible Delayed Adverse Effects:** Not defined at present.

▷ **Adverse Effects That May Mimic Natural Diseases or Disorders:**
  Rapid heart rate may mimic heart disease.
Bronchospasm may mimic asthma.

▷ *CAUTION*
  1. The use of salmeterol by inhalation with beclomethasone aerosol (Beclovent, Vanceril) may increase the risk of fluorocarbon propellant toxicity. Use salmeterol aerosol 20 to 30 minutes BEFORE beclomethasone aerosol to reduce toxicity and enhance the penetration of beclomethasone into the lungs.
  2. Serious heart rhythm problems or cardiac arrest can result from excessive and prolonged use of this drug.
  3. Call your doctor if your symptoms become more frequent, or if you increase your use of the immediate bronchodilator that was prescribed for you.
  4. Safety and effectiveness of this drug for those under 12 years old have not been established.
  5. Those over 60 should avoid increased use of this drug. If your

asthma is not as controlled as it had been in the past, call your doctor.

Advisability of Use During Pregnancy or If Breast-Feeding:
Pregnancy Category: C. Ask your doctor for guidance. Present in breast milk; avoid taking this drug or refrain from nursing.

▷ **Overdose Symptoms:**   Exaggeration of pharmacologic effects: tachycardia and/or arrhythmia, muscle cramps, cardiac arrest, and death.

▷ **Suggested Periodic Examinations While Taking This Drug:** (at doctor's discretion)
Blood pressure checks, evaluations of heart status.

▷ **While Taking This Drug the Following Apply:**
Beverages: Avoid excessive caffeine as in coffee, tea, cola, and chocolate.
Other Drugs:
Salmeterol *taken concurrently* with
- MAO type A inhibitors can cause extreme increases in blood pressure and heart stimulation.

The following drugs may *increase* the effects of salmeterol
- tricyclic antidepressants.
- methylxanthines such as caffeine or theophylline.

Driving, Hazardous Activities: May cause nervousness or dizziness. Restrict your activities as necessary.
Heavy Exercise or Exertion: Use caution; these may stress the protective effects of this drug.

▷ **Saving Money When Using This Medicine:**
- Many new drugs are available to treat asthma. Ask your doctor if this medicine offers the best balance of cost and outcome for you.
- Ask your doctor if this drug can be stopped after you have experienced a significant asthma-free period.
- Talk with your doctor about using nebulized lidocaine, or nedocromil or cromolyn in order to further help prevent asthmatic attacks.

SELEGILINE (se LEDGE i leen)

Other Name: Deprenyl

Prescription Needed: Yes   **Controlled Drug:** No   **Generic:** No

Brand Name: Eldepryl

```
┌─────────────────────────────────────────────────────────────┐
│              Overview of BENEFITS versus RISKS                │
│        Possible Benefits              Possible Risks          │
│  EFFECTIVE INITIAL              ABNORMAL INVOLUNTARY          │
│     TREATMENT OF                   MOVEMENTS                   │
│     PARKINSON'S DISEASE         HALLUCINATIONS                │
│     when started at the onset   INITIAL FALL IN BLOOD         │
│     of symptoms                    PRESSURE/ORTHOSTATIC       │
│  ADDITIVE RELIEF OF                HYPOTENSION                │
│     SYMPTOMS OF                                                │
│     PARKINSON'S DISEASE                                        │
│     (used concurrently with                                   │
│     levodopa/carbidopa                                        │
│     [Sinemet])                                                │
│  PERMITS UP TO 30%                                            │
│     REDUCTION IN SINEMET                                      │
│     DOSAGE with resultant                                     │
│     decrease in adverse effects                              │
└─────────────────────────────────────────────────────────────┘
```

▷ **Illness This Medication Treats:**

Parkinson's disease (soon after onset of symptoms), thus delaying the use of levodopa/carbidopa. Also used as an adjunct to levodopa/carbidopa treatment of Parkinson's disease for people who experience intolerable abnormal movements (dyskinesia) and/or increasing on-off episodes due to the loss of levodopa's effectiveness. The addition of selegiline: (1) permits reduction of the daily dose of levodopa (by 25–30%) with consequent lessening of dyskinesia and erratic drug response, and (2) provides additional relief of parkinsonian symptoms.

▷ **Typical Dosage Range:** (Dosage or schedule must be determined by the doctor for each individual.)

5 mg once or twice daily. The usual maintenance dose is 5 mg after breakfast and 5 mg after lunch. A total daily dose of 10 mg is adequate to achieve optimal benefit from this drug. Higher doses do not result in further improvement and are not advised.

During gradual introduction, the concurrent dose of levodopa/carbidopa (Sinemet) may be cautiously decreased in accord with your doctor's instructions. Concurrent Sinemet dosage should be reduced by 10 to 20% when selegiline is started.

▷ **Conditions Requiring Dosing Adjustments:**

Liver function: This drug is extensively metabolized in the liver to form methamphetamine and amphetamine. Patients with liver compromise should be followed closely.

Kidney function: The kidney does not have a major role in the elimination of this medication. Patients with urine outflow problems should use this drug with caution.

▷ **How Best to Take This Medicine:**   Take with food or milk to reduce stomach irritation. The tablet may be crushed.

▷ **How Long This Medicine Is Usually Taken:**   Use on a regular schedule for 4 to 6 weeks usually determines the effectiveness of this drug in controlling the symptoms of Parkinson's disease and permitting reduction of levodopa/carbidopa dosage. Long-term use (months to years) requires periodic evaluation of response and dosage adjustment. See your doctor regularly.

▷ **Tell Your Doctor Before Taking This Medicine If You:**
- ever had an allergic reaction to it.
- have Huntington's disease, hereditary (essential) tremor, or tardive dyskinesia.
- are pregnant or breast-feeding.
- have constitutionally low blood pressure.
- have peptic ulcer disease.
- have a history of heart rhythm disorder.
- are taking any antihypertensive or antipsychotic drugs.

▷ **Possible Side Effects:**   Weakness, orthostatic hypotension, dry mouth, insomnia.

▷ **Possible Adverse Effects:**
If any of the following develop, call your doctor promptly for guidance.
Some Mild Problems Drug Can Cause
   Headache, dizziness, agitation.
   Palpitations, fainting.
   Altered taste, nausea and vomiting, stomach pain.
   Vivid dreams.
Some Serious Problems Drug Can Cause
   Dyskinesias: abnormal involuntary movements.
   Confusion and hallucinations, depression, psychosis.
   Aggravation of peptic ulcer, gastrointestinal bleeding.

▷ **Possible Effects on Sex Life:**   Increased libido may occur. Rare reports of decreased penile sensation or anorgasmia have occurred with doses over 10 mg per day.

▷ **Adverse Effects That May Mimic Natural Diseases or Disorders:**   Effects on mental function and behavior may resemble psychotic disorders.

▷ *CAUTION*
1. This drug can initiate dyskinesias and intensify existing dyskinesias. Observe carefully for and promptly report the development of tremors, twitching, or abnormal, involuntary movements.
2. This drug potentiates the effects of levodopa. Added to current

levodopa treatment, selegiline may produce or intensify adverse effects of levodopa. Reduce the dose of levodopa by 10 to 20% when treatment with selegiline begins.

3. Tell your doctor promptly if you become pregnant or plan pregnancy. The manufacturer does not recommend use of this drug during pregnancy.
4. Do not use this drug in infants and children.
5. This drug is usually well tolerated by the elderly. Observe closely for any tendency to light-headedness or faintness, especially on arising from a lying or sitting position.

Advisability of Use During Pregnancy or If Breast-Feeding:

Pregnancy Category: C. The manufacturer advises against use of this drug during pregnancy. Presence in breast milk is unknown; avoid taking this drug or refrain from nursing.

▷ **Overdose Symptoms:** Nausea, vomiting, palpitations, low blood pressure, agitation, severe involuntary movements, hallucinations.

▷ **Suggested Periodic Examinations While Taking This Drug:** (at doctor's discretion)

Regular evaluation of drug response, heart function, and blood pressure status.

▷ **While Taking This Drug the Following Apply:**

Beverages: May be taken with milk.

Alcohol: Use caution until the combined effects have been determined. Alcohol may exaggerate this drug's blood pressure–lowering and sedative effects.

Other Drugs:

Selegiline *taken concurrently* with

- albuterol (Ventolin, others) may lead to increased adverse vascular effects.
- amphetamine (Dexodrine) can lead to a severe increase in blood pressure.
- antihypertensives (and other drugs that can lower blood pressure) requires careful monitoring for excessive drops in pressure. Dosage adjustments may be necessary.
- benzodiazepines (see Drug Classes) can increase sedation.
- buspirone (BuSpar) can lead to increased blood pressure.
- dextromethorphan (various "DM" cough medicines) can be toxic; these should not be combined.
- ephedrine may lead to severe increases in temperature.
- fluoxetine (Prozac) may cause serotonin syndrome.
- fluvoxamine (Luvox) may result in extreme agitation and excessive temperatures. DO NOT COMBINE.
- lithium (Lithobid) can lead to serotonin syndrome.

- meperidine (Demerol) may cause a life-threatening reaction of unknown cause; avoid this combination.
- oral hypoglycemic agents (see Drug Classes) can cause very low blood sugars.
- paroxetine (Paxil) can lead to central nervous system toxicity.
- phenothiazines (see Drug Classes) may increase the risk of movement problems.
- phenylpropanolamine or pseudoephedrine can lead to severe increases in temperature or blood pressure.
- sertraline (Zoloft) can lead to central nervous system toxicity.
- tryptophan can cause a fatal serotonin syndrome.
- venlafaxine (Effexor) can result in nervous system toxicity.

The following drugs may *decrease* the effects of selegiline and diminish its effectiveness:

- chlorprothixene (Taractan).
- haloperidol (Haldol).
- metoclopramide (Reglan).
- phenothiazines (see Drug Classes).
- reserpine (Ser-Ap-Es, etc.), in high doses.
- thiothixene (Navane).

Driving, Hazardous Activities: May cause dizziness, drowsiness, impaired coordination, or fainting. Restrict your activities as necessary.

Exposure to Heat: Use caution until the combined effects have been determined. Hot environments can cause lowering of blood pressure.

Discontinuation: Do not stop taking this drug abruptly. Sudden withdrawal can cause a prompt increase in parkinsonian symptoms and deterioration of control. Talk with your doctor about developing a schedule for gradual withdrawal and concurrent adjustment of Sinemet or other appropriate drugs.

▷ **Saving Money When Using This Medicine:**

- Several drugs are available to treat Parkinson's. Ask your doctor if this medicine offers the best balance of cost and outcome for you.
- Several interesting new medicines are being researched; talk with your doctor about these.
- This drug may lose its effectiveness as your disease progresses. Ask your doctor when you should change medications.

SERTRALINE (SER tra leen)

Prescription Needed: Yes   **Controlled Drug:** No   **Generic:** No

Brand Name: Zoloft

Overview of BENEFITS versus RISKS

Possible Benefits	*Possible Risks*
EFFECTIVE TREATMENT OF MAJOR DEPRESSIVE DISORDERS	Impaired sexual function
	Conversion of depression to mania in manic-depressive disorders
Possibly effective in relieving the symptoms of obsessive-compulsive disorder	Rare seizures

---

▷ **Illness This Medication Treats:**

Treats major forms of depression that have not responded to other therapies. This drug should be used only with a diagnosis of a true, primary depression of significant degree.

▷ **Typical Dosage Range:** (Dosage or schedule must be determined by the doctor for each individual.)

Infants and Children: Dosage not established.

12 to 60 Years of Age: Initially 50 mg once daily, taken in the morning or evening. Increase dose gradually, as needed and tolerated, in increments of 50 mg at intervals of 1 week. The total daily dosage should not exceed 200 mg.

Over 60 Years of Age: Same as for 12 to 60 years of age. Adjust dosage as appropriate for impaired liver or kidney function.

▷ **Conditions Requiring Dosing Adjustments:**

Liver function: This drug is a rare cause of liver damage, and patients should be followed closely.

Kidney function: The role of the kidneys in eliminating this drug is unknown. This drug can be a cause of urinary retention and should be used with caution by patients with urine outflow problems.

▷ **How Best to Take This Medicine:**   Preferably taken with food to enhance absorption, but may be taken with or without food. The tablet may be crushed.

▷ **How Long This Medicine Is Usually Taken:**   Use on a regular schedule for 4 to 8 weeks usually determines (1) the effectiveness of this drug in relieving depression; (2) the pattern of favorable and unfavorable effects. Long-term use (months to years) requires periodic evaluation of response and dosage adjustment. See your doctor regularly.

▷ **Tell Your Doctor Before Taking This Medicine If You:**

- ever had an allergic reaction to it.
- are currently taking, or have taken within the past 14 days, any MAO type A inhibitor.
- have experienced any adverse effects from antidepressant drugs used in the past.

- have impaired liver or kidney function.
- have Parkinson's disease, heart disease, or have had a heart attack.
- have a seizure disorder.
- are pregnant or planning pregnancy.

▷ **Possible Side Effects:**   Decreased appetite, weight loss (average 1 to 2 lbs).

▷ **Possible Adverse Effects:**
If any of the following develop, call your doctor promptly for guidance.
Some Mild Problems Drug Can Cause
Allergic reactions: skin rash, itching.
Headache, insomnia, drowsiness, tremor, dizziness, impaired concentration, abnormal vision, numbness and tingling, hallucinations.
Dry mouth, altered taste, indigestion, nausea, vomiting, diarrhea.
Some Serious Problems Drug Can Cause
Allergic reactions: dermatitis.
Drug-induced seizures.
Rare anemia.

▷ **Possible Effects on Sex Life:**   Male sexual dysfunction: delayed ejaculation. Female sexual dysfunction: inhibited orgasm. Swelling and tenderness of the male breast tissue (gynecomastia).

▷ *CAUTION*
1. If any type of skin reaction develops (rash, hives, etc.), discontinue this drug and tell your doctor promptly.
2. If dryness of the mouth develops and persists for more than 2 weeks, consult your dentist for guidance.
3. Ask your doctor before taking any other prescription or over-the-counter drug while taking this drug.
4. If you are advised to take any MAO type A inhibitor, allow an interval of 5 weeks after discontinuing sertraline before starting it.
5. It is advisable to withhold this drug if electroconvulsive therapy is to be used for your depression.
6. Safety and effectiveness of this drug for those under 12 years old have not been established.
7. For people over 60, the lowest effective dose should be determined for maintenance treatment. The dose must be adjusted as necessary for reduced kidney function.

Advisability of Use During Pregnancy or If Breast-Feeding:
Pregnancy Category: B. Use this drug only if clearly needed. Ask your doctor for guidance. Presence in breast milk is unknown; avoid taking this drug or refrain from nursing.

▷ **Overdose Symptoms:** Agitation, restlessness, excitement, nausea, vomiting, seizures.

▷ **While Taking This Drug the Following Apply:**
Beverages: May be taken with milk.
Alcohol: Avoid completely.
Other Drugs:
Sertraline may *increase* the effects of
- diazepam (Valium).
- tolbutamide (Orinase).
- warfarin (Coumadin) and related oral anticoagulants. More frequent INR (prothrombin time) testing is needed.

Sertraline *taken concurrently* with
- antidiabetic drugs (insulin, oral hypoglycemics) may increase the risk of hypoglycemic reactions; monitor blood and urine sugar levels carefully.
- MAO type A inhibitors may cause confusion, agitation, high fever, seizures, and dangerous elevations of blood pressure. Avoid the concurrent use of these drugs.

Driving, Hazardous Activities: May cause drowsiness, dizziness, impaired judgment, and altered vision. Restrict your activities as necessary.
Exposure to Sun: Use caution until the full effect is known. This drug may rarely cause photosensitivity.
Discontinuation: Slow elimination of this drug from the body makes withdrawal effects from abrupt discontinuation unlikely. However, talk with your doctor if you plan to discontinue this drug for any reason.

▷ **Saving Money When Using This Medicine:**
- Many new drugs are available to treat depression. Ask your doctor if this medicine offers the best balance of cost and outcome for you.
- Depression has recently been associated with an increased risk of osteoporosis. Talk with your doctor about exercise, calcium supplements, risk factors, and need for bone mineral density testing based on risk factors.

SIMVASTATIN (sim vah STA tin)

Prescription Needed: Yes   **Controlled Drug:** No   **Generic:** No

Brand Name: Zocor

```
┌─────────────────────────────────────────────────────┐
│              Overview of BENEFITS versus RISKS       │
│     Possible Benefits            Possible Risks      │
│  EFFECTIVE REDUCTION OF      Rare drug-induced hepatitis │
│    TOTAL BLOOD                 without jaundice       │
│    CHOLESTEROL AND LDL       Rare drug-induced myositis │
│    CHOLESTEROL in selected                            │
│    individuals                                        │
└─────────────────────────────────────────────────────┘
```

▷ **Illness This Medication Treats:**
(1) High total blood cholesterol levels (in individuals with Types IIa and IIb hypercholesterolemia) due to increased fractions of LDL cholesterol; simvastatin reduces deaths from heart disease and also decreases the number of nonfatal heart attacks, in conjunction with a cholesterol-lowering diet. This drug should not be used until an adequate trial of nondrug methods for lowering cholesterol has proved to be ineffective. (2) Stops the progression and decreases the number of deaths in patients with coronary artery disease.

▷ **Typical Dosage Range:** (Dosage or schedule must be determined by the doctor for each individual.)
Infants and Children: Under 2 years old: Do not use this drug.
2 to 20 years old: Dosage not established.
20 to 60 Years of Age: Initially 5 to 10 mg daily taken at bedtime. The dose is increased as needed and tolerated to reach the desired cholesterol goals. Increase dose, as needed and tolerated, by increments of 5 to 10 mg at intervals of 4 weeks. The total daily dose should not exceed 40 mg.
Over 60 Years of Age:
Initially 5 mg daily. Increase dose as needed and tolerated by increments of 5 mg, at intervals of 4 weeks. The total daily dose should not exceed 20 mg.

▷ **Conditions Requiring Dosing Adjustments:**
Liver function: This drug achieves a high concentration in the liver, and is subsequently eliminated in the bile. It can be a rare cause of liver damage, and patients should be followed closely.
Kidney function: For patients with severe kidney failure the dose should be started at 5 mg, and the patient closely followed.

▷ **How Best to Take This Medicine:**   Can be taken without regard to eating; preferably at bedtime (the highest rates of cholesterol production occur between midnight and 5 A.M.). The tablet may be crushed.

▷ **How Long This Medicine Is Usually Taken:**   Continual use on a regular schedule for 4 to 6 weeks usually shows the effectiveness of this drug in reducing blood levels of total and LDL cholesterol.

Long-term use (months to years) requires periodic evaluation of response and dosage adjustment. See your doctor regularly.

▷ **Tell Your Doctor Before Taking This Medicine If You:**
- ever had an allergic reaction to it.
- have active liver disease.
- are pregnant or breast-feeding.
- have previously taken any other drugs in this class such as lovastatin (Mevacor) or pravastatin (Pravachol).
- have a history of liver disease or impaired liver function.
- are not using any method of birth control, or are planning pregnancy.
- regularly consume substantial amounts of alcohol.
- have cataracts or impaired vision.
- have any type of chronic muscular disorder.
- plan to have major surgery soon.

▷ **Possible Side Effects:** Development of abnormal liver function tests without associated symptoms.

▷ **Possible Adverse Effects:**
If any of the following develop, call your doctor promptly for guidance.

Some Mild Problems Drug Can Cause
Headache.
Nausea, excessive gas, constipation, diarrhea.

Some Serious Problems Drug Can Cause
Marked and persistent abnormal liver function tests with focal hepatitis, without jaundice.
Rare acute myositis (long-term use).
Rare depression, protein in the urine, or skin rash.

▷ *CAUTION*
1. If pregnancy occurs while taking this drug, discontinue taking it immediately and call your doctor.
2. Report promptly any muscle pain or tenderness, especially if accompanied by fever or malaise.
3. Report promptly any altered or impaired vision so that an appropriate evaluation can be made.
4. Safety and effectiveness of this drug for those under 20 years old have not been established.
5. Those over 60 should tell their doctor about any personal or family history of cataracts. Comply with all recommendations regarding periodic eye examinations. Report promptly any alterations in vision.

Advisability of Use During Pregnancy or If Breast-Feeding:
Pregnancy Category: X. Avoid using this drug during entire pregnancy. Presence in breast milk is unknown; avoid taking this drug or refrain from nursing.

▷ **Overdose Symptoms:**   Increased indigestion, stomach distress, nausea, diarrhea.

▷ **Possible Effects of Long-Term Use:**   Abnormal liver function with focal hepatitis.

▷ **Suggested Periodic Examinations While Taking This Drug:** (at doctor's discretion)

Blood cholesterol studies: total cholesterol, HDL and LDL fractions.

Liver function tests before treatment, every 6 weeks during the first 3 months of use, every 8 weeks for the rest of the first year, and at 6-month intervals thereafter.

Complete eye examination at the beginning of treatment and any time a significant change in vision occurs. Ask your doctor for guidance.

▷ **While Taking This Drug the Following Apply:**

Foods: Follow a standard low-cholesterol diet.

Beverages: May be taken with milk.

Alcohol: No interactions expected. Use sparingly.

Other Drugs:

Simvastatin may ***increase*** the effects of

• digoxin (Lanoxin).
• warfarin (Coumadin); monitor INR (prothrombin time) and adjust dosing to results.

Simvastatin ***taken concurrently*** with

• clofibrate (Atromid-S) may increase the risk of serious muscle damage.
• gemfibrozil (Lopid) may alter the absorption and excretion of simvastatin; these should not be taken concurrently.
• cyclosporine (Sandimmune) can result in kidney failure and myopathy.
• niacin may increase risk of muscle problems (myopathy).

The following drug may ***decrease*** the effects of simvastatin

• cholestyramine (Questran) may reduce the absorption of simvastatin; take simvastatin 1 hour before or 4 hours after cholestyramine.

Discontinuation: Do not discontinue taking this drug without your doctor's knowledge and guidance. A significant increase in blood cholesterol levels may follow discontinuation.

▷ **Saving Money When Using This Medicine:**

• Many new drugs are available to treat elevated cholesterol. Ask your doctor if this medicine offers the best balance of cost and outcome for you.
• Ask your doctor about the advisability of taking aspirin every other day in order to help prevent a heart attack.

SPIRONOLACTONE (speer on oh LAK tohn)

Prescription Needed: Yes · **Controlled Drug:** No · **Generic:** Yes

Brand Names: Alatone, Aldactazide [CD], Aldactone, Spironazide

Overview of BENEFITS versus RISKS	
Possible Benefits	*Possible Risks*
EFFECTIVE PREVENTION OF POTASSIUM LOSS when used adjunctively with other diuretics	ABNORMALLY HIGH BLOOD POTASSIUM LEVEL with excessive use
EFFECTIVE DIURETIC IN REFRACTORY CASES OF FLUID RETENTION when used adjunctively with other diuretics	Enlargement of male breast tissue
	Masculinization effects in women: excessive hair growth, deepening of the voice
	Rare hepatitis

▷ **Illness This Medication Treats:**
(1) Helps in congestive heart failure and disorders of the liver and kidney that cause an abnormal accumulation of fluid; (2) used in conjunction with other measures in treating high blood pressure, primarily in situations where prevention of potassium loss is advisable.

▷ **Typical Dosage Range:** (Dosage or schedule must be determined by the doctor for each individual.)
For edema: Initially 100 mg in one dose or divided into several doses. The ongoing dose is then adjusted to individual response. The usual maintenance dose is 50 to 200 mg daily, divided into two to four doses. If response is not adequate after 5 days, a second fluid medicine (diuretic) is added.

▷ **Conditions Requiring Dosing Adjustments:**
Liver function: This drug can be a rare cause of liver damage, and patients should be followed closely.
Kidney function: For patients with mild kidney failure, this drug can be taken every 12 hours in the usual dose. For patients with moderate kidney failure, this drug can be taken every 12 to 24 hours in the usual dose. This drug should NOT be used by patients with severe kidney failure or acute kidney failure.

▷ **How Best to Take This Medicine:** May be taken with or following meals to promote absorption and to reduce stomach irritation. The tablet may be crushed. Intermittent or alternate-day use is recommended to minimize the possibility of sodium and potassium imbalance.

▷ **How Long This Medicine Is Usually Taken:**   Continual use on a regular schedule for 5 to 10 days is usually necessary to determine the effectiveness of this drug in clearing edema, and for 2 to 3 weeks to determine its effect on hypertension. Long-term use (months to years) requires physician supervision.

▷ **Tell Your Doctor Before Taking This Medicine If You:**
- ever had an allergic reaction to it.
- have severely impaired liver or kidney function or a history of liver or kidney disease.
- have diabetes.
- are taking an anticoagulant, antihypertensives, a digitalis preparation, another diuretic, lithium, or a potassium preparation.
- plan to have surgery under general anesthesia soon.

▷ **Possible Side Effects:**   Abnormally high blood potassium levels, abnormally low blood sodium levels, dehydration.

▷ **Possible Adverse Effects:**
If any of the following develop, call your doctor promptly for guidance.
Some Mild Problems Drug Can Cause
   Allergic reactions: skin rash, itching, drug fever.
   Headache, dizziness, weakness, drowsiness, confusion.
   Dry mouth, nausea, vomiting, diarrhea.
Some Serious Problems Drug Can Cause
   Allergic reaction: abnormally low blood platelet count (rare).
   Symptomatic potassium excess: confusion, numbness and tingling in lips and extremities, shortness of breath, slow heart rate, low blood pressure.
   Masculine pattern of hair growth and deepening of the voice in women.
   Rare systemic lupus erythematosus–like syndrome, porphyria, or thinning of the bones.
   Stomach ulceration with bleeding (rare).

▷ **Possible Effects on Sex Life:**   Decreased libido, impaired erection, or impotence.
Male breast enlargement and tenderness.
Female breast enlargement, altered timing and pattern of menstruation; postmenopausal bleeding.
Decreased vaginal secretion.

▷ *CAUTION*
1. Do not take potassium supplements or increase your intake of potassium-rich foods while taking this drug.
2. Do not abruptly discontinue this drug unless abnormally high blood levels of potassium develop.

3. Ordinary doses of aspirin (600 mg) may reverse this drug's diuretic effect. Observe your response to this combination.

4. Avoid the excessive use of salt substitutes containing potassium; these are a potential cause of potassium excess.

5. Limit continual use of this drug in children to 1 month. Observe closely for indications of potassium accumulation.

6. The natural decline in kidney function in those over 60 may predispose them to potassium retention in the body. Limit continual use of this drug to periods of 2 to 3 weeks. Look for indications of potassium excess: slow heart rate, irregular heart rhythms, low blood pressure, confusion, drowsiness. The excessive use of diuretics can cause harmful loss of body water (dehydration), increased viscosity of the blood, and an increased tendency to blood-clotting—predisposing to stroke, heart attack, or thrombophlebitis.

Advisability of Use During Pregnancy or If Breast-Feeding:

Pregnancy Category: B. This drug should not be used during pregnancy except for a very serious complication of pregnancy for which it is significantly beneficial. A metabolic byproduct (canrenone) is present in breast milk; avoid taking this drug or refrain from nursing.

▷ **Overdose Symptoms:** Thirst, drowsiness, fatigue, weakness, nausea, vomiting, confusion, irregular heart rhythm, low blood pressure.

▷ **Suggested Periodic Examinations While Taking This Drug:** (at doctor's discretion)
Measurements of blood sodium, potassium, and chloride levels. Kidney function tests.

▷ **While Taking This Drug the Following Apply:**

Foods: Avoid excessive restriction of salt.

Beverages: May be taken with milk.

Alcohol: Use with caution until the combined effects have been determined. Alcohol may enhance the drowsiness and blood pressure–lowering effect of this drug.

Other Drugs:

Spironolactone may *increase* the effects of
• digoxin (Lanoxin).

Spironolactone may *decrease* the effects of
• anticoagulants (Coumadin, etc.). Increased INR (prothrombin time) testing is needed.

Spironolactone *taken concurrently* with
• captopril (Capoten) may cause excessively high blood potassium levels.
• cyclosporine (Sandimmune) may lead to severe increases in potassium levels.

- digitoxin (Crystodigin) may cause either increased or decreased digitoxin effects (unpredictable).
- lithium may cause the accumulation of lithium to toxic levels.
- potassium preparations may cause excessively high blood potassium levels.

The following drugs may **decrease** the effects of spironolactone

- aspirin or other NSAIDs (see Drug Classes); these may reduce its diuretic effectiveness.

Driving, Hazardous Activities: May cause dizziness and drowsiness. Restrict your activities as necessary.

Discontinuation: With high dosage or prolonged use, withdraw this drug gradually. Ask your doctor for guidance.

▷ **Saving Money When Using This Medicine:**

- Many drugs are available to treat high blood pressure. Ask your doctor if this medicine offers the best balance of cost and outcome for you.
- Ask your doctor if a magnesium level can be checked with your next laboratory work.
- A generic form can be substituted for the brand name.

STAVUDINE (STAV you dine)

Other Name: d4T

Prescription Needed: Yes   **Controlled Drug:** No   **Generic:** No

Brand Name: Zerit

Overview of BENEFITS versus RISKS	
Possible Benefits	*Possible Risks*
INCREASED CD4 COUNTS IN ADULTS WITH ADVANCED HIV THERAPEUTIC OPTION FOR THOSE INTOLERANT OF AZT OR DIDANOSINE	PERIPHERAL NEUROPATHY Rare pancreatitis

▷ **Illness This Medication Treats:**

HIV in adults who failed to respond to or are intolerant of AZT or didanosine.

Other (unlabeled) generally accepted uses: (1) used in a small number of children; (2) many clinicians are now advocates of combination therapy with two or more medicines.

▷ **Typical Dosage Range:** (Dosage or schedule must be determined by the doctor for each individual.)

Infants and Children: Safety and efficacy of this drug are not established.

18 to 60 Years of Age: Patients who weigh 60 kg (132 lb) or more should be given 40 mg twice daily. Patients who weigh less than 60 kg should be given 30 mg twice daily.

For those who have had to stop this medicine because of peripheral neuropathy (with complete resolution of symptoms):

20 mg twice daily for patients who weigh 60 kg or more.

15 mg twice daily for those who weigh less than 60 kg.

Over 65 Years of Age: Use of this drug has NOT been studied in those over 65.

▷ **Conditions Requiring Dosing Adjustments:**

Liver function: Liver involvement in elimination of this drug has not been studied in humans.

Kidney function: Patients with mild kidney compromise (creatinine clearance greater than 50 ml/min) may take the usual weight-adjusted dose for adults. Those with mild to moderate kidney failure (creatinine clearance 26–50 ml/min) should take one-half of the usual weight-adjusted dose every 12 hours. Those with severe kidney compromise (creatinine clearance 10–25 ml/min) should take one-half the usual weight-adjusted dose every 24 hours.

▷ **How Best to Take This Medicine:**   May be taken without regard to food.

▷ **How Long This Medicine Is Usually Taken:** Use on a regular schedule for several months usually determines the effectiveness of this drug in slowing AIDS progression and increasing CD4 counts. Long-term use (months to years) requires periodic physician evaluation of response (often with CD4 or viral burden) and dosage adjustment.

▷ **Tell Your Doctor Before Taking This Medicine If You:**
- have had peripheral neuropathy caused by other drugs before.
- have vitamin B12 or folic acid deficiency.
- have kidney or liver compromise.
- have had pancreatitis.

▷ **Possible Adverse Effects:**
If any of the following develop, call your doctor promptly for guidance.

Some Mild Problems Drug Can Cause
Allergic reactions: skin rash.
Nausea and vomiting.
Abdominal pain.

Some Serious Problems Drug Can Cause
Allergic reactions: rare anaphylactic reactions.
Peripheral neuropathy.

Pancreatitis.

Liver toxicity.

Low white blood cell and platelet counts (rare).

▷ **Possible Effects on Sex Life:**   Rare impotence.

▷ **Adverse Effects That May Mimic Natural Diseases or Disorders:**
Increased liver function tests may mimic hepatitis.

▷ *CAUTION*
1. Stavudine has NOT been shown to decrease the risk of transmitting HIV to others through sexual contact or blood contamination.
2. Promptly report the development of stomach pain and vomiting; this could indicate pancreatitis.
3. Report development of pain, numbness, tingling, or burning in the hands or feet, which may be peripheral neuropathy.
4. Safety and effectiveness of this drug for those under 18 years old are not established.

Advisability of Use During Pregnancy or If Breast-Feeding:
Pregnancy Category: C. Ask your doctor for guidance. Present in breast milk; avoid taking this drug or refrain from nursing.

▷ **Overdose Symptoms:**   Adults treated with 12 to 24 times the recommended daily dose revealed no acute toxicity.

▷ **Possible Effects of Long-Term Use:**   Peripheral neuropathy and hepatic toxicity.

▷ **Suggested Periodic Examinations While Taking This Drug:** (at doctor's discretion)
Liver function tests, amylase and complete blood counts. CD4 tests and viral load measurement are often used to judge the success of therapy.

▷ **While Taking This Drug the Following Apply:**
Other Drugs:
Stavudine *taken concurrently* with
- other medicines—such as metronidazole (Flagyl), which can cause peripheral neuropathy—should be avoided if possible.

Stavudine may *increase* the effects of
- didanosine (Videx) at specific drug concentration ratios.
- zidovudine (AZT) at specific drug concentration ratios.

Stavudine may *decrease* the effects of
- didanosine (Videx) at specific drug concentration ratios.
- zidovudine (AZT) at specific drug concentration ratios.

Driving, Hazardous Activities: May cause dizziness. Restrict your activities as necessary.

Discontinuation: Do not stop taking this drug without your doctor's knowledge and guidance.

▷ **Saving Money When Using This Medicine:**
- Four drugs are available to treat AIDS. Ask your doctor if this medicine offers the best balance of cost and outcome for you.
- Talk with your doctor about combination therapy if you are not already taking it. Also ask about using viral load in addition to CD4 to check the continued success of treatment.
- This drug should NOT be used by people with compromised kidneys.

STRONTIUM-89 CHLORIDE (STRON tee um)

Prescription Needed: Yes **Controlled Drug:** No **Generic:** No

Brand Name: Metastron

Overview of BENEFITS versus RISKS	
Possible Benefits	*Possible Risks*
EFFECTIVE RELIEF OF PRIMARY OR METASTATIC BONE CANCER PAIN	BONE MARROW TOXICITY (decreased white blood cells and platelets)
	Transient increase in bone pain

▷ **Illness This Medication Treats:**
Primary or metastatic bone cancer pain.

▷ **Typical Dosage Range:** (Dosage or schedule must be determined by the doctor for each individual.)
Infants and Children: Safety and efficacy of this drug for those less than 18 years old have not been established.
18 to 60 Years of Age: A dose of 4 mCi (148 MBq) is given intravenously over 1 to 2 minutes. The dose may also be calculated using 40 to 60 mcCI per kilogram of body weight. The dose may be repeated at 90-day intervals if needed.
Over 60 Years of Age: Same as for 18 to 60 years of age.

▷ **Conditions Requiring Dosing Adjustments:**
Liver function: Dosing changes for patients with liver compromise do not appear to be needed.
Kidney function: This agent is primarily removed by the kidneys; however, decreases in dose are not presently defined

▷ **How Best to Take This Medicine:** You may eat and drink as you normally would. During the first week after injection, strontium-89 is present in the blood and urine. A normal toilet should be used in preference to a urinal.

▷ **How Long This Medicine Is Usually Taken:**   Use of previously prescribed pain medicine is expected for 7 to 20 days after the injection.
A maximum of 20 days after injection has been needed to determine
peak effectiveness of this drug in controlling bone cancer pain. The
dose may be repeated (if blood tests are acceptable) 90 days after the
prior dose. See your doctor regularly.

▷ **Tell Your Doctor Before Taking This Medicine If You:**
- ever had an allergic reaction to it.
- have cancer that does NOT involve the bone.
- have a history of low platelets or white blood cell counts.
- take other drugs that may lower white cells or platelets.

▷ **Possible Side Effects:**   May cause a calciumlike flushing when injected.
May cause a transient (up to 72 hours) increase in bone pain.

▷ **Possible Adverse Effects:**
If any of the following develop, call your doctor promptly for guid-
ance.
Some Mild Problems Drug Can Cause
Allergic reactions: chills and fever.
Mild calciumlike flushing upon injection.
Transient (up to 72 hours) increase in bone pain.
Some Serious Problems Drug Can Cause
Bone marrow toxicity: low white blood cell counts and low platelets.
Very rare bacterial infection of the blood following drug-induced
decreases in white blood cells.

▷ **Possible Delayed Adverse Effects:**   Lowering of white blood cells
(recovery in up to 6 months) and blood platelets (lowest count 12 to
16 weeks after therapy).

▷ *CAUTION*
1. Promptly report any signs of infection (lethargy, temperature,
   sore throat).
2. It may take up to 20 days for this agent to work. Use of narcotics
   will need to be continued.
3. Your blood and urine will contain radioactive strontium for 7
   days after injection. Ask your doctor for help regarding appropriate disposal.
4. This drug is a potential carcinogen.
5. Promptly report any abnormal bleeding or bruising.
6. Safety and effectiveness of this drug for those under 18 years old
   are not established.

Advisability of Use During Pregnancy or If Breast-Feeding:
Pregnancy Category: D. May cause fetal harm. Ask your doctor for advice. Present in breast milk; avoid taking this drug or refrain from nursing.

▷ **Overdose Symptoms:** May result in acute radiation syndrome, with initial nausea and vomiting followed by depressed white cells, platelets, and tendency to infections. Careful dosage calculations are indicated, as this drug emits beta radiation.

▷ **Suggested Periodic Examinations While Taking This Drug:** (at doctor's discretion)
Complete blood counts should be tested once every other week during therapy.

▷ **While Taking This Drug the Following Apply:**
Other Drugs:
Strontium-89 *taken concurrently* with
• medications that lower white blood cells or platelets may result in severe decreases.
Driving, Hazardous Activities: May cause a transient increase in bone pain. Restrict your activities as necessary.
Discontinuation: Dosing may be repeated if blood counts are acceptable.

▷ **Saving Money When Using This Medicine:**
• This medicine is very expensive. Ask your doctor if it offers the best balance of cost and outcome for you.
• Ask your doctor if a visit to a specialized chronic pain center is advisable.

SUCRALFATE (soo KRAL fayt)

Prescription Needed: Yes   **Controlled Drug:** No   **Generic:** No

Brand Name: Carafate

Overview of BENEFITS versus RISKS	
Possible Benefits	*Possible Risks*
EFFECTIVE TREATMENT IN DUODENAL ULCER DISEASE	Constipation
	Skin rash, hives, itching
No serious adverse effects	
No significant drug interactions	

▷ **Illness This Medication Treats:**
Recurrent duodenal ulcer disease. This drug is effective when used alone, but may be used with antacids for pain relief.

▷ **Typical Dosage Range:** (Dosage or schedule must be determined by the doctor for each individual.)
1 g four times daily.

▷ **How Best to Take This Medicine:** Take with water on an empty stomach at least 1 hour before or 2 hours after each meal and at bedtime. Swallow the tablets whole; do not alter or chew. Take the full course prescribed.

▷ **How Long This Medicine Is Usually Taken:** Continual use on a regular schedule for 6 to 8 weeks is usually needed for peak effect in promoting the healing of ulcers. Use beyond 8 weeks must be determined by your doctor.

▷ **Tell Your Doctor Before Taking This Medicine If You:**
- ever had an allergic reaction to it.
- have chronic constipation or kidney failure.
- are taking any other drugs at this time.

▷ **Possible Side Effects:** Constipation.

▷ **Possible Adverse Effects:**
If any of the following develop, call your doctor promptly for guidance.
Some Mild Problems Drug Can Cause
  Allergic reactions: skin rash, itching.
  Dizziness, light-headedness, drowsiness.
  Dry mouth, indigestion, nausea, cramping, diarrhea.
Some Serious Problems Drug Can Cause
  Increased risk of aluminum toxicity.
  Increased bezoar risk (food clump in the esophagus).

▷ *CAUTION*
1. If antacids are needed to relieve ulcer pain, do not take them within half an hour before or 2 hours after the dose of sucralfate.
2. This drug may impair the absorption of other drugs if they are taken close together. Avoid taking any other drugs within 2 hours of taking sucralfate. This applies especially to cimetidine (Tagamet), phenytoin (Dilantin), and tetracyclines.

Advisability of Use During Pregnancy or If Breast-Feeding:
Pregnancy Category: B. Use this drug only if clearly needed. Ask your doctor for guidance. Presence in breast milk is unknown. Watch the nursing infant closely and stop taking this drug or nursing if adverse effects develop.

▷ **Overdose Symptoms:** Nausea, stomach cramping, possible diarrhea.

▷ **While Taking This Drug the Following Apply:**

Foods: Follow the diet prescribed by your doctor. Vitamins A, D, E, and K may become a deficiency problem.

Beverages: Preferably taken with water.

Alcohol: No interactions expected. However, alcohol is best avoided because of its irritant effect on the stomach.

Tobacco Smoking: Nicotine can delay ulcer healing and reduce the effectiveness of this drug. Avoid all forms of tobacco.

Other Drugs:

Sucralfate may **decrease** the effects of
- cimetidine (Tagamet).
- ciprofloxacin (Cipro).
- digoxin (Lanoxin).
- enoxacin (Penetrex).
- fleroxacin (Megalone).
- ketoconazole (Nizoral).
- norfloxacin (Noroxin).
- ofloxacin (Floxin).
- quinidine (Quinaglute).
- phenytoin (Dilantin, etc.).
- tetracycline (Achromycin, Tetracyn, etc.).
- warfarin (Coumadin, etc.), reducing its anticoagulant effect. Increased INR (prothrombin time) testing is needed, with dosing adjusted to test results.

Driving, Hazardous Activities: May cause dizziness or drowsiness. Restrict your activities as necessary.

▷ **Saving Money When Using This Medicine:**
- Many new drugs are available to treat ulcers. Ask your doctor if this medicine offers the best balance of cost and outcome for you.
- Ulcers, especially recurrent ulcers, are now thought to be infections. Talk to your doctor about usage of the combination of clarithromycin and omeprazole for ulcers.

SULFADIAZINE   (sul fa DI a zeen)

Prescription Needed: Yes   **Controlled Drug:** No   **Generic:** Yes

Brand Names: Microsulfon, Trisem [CD], Trisoralen [CD]

Overview of BENEFITS versus RISKS

Possible Benefits	*Possible Risks*
EFFECTIVE TREATMENT OF A BROAD SPECTRUM OF INFECTIONS DUE TO SUSCEPTIBLE MICROORGANISMS	BONE MARROW DEPRESSION DRUG-INDUCED HEPATITIS SEVERE ALLERGIC REACTIONS
Effective treatment of AIDS-related paracoccidioidomycosis	Drug-induced kidney damage
Effective adjunctive treatment of AIDS-related toxoplasmosis	
Effective adjunctive treatment of certain types of malaria	

▷ **Illness This Medication Treats:**

Treatment of urinary infections.

Other (unlabeled) generally accepted uses: (1) chancroid, inclusion conjunctivitis, meningococcal meningitis, nocardiosis, rheumatic fever, trachoma; (2) adjunctively with other anti-infectives for certain types of malaria, *H. influenzae* meningitis, acute otitis media; (3) with pyrimethamine in treatment of AIDS-related cerebral toxoplasmosis.

Author's note: The information on this medicine has been abbreviated in order to allow room for medicines that are more widely used.

SULFAMETHOXAZOLE   (sul fa meth OX a zohl)

Prescription Needed: Yes   **Controlled Drug:**   No   **Generic:** Yes

Brand Names: Azo Gantanol [CD], Bactrim [CD], Bactrim DS [CD], Bethaprim [CD], Comoxol [CD], Cotrim [CD], Gantanol, Septra [CD], Septra DS [CD], Uroplus DS [CD], Uroplus SS [CD], Vagitrol

---

Overview of BENEFITS versus RISKS

Possible Benefits	*Possible Risks*
EFFECTIVE ANTIMICROBIAL ACTION against susceptible bacteria and protozoa	Allergic reactions: mild to severe skin reactions, anaphylaxis, myocarditis
Effective adjunctive prevention and treatment of *Pneumocystis carinii* pneumonia associated with AIDS	Rare blood cell disorders: aplastic anemia, hemolytic anemia, abnormally low white cell and platelet counts
	Drug-induced liver damage
	Drug-induced kidney damage

▷ **Illness This Medication Treats:**
(1) A variety of bacterial and protozoal infections: chancroid, cystitis, and other urinary tract infections; (2) combined with trimethoprim (co-trimoxazole) to treat middle ear infections.

As *Combination Drug Product* [CD]: This drug is available in combination with phenazopyridine, an analgesic. This combination provides early symptomatic relief while the underlying infection is being treated. This drug is also available in combination with trimethoprim; in some countries this combination is given the generic name co-trimoxazole. This combination is quite effective in the treatment of certain types of middle ear infections, bronchitis, pneumonia, and certain infections of the intestinal tract and urinary tract. It is now used as primary prevention and treatment for *Pneumocystis carinii* pneumonia associated with AIDS.

▷ **Typical Dosage Range:** (Dosage or schedule must be determined by the doctor for each individual.)
Initially 2 g, then 1 g every 8 to 12 hours, depending upon the severity of the infection. The total daily dosage should not exceed 3 g. Discuss co-trimoxazole dosing with your doctor.

▷ **Conditions Requiring Dosing Adjustments:**
Liver function: This drug is metabolized in the liver. Patients with compromised livers should be followed closely; however, no specific guidelines for decreasing doses are defined.
Kidney function: The dose should be decreased for patients with compromised kidneys. For patients with moderate failure, 50% of the usual dose can be taken at the normal interval.

▷ **How Best to Take This Medicine:** Preferably taken on an empty stomach, 1 hour before or 2 hours after eating. However, it may be taken with or following food to reduce stomach irritation. The tablet may be crushed for administration.

▷ **How Long This Medicine Is Usually Taken:** Continual use on a regular schedule for 4 to 7 days is usually necessary to determine the effectiveness of this drug in controlling responsive infections. Treatment should be continued until the patient is free of symptoms for 48 hours. Limit treatment to no more than 14 days if possible.

▷ **Tell Your Doctor Before Taking This Medicine If You:**
• are allergic to any sulfonamide drug or to any sulfonamide derivative: acetazolamide, thiazide diuretics, sulfonylurea antidiabetics.
• are in the last month of pregnancy or are breast-feeding.
• are allergic by nature: history of hay fever, asthma, hives, eczema.
• have impaired liver or kidney function.
• have a personal or family history of porphyria.

- have had a drug-induced blood cell or bone marrow disorder in the past.
- are currently taking any oral anticoagulant, antidiabetic, or phenytoin.
- plan to have surgery under pentothal anesthesia soon.

▷ **Possible Side Effects:**   Brownish coloration of the urine, of no significance.

Superinfections, bacterial or fungal.

▷ **Possible Adverse Effects:**

If any of the following develop, call your doctor promptly for guidance.

Some Mild Problems Drug Can Cause

Allergic reactions: skin rashes, itching, localized swellings, reddened eyes.

Headache, dizziness, unsteadiness, ringing in the ears.

Loss of appetite, irritation of the mouth and tongue, nausea, vomiting, abdominal pain, diarrhea.

Some Serious Problems Drug Can Cause

Allergic reactions: drug fever, swollen glands, painful joints, anaphylaxis. Allergic reaction in the heart muscle (myocarditis), allergic pneumonitis, allergic hepatitis. Severe skin reactions.

Idiosyncratic reaction: hemolytic anemia.

Bone marrow depression: fatigue, weakness, fever, sore throat, abnormal bleeding or bruising.

Rare methemoglobinemia, drug-induced lupus erythematosus, low blood clotting.

Pancreatitis; kidney damage: bloody or cloudy urine, reduced urine volume.

Psychotic reactions, hallucinations, seizures, hearing loss, peripheral neuropathy.

▷ **Adverse Effects That May Mimic Natural Diseases or Disorders:**

Liver reactions may suggest viral hepatitis.

Lung reactions may suggest an infectious pneumonia.

▷ *CAUTION*

1. A large intake of water (up to 2 qt daily) is necessary to ensure an adequate volume of urine.
2. Shake liquid dosage forms thoroughly before measuring each dose.
3. This drug should not be used in infants under 2 months old.
4. For those over 60, small doses taken at longer intervals often achieve adequate blood and tissue drug levels. Watch for reduced urine volume, fever, sore throat, abnormal bleeding or bruising, or skin irritation with itching, particularly in the anal or genital regions.

Advisability of Use During Pregnancy or If Breast-Feeding:

Pregnancy Category: C, however, this drug SHOULD NOT be given near the time of the birth of the baby. Avoid use of this drug during the last month of pregnancy because of possible adverse effects on the newborn infant. Present in breast milk; avoid taking this drug or refrain from nursing.

▷ **Overdose Symptoms:**   Headache, dizziness, nausea, vomiting, abdominal cramping, toxic fever, coma, jaundice, kidney failure.

▷ **Suggested Periodic Examinations While Taking This Drug:** (at doctor's discretion)

Complete blood cell counts, weekly for the first 8 weeks.

Urine analysis weekly.

Liver and kidney function tests.

▷ **While Taking This Drug the Following Apply:**

Beverages: May be taken with milk.

Alcohol: Use caution—sulfonamide drugs can increase the intoxicating effects of alcohol.

Other Drugs:

Sulfamethoxazole may *increase* the effects of

- amantadine (Symmetrel), causing abnormal heart rhythms and central nervous system stimulation (disorientation).
- anticoagulants (Coumadin, etc.), increasing the risk of bleeding. More INR (prothrombin time) testing is needed.
- methotrexate (Mexate), causing severe toxicity.
- sulfonylureas (see Drug Classes), increasing the risk of hypoglycemia.
- zidovudine (AZT) and lead to zidovudine toxicity.

Sulfamethoxazole may *decrease* the effects of

- cyclosporine (Sandimmune), reducing its immunosuppressive effect.
- oral contraceptives (birth control pills) and lead to unwanted pregnancy.
- penicillins (see Drug Classes).

Driving, Hazardous Activities: May cause dizziness. Restrict your activities as necessary.

Exposure to Sun: Use caution until your sensitivity has been determined. Some sulfonamides can cause photosensitivity.

▷ **Saving Money When Using This Medicine:**

- Many drugs are available to treat infections. Ask your doctor if this medicine offers the best balance of cost and outcome for you.
- A generic form can be substituted for the brand name.
- Ask your doctor if the power of this antibiotic matches the severity of your infection.

SULFASALAZINE (sul fa SAL a zeen)

Prescription Needed: Yes   **Controlled Drug:** No   **Generic:** Yes

Brand Names: Azaline, Azulfidine, Azulfidine EN-tabs, SAS-500

Overview of BENEFITS versus RISKS

Possible Benefits	*Possible Risks*
EFFECTIVE SUPPRESSION OF INFLAMMATORY BOWEL DISEASE SYMPTOMATIC RELIEF IN TREATMENT OF REGIONAL ENTERITIS AND ULCERATIVE COLITIS	Allergic reactions: mild to severe skin reactions Rare blood cell disorders: aplastic anemia, hemolytic anemia, abnormally low white cell and platelet counts Drug-induced liver damage Drug-induced kidney damage Rare seizures

---

▷ **Illness This Medication Treats:**
   Treats inflammatory disease of the lower intestinal tract: regional enteritis (Crohn's disease) and ulcerative colitis; usually taken by mouth, but may also be used in retention enemas.

▷ **Typical Dosage Range:** (Dosage or schedule must be determined by the doctor for each individual.)
   For ulcerative colitis: Initially 1 to 2 g every 6 to 8 hours until symptoms are adequately controlled. For maintenance, 500 mg/6 hr. The total daily dosage should not exceed 12 g.

▷ **Conditions Requiring Dosing Adjustments:**
   Liver function: This drug can cause liver damage, and patients should be followed closely.
   Kidney function: Decreases in doses should be considered. This drug should be used with caution by patients with renal compromise.

▷ **How Best to Take This Medicine:** Best taken with 8 oz of water on an empty stomach, 1 hour before or 2 hours after eating. However, it may be taken with or following food to reduce stomach irritation. Intervals between doses (day and night) should be no longer than 8 hours. The regular tablet may be crushed; the enteric-coated tablet should be swallowed whole without alteration.

▷ **How Long This Medicine Is Usually Taken:** Use on a regular schedule for 1 to 3 weeks usually determines the effectiveness of this drug in controlling the symptoms of regional enteritis or ulcerative colitis. Long-term use (months to years) requires supervision and periodic evaluation. See your doctor regularly.

▷ **Tell Your Doctor Before Taking This Medicine If You:**
- are allergic to *any* sulfonamide or sulfonamide derivative: acetazol-amide, thiazide diuretics, sulfonylurea antidiabetics; or to aspirin (or other salicylates).
- are in the last month of pregnancy or are breast-feeding.
- are allergic by nature: history of hay fever, asthma, hives, eczema.
- have impaired liver or kidney function.
- have a personal or family history of porphyria.
- had a drug-induced blood cell or bone marrow disorder in the past.
- have a G6PD deficiency.
- are currently taking any oral anticoagulant, antidiabetic, or pheny-toin.
- plan to have surgery under pentothal anesthesia soon.

▷ **Possible Side Effects:**   Brownish coloration of the urine, of no sig-nificance.
Superinfections, bacterial or fungal.

▷ **Possible Adverse Effects:**
If any of the following develop, call your doctor promptly for guid-ance.
Some Mild Problems Drug Can Cause
Allergic reactions: skin rashes, itching.
Headache, dizziness.
Loss of appetite, irritation of the mouth and tongue, nausea, vomit-ing, diarrhea.
Some Serious Problems Drug Can Cause
Allergic reactions: drug fever, swollen glands, painful joints, ana-phylaxis. Allergic pneumonitis, allergic hepatitis. Severe skin re-actions.
Idiosyncratic reaction: hemolytic anemia.
Bone marrow depression, fatigue, weakness, fever, sore throat, ab-normal bleeding or bruising.
Pancreatitis; kidney damage: bloody or cloudy urine, reduced urine volume.
Inflammation of tissue around the heart.
Rare lupus erythematosus or myopathy.
Peripheral neuropathy.

▷ **Possible Effects on Sex Life:**   Decreased production of sperm, re-versible infertility.

▷ **Adverse Effects That May Mimic Natural Diseases or Disorders:**
Liver reactions may suggest viral hepatitis.
Lung reactions may suggest an infectious pneumonia.

▷ *CAUTION*

1. A large intake of water (up to 2 qt daily) is necessary to ensure an adequate volume of urine.
2. Shake liquid dosage forms thoroughly before measuring each dose.
3. Safety and effectiveness of this drug for those under 2 years old have not been established.
4. Those over 60 should watch for reduced urine volume, fever, sore throat, abnormal bleeding or bruising, or skin irritation with itching, particularly in the anal or genital regions.

Advisability of Use During Pregnancy or If Breast-Feeding:

Pregnancy Category: B, however, this drug SHOULD NOT be used near the time of the birth of the baby. Avoid during the last month of pregnancy because of possible adverse effects on the newborn infant. Present in breast milk; avoid taking this drug or refrain from nursing.

▷ **Overdose Symptoms:**   Headache, dizziness, nausea, vomiting, toxic fever, coma, jaundice, kidney failure.

▷ **Suggested Periodic Examinations While Taking This Drug:** (at doctor's discretion)

Complete blood cell counts, weekly for the first 8 weeks.

Urine analysis weekly.

Liver and kidney function tests.

▷ **While Taking This Drug the Following Apply:**

Foods: Follow the prescribed diet.

Beverages: May be taken with milk.

Alcohol: Use caution until the combined effect has been determined. Sulfonamides can increase the intoxicating effects of alcohol.

Other Drugs:

Sulfasalazine may *increase* the effects of

- anticoagulants (Coumadin, etc.), increasing the risk of bleeding. More INR (prothrombin time) tests are needed.
- sulfonylureas, increasing the risk of hypoglycemia.

Sulfasalazine may *decrease* the effects of

- digoxin (Lanoxin).

Sulfasalazine *taken concurrently* with

- ampicillin and perhaps other penicillins may blunt the therapeutic effects of sulfasalazine.
- calcium supplements (gluconate) may blunt sulfasalazine's benefits.
- iron salts may blunt sulfasalazine's effects.
- some barbiturates (see Drug Classes) may blunt sulfasalazine's benefits.

Driving, Hazardous Activities: May cause dizziness. Restrict your activities as necessary.

Exposure to Sun: Use caution until your sensitivity has been determined. Some sulfonamides can cause photosensitivity.

▷ **Saving Money When Using This Medicine:**
- Ask your doctor if this medicine offers the best balance of cost and outcome for you.
- A generic form can be substituted for the brand name.

SULFISOXAZOLE (sul fi SOX a zohl)

Prescription Needed: Yes   **Controlled Drug:** No   **Generic:** Yes

Brand Names: Azo Gantrisin [CD], Eryzole [CD], Gantrisin, Lipo Gantrisin, Pediazole [CD], SK-Soxazole

Overview of BENEFITS versus RISKS	
Possible Benefits	*Possible Risks*
EFFECTIVE ANTIMICROBIAL ACTION against susceptible bacteria and protozoa	Allergic reactions: mild to severe skin reactions, anaphylaxis
	Rare blood cell disorders: aplastic anemia, hemolytic anemia, abnormally low white cell and platelet counts
	Drug-induced liver damage
	Drug-induced kidney damage

▷ **Illness This Medication Treats:**
A variety of bacterial and protozoal infections, most commonly for certain infections of the urinary tract.

As Combination Drug Product [CD]: In combination with phenazopyridine, an analgesic that relieves the discomfort associated with acute infections of the urinary bladder and urethra, sulfisoxazole provides early symptomatic relief while the underlying infection is being eradicated.

▷ **Typical Dosage Range:** (Dosage or schedule must be determined by the doctor for each individual.)
Initially 2 to 4 g, then 750 to 1500 mg (1.5 g) every 4 hours, or 1 to 2 g every 6 hours, depending on the severity of the infection. The total daily dosage should not exceed 12 g.

▷ **Conditions Requiring Dosing Adjustments:**
Liver function: This drug is a rare cause of liver damage, and patients should be followed closely.
Kidney function: For patients with mild to moderate kidney failure,

sulfisoxazole can be taken every 6 hours in the usual dose. For those with moderate to severe failure, it can be taken every 12 to 24 hours in the usual dose. For patients with severe kidney failure, it can be taken once a day. This drug should be used with caution by patients with renal compromise.

▷ **How Best to Take This Medicine:**   Preferably taken with 8 oz of water on an empty stomach, 1 hour before or 2 hours after eating. However, it may be taken with or following food to reduce stomach irritation. The tablet may be crushed.

▷ **How Long This Medicine Is Usually Taken:**   Use on a regular schedule for 7 to 10 days usually determines the effectiveness of this drug in controlling responsive infections. Treatment should be continued until the patient is symptom-free for 48 hours. Limit treatment to 14 days if possible.

▷ **Tell Your Doctor Before Taking This Medicine If You:**
- are allergic to *any* sulfonamide (see Drug Classes) or sulfonamide derivative: acetazolamide, thiazide diuretics, sulfonylurea antidiabetics.
- are allergic by nature: history of hay fever, asthma, hives, eczema.
- are in the last month of pregnancy or are breast-feeding.
- have impaired liver or kidney function.
- have a personal or family history of porphyria.
- had a drug-induced blood cell or bone marrow disorder in the past.
- have a G6PD deficiency.
- are currently taking any oral anticoagulant, antidiabetic, or phenytoin.
- plan to have surgery under pentothal anesthesia soon.

▷ **Possible Side Effects:**   Brownish coloration of the urine, of no significance.
Superinfections, bacterial or fungal.

▷ **Possible Adverse Effects:**
If any of the following develop, call your doctor promptly for guidance.
Some Mild Problems Drug Can Cause
Allergic reactions: skin rashes, itching, localized swellings, reddened eyes.
Headache, dizziness, ringing in the ears.
Loss of appetite, irritation of the mouth and tongue, nausea, vomiting, abdominal pain, diarrhea.
Some Serious Problems Drug Can Cause
Allergic reactions: drug fever, swollen glands, painful joints, anaphylaxis. Allergic hepatitis. Severe skin reactions.

Idiosyncratic reaction: hemolytic anemia.

Bone marrow depression: fatigue, weakness, fever, sore throat, abnormal bleeding or bruising.

Rare drug-induced systemic lupus erythematosus, parotitis, or disulfiramlike reaction.

Kidney damage: bloody or cloudy urine, reduced urine volume.

Peripheral neuropathy.

▷ **Adverse Effects That May Mimic Natural Diseases or Disorders:**
Liver reactions may suggest viral hepatitis.

▷ *CAUTION*
1. A large intake of water (up to 2 qt daily) is necessary to ensure an adequate volume of urine and avoid harmful crystal formation in the urine.
2. Shake liquid dosage forms thoroughly before measuring each dose.
3. This drug should not be used in infants under 2 months old.
4. Those over 60 should take small doses at longer intervals, which often achieve adequate blood and tissue drug levels. Watch for reduced urine volume, fever, sore throat, abnormal bleeding or bruising, or skin irritation with itching, particularly in the anal or genital regions.

Advisability of Use During Pregnancy or If Breast-Feeding:
Pregnancy Category: C. Avoid using this drug during the last month of pregnancy because of possible adverse effects on the newborn infant. Present in breast milk; avoid taking this drug or refrain from nursing.

▷ **Overdose Symptoms:** Headache, dizziness, nausea, vomiting, abdominal cramping, toxic fever, coma, jaundice, kidney failure.

▷ **Suggested Periodic Examinations While Taking This Drug:** (at doctor's discretion)
Complete blood cell counts, weekly for the first 8 weeks.
Urine analysis weekly.
Liver and kidney function tests.

▷ **While Taking This Drug the Following Apply:**
Beverages: May be taken with milk.
Alcohol: Use caution until the combined effect has been determined. Sulfonamides can increase the intoxicating effects of alcohol.
Other Drugs:
Sulfisoxazole may *increase* the effects of
• anticoagulants (Coumadin, etc.), increasing the risk of bleeding. More INR (prothrombin time) tests are needed.

- methotrexate (Mexate), causing serious toxicity.
- sulfonylureas, increasing the risk of hypoglycemia.

Sulfisoxazole may *decrease* the effects of

- oral contraceptives (birth control pills).
- penicillins.

Driving, Hazardous Activities: May cause dizziness. Restrict your activities as necessary.

Exposure to Sun: Use caution until your sensitivity has been determined. Some sulfonamide drugs can cause photosensitivity.

▷ **Saving Money When Using This Medicine:**

- Ask your doctor if this medicine offers the best balance of cost and outcome for you.
- Ask your doctor if the power of this antibiotic matches the severity of your infection.
- The dose MUST be adjusted for patients with kidney compromise.
- A generic form can be substituted for the brand name.

SULINDAC (sul IN dak)

Prescription Needed: Yes   **Controlled Drug:** No   **Generic:** Yes

Brand Name: Clinoril

Overview of BENEFITS versus RISKS	
Possible Benefits	*Possible Risks*
EFFECTIVE RELIEF OF MILD TO MODERATE PAIN AND INFLAMMATION	Rare gastrointestinal pain, ulceration, bleeding
	Rare liver damage
	Rare kidney damage
	Rare bone marrow depression (aplastic anemia)
	Rare pancreatitis

See the acetic acids (NSAIDs) drug profile for further information.

SUMATRIPTAN (soo ma TRIP tan)

Prescription Needed: Yes   **Controlled Drug:** No   **Generic:** No

Brand Name: Imitrex

```
┌─────────────────────────────────────────────────────────┐
│              Overview of BENEFITS versus RISKS          │
│       Possible Benefits              Possible Risks     │
│  RAPID AND EFFECTIVE          SYNCOPE (fainting) (rare)  │
│     RELIEF OR PREVENTION      Very rare heart attack     │
│     OF NONBASILAR,            Seizures (rare)            │
│     NONHEMIPLEGIC             Abnormal heartbeats (rare) │
│     MIGRAINE HEADACHES                                   │
│  USUALLY WELL TOLERATED                                  │
│     RELATIVE TO OTHER                                    │
│     AVAILABLE TREATMENTS                                 │
│  Relieves photophobia,                                   │
│     phonophobia, nausea, and                             │
│     vomiting often associated                            │
│     with migraine attacks                                │
└─────────────────────────────────────────────────────────┘
```

▷ **Illness This Medication Treats:**
Acute treatment of migraine with or without aura.

▷ **Typical Dosage Range:** (Dosage or schedule must be determined by the doctor for each individual.)

Infants and Children: Safety and effectiveness of this drug in pediatrics have NOT been determined.

18 to 60 Years of Age: Subcutaneous: Maximum adult dose is 6 mg, and should be given as soon as possible once symptoms of acute migraine are recognized. Controlled clinical trials have failed to demonstrate a benefit of repeat injections if the initial injection does not work. If symptoms return, a second 6-mg injection may be given 12 hours after the first injection. If side effects occur, use the lowest effective dose in the approved dosage range.

Oral form: 25 mg taken as soon as headache pain starts. If symptoms don't improve in 2 hours, another 25 mg may be taken. Maximum oral dose is 100 mg, but data do not show that this gives better results.

Over 65 Years of Age: Safety and effectiveness of this drug have NOT been evaluated in this age group. Since declines in renal and hepatic function and coronary artery disease are more common in those over 65, the possibility of an increase in side effects would be expected.

▷ **Conditions Requiring Dosing Adjustments:**
Liver function: The effect of this drug on patients with hepatic impairment has not been specifically studied, and no dosage or interval adjustments have been established.

▷ **How Best to Take This Medicine:** The injection form must be given subcutaneously, **NOT INTRAVENOUSLY.** Intravenous injection must be avoided because of its potential to cause coronary vaso-spasm (constriction of the blood vessels that supply the heart). The medicine should be colorless to pale yellow and clear. Particles or precipitation should never be present. Extensive information on self-injection is available from your doctor or pharmacist. The tablet form may take an hour to work. Tablets may be taken with food.

▷ **How Long This Medicine Is Usually Taken:**   The maximum dose is two 6-mg doses in 24 hours. This medication relieves existing migraines, and will not change the frequency or number of attacks. Recurring use will be needed. If your migraines increase in frequency or severity, or if this medicine does not help, consult your doctor.

▷ **Tell Your Doctor Before Taking This Medicine If You:**
- ever had an allergic reaction to it.
- have ischemic heart disease with symptoms such as angina pectoris or silent ischemia, or a history of myocardial infarction.
- have Prinzmetal's angina, chest pain, heart disease, or irregular heartbeats.
- have uncontrolled hypertension.
- have basilar or hemiplegic migraine.
- have taken an ergotamine preparation within 24 hours.
- are pregnant, planning pregnancy, or are breast-feeding.
- have taken an MAO inhibitor (see Drug Classes) in the last 2 weeks.
- have had a heart attack.
- have taken or have prescriptions for other migraine medications.
- have allergies or trouble taking other medication.
- have liver or kidney disease.
- take other prescription or over-the-counter medicines that were not discussed when sumatriptan was prescribed.
- have Raynaud's syndrome.

▷ **Possible Side Effects:**   Excessive thirst and frequent urination. Transient rises in blood pressure.

▷ **Possible Adverse Effects:**
If any of the following develop, call your doctor promptly for guidance.
Some Mild Problems Drug Can Cause
  Allergic reactions: red itching skin, skin rash, and tenderness.
  Rare tingling and numbness, confusion, or dizziness.
  Rare pain at the injection site or joint pain.
Some Serious Problems Drug Can Cause
  Allergic reactions: rare anaphylactic reaction.
  Rare syncope (fainting), cerebrovascular accident, dysphasia, or seizure.

Rare serious changes in heart rhythm.
Rare Raynaud's syndrome or dyspnea (difficulty breathing).
Very rare kidney problems or heart attack.

▷ **Possible Effects on Sex Life:** Dysmenorrhea, difficulties with erection.

▷ **Adverse Effects That May Mimic Natural Diseases or Disorders:**
Changes in heart rate and rhythm may mimic a number of cardiac conditions. Drug-induced acute renal failure (ARF) may mimic non-drug-induced ARF. Drug-induced hypertension may mimic hypertension from other causes.
Urological symptoms may mimic benign prostatic hypertrophy. Effects can mimic Raynaud's syndrome.

▷ *CAUTION*
1. Do not use this drug if you are pregnant.
2. Call your doctor if you have any pain or tightness in the chest or throat when you use this medicine.
3. Do not use this drug if you have used an ergotamine preparation within the last 24 hours.
4. This medication is NOT to be used intravenously. Discuss this with your doctor if you are unfamiliar with the subcutaneous route. Particular care must be taken to avoid intravenous use, because this may lead to coronary vasospasm.
5. If you are diagnosed as having ischemic heart disease after sumatriptan has been prescribed for you, do not use this medicine again.
6. Safety and effectiveness of this drug for those under 18 years old have not been established.

Advisability of Use During Pregnancy or If Breast-Feeding:
Pregnancy Category: C. Ask your doctor for guidance. Present in breast milk of animals, unknown in humans; use of this drug by nursing mothers requires a benefit-to-risk decision by your doctor.

▷ **Overdose Symptoms:** Patients have received doses of 8 to 12 mg without adverse effects. Healthy volunteers have taken up to 16 mg subcutaneously without serious adverse events. Coronary vasospasm has resulted from intravenous administration of normal doses. Animal data includes reactions such as convulsions, tremor, flushing, decreased breathing and activity, cyanosis, ataxia, and paralysis.

▷ **Suggested Periodic Examinations While Taking This Drug:** (at doctor's discretion)
Liver function tests, electrocardiograms.

▷ **While Taking This Drug the Following Apply:**

Alcohol: May cause additive sedation.

Marijuana Smoking: May cause additive dizziness, drowsiness, and lethargy; additive increases in blood pressure.

Other Drugs:

Sumatriptan *taken concurrently* with

- ergotamine-containing preparations may result in additive vasospasm (prolonged constriction of the blood vessels).
- monoamine oxidase inhibitors (MAOIs) may lead to toxicity. DO NOT COMBINE.

Driving, Hazardous Activities: May cause dizziness and drowsiness. Restrict your activities as necessary.

Exposure to Cold: Use caution until your tolerance is determined. Cold environments may enhance this drug's vasoconstrictive action.

Special Storage Instructions: KEEP OUT OF REACH OF CHILDREN. Store at room temperature where the temperature will not exceed 86° F. Keep this drug away from heat and light.

Observe the Following Expiration Times: An expiration date is printed on the treatment package. Throw the medication away if it has expired. The autoinjector may be used again.

▷ **Saving Money When Using This Medicine:**

- Ask your doctor if this medicine offers the best balance of cost and outcome for you.
- Talk with your doctor about the medicines used to help PREVENT migraine attacks.
- Once you start sumatriptan, keep a record of how many times you go to the hospital for migraines, and then compare it to the records of your hospitalizations for the previous year.

TACRINE (TA kreen)

Prescription Needed: Yes   **Controlled Drug:** No   **Generic:** No

Brand Name: Cognex

Overview of BENEFITS versus RISKS	
Possible Benefits	*Possible Risks*
IMPROVEMENT OF MEMORY IN MILD TO MODERATE ALZHEIMER'S DISEASE	LIVER TOXICITY Hallucinations

▷ **Illness This Medication Treats:**

Mild to moderate Alzheimer's disease.

Other (unlabeled) generally accepted uses: (1) significant increases in protective white blood cells (CD4 lymphocytes) occurred when tacrine was used to treat AIDS dementia; (2) early data indicated a benefit in movement disorders (tardive dyskinesia).

▷ **Typical Dosage Range:** (Dosage or schedule must be determined by the doctor for each individual.)

Infants and Children: No data are available on use of this drug in infants and children.

18 to 60 Years of Age: Adult starting dose is 10 mg taken four times a day. The dose can be increased at 6-week intervals if needed. Maximum daily dose is 160 mg.

Over 60 Years of Age: Same as for 12 to 60 years of age.

▷ **Conditions Requiring Dosing Adjustments:**

Liver function: Patients with liver compromise should use this drug with great caution.

Kidney function: Dose decreases for patients with kidney compromise are not presently indicated.

▷ **How Best to Take This Medicine:**   Tablet may be crushed; it is best taken 1 hour before meals.

▷ **How Long This Medicine Is Usually Taken:**   Use of this drug on a regular schedule for 1 to 4 weeks is usually needed to see clinical improvement. Dose increases are made at 6-week intervals. Long-term use (months to years) requires your doctor's periodic evaluation of response and dosage adjustment.

▷ **Tell Your Doctor Before Taking This Medicine If You:**

- ever had an allergic reaction to it.
- have had tacrine-caused hepatoxicity and blood bilirubin levels greater than 3 mg/dl.
- have bronchial asthma.
- have a slow heartbeat (bradycardia), an abnormal electrical conduction system in your heart, or excessively low blood pressure.
- have an overly active thyroid.
- have peptic ulcer disease.
- have an intestinal or urinary tract obstruction.
- have a history of seizure disorder.
- have had liver disease.
- take an NSAID.
- take muscle relaxants.

▷ **Possible Adverse Effects:**

If any of the following develop, call your doctor promptly for guidance.

Some Mild Problems Drug Can Cause
    Allergic reactions: skin rash.
    Increased sweating.
    Muscle aches.
    Nausea or vomiting, diarrhea, decreased appetite.
    Dizziness, confusion and insomnia.
Some Serious Problems Drug Can Cause
    Allergic reactions: anaphylactic reactions.
    Liver toxicity starts within 6 to 8 weeks after therapy is begun.
    Agitation, hallucinations.
    Purpura.
    Excessive urination.
    Respiratory compromise.
    Slow heart rate or abnormal rhythm.
    Low white blood cell count.

▷ **Possible Effects on Sex Life:**   Very rare effect: starting of lactation.

▷ **Possible Delayed Adverse Effects:**   Liver toxicity, rash, low white
    blood cell count.

▷ **Adverse Effects That May Mimic Natural Diseases or Disorders:**
    Liver toxicity may mimic acute hepatitis.

▷ *CAUTION*
    1. Tacrine should NOT be stopped abruptly, as acute deterioration
       of cognitive abilities may result.
    2. Changes in the color of stools (light or very black) should be
       promptly reported to your doctor.
    3. This drug does NOT alter the course of Alzheimer's disease. Over
       time its benefits may be lost.
    4. The dose MUST be decreased by 40 mg/day if the liver function
       levels (transaminases) rise to three to five times the upper normal
       value.
    5. Blood levels achieved by females are 50% higher than those in
       men. Dose-related side effects may occur sooner (with lower
       doses) in women than in men. Therapeutic doses may be lower for
       women than men.
    6. Safety and effectiveness of this drug for those under 18 years old
       are not established.
    7. No specific dose changes are presently indicated for those over 60.

Advisability of Use During Pregnancy or If Breast-Feeding:
Pregnancy Category: C. Consult your doctor. Presence in breast milk is
    unknown. Monitor the nursing infant closely and discontinue tak-
    ing this drug or nursing if adverse effects develop.

▷ **Overdose Symptoms:**   Tacrine may precipitate a cholinergic crisis:
    severe nausea and vomiting, slow heartbeat, low blood pressure, ex-
    treme muscle weakness, collapse, and convulsions.

▷ **Suggested Periodic Examinations While Taking This Drug:** (at doctor's discretion)

Assessment of mental status: checked periodically for the benefit of therapy and potential loss of this drug's effectiveness as the underlying disease progresses.

Liver function tests: should be checked weekly for the first 18 weeks of therapy, then every 3 weeks if the same dose is maintained. If the dose is increased, liver function tests should be checked weekly for 7 weeks.

Complete blood count: checked periodically or if symptoms of low blood count occur.

▷ **While Taking This Drug the Following Apply:**

Foods: This drug is best NOT taken with food.

Alcohol: Occasional small amounts of alcohol are acceptable. Frequent use of alcohol may worsen memory impairment and adversely effect liver enzymes.

Marijuana Smoking: Additive dizziness may occur.

Other Drugs:

Tacrine may *increase* the effects of
- bethanechol (Duvoid, others).
- theophylline (Theo-Dur, others) by doubling the drug level.
- succinylcholine (Anectine, others).

Tacrine may *decrease* the effects of
- anticholinergic medications.

The following drug may *increase* the effects of tacrine
- cimetidine (Tagamet).

Driving, Hazardous Activities: May cause confusion. Restrict your activities as necessary.

Exposure to Heat: Increased sweating may routinely occur with this drug. The combination of increased sweating and hot environments may lead to more rapid dehydration.

Discontinuation: This drug should NOT be stopped abruptly. Some dose-related adverse effects may abate if the dose is decreased. Slow withdrawal is indicated if tacrine is not tolerated and must be stopped.

▷ **Saving Money When Using This Medicine:**
- Ask your doctor if this medicine offers the best balance of cost and outcome for you.
- This drug should be used only with great caution by those with liver compromise.
- Ask your doctor about investigational agents for this condition.
- If a loved one has Alzheimer's, find out as much as possible about it. *The Essential Guide To Chronic Illness* is a great resource.

TAMOXIFEN (ta MOX i fen)

Prescription Needed: Yes   **Controlled Drug:** No   **Generic:** No

Brand Name: Nolvadex

Overview of BENEFITS versus RISKS

Possible Benefits	*Possible Risks*
EFFECTIVE ADJUNCTIVE TREATMENT FOR ADVANCED BREAST CANCER	Severe increase in tumor or bone pain (transient)
	Thrombophlebitis, pulmonary embolism
	Uterine cancer (risk may be increased)
	Abnormally high blood calcium levels
	Eye changes: corneal opacities, retinal injury

▷ **Illness This Medication Treats:**

Alternative to estrogens and androgens (male sex hormones) for treatment of advanced breast cancer in postmenopausal women, including cancer spread from a prior site.

Other (unlabeled) generally accepted use: to stimulate ovulation in premenopausal women with infertility.

▷ **Typical Dosage Range:** (Dosage or schedule must be determined by the doctor for each individual.)

10 to 20 mg twice daily, morning and evening. This treatment may continue for years.

▷ **Conditions Requiring Dosing Adjustments:**

Kidney function: The kidney plays a minor role in the elimination of this drug; however, this drug should be used with caution by patients with renal compromise.

▷ **How Best to Take This Medicine:** May be taken either on an empty stomach or with food. The tablet may be crushed for administration.

▷ **How Long This Medicine Is Usually Taken:** Use on a regular schedule for 4 to 10 weeks usually determines the effectiveness of this drug in controlling advanced breast cancer. In the presence of bone involvement, treatment for several months may be required to evaluate its effectiveness. Long-term use (months to years) requires physician supervision.

▷ **Tell Your Doctor Before Taking This Medicine If You:**
- ever had an allergic reaction to it before.
- have active phlebitis or a history of thrombophlebitis or pulmonary embolism.
- have a significant deficiency of white blood cells or blood platelets.
- have a history of abnormally high blood calcium levels.
- have a history of any type of blood cell or bone marrow disorder.
- have cataracts or other visual impairment.
- have impaired liver function.
- plan to have surgery in the near future.

▷ **Possible Side Effects:**   Hot flashes, fluid retention, weight gain.

▷ **Possible Adverse Effects:**
If any of the following develop, call your doctor promptly for guidance.

Some Mild Problems Drug Can Cause
  Allergic reaction: skin rash.
  Headache, dizziness, drowsiness, depression, confusion.
  Nausea, vomiting, itching in genital area, loss of hair.

Some Serious Problems Drug Can Cause
  Initial flare of severe pain in tumor or involved bone.
  Development of thrombophlebitis, risk of pulmonary embolism.
  Eye changes: corneal opacities, retinal injury.
  Development of abnormally high blood calcium levels.
  Transient decreases in white blood cells and blood platelets.
  Rare liver toxicity or delusions.

▷ **Possible Effects on Sex Life:**   Premenopausal: altered timing and pattern of menstruation.
Postmenopausal: vaginal bleeding.
May be effective in treating male infertility due to abnormally low sperm counts; male breast enlargement and tenderness; chronic female breast pain (mastodynia).

▷ *CAUTION*
  1. If this drug is used prior to your menopause, it may induce ovulation and predispose you to pregnancy. Because this drug should not be used during pregnancy, some method of contraception (other than oral contraceptives) is advised.
  2. Do not take any form of estrogen while taking this drug; estrogens can inhibit its effectiveness.

Advisability of Use During Pregnancy or If Breast-Feeding:
Pregnancy Category: D. Can have estrogenic effects. This drug should not be used during pregnancy. Presence in breast milk is unknown; avoid taking this drug or refrain from nursing.

▷ **Suggested Periodic Examinations While Taking This Drug:** (at doctor's discretion)
Complete blood cell counts, measurements of blood calcium levels.
Complete eye examinations if impaired vision occurs.

▷ **While Taking This Drug the Following Apply:**
Beverages: May be taken with milk.
Other Drugs:
The following drugs may ***decrease*** the effects of tamoxifen
- estrogens.
- oral contraceptives (birth control pills containing estrogens).
Tamoxifen ***taken concurrently*** with
- allopurinol (Zyloprim) may worsen allopurinol's liver toxicity risk.
- cyclosporine (Sandimmune) may lead to toxicity.
- mitomycin increases the risk of hemolytic uremic syndrome.
- pneumococcal and perhaps other vaccines can decrease the protective benefits of the vaccine.
- warfarin (Coumadin) increases the risk of bleeding. More frequent INR (prothrombin time) tests are needed.
Driving, Hazardous Activities: May cause dizziness or drowsiness. Restrict your activities as necessary.

▷ **Saving Money When Using This Medicine:**
- Many new drugs are available to treat cancer. Ask your doctor if this medicine offers the best balance of cost and outcome for you.
- Some liposomally encapsulated or lipid-associated medicines are under research. Ask your doctor about them.

TERAZOSIN   (ter AY zoh sin)

Prescription Needed: Yes   **Controlled Drug:** No   **Generic:** No

Brand Name: Hytrin

Overview of BENEFITS versus RISKS	
Possible Benefits	*Possible Risks*
EFFECTIVE TREATMENT OF MILD TO MODERATE HYPERTENSION when used alone or in combination with other antihypertensives	Rare first-dose drop in blood pressure with fainting
	Fluid retention
	Rapid heart rate
TREATMENT OF PROSTATIC HYPERPLASIA	

▷ **Illness This Medication Treats:**
(1) Step 1 antihypertensive in treatment of mild to moderate hypertension. Also used in combination with other drugs for moderate to severe hypertension. (2) Treatment of symptomatic benign prostatic hyperplasia (BPH).

▷ **Typical Dosage Range:** (Dosage or schedule must be determined by the doctor for each individual.)
Hypertension: Start with a test dose of 1 mg and observe the response for 2 hours. If tolerated, the dose can be slowly (as needed and tolerated) increased up to 5 mg/24 hr. Maximum daily dosage should not exceed 20 mg.
Prostatic hyperplasia: 1 mg taken at bedtime and then increased as needed for symptom relief. Many people need 10 mg.

▷ **Conditions Requiring Dosing Adjustments:**
Liver function: The dose should be decreased for patients with severe liver problems.
Kidney function: The dose should be decreased for patients with severe kidney failure.

▷ **How Best to Take This Medicine:** Take at bedtime to avoid orthostatic hypotension. This drug may be taken without regard to food. The tablet may be crushed.

▷ **How Long This Medicine Is Usually Taken:** Use on a regular schedule for 6 to 8 weeks is usually necessary to determine the effectiveness of this drug in controlling hypertension; 4 to 6 weeks of scheduled use is needed for benign prostatic hyperplasia (BPH). See your doctor regularly.

▷ **Tell Your Doctor Before Taking This Medicine If You:**
- ever had an allergic reaction to it.
- are experiencing or have a history of mental depression.
- have angina (active coronary artery disease) and are not taking a beta-blocker.
- have experienced orthostatic hypotension.
- have impaired circulation to the brain or a history of stroke.
- have a job that requires alertness or dexterity
- have coronary artery disease.
- have impaired liver or kidney function.
- plan to have surgery under general anesthesia soon.

▷ **Possible Side Effects:** Orthostatic hypotension, drowsiness, salt and water retention, dry mouth, nasal congestion, constipation.

▷ **Possible Adverse Effects:**
If any of the following develop, call your doctor promptly for guidance.

Some Mild Problems Drug Can Cause
   Allergic reaction: skin rash.
   Headache, dizziness, weakness, nervousness, sweating, numbness
     and tingling, blurred vision.
   Palpitation, rapid heart rate, shortness of breath.
   Nausea, vomiting, diarrhea, abdominal pain.
Some Serious Problems Drug Can Cause
   Rare mental depression.

▷ **Possible Effects on Sex Life:**   Impotence.

▷ *CAUTION*
   1. A first-dose precipitous drop in blood pressure, with or without
      fainting, can happen (usually within 30 to 90 minutes). Limit ini-
      tial doses to 1 mg taken at bedtime (for first 3 days); remain prone
      after taking trial doses.
   2. Call your doctor if you plan to use over-the-counter remedies for
      allergic rhinitis or head colds. Serious drug interactions are possi-
      ble.
   3. Safety and effectiveness of this drug for those under 12 years old
      have not been established.
   4. Those over 60 should begin treatment with no more than 1 mg/
      day for the first 3 days. Any dose increases must be very gradual
      and closely supervised. Orthostatic hypotension can cause falls
      and injury. Sit or lie down promptly if you feel light-headed or
      dizzy. Report dizziness or chest pain promptly.
   5. The dose MUST be decreased for patients with liver or kidney
      compromise.
   Advisability of Use During Pregnancy or If Breast-Feeding:
   Pregnancy Category: C. Use this drug only if clearly needed. Ask your
      doctor for guidance. Presence in breast milk is unknown. Watch the
      nursing infant closely and stop taking this drug or nursing if adverse
      effects start.

▷ **Overdose Symptoms:**   Orthostatic hypotension, headache, flushing,
      fast heart rate, extreme weakness, irregular heart rhythm, circula-
      tory collapse.

▷ **While Taking This Drug the Following Apply:**
   Foods: Avoid excessive salt intake.
   Beverages: May be taken with milk.
   Alcohol: Alcohol can exaggerate this drug's blood pressure–lowering
      actions, causing excessive reduction. Use with extreme caution.
   Tobacco Smoking: Nicotine can intensify this drug's ability to worsen
      coronary insufficiency. All forms of tobacco should be avoided.

Other Drugs:

The following drugs may **_increase_** the effects of terazosin

- beta-adrenergic-blockers (see Drug Classes); severity and duration of the first-dose response may be increased.
- verapamil (Verelan); can cause additive lowering of blood pressure. Care must be taken to avoid excessive lowering.

The following drugs may **_decrease_** the effects of terazosin

- estrogens.
- indomethacin (Indocin) or other NSAIDs.

Driving, Hazardous Activities: May cause dizziness or drowsiness. Restrict your activities as necessary.

Exposure to Cold: Cold environments may increase this drug's ability to cause coronary insufficiency (angina) and hypothermia. Use caution.

Heavy Exercise or Exertion: Excessive exertion can increase the likelihood of chest pain.

Discontinuation: Do not stop taking this drug abruptly in treatment of congestive heart failure. Ask your doctor for guidance.

▷ **Saving Money When Using This Medicine:**

- Many new drugs are available to treat high blood pressure. Ask your doctor if this medicine offers the best balance of cost and outcome for you. Ask how often your blood pressure should be checked.
- Ask your doctor if taking aspirin every other day makes sense for you.
- Talk with your doctor about stress management or exercise programs available in your community.
- Talk with your doctor or pharmacist BEFORE taking any other nonprescription or prescription medicines.

TERBUTALINE (ter BYU ta leen)

Prescription Needed: Yes   **Controlled Drug:** No   **Generic:** No

Brand Names: Brethaire, Brethine, Bricanyl

Overview of BENEFITS versus RISKS	
Possible Benefits	*Possible Risks*
VERY EFFECTIVE RELIEF OF BRONCHOSPASM	Increased blood pressure
	Fine hand tremor
	Irregular heart rhythm (with excessive use)

▷ **Illness This Medication Treats:**
  (1) Relieves acute bronchial asthma and reduces frequency and severity of chronic, recurrent asthmatic attacks; (2) also relief of reversible bronchospasm associated with chronic bronchitis and emphysema.
  Other (unlabeled) generally accepted uses: (1) help in stopping premature labor; (2) easing fetal distress.

▷ **Typical Dosage Range:** (Dosage or schedule must be determined by
  the doctor for each individual.)
  Aerosol: 0.4 mg taken in two separate inhalations 1 minute apart; repeat every 4 to 6 hours as needed. Tablets: 2.5 to 5 mg taken three
  times daily, 6 hours apart. The total daily dosage should not exceed
  15 mg.

▷ **Conditions Requiring Dosing Adjustments:**
  Liver function: This drug is extensively changed in the liver. Guidelines
  for dosing changes for patients with compromised livers are not
  available.
  Kidney function: For patients with moderate to severe kidney failure,
  50% of the usual dose can be taken at the usual interval. This drug
  should not be used by patients with severe kidney failure.

▷ **How Best to Take This Medicine:**   May be taken on empty stomach
  or with food or milk. Tablets may be crushed for administration.
  For aerosol, follow the written instructions carefully. Do not overuse.

▷ **How Long This Medicine Is Usually Taken:**   According to individual requirements. Do not use this drug beyond the time necessary to
  terminate episodes of asthma.

▷ **Tell Your Doctor Before Taking This Medicine If You:**
  • ever had an allergic reaction to it.
  • currently have an irregular heart rhythm.
  • are taking, or have taken within the past 2 weeks, any MAO type A
    inhibitor (see Drug Classes).
  • are overly sensitive to drugs that stimulate the sympathetic nervous
    system.
  • are currently using epinephrine (Adrenalin, Primatene Mist, etc.) to
    relieve asthmatic breathing.
  • have a seizure disorder.
  • have any type of heart or circulatory disorder, especially high blood
    pressure or coronary heart disease.
  • have diabetes or an overactive thyroid gland.
  • are taking any form of digitalis or stimulant.

▷ **Possible Side Effects:**   Aerosol: dryness or irritation of mouth or
  throat, altered taste. Tablet: nervousness, tremor, palpitation.

▷ **Possible Adverse Effects:**

If any of the following develop, call your doctor promptly for guidance.

Some Mild Problems Drug Can Cause

Headache, dizziness, drowsiness, insomnia.

Rapid, pounding heartbeat; increased sweating; muscle cramps in arms and legs.

Increased blood sugar.

Nausea, heartburn, vomiting.

Some Serious Problems Drug Can Cause

Rapid or irregular heart rhythm, intensification of angina, increased blood pressure.

Very rare liver toxicity.

▷ *CAUTION*

1. Concurrent use of terbutaline by aerosol inhalation with beclomethasone aerosol (Beclovent, Vanceril) may increase the risk of toxicity due to fluorocarbon propellants. Use this aerosol 20 to 30 minutes *before* beclomethasone aerosol to reduce the risk of toxicity and enhance the penetration of beclomethasone.

2. *Avoid excessive use of aerosol inhalation.* Excessive or prolonged use by inhalation can reduce this drug's effectiveness and cause serious heart rhythm disturbances, including cardiac arrest.

3. Do not use this drug concurrently with epinephrine. These two drugs may be used alternately, with an interval of 4 hours between doses.

4. If you do not respond to your usually effective dose, do not increase the size or frequency of the dose without your doctor's approval.

5. Safety and effectiveness of this drug for those under 12 years old have not been established.

6. Those over 60 should avoid excessive and continual use of this drug. If acute asthma is not relieved promptly, try other drugs. Observe for nervousness, palpitations, irregular heart rhythm, and muscle tremors. Use this drug with extreme caution if you have hardening of the arteries, heart disease, or high blood pressure.

7. The dose MUST be decreased for patients with kidney or liver compromise.

Advisability of Use During Pregnancy or If Breast-Feeding:

Pregnancy Category: B. Use this drug only if clearly needed. Ask your doctor for guidance. Present in breast milk. Monitor the nursing infant closely and discontinue taking this drug or nursing if adverse effects develop.

▷ **Overdose Symptoms:** Nervousness, palpitation, rapid heart rate, sweating, headache, tremor, vomiting, chest pain.

▷ **While Taking This Drug the Following Apply:**

Beverages: Avoid excessive use of caffeine-containing beverages: coffee, tea, cola, chocolate.

Other Drugs:

Terbutaline *taken concurrently* with

- MAO type A inhibitors may cause an excessive increase in blood pressure and undesirable heart stimulation.
- theophylline (Theo-Dur, others) may blunt theophylline's benefits.

The following drugs may *decrease* the effects of terbutaline

- beta-blockers (see Drug Classes); may impair terbutaline's effectiveness.

Driving, Hazardous Activities: Use caution if excessive nervousness or dizziness occurs.

Heavy Exercise or Exertion: Use caution. Excessive exercise can induce asthma in sensitive individuals.

▷ **Saving Money When Using This Medicine:**

- Many drugs are available to treat asthma. Ask your doctor if this medicine offers the best balance of cost and outcome for you.
- Talk with your doctor about using nedocromil or cromolyn to help decrease the frequency of acute asthma. Also ask about usage of nebulized lidocaine.

TERFENADINE (ter FEN a deen)

Prescription Needed: Yes   **Controlled Drug:** No   **Generic:** No

Brand Names: Seldane, Seldane-D

Overview of BENEFITS versus RISKS	
Possible Benefits	*Possible Risks*
EFFECTIVE RELIEF OF ALLERGIC RHINITIS AND ALLERGIC SKIN DISORDERS	RARE HEART RHYTHM DISTURBANCES Infrequent headache Minor digestive disturbances Slight atropinelike effects

▷ **Illness This Medication Treats:**

Symptomatic relief for allergic and related disorders: seasonal and perennial allergic rhinitis (hay fever), allergic conjunctivitis, and vasomotor rhinitis.

▷ **Typical Dosage Range:** (Dosage or schedule must be determined by the doctor for each individual.)

For those 12 to 60 years old: 60 mg every 12 hours as needed. The total daily dosage should not exceed 120 mg.

▷ **Conditions Requiring Dosing Adjustments:**

Liver function: This drug is extensively metabolized in the liver; this drug should NOT BE TAKEN by patients with liver compromise.

Kidney function: This drug's metabolites are only partially eliminated in the urine, and changes in dosing do not appear to be needed for patients with renal compromise.

▷ **How Best to Take This Medicine:**　May be taken with food or milk to prevent stomach irritation. The tablet may be crushed.

▷ **How Long This Medicine Is Usually Taken:**　Use of this drug on a regular schedule for 2 to 3 days usually shows its benefits in relieving the symptoms of allergic rhinitis and dermatosis. It may be necessary to take this drug throughout the pollen season. However, antihistamines should not be taken continually (without interruption) for long-term use. Limit their use to periods that require symptomatic relief. See your doctor regularly.

▷ **Tell Your Doctor Before Taking This Medicine If You:**
- ever had an allergic reaction to it.
- are currently undergoing allergy skin tests.
- have severely impaired liver function or a history of liver disease.
- are taking any form of erythromycin, itraconazole, ketoconazole, or troleandomycin.
- have had any allergic reactions or unfavorable responses to antihistamines.
- have a history of heart rhythm disorders.

▷ **Possible Side Effects:**　Dry nose, mouth, or throat.

▷ **Possible Adverse Effects:**

If any of the following develop, call your doctor promptly for guidance.

Some Mild Problems Drug Can Cause

Allergic reactions: skin rash, itching.

Headache, nervousness, fatigue.

Increased appetite, nausea, vomiting.

Some Serious Problems Drug Can Cause

Significant heart rhythm disorders (resulting from excessive dosage or drug interactions).

Rare liver toxicity or lowered platelet counts.

▷ **Possible Effects on Sex Life:**　Altered timing and pattern of menstruation.

Female breast enlargement with milk production.

▷ **CAUTION**

1. Do not exceed recommended doses; high blood levels may cause serious heart rhythm disturbances.
2. Do not take this drug concurrently with any form of erythromycin, ketoconazole (Nizoral), or troleandomycin (Tao).
3. Report promptly any faintness, dizziness, heart palpitation, or chest pain.
4. Discontinue taking this drug 4 days before diagnostic skin testing procedures to prevent false-negative test results.
5. Do not use this drug if you have active bronchial asthma, bronchitis, or pneumonia; it may thicken bronchial mucus and make it more difficult to remove (by absorption or coughing).
6. Safety and effectiveness of this drug for those under 12 years old have not been established.
7. Those over 60 may be more susceptible to headache and fatigue. Use smaller doses at longer intervals if necessary.
8. This drug should NOT be used by patients with compromised livers.

Advisability of Use During Pregnancy or If Breast-Feeding:

Pregnancy Category: C. Use this drug only if clearly needed. Ask your doctor for guidance. Presence in breast milk is unknown; avoid taking this drug or refrain from nursing.

▷ **Overdose Symptoms:** Possible development of serious heart rhythm disturbances.

▷ **Suggested Periodic Examinations While Taking This Drug:** (at doctor's discretion)

Electrocardiograms for those with heart disorders.

▷ **While Taking This Drug the Following Apply:**

Beverages: DO NOT take with grapefruit juice. This can increase this drug's blood levels and cause toxicity. This drug may be taken with milk.

Other Drugs:

Terfenadine *taken concurrently* with

- amiodarone (Cordarone) can lead to heart toxicity.
- carbamzepine (Tegretol) can result in carbamazepine toxicity.
- ciprofloxacin (Cipro) can increase the risk of cardiovascular effects.
- disopyramide (Norpace) can increase the risk of adverse heart effects.
- fluoxetine (Prozac) or fluvoxamine (Luvox) may result in terfenadine toxicity.
- ketoconazole (Nizoral), itraconazole (Sporanox), or miconazole (Monistat) may cause increased blood levels of terfenadine, resulting in serious heart rhythm disorders.
- macrolide antibiotics (erythromycin, azithromycin, troleandomy-

cin, others) may cause increased blood levels of terfenadine, resulting in serious heart rhythm disorders.

- paroxetine (Paxil) can lead to terfenadine toxicity.
- sotalol (Betapace) can cause serious heart rhythm changes.
- tricyclic antidepressants can increase the risk of heart problems.

▷ **Saving Money When Using This Medicine:**
- There are several nonsedating antihistamines. Ask your doctor if this medicine offers the best balance of cost and outcome for you.

Author's note: This medicine has life-threatening drug interactions and the FDA is removing the product.

TETRACYCLINE   (te trah SI kleen)

Prescription Needed: Yes   **Controlled Drug:** No   **Generic:** Yes

Brand Names: Achromycin, Achromycin V, Actisite, Cyclopar, Mysteclin-F [CD], Nor-Tet, Panmycin, Retet, Robitet, Sumycin, Tetra-C, Tetracyn, Tetralan, Tetram, Tropicycline

Overview of BENEFITS versus RISKS	
Possible Benefits	*Possible Risks*
EFFECTIVE TREATMENT OF INFECTIONS due to susceptible bacteria and protozoa	ALLERGIC REACTIONS, mild to severe: ANAPHYLAXIS, DRUG-INDUCED HEPATITIS (rare)
	Drug-induced colitis
	Superinfections (bacterial or fungal)
	Rare blood cell disorders: hemolytic anemia, abnormally low white cell and platelet counts

▷ **Illness This Medication Treats:**
(1) A broad range of infections caused by susceptible bacteria and protozoa (short-term use); (2) severe, resistant pustular acne (long-term use); and (3) in a sustained-release form (Actisite) gum disease (periodontitis) in adults.

Other (unlabeled) generally accepted uses: combination antibiotic treatment of duodenal ulcers caused by *Helicobacter pylori*; early Lyme disease.

As Combination Drug Product [CD]: This drug is available in combination with amphotericin B, an antifungal antibiotic that reduces the risk of yeast overgrowth (superinfection) of the gastrointestinal tract.

▷ **Typical Dosage Range:** (Dosage or schedule must be determined by the doctor for each individual.)

250 to 500 mg every 6 hours, or 500 to 1000 mg every 12 hours. The total daily dosage should not exceed 4000 mg (4 g).

▷ **Conditions Requiring Dosing Adjustments:**

Liver function: This drug is a cause of liver toxicity. A benefit-to-risk decision—whether patients with compromised livers should use this drug—should be made.

Kidney function: Patients with mild kidney failure can take the usual dose every 8 to 12 hours. Those with moderate to severe kidney failure can take the usual dose every 12 to 24 hours. This drug SHOULD NOT BE USED by patients with severe kidney failure (creatinine clearance is less than 10 ml/min), and only with caution by patients with kidney compromise.

▷ **How Best to Take This Medicine:**   Best taken on an empty stomach, 1 hour before or 2 hours after eating. However, to reduce stomach irritation it may be taken with crackers that contain insignificant amounts of iron, calcium, magnesium, or zinc. Avoid all dairy products for 2 hours before and after taking this drug. Take it at the same time each day, with a full glass of water. Take the full course prescribed. The tablet may be crushed and the capsule opened.

▷ **How Long This Medicine Is Usually Taken:**   This drug should be taken for the time required to control acute infection and be free of fever and symptoms for 48 hours. This varies with the nature of the infection. Long-term use (months to years, as for treatment of acne) requires supervision and periodic evaluation. See your doctor regularly.

▷ **Tell Your Doctor Before Taking This Medicine If You:**
- are allergic to any tetracycline drug.
- are pregnant or breast-feeding.
- are given a prescription for a child under 8 years of age.
- have a history of liver or kidney disease.
- have systemic lupus erythematosus.
- are taking any penicillin drug.
- are taking any anticoagulant drugs.
- plan to have surgery under general anesthesia soon.

▷ **Possible Side Effects:**   Superinfections, often due to yeast organisms. These can occur in the mouth, intestinal tract, rectum, and/or vagina, resulting in rectal and vaginal itching.

▷ **Possible Adverse Effects:**

If any of the following develop, call your doctor promptly for guidance.

Some Mild Problems Drug Can Cause
>   Allergic reactions: skin rash, itching of hands and feet, swelling of face or extremities.
>   Loss of appetite, nausea, vomiting, diarrhea.
>   Irritation of mouth or tongue, black tongue, sore throat, abdominal cramping or pain.

Some Serious Problems Drug Can Cause
>   Allergic reactions: anaphylactic reaction, asthma, fever, swollen joints and lymph glands.
>   Drug-induced hepatitis with jaundice.
>   Permanent discoloration and/or malformation of teeth in those under 8 years old, including unborn children and infants.
>   Impaired vision, increased intracranial pressure.
>   Drug-induced colitis.
>   Rare blood cell disorders: hemolytic anemia; abnormally low white blood cell count, causing fever, sore throat, and infections; abnormally low blood platelet count, causing abnormal bleeding or bruising.
>   Rare pancreatitis or kidney problems.

▷ **Possible Effects on Sex Life:**   Decreased effectiveness of oral contraceptives taken concurrently (several reports of pregnancy).

▷ **Adverse Effects That May Mimic Natural Diseases or Disorders:**
  Drug-induced hepatitis may suggest viral hepatitis.

▷ *CAUTION*
  1. Antacids, dairy products, and preparations containing aluminum, bismuth, calcium, iron, magnesium, or zinc can prevent adequate absorption of this drug and reduce its effectiveness significantly.
  2. Troublesome and persistent diarrhea can develop in sensitive individuals. If diarrhea persists for more than 24 hours, discontinue this drug and call your doctor.
  3. If surgery under general anesthesia is required while taking this drug, the choice of anesthetic agent must be considered carefully to prevent serious kidney damage.
  4. If possible, tetracyclines should not be given to children under 8 years old because of the risk of permanent discoloration and deformity of the teeth. Rarely, young infants may develop increased intracranial pressure within the first 4 days of receiving this drug. This drug may inhibit normal bone growth and development.
  5. Dosage must be carefully individualized and based on kidney function determinations. Natural skin changes in those over 60 may predispose them to severe and prolonged itching reactions in the genital and anal regions.

Advisability of Use During Pregnancy or If Breast-Feeding:
Pregnancy Category: D. Avoid using this drug completely during entire pregnancy. Present in breast milk; avoid taking this drug or refrain from nursing.

▷ **Overdose Symptoms:** Stomach burning, nausea, vomiting, diarrhea.

▷ **Suggested Periodic Examinations While Taking This Drug:** (at doctor's discretion)
Complete blood cell counts, liver and kidney function tests.
During extended use, sputum and stool examinations may detect early yeast superinfection.

▷ **While Taking This Drug the Following Apply:**
Foods: Avoid cheeses, yogurt, ice cream, iron-fortified cereals and supplements, and meats for 2 hours before and after taking this drug. Calcium and iron can combine with this drug and reduce its absorption significantly.
Beverages: Avoid all forms of milk for 2 hours before and after taking this drug.
Alcohol: No interactions are expected. However, it is best that those with active liver disease avoid using alcohol.
Other Drugs:
Tetracyclines may *increase* the effects of
- oral anticoagulants, making their dosage reduction necessary.
- digoxin (Lanoxin), causing digitalis toxicity.
- lithium (Eskalith, Lithane, etc.), increasing the risk of lithium toxicity.

Tetracyclines may *decrease* the effects of
- oral contraceptives (birth control pills), impairing their effectiveness in preventing pregnancy.
- penicillins, impairing their effectiveness in treating infections.

Tetracyclines *taken concurrently* with
- furosemide (Lasix) may increase the blood urea nitrogen (BUN).
- isotretinoin (Accutane) may increase the risk of elevated pressure in the head.
- methoxyflurane anesthesia may impair kidney function.
- theophylline (Theo-Dur) may change blood levels. Increased theophylline blood level testing is needed.
- warfarin (Coumadin) poses an increased risk of bleeding. INR (promthrombin time) testing should be used to guide dosing.

The following drugs may *decrease* the effects of tetracyclines
- antacids (aluminum and magnesium preparations, sodium bicarbonate, etc.); reduces its drug absorption.
- bismuth subsalicylate (Pepto-Bismol, others).
- calcium supplements.

- cholestyramine (Questran) or other resins.
- colestipol (Colestid).
- iron and mineral preparations; reduces drug absorption.
- sucralfate (Carafate).

Driving, Hazardous Activities: May cause nausea or diarrhea. Restrict your activities as necessary.

Exposure to Sun: Use caution until your sensitivity has been determined. Some tetracyclines can cause photosensitivity.

▷ **Saving Money When Using This Medicine:**
- Ask your doctor if this medicine offers the best balance of cost and outcome for you. Ask if the strength of this medicine matches the severity of your infection.
- A generic form can be substituted for the brand name.

THEOPHYLLINE (thee OFF i lin)

Prescription Needed: Yes   **Controlled Drug:** No   **Generic:** Yes

Brand Names: Accurbron, Bronkaid Tablets [CD], Bronkodyl, Bronkolixir [CD], Bronkotabs [CD], Constant-T, Elixicon, Elixophyllin, Lodrane, Lodrane CR, Marax [CD], Marax DF [CD], Mudrane GG Elixir [CD], Quadrinal [CD], Quibron [CD], Quibron-300 [CD], Quibron Plus [CD], Quibron-T Dividose, Quibron-T/SR, Respbid, Slo-bid, Slo-bid Gyrocaps, Slo-Phyllin, Slo-Phyllin GG [CD], Slo-Phyllin Gyrocaps, Sustaire, Tedral [CD], Tedral SA [CD], Theobid Duracaps, Theochron, Theo-Dur, Theolair, Theophyl-SR, Theo-24, Theovent, Theo-X

Overview of BENEFITS versus RISKS	
Possible Benefits	*Possible Risks*
EFFECTIVE PREVENTION AND RELIEF OF ACUTE BRONCHIAL ASTHMA	NARROW TREATMENT RANGE
MODERATELY EFFECTIVE CONTROL OF CHRONIC, RECURRENT BRONCHIAL ASTHMA	FREQUENT STOMACH DISTRESS
	Gastrointestinal bleeding
Moderately effective symptomatic relief in chronic bronchitis and emphysema	Central nervous system toxicity, seizures
	Heart rhythm disturbances

▷ **Illness This Medication Treats:**
(1) Relief of shortness of breath and wheezing characteristic of acute bronchial asthma, and prevention of the recurrent asthmatic epi-

sodes; (2) also relief of asthmaticlike symptoms associated with some types of chronic bronchitis and emphysema.

As Combination Drug Product [CD]: This drug is available in combination with several other drugs that are beneficial in managing bronchial asthma and related conditions. Ephedrine enhances the bronchodilator effects; guaifenesin provides an expectorant effect to thin bronchial mucus secretions; mild sedatives such as phenobarbital allay the anxiety often accompanying acute attacks of asthma.

▷ **Typical Dosage Range:** (Dosage or schedule must be determined by the doctor for each individual.)

Infants and Children: For acute attack of asthma (not currently taking theophylline): Loading dose of 5 to 6 mg per kilogram of body weight.

For acute attack while currently taking theophylline: A single dose of 2.5 mg per kilogram of body weight, if there are no indications of theophylline toxicity. Monitor blood levels of theophylline.

For maintenance during acute attack, dosage based on age:

Up to 6 months—0.07 per week of age + 1.7 = milligram per kilogram of body weight, given every 8 hours.

6 months to 1 year—0.05 per week of age + 1.25 = milligram per kilogram of body weight, given every 6 hours.

1 to 9 years—5 milligram per kilogram of body weight, given every 6 hours.

9 to 12 years—4 mg per kilogram of body weight, given every 6 hours.

12 to 16 years—3 mg per kilogram of body weight, given every 6 hours.

For chronic treatment to prevent recurrence of asthma: Dosage based on age: Initially 16 mg per kilogram of body weight, in three or four divided doses at 6- to 8-hour intervals; up to a maximum of 400 mg daily. Increase dose as needed and tolerated by increments of 25% every 2 to 3 days. Limit total daily dosage as follows:

Up to 1 year of age—0.3 for each week of age + 8.0 = milligram per kilogram of body weight, per day.

1 to 9 years—22 mg per kilogram of body weight per day.

9 to 12 years—20 mg per kilogram of body weight per day.

12 to 16 years—18 mg per kilogram of body weight per day.

16 years and over—13 mg per kilogram of body weight per day or 900 mg/day, whichever is less.

Note: It is advisable to measure drug blood levels periodically during chronic therapy.

16 to 60 Years of Age: For acute attack of asthma (not currently taking theophylline): Loading dose of 5 to 6 mg per kilogram of body weight.

For acute attack while currently taking theophylline: A single dose of 2.5 mg per kilogram of body weight, if there are no indications of theophylline toxicity. Monitor blood levels of theophylline.

For maintenance during acute attack: For nonsmokers: 3 mg per kilogram of body weight, every 8 hours. For smokers: 4 mg per kilogram of body weight every 6 hours.

For chronic treatment to prevent recurrence of asthma: Initially 6 to 8 mg per kilogram of body weight, in three or four divided doses at 6- to 8-hour intervals, up to a maximum of 400 mg daily. Increase dose as needed and tolerated by increments of 25% every 2 to 3 days. The total daily dosage should not exceed 13 mg per kilogram of body weight or 900 mg, whichever is less.

Prolonged formulations may allow twice-daily dosing with good results.

Over 60 Years of Age: For acute attack: Same as for 16 to 60 years of age.

For maintenance during acute attack: 2 mg per kilogram of body weight, every 8 hours.

▷ **Conditions Requiring Dosing Adjustments:**

Liver function: The dose **must** be lowered, and blood levels obtained frequently.

Kidney function: Drug levels should be followed closely in patients with severe kidney failure.

▷ **How Best to Take This Medicine:**   May be taken with or following food to reduce stomach irritation. The regular capsules may be opened and the regular tablets crushed for administration. The prolonged-action dosage forms should be swallowed whole and not altered. Shake the oral suspension well before measuring each dose. Do not refrigerate any liquid dosage forms.

▷ **How Long This Medicine Is Usually Taken:**   Continual use on a regular schedule for 48 to 72 hours usually determines the effectiveness of this drug in controlling bronchial asthma and chronic lung disease. Long-term use (months to years) requires physician supervision.

▷ **Tell Your Doctor Before Taking This Medicine If You:**

- ever had an allergic reaction to it or to aminophylline, dyphylline, or oxtriphylline.
- have active peptic ulcer disease or a history of peptic ulcer disease.
- have an uncontrolled seizure disorder.
- have had an unfavorable reaction to any xanthine drug (see Drug Classes).
- have impaired liver or kidney function.
- have hypertension, heart disease, or any type of heart rhythm disorder.

▷ **Possible Side Effects:**   Nervousness, insomnia, rapid heart rate, increased urine volume.

▷ **Possible Adverse Effects:**

If any of the following develop, call your doctor promptly for guidance.

Some Mild Problems Drug Can Cause

Allergic reactions: skin rash, hives.

Headache, dizziness, irritability, tremor, weakness.

Nausea, vomiting, diarrhea, excessive thirst.

Flushing of face.

Some Serious Problems Drug Can Cause

Idiosyncratic reactions: marked anxiety, confusion, behavioral disturbances.

Rare drug-induced porphyria or excessive urination.

Central nervous system toxicity: muscle twitching, seizures.

Heart rhythm abnormalities, rapid breathing, low blood pressure.

Gastrointestinal bleeding.

▷ *CAUTION*

1. Do not take this drug concurrently with other antiasthmatic drugs unless you are directed to do so by your doctor. Serious overdosage could result.

2. Influenza vaccine may delay elimination of this drug and cause its accumulation to toxic levels.

3. Do not exceed recommended doses. Observe for indications of toxicity: irritability, agitation, tremors, lethargy, fever, vomiting, rapid heart rate and breathing, or seizures. Monitor blood levels during long-term use.

4. Those over 60 should start treatment with small doses until their tolerance has been determined. They may be more susceptible to stomach irritation, nausea, vomiting, or diarrhea. Concurrent use with coffee (caffeine) or nasal decongestants may cause excessive stimulation and a hyperactivity syndrome.

5. The dose must be decreased, and blood levels obtained, for patients with compromised livers or kidneys.

Advisability of Use During Pregnancy or If Breast-Feeding:

Pregnancy Category: C. Avoid using this drug during the first 3 months. Use it otherwise only if clearly needed. Ask your doctor for guidance. Present in breast milk; avoid taking this drug or refrain from nursing.

▷ **Overdose Symptoms:**   Nausea, vomiting, restlessness, irritability, confusion, delirium, seizures, high fever, weak pulse, coma.

▷ **Suggested Periodic Examinations While Taking This Drug:** (at doctor's discretion)

Measurement of blood theophylline levels, especially with high dosage or long-term use.

Sample blood: 2 hours after regular (standard) dosage forms; 5 hours after sustained-release dosage forms.
Recommended therapeutic range: 10—20 mcg/ml.

▷ **While Taking This Drug the Following Apply:**

Beverages: Avoid excessive use of caffeine-containing beverages: coffee, tea, cola, chocolate; this combination could cause nervousness and insomnia.

Alcohol: May have additive effect on stomach irritation.

Tobacco Smoking: May hasten elimination and reduce this drug's effectiveness. Higher doses may be necessary to maintain a therapeutic blood level.

Other Drugs:

Theophylline may ***decrease*** the effects of

- lithium (Lithane, Lithobid, etc.), reducing its effectiveness.

Theophylline ***taken concurrently*** with

- halothane (anesthesia) may cause heart rhythm abnormalities.
- phenytoin (Dilantin) may decrease the effects of both drugs. Monitor blood levels and adjust dosages as appropriate.

The following drugs may ***increase*** the effects of theophylline

- allopurinol (Lopurin, Zyloprim).
- amiodarone (Cordarone).
- cimetidine (Tagamet).
- ciprofloxacin (Cipro).
- clarithromycin (Biaxin).
- disulfiram (Antabuse).
- doxycycline or other tetracyclines.
- enoxacin (Penetrex).
- ephedrine.
- erythromycin (E-Mycin, Erythrocin, etc.).
- famotidine (Pepcid).
- fluvoxamine (Luvox).
- furosemide (Lasix).
- interferon alfa.
- methotrexate (Mexate).
- mexiletine (Mexitil).
- nicotine (Nicorette, others).
- norfloxacin (Noroxin).
- oral contraceptives.
- ranitidine (Zantac).
- tacrine (Cognex).
- ticlopidine (Ticlid).
- troleandomycin (Tao).
- verapamil (Calan).
- viloxazine.

The following drugs may *decrease* the effects of theophylline

- barbiturates (phenobarbital, etc.).
- beta-blockers (see Drug Classes).
- carbamazepine (Tegretol).
- isoproterenol.
- primidone (Mysoline).
- rifampin.(Rifadin, Rimactane, etc.).
- sulfinpyrazone (Anturane).

Driving, Hazardous Activities: May cause dizziness. Restrict your activities as necessary.

Occurrence of Unrelated Illness: Acute viral respiratory infections can significantly delay elimination of this drug. Observe closely for indications of toxicity and the need to reduce dosage or lengthen the dosage interval.

Discontinuation: Avoid prolonged and unnecessary use of this drug. When you have achieved an asthma-free state, ask your doctor if usage of this drug can be stopped.

▷ **Saving Money When Using This Medicine:**

- Many drugs are available to treat or prevent asthma. Ask your doctor if this medicine offers the best balance of cost and outcome for you.
- Talk with your doctor about using nedocromil or cromolyn to help prevent asthmatic attacks. Also ask about using nebulized lidocaine.
- A generic form can be substituted for the brand name.
- Drug levels are expensive. Make sure levels are obtained at prudent, not excessive, intervals.

THIAZIDE DIURETICS

Bendroflumethiazide (ben droh flu meh THI a zide)
Chlorothiazide (klor oh THI a zide)
Chlorthalidone (klor THAL i dohn)
Hydrochlorothiazide (hi droh klor oh THI a zide)
Methyclothiazide (METHI klo thi a zide)
Metolazone (me TOHL a zohn)
Trichlormethiazide (try klor me THI azide)

Prescription Needed: Yes   **Controlled Drug:** No   **Generic:** Yes

Brand Names:
Bendroflumethiazide: Naturetin
Chlorothiazide: Aldoclor [CD], Diachlor, Diupres [CD], Diurigen, Diuril

Chlorthalidone: Combipres [CD], Demi-Regroton [CD], Hygroton, Hylidone, Thalitone, Tenoretic

Hydrochlorothiazide: Aldactazide [CD], Aldoril—15/25 [CD], Aldoril D30/D50 [CD], Apresazide [CD], Apresoline-Esidrix [CD], Capozide [CD], Dyazide [CD], Esidrix, HydroDIURIL, Hydropres [CD], Hydro-Z-50, Inderide [CD], Inderide LA [CD], Lopressor HCT [CD], Maxzide [CD], Maxzide-25 [CD], Moduretic [CD], Normozide [CD], Oretic, Oreticyl [CD], Prinzide [CD], Ser-Ap-Es [CD], Serpasil-Esidrix [CD], Thiuretic, Timolide [CD], Trandate HCT [CD], Unipres [CD], Vaseretic [CD], Zestoretic [CD], Zide

Methyclothiazide: Aquatensen, Enduron

Metolazone: Diulo, Mykrox, Zaroxolyn

Trichlormethiazide: Diurese, Metahyrdin, Naqua

Overview of BENEFITS versus RISKS

Possible Benefits	*Possible Risks*
EFFECTIVE, WELL-TOLERATED DIURETIC	Loss of body potassium and magnesium
	Increased blood sugar
POSSIBLY EFFECTIVE FOR MILD HYPERTENSION	Increased blood uric acid
	Increased blood calcium
ENHANCES EFFECTIVENESS OF OTHER ANTIHYPERTENSIVES	Blood cell disorders (rare)
Beneficial in treatment of diabetes insipidus	

▷ **Illness This Medication Treats:**

(1) Increases urine volume (diuresis) to correct fluid retention (edema) in congestive heart failure and certain types of liver and kidney disease; and (2) starting therapy for high blood pressure.

Other (unlabeled) generally accepted uses: (1) prevention of kidney stones that contain calcium; (2) may help in decreasing the frequency of hip fractures in the elderly.

As Combination Drug Product [CD]: If this drug fails to reduce the blood pressure adequately, a second antihypertensive is added to be taken concurrently, or a combined product is used.

▷ **Typical Dosage Range:** (Dosage or schedule must be determined by the doctor for each individual.)

Bendroflumethiazide as antihypertensive: 2.5 to 5 mg daily. As a diuretic: 5 mg in the morning to start; up to 15 mg once daily.

Chlorothiazide as antihypertensive: 500 to 1000 mg daily to start and 500 to 2000 mg daily as a maintenance dose. As a diuretic: 500 to 2000 mg daily, with the smallest effective dose used as an ongoing dose. Daily maximum is 2000 mg.

Chlorthalidone as antihypertensive: 25 to 50 mg daily, then ongoing dosing with the smallest effective dose. Daily maximum is 200 mg; however, this may change with recently published data.

Hydrochlorothiazide as antihypertensive: Initially 50 to 100 mg daily; 50 to 200 mg daily for maintenance. As diuretic: Initially 50 to 200 mg daily; the smallest effective dose should be determined. The total daily dose should not exceed 200 mg.

Methyclothiazide as antihypertensive or diuretic: 2.5 to 5 mg daily. Maximum daily diuretic dose is 10 mg. Pediatric dose: 0.05 to 0.2 mg per kilogram of body weight daily.

Trichlormethiazide as antihypertensive or diuretic: May start with 1 to 4 mg twice daily. Usual ongoing dose is 1 to 4 mg once daily.

▷ **Conditions Requiring Dosing Adjustments:**

Liver function: Electrolyte balance is critical in hepatic failure, and these drugs may precipitate encephalopathy. Hydrochlorothiazide and chlorothiazide are also rare causes of cholestatic jaundice and should be used with caution by patients with liver compromise.

Kidney function: These drugs should be used with caution by patients with mild kidney failure; they are not effective in patients with moderate failure. These drugs are contraindicated for patients with severe kidney failure and are a rare cause of kidney damage.

▷ **How Best to Take This Medicine:**   The tablet may be crushed and taken with or following meals to reduce stomach irritation. These drugs are best taken in the morning to avoid nighttime urination.

▷ **How Long This Medicine Is Usually Taken:**   Use on a regular schedule for 2 to 3 weeks determines the effectiveness of these drugs in lowering high blood pressure. Long-term use (months to years) requires your doctor's periodic evaluation.

▷ **Tell Your Doctor Before Taking This Medicine If You:**
  • ever had an allergic reaction to it.
  • know your kidneys are not making urine.
  • are allergic to any form of sulfa drug.
  • are pregnant or planning pregnancy.
  • have a history of kidney or liver disease.
  • have a history of pancreatitis.
  • have diabetes, gout, or lupus erythematosus.
  • take any form of cortisone, digitalis, oral antidiabetic, or insulin.
  • plan to have surgery under general anesthesia soon.

▷ **Possible Side Effects:**   Light-headedness on arising from sitting or lying position.
Increase in blood sugar level, affecting control of diabetes.
Increase in blood uric acid level, affecting control of gout.

Decrease in blood potassium level, causing muscle weakness and cramping.

Decreased potassium coupled with loss of magnesium; if this is not corrected, it may lead to an increased risk of serious heart problems.

▷ **Possible Adverse Effects:**
If any of the following develop, call your doctor promptly for guidance.

Some Mild Problems These Drugs Can Cause
Allergic reactions: skin rashes, drug fever.
Headache, dizziness, blurred or yellow vision.
Reduced appetite, nausea, vomiting, diarrhea.

Some Serious Problems These Drugs Can Cause
Allergic reactions: hepatitis with jaundice, anaphylactic reaction, severe skin reactions.
Inflammation of the pancreas—severe abdominal pain.
Bone marrow depression—weakness, fever, sore throat, abnormal bleeding or bruising.
Data from studies of hydrochlorothiazide and chlorthalidone suggest that the loss of potassium and magnesium (if not corrected) may increase the risk of sudden cardiac death.

▷ **Possible Effects on Sex Life:** Decreased libido; impotence by some members of this class.

▷ **Adverse Effects That May Mimic Natural Diseases or Disorders:**
Liver reaction may suggest viral hepatitis.

▷ *CAUTION*
1. Take these drugs exactly as prescribed. Excessive loss of sodium and potassium can lead to loss of appetite, nausea, fatigue, weakness, confusion, and tingling in the extremities. One study found that higher doses of hydrochlorothiazide or chlorthalidone can cause the loss of magnesium as well as potassium, and can increase the risk of sudden cardiac death if not corrected.
2. If you take digitalis (digitoxin, digoxin), adequate potassium is critical. Periodic testing and high-potassium foods may be needed to prevent potassium deficiency—a potential cause of digitalis toxicity.
3. The overdose of these drugs could cause serious dehydration in infants and children. Significant potassium loss can occur within the first 2 weeks of use.
4. Those over 60 should take starting doses as low as 12.5 mg. They have an increased risk of impaired thinking, orthostatic hypotension, potassium loss, and blood sugar increase. An overdose or extended use of these drugs can cause excessive loss of body water, thickening of blood, and increased tendency for blood clotting—predisposing to stroke, heart attack, or thrombophlebitis.

5. Lower doses may be extremely effective for older people and may avoid much of the potassium loss that can occur.

6. These drugs should NOT be used by patients with severe kidney failure.

Advisability of Use During Pregnancy or If Breast-Feeding:

Pregnancy Category: Metolazone: B (by the manufacturer), D (by independent researchers); all other thiazides in this class, D. These drugs should not be used during pregnancy unless a very serious complication occurs for which these are significantly beneficial. Ask your doctor for guidance. Present in breast milk; avoid taking these drugs or refrain from nursing.

▷ **Overdose Symptoms:** Dry mouth, thirst, lethargy, weakness, muscle cramping, nausea, vomiting, drowsiness progressing to stupor or coma.

▷ **Suggested Periodic Examinations While Taking This Drug:** (at doctor's discretion)

Complete blood cell counts, measurements of blood levels of sodium, potassium, chloride, sugar, and uric acid.

Kidney and liver function tests.

▷ **While Taking This Drug the Following Apply:**

Foods: Ask your doctor if you need to eat foods rich in potassium (see Table 11, "High-Potassium Foods," Section Six). Follow your doctor's advice regarding the use of salt.

Beverages: May be taken with milk.

Alcohol: Use with caution—alcohol may exaggerate the blood pressure–lowering effects of these drugs and cause orthostatic hypotension.

Other Drugs:

Thiazide diuretics may ***increase*** the effects of

- other antihypertensives; dosage adjustments may be necessary to prevent excessive lowering of blood pressure.
- lithium, causing lithium toxicity.

Thiazide diuretics may ***decrease*** the effects of

- oral anticoagulants (warfarin); dose adjustments may be required. More frequent INR (prothrombin time) tests are needed, with dosing adjusted to results.
- oral antidiabetic drugs (sulfonylureas); dosage adjustments may be necessary for proper control of blood sugar.

Thiazide diuretics ***taken concurrently*** with

- allopurinol (Zyloprim) may decrease kidney function.
- amphotericin B (Fungizone) may result in additive potassium loss.
- calcium may result in the milk-alkali syndrome: increased calcium, alkalosis, and kidney failure.

- carbamazepine (Tegretol) may result in low sodium levels and symptomatic hyponatremia.
- cortisone may result in excessive potassium loss with resultant heart rhythm changes and lethargy.
- digitalis preparations (digitoxin, digoxin) require careful monitoring and dose changes to prevent low potassium levels and serious heart rhythm disturbances.
- nonsteroidal anti-inflammatory drugs (NSAIDs) such as sulindac (Clinoril) and naproxen (Naprosyn, Aleve, Anaprox, others) may result in decreased thiazide effectiveness.

The following drugs may *decrease* the effects of thiazide diuretics

- cholestyramine (Cuemid, Questran); may interfere with thiazide absorption.
- colestipol (Colestid); may interfere with thiazide absorption.

Take cholestyramine and colestipol 1 hour before any oral diuretic.

Driving, Hazardous Activities: Use caution until the possible occurrence of orthostatic hypotension, dizziness, or impaired vision has been determined.

Exposure to Sun: Use caution until your sensitivity has been determined. These drugs can cause photosensitivity.

Exposure to Heat: Caution—excessive perspiring could cause additional loss of salt and water.

Heavy Exercise or Exertion: Avoid exertion that produces light-headedness, excessive fatigue, or muscle cramping. Isometric exercises can raise blood pressure significantly. Ask your doctor for help.

Occurrence of Unrelated Illness: Vomiting or diarrhea can produce a serious body chemistry imbalance. Ask your doctor for guidance.

Discontinuation: These drugs should not be stopped abruptly following long-term use; sudden discontinuation can cause serious thiazide-withdrawal fluid retention (edema). Reduce dose gradually. It may be advisable to discontinue these drugs 5 to 7 days before major surgery. Ask your doctor, surgeon, and/or anesthesiologist for guidance.

▷ **Saving Money When Using This Medicine:**
- Many new drugs are available to treat high blood pressure. Ask your doctor if this medicine offers the best balance of cost and outcome for you.
- Talk with your doctor about checking a magnesium level with the next laboratory tests ordered, as this medicine can also deplete magnesium.
- Some generic forms can be substituted for the brand names.

THIORIDAZINE (thi oh RID a zeen)

Prescription Needed: Yes   **Controlled Drug:** No   **Generic:** Yes

Brand Names: Mellaril, Mellaril-S, Millazine, SK-Thioridazine

---

Overview of BENEFITS versus RISKS

Possible Benefits	*Possible Risks*
EFFECTIVE CONTROL OF ACUTE MENTAL DISORDERS in most patients: beneficial effects on thinking, mood, and behavior	SERIOUS TOXIC EFFECTS ON BRAIN (long-term use)
Relief of anxiety, agitation, and tension	Liver damage with jaundice (infrequent)
Possibly effective in managing hyperactivity syndrome in children	Blood cell disorders: abnormally low white blood cell count (rare)

▷ **Illness This Medication Treats:**

(1) Moderate to marked depression with significant anxiety and nervous tension; agitation, anxiety, depression, and exaggerated fears in the elderly; (2) severe behavioral problems in children characterized by hyperexcitability, combativeness, short attention span, and rapid mood swings.

▷ **Typical Dosage Range:** (Dosage or schedule must be determined by the doctor for each individual.)

Initially 25 to 100 mg three times daily. Dose may be increased by 25 to 50 mg at 3- to 4-day intervals, as needed and tolerated. Usual dosage range is 200 to 800 mg daily, divided into two to four doses. The total daily dosage should not exceed 800 mg.

▷ **Conditions Requiring Dosing Adjustments:**

Liver function: This drug should be used with caution by patients with liver compromise, and monitored closely.

Kidney function: Patients with compromised kidneys should be closely monitored.

▷ **How Best to Take This Medicine:** May be taken with or following meals to reduce stomach irritation. The tablets may be crushed.

▷ **How Long This Medicine Is Usually Taken:** Use on a regular schedule for 3 to 4 weeks usually determines the effectiveness of this drug in controlling psychotic disorders. If not significantly beneficial within 6 weeks, use of this drug should be stopped. Long-term use (months to years) requires periodic physician evaluation, and consideration of continued need.

▷ **Tell Your Doctor Before Taking This Medicine If You:**
- ever had an allergic reaction to it.
- have active liver disease, or impaired liver or kidney function.
- have cancer of the breast.
- have a current blood cell or bone marrow disorder.
- are allergic or abnormally sensitive to any phenothiazine drug (see Drug Classes).
- have any type of seizure disorder.
- have diabetes, glaucoma, or heart disease.
- have a history of lupus erythematosus.
- are taking any drug with sedative effects.
- plan to have surgery under general or spinal anesthesia soon.

▷ **Possible Side Effects:** Drowsiness (usually during the first 2 weeks), orthostatic hypotension, blurred vision, dry mouth, nasal congestion, constipation, impaired urination.
Pink or purple coloration of urine, of no significance.

▷ **Possible Adverse Effects:**
If any of the following develop, call your doctor promptly for guidance.
Some Mild Problems Drug Can Cause
Allergic reactions: skin rash, low-grade fever.
Lowering of body temperature, especially in the elderly.
Increased appetite and weight gain.
Weakness, agitation, insomnia, impaired day and night vision.
Chronic constipation, fecal impaction.
Some Serious Problems Drug Can Cause
Allergic reactions: hepatitis with jaundice, severe skin reactions.
Idiosyncratic reactions: neuroleptic malignant syndrome.
Depression, disorientation, seizures, loss of peripheral vision.
Rapid heart rate, heart rhythm disorders.
Blood cell disorders: reduced white blood cell count (more common in the elderly).
Rare liver toxicity.
Nervous system reactions: Parkinson-like disorders, severe restlessness, muscle spasms involving the face and neck, tardive dyskinesia.

▷ **Possible Effects on Sex Life:** Decreased male and female libido, inhibited ejaculation, impotence, impaired female orgasm, priapism.
Male breast enlargement and tenderness.
Female breast enlargement with milk production.
Altered timing and pattern of menstruation.
False-positive pregnancy test results.

▷ **Adverse Effects That May Mimic Natural Diseases or Disorders:**
Nervous system reactions may suggest true Parkinson's disease.
Liver reactions may suggest viral hepatitis.
Reactions resembling systemic lupus erythematosus can occur.

▷ *CAUTION*
1. Many over-the-counter medications for allergies, colds, and coughs contain drugs that can interact unfavorably with this drug. Ask your doctor or pharmacist for guidance before using any such medications.
2. Antacids that contain aluminum and/or magnesium can prevent absorption and reduce the effectiveness of this drug.
3. Obtain prompt evaluation of any change or disturbance of vision.
4. Use of this drug is not recommended in children under 2 years old. Do not use this drug in the presence of symptoms suggestive of Reye's syndrome. Children with acute infectious diseases (flu-like infections, chickenpox, measles, etc.) are more prone to develop muscular spasms of the face, back, and extremities when this drug is given for any reason.
5. For those over 60, small doses are advisable until individual response has been determined. The elderly may be more susceptible to drowsiness, lethargy, constipation, lowering of body temperature, and orthostatic hypotension. This drug can enhance existing prostatism. Susceptibility to Parkinson-like reactions and/or tardive dyskinesia are also increased in this population. These reactions must be recognized early, as they may become unresponsive to treatment and irreversible.
6. This drug should be used in decrease doses by those with liver compromise.

Advisability of Use During Pregnancy or If Breast-Feeding:
Pregnancy Category: C. Avoid using this drug during the first 3 months. Use otherwise only if clearly needed. Ask your doctor for guidance. Present in breast milk in minute amounts. Monitor the nursing infant closely and discontinue taking this drug or nursing if adverse effects develop.

▷ **Overdose Symptoms:**   Marked drowsiness, weakness, tremor, agitation, unsteadiness, deep sleep, coma, convulsions.

▷ **Suggested Periodic Examinations While Taking This Drug:** (at doctor's discretion)
Complete blood cell counts, especially between the fourth and tenth weeks of treatment.
Liver function tests, electrocardiograms.
Complete eye examinations—eye structures and vision.

Careful inspection of the tongue for early evidence of fine, involuntary, wavelike movements that could indicate the beginning of tardive dyskinesia.

▷ **While Taking This Drug the Following Apply:**

Nutritional Support: A riboflavin (vitamin B2) supplement should be taken with long-term use.

Beverages: May be taken with milk.

Alcohol: Avoid completely. Alcohol can increase this drug's sedative action and accentuate its depressant effects on brain function and blood pressure. Phenothiazines can increase the intoxicating effects of alcohol.

Tobacco Smoking: Possible reduction of drowsiness from this drug.

Marijuana Smoking: Moderate increase in drowsiness; accentuation of orthostatic hypotension; increased risk of precipitating latent psychoses, confusing the interpretation of mental status and drug responses.

Other Drugs:

Thioridazine may *increase* the effects of
- all sedatives, especially meperidine (Demerol), causing excessive sedation.
- all atropinelike drugs, causing nervous system toxicity.

Thioridazine may *decrease* the effects of
- bromocriptine (Parlodel).
- guanethidine (Ismelin, Esimil), reducing its effectiveness in lowering blood pressure.
- oral hypoglycemic agents (see Drug Classes).

Thioridazine *taken concurrently* with
- ascorbic acid (vitamin C) may blunt thioridazine's benefits.
- lithium (Lithobid, Lithotabs) may impair the effectiveness of lithium and cause nervous system toxicity.
- phenytoin (Dilantin) may change phenytoin blood levels.

The following drugs may *decrease* the effects of thioridazine
- antacids containing aluminum and/or magnesium.
- barbiturates.
- benztropine (Cogentin).
- disulfiram (Antabuse).
- trihexyphenidyl (Artane).

Driving, Hazardous Activities: Can impair mental alertness, judgment, and physical coordination. Avoid hazardous activities.

Exposure to Sun: Use caution until your sensitivity has been determined. Some phenothiazines can cause photosensitivity.

Exposure to Heat: Use caution and avoid excessive heat as much as possible. This drug may impair the body temperature regulation and increase the risk of heatstroke.

Exposure to Cold: Use caution and dress warmly. This drug can increase the risk of hypothermia in the elderly.

Discontinuation: After a period of long-term use, do not suddenly discontinue taking this drug. Gradual withdrawal over 2 to 3 weeks under your doctor's supervision is recommended. Do not discontinue this drug without your doctor's knowledge and approval.

▷ **Saving Money When Using This Medicine:**
- Many drugs are available to treat mental problems. Ask your doctor if this medicine offers the best balance of cost and outcome for you.
- A generic form can be substituted for the brand name.
- A new medicine with a novel form, olanzapine, has been approved that does not appear to have any of the Parkinson-like side effects.

THIOTHIXENE (thi oh THIX een)

Prescription Needed: Yes   **Controlled Drug:** No   **Generic:** Yes

Brand Name: Navane

Overview of BENEFITS versus RISKS	
Possible Benefits	*Possible Risks*
EFFECTIVE CONTROL OF ACUTE MENTAL DISORDERS	SERIOUS TOXIC EFFECTS ON BRAIN with long-term use
Beneficial effects on thinking, mood, and behavior	Liver damage with jaundice (rare)
	Blood cell disorders: abnormally low white blood cell count (rare)

▷ **Illness This Medication Treats:**
Psychotic thinking and behavior associated with acute psychoses of unknown nature, episodes of mania and paranoia, and acute schizophrenia.

▷ **Typical Dosage Range:** (Dosage or schedule must be determined by the doctor for each individual.)
Initially 2 to 5 mg two or three times daily. Dose may be increased by 2 mg at 3- to 4-day intervals, as needed and tolerated. Usual dosage range is 20 to 30 mg daily. The total daily dosage should not exceed 60 mg.

▷ **Conditions Requiring Dosing Adjustments:**
Liver function: This drug is extensively metabolized in the liver and eliminated in the urine. This drug should be used with caution by patients with liver compromise, and the effects closely monitored.

Kidney function: Patients with compromised kidneys should be closely monitored.

▷ **How Best to Take This Medicine:**   May be taken with or following meals to reduce stomach irritation. The capsules may be opened for administration. The liquid concentrate must be diluted just before administration by adding it to 8 oz of water, milk, fruit juice, or carbonated beverage.

▷ **How Long This Medicine Is Usually Taken:**   Continual use on a regular schedule for several weeks is usually necessary to determine the effectiveness of this drug in controlling psychotic disorders. If this drug is not significantly beneficial within 6 weeks, discontinue taking it. Long-term use (months to years) requires periodic physician evaluation of response.

▷ **Tell Your Doctor Before Taking This Medicine If You:**
- ever had an allergic reaction to it.
- have active liver disease.
- have cancer of the breast.
- have a current blood cell or bone marrow disorder.
- are allergic or abnormally sensitive to other thioxanthenes or any phenothiazine (see Drug Classes).
- have impaired liver or kidney function.
- have any type of seizure disorder.
- have diabetes, glaucoma, or heart disease.
- have a history of lupus erythematosus.
- are taking any drug with sedative effects.
- drink alcohol daily.
- have Parkinson's disease.
- plan to have surgery under general or spinal anesthesia soon.

▷ **Possible Side Effects:**   Mild drowsiness (usually during the first 2 weeks), orthostatic hypotension, blurred vision, dry mouth, nasal congestion, constipation, impaired urination.

▷ **Possible Adverse Effects:**
If any of the following develop, call your doctor promptly for guidance.
Some Mild Problems Drug Can Cause
Allergic reactions: skin rash, itching.
Lowering of body temperature, especially in the elderly.
Fluid retention, weight gain.
Dizziness, weakness, agitation, insomnia, impaired vision.
Nausea, vomiting.
Some Serious Problems Drug Can Cause
Allergic reactions: rare hepatitis with jaundice, anaphylactic reaction.

Idiosyncratic reactions: paradoxical worsening of psychotic symptoms, development of neuroleptic malignant syndrome.

Depression, disorientation, seizures, deposits in cornea and lens.

Rare lupus erythematosus, deposits in the cornea or lens of the eye.

Rapid heart rate, heart rhythm disorders.

Blood cell disorders: reduced white blood cell count.

Nervous system reactions: Parkinson-like disorders, severe restlessness, muscle spasms involving the face and neck, tardive dyskinesia.

▷ **Possible Effects on Sex Life:** Altered timing and pattern of menstruation.

Impotence (rare).

Male breast enlargement and tenderness.

Female breast enlargement with milk production.

▷ **Adverse Effects That May Mimic Natural Diseases or Disorders:** Nervous system reactions may suggest true Parkinson's disease or Reye's syndrome.

Liver reactions may suggest viral hepatitis.

▷ *CAUTION*

1. Many over-the-counter medications for allergies, colds, and coughs contain drugs that can interact unfavorably with this drug. Ask your doctor or pharmacist for guidance before using any such medications.

2. Antacids that contain aluminum and/or magnesium may prevent absorption of this drug and reduce its effectiveness.

3. Obtain prompt evaluation of any change or disturbance of vision.

4. Use of this drug is not recommended in children under 12 years old. Do not use thiothixene in the presence of symptoms suggestive of Reye's syndrome. Children with acute infectious diseases (flu-like infections, chickenpox, measles, etc.) are more prone to develop muscular spasms of the face, back, and extremities.

5. Small doses of this drug are advisable until individual response has been determined for those over 60. The elderly may be more susceptible to drowsiness, lethargy, constipation, lowering of body temperature, and orthostatic hypotension. This drug can enhance existing prostatism. Susceptibility to Parkinson-like reactions and/or tardive dyskinesia is also increased in this population. These reactions must be recognized early since they may become unresponsive to treatment and irreversible.

Advisability of Use During Pregnancy or If Breast-Feeding:

Pregnancy Category: C. Avoid using this drug during the first 3 months if possible. Avoid during the last month because of possible effects on the newborn infant. Present in breast milk in small amounts; avoid taking this drug or refrain from nursing.

▷ **Overdose Symptoms:**   Marked drowsiness, weakness, tremor, agitation, unsteadiness, deep sleep, coma, convulsions.

▷ **Possible Effects of Long-Term Use:**   Opacities in the cornea or lens, pigmentation of the retina. Tardive dyskinesia.

▷ **Suggested Periodic Examinations While Taking This Drug:** (at doctor's discretion)

Complete blood cell counts, especially between the fourth and tenth weeks of treatment.

Liver function tests, electrocardiograms.

Complete eye examinations—eye structures and vision.

Careful inspection of the tongue for early evidence of fine, involuntary, wavelike movements that could indicate the beginning of tardive dyskinesia.

▷ **While Taking This Drug the Following Apply:**

Beverages: May be taken with milk.

Alcohol: Avoid completely. Alcohol can increase this drug's sedative action and accentuate its depressant effects on brain function and blood pressure. Thiothixene can increase the intoxicating effects of alcohol.

Marijuana Smoking: Moderate increase in drowsiness; accentuation of orthostatic hypotension; increased risk of precipitating latent psychoses, confusing the interpretation of mental status and drug responses.

Other Drugs:

Thiothixene may *increase* the effects of

• all sedatives, especially barbiturates and narcotic analgesics, causing excessive sedation.

• all atropinelike drugs, causing nervous system toxicity.

Thiothixene may *decrease* the effects of

• guanethidine (Ismelin, Esimil), reducing its effectiveness in lowering blood pressure.

Thiothixene *taken concurrently* with

• ketorolac (Toradol) may result in hallucinations.

• lithium (Lithobid, others) may exaggerate nerve toxicity.

• monoamine oxidase inhibitors (MAOIs) may result in worsening of the central nervous system and breathing depressive effects of thiothixene.

The following drugs may *decrease* the effects of thiothixene

• antacids containing aluminum and/or magnesium.

• barbiturates.

• benztropine (Cogentin)

• trihexyphenidyl (Artane).

Driving, Hazardous Activities: Can impair mental alertness, judgment, and physical coordination. Avoid hazardous activities.

Exposure to Sun: Use caution until your sensitivity has been determined. This drug can cause photosensitivity.

Exposure to Heat: Use caution and avoid excessive heat as much as possible. This drug may impair body temperature regulation and increase the risk of heatstroke.

Exposure to Cold: Use caution and dress warmly. This drug can increase the risk of hypothermia in the elderly.

Discontinuation: After a period of long-term use, do not suddenly discontinue taking this drug. Gradual withdrawal over 2 to 3 weeks under your doctor's supervision is recommended. Do not discontinue taking thiothixene without your doctor's knowledge and approval. The relapse rate of schizophrenia after discontinuation is 50 to 60%.

▷ **Saving Money When Using This Medicine:**

- Many new drugs are available to treat mental problems. Ask your doctor if this medicine offers the best balance of cost and outcome for you.
- A generic form can be substituted for the brand name.
- A new medicine called olanzapine has been approved, which does not appear to have as many side effects as older agents. Talk to your doctor about this if side effects become a problem.

TICLOPIDINE (ti KLOH pi deen)

Prescription Needed: Yes   **Controlled Drug:** No   **Generic:** No

Brand Name: Ticlid

Overview of BENEFITS versus RISKS	
Possible Benefits	*Possible Risks*
SIGNIFICANT REDUCTION IN THE RISK OF STROKE FOR THOSE WITH TRANSIENT ISCHEMIC ATTACK (TIA) OR A PREVIOUS STROKE	SIGNIFICANT REDUCTION IN WHITE BLOOD CELL COUNTS
	Increase (8–10%) in total blood cholesterol level
	Drug-induced hepatitis with jaundice (rare)

▷ **Illness This Medication Treats:**
Prevention of recurrent stroke following initial thrombotic stroke.

▷ **Typical Dosage Range:** (Dosage or schedule must be determined by the doctor for each individual.)
Infants and Children: Dosage not established.

18 to 60 Years of Age: 250 mg twice daily, 12 hours apart, taken with food.

Over 60 Years of Age: Same as for 18 to 60 years of age.

▷ **Conditions Requiring Dosing Adjustments:**

Liver function: This drug is contraindicated for patients with severe hepatic impairment.

Kidney function: Changes in dosing of this drug do not appear to be needed for patients with compromised kidneys.

▷ **How Best to Take This Medicine:**   Recommended with meals to enhance absorption and reduce stomach irritation. The tablet may be crushed.

▷ **How Long This Medicine Is Usually Taken:**   Continual use on a regular schedule for 6 to 12 months is usually necessary to determine the effectiveness of this drug in preventing stroke. Long-term use (months to years) requires periodic evaluation of response and dosage adjustment. See your doctor regularly.

▷ **Tell Your Doctor Before Taking This Medicine If You:**

- ever had an allergic reaction to it.
- currently have a bone marrow, blood cell, or bleeding disorder or a history of drug-induced bone marrow depression or blood cell disorders.
- have active peptic ulcer disease, Crohn's disease, or ulcerative colitis.
- are taking aspirin, anticoagulants, or cortisonelike drugs.
- have impaired liver or kidney function.
- plan to have surgery soon.

▷ **Possible Side Effects:**   Spontaneous bruising (purpura).

▷ **Possible Adverse Effects:**

If any of the following develop, call your doctor promptly **for guidance.**

Some Mild Problems Drug Can Cause

Allergic reactions: rash, itching.

Dizziness.

Nausea, vomiting, diarrhea.

Some Serious Problems Drug Can Cause

Allergic reactions: drug-induced hepatitis with jaundice (rare), usually during the first 4 months of treatment.

Idiosyncratic reactions: decreased production of white blood cells (neutrophils and granulocytes); fever, sore throat, susceptibility to infection.

Very rare aplastic anemia.

Rare lupus erythematosus.

▷ **Adverse Effects That May Mimic Natural Diseases or Disorders:**
Drug-induced hepatitis may suggest viral hepatitis.

▷ *CAUTION*

1. A significant reduction in white blood cell counts; usually begins between 3 weeks and 3 months after treatment with this drug starts. Complete blood cell counts every 2 weeks from the second week to the end of the third month of drug administration are mandatory.
2. Report promptly any indications of infection: fever, chills, sore throat, cough.
3. Report promptly any abnormal or unusual bleeding or bruising.
4. Do not take any type of aspirin or anticoagulant drug without your doctor's approval while using ticlopidine.
5. Tell all doctors and dentists who provide your care that you are taking this drug.
6. Safety and effectiveness of this drug for those under 18 years old have not been established.
7. Those over 60 may be more susceptible to bone marrow depression and blood cell decreases. Observe carefully for and report promptly any tendency to infections or unusual bleeding or bruising.

Advisability of Use During Pregnancy or If Breast-Feeding:
Pregnancy Category: B. Use this drug only if clearly needed. Ask your doctor for guidance. Presence in breast milk is unknown; avoid taking this drug or refrain from nursing.

▷ **Overdose Symptoms:** Abnormal bleeding or bruising, dizziness, nausea, diarrhea.

▷ **Suggested Periodic Examinations While Taking This Drug:** (at doctor's discretion)
Complete blood cell counts. See "CAUTION," above.
Liver function tests.

▷ **While Taking This Drug the Following Apply:**
Foods: High-fat meals may increase absorption of this drug by 20%.
Beverages: May be taken with milk.
Alcohol: No interactions expected. Avoid alcohol if you have active peptic ulcer disease.
Other Drugs:
Ticlopidine may *increase* the effects of
- aspirin.
- theophylline (Theo-Dur, others).
- warfarin (Coumadin); may increase the risk of hepatitis.
Ticlopidine may *decrease* the effects of
- cyclosporine (Sandimmune), decreasing its effectiveness.

The following drug may *increase* the effects of ticlopidine
- cimetidine (Tagamet).

The following drugs may *decrease* the effects of ticlopidine
- antacids; decreases absorption of ticlopidine.

Driving, Hazardous Activities: May cause dizziness. Restrict your activities as necessary.

Discontinuation: To be determined and guided by your doctor. This drug should be discontinued 10 to 14 days prior to surgery.

▷ **Saving Money When Using This Medicine:**
- Ask your doctor if this medicine offers the best balance of cost and outcome for you.

TIMOLOL (TI moh lohl)

Prescription Needed: Yes   **Controlled Drug:** No   **Generic:** Yes

Brand Names: Betimol, Blocadren, Timolide [CD], Timoptic, Timoptic in Ocudose, Timoptic-XE

Overview of BENEFITS versus RISKS	
Possible Benefits	*Possible Risks*
EFFECTIVE, WELL-TOLERATED ANTIANGINAL DRUG for effort-induced angina; ANTIGLAUCOMA DRUG for open-angle glaucoma; antihypertensive for mild to moderate hypertension	CONGESTIVE HEART FAILURE in advanced heart disease
EFFECTIVE PREVENTION OF MIGRAINE HEADACHES	Worsening of angina in coronary heart disease (if abruptly withdrawn)
Effective adjunct for prevention of recurrent heart attack (myocardial infarction)	Masking of low blood sugar in drug-treated diabetes
EFFECTIVE LOWERING OF INCREASED EYE PRESSURE IN GLAUCOMA	Provocation of asthma

▷ **Illness This Medication Treats:**
(1) Classical effort-induced angina, certain types of heart rhythm disturbance, and high blood pressure; (2) lowers increased internal eye pressure in chronic open-angle glaucoma; (3) beneficial in prevent-

ing recurrent heart attacks (myocardial infarction); (4) reduction of the frequency and severity of migraine headaches.

As Combination Drug Product [CD]: Combined with hydrochlorothiazide for the treatment of hypertension; includes two step 1 drugs with different mechanisms of action for greater effectiveness and convenience for long-term use.

▷ **Typical Dosage Range:** (Dosage or schedule must be determined by the doctor for each individual.)

Varies with indication.

Antianginal and antihypertensive: Initially 10 mg twice daily; increase dose gradually every 7 days, as needed and tolerated. Usual maintenance dose is 10 to 20 mg twice daily. The total daily dosage should not exceed 60 mg.

Migraine headache prevention: Initially 10 mg twice daily; increase dose as needed to 10 mg in the morning and 20 mg at night.

Recurrent heart attack prevention: 10 mg twice daily.

Antiglaucoma: One drop in affected eye every 12 to 24 hours.

▷ **Conditions Requiring Dosing Adjustments:**

Liver function: This drug is extensively metabolized in the liver. An empirical decrease of the dose must be considered for patients with compromised livers.

Kidney function: Patients with renal compromise should be followed closely, and their dose decreased if the medication accumulates.

▷ **How Best to Take This Medicine:**   Preferably taken 1 hour before eating to maximize absorption. The tablet may be crushed. Do not abruptly discontinue taking this drug.

▷ **How Long This Medicine Is Usually Taken:**   Use on a regular schedule for 10 to 14 days determines the effectiveness of this drug in preventing angina, controlling heart rhythm disorders, and lowering blood pressure. Peak benefit may require continual use for 6 to 8 weeks. Long-term use (months to years) is determined by the course of symptoms over time and your response to the overall treatment program (weight reduction, salt restriction, smoking cessation, etc.). See your doctor regularly.

▷ **Tell Your Doctor Before Taking This Medicine If You:**

- ever had an allergic reaction to it.
- have asthma.
- have Prinzmetal's variant angina (coronary artery spasm).
- have congestive heart failure or a history of serious heart disease, with or without episodes of heart failure.
- have an abnormally slow heart rate or a serious form of heart block.
- are taking, or have taken within the past 14 days, any MAO type A inhibitor.

- had an adverse reaction to any beta-blocker in the past.
- have a history of hay fever, asthma, chronic bronchitis, or emphysema.
- have a history of overactive thyroid function.
- have a history of low blood sugar.
- have impaired liver or kidney function.
- have diabetes or myasthenia gravis.
- are currently taking any form of digitalis, quinidine, or reserpine, or any calcium blocker.
- plan to have surgery under general anesthesia soon.

▷ **Possible Side Effects:** Lethargy and fatigability, cold extremities, slow heart rate, light-headedness in upright position.

▷ **Possible Adverse Effects:**
If any of the following develop, call your doctor promptly for guidance.

Some Mild Problems Drug Can Cause
Allergic reactions: skin rash, itching.
Loss of hair involving the scalp, eyebrows, and/or eyelashes. This effect can occur with use of the oral tablets or the eyedrops (for glaucoma). Regrowth occurs with the discontinuation of this drug.
Headache, dizziness, visual disturbances, vivid dreams.
Nausea, vomiting, diarrhea.
Numbness and tingling in extremities.

Some Serious Problems Drug Can Cause
Allergic reactions: laryngospasm, severe dermatitis.
Idiosyncratic reactions: acute behavioral disturbances, depression, hallucinations.
Chest pain, shortness of breath, precipitation of congestive heart failure.
Induction of bronchial asthma (in asthmatic individuals).
Masked warning signs of impending low blood sugar in drug-treated diabetes.

▷ **Possible Effects on Sex Life:** Decreased libido, impaired erection, impotence.
Note: All of these effects can occur with the use of timolol eyedrops at the recommended dosage.

▷ **Adverse Effects That May Mimic Natural Diseases or Disorders:**
Reduced blood flow to extremities may resemble Raynaud's phenomenon.

▷ *CAUTION*
1. ***Do not suddenly stop taking this drug*** without the knowledge and guidance of your doctor. Carry a personal identification card that states you are taking this drug.

2. Ask your doctor or pharmacist before using nasal decongestants, which are usually present in over-the-counter cold preparations and nose drops. These can cause sudden increases in blood pressure when taken concurrently with beta-blockers.

3. Report the development of any tendency to emotional depression (rare).

4. Safety and effectiveness of this drug for those under 12 years old have not been established. However, if this drug is used, observe for low blood sugar during periods of reduced food intake.

5. Those over 60 should proceed *cautiously* with all antihypertensives. Unacceptably high blood pressure should be reduced without the risks associated with excessively low blood pressure. Start treatment with small doses, and monitor the blood pressure response frequently. Sudden, rapid, and excessive reduction of blood pressure can predispose to stroke or heart attack. Observe for dizziness, unsteadiness, tendency to fall, confusion, hallucinations, depression, or urinary frequency.

Advisability of Use During Pregnancy or If Breast-Feeding:
Pregnancy Category: C. Avoid using this drug during the first 3 months if possible. Use only if clearly needed. Ask your doctor for guidance. Present in breast milk. Monitor the nursing infant closely and taper this drug or stop nursing if adverse effects develop.

▷ **Overdose Symptoms:** Weakness, slow pulse, low blood pressure, fainting, cold and sweaty skin, congestive heart failure, possible coma, and convulsions.

▷ **Suggested Periodic Examinations While Taking This Drug:** (at doctor's discretion)
Complete blood cell counts (because of adverse effects of other drugs of this class).
Measurements of blood pressure, evaluation of heart function.

▷ **While Taking This Drug the Following Apply:**
Foods: Avoid excessive salt intake.
Beverages: May be taken with milk.
Alcohol: Alcohol may exaggerate this drug's ability to lower blood pressure and increase its mild sedative effect.
Tobacco Smoking: Nicotine may reduce this drug's effectiveness in treating angina, heart rhythm disorders, and high blood pressure. In addition, high doses of timolol may potentiate the constriction of the bronchial tubes caused by regular smoking.
Other Drugs:
Timolol may *increase* the effects of
• other antihypertensives, causing excessive lowering of blood pressure. Dosage adjustments may be necessary.
• amiodarone (Cordarone), causing cardiac arrest.

- lidocaine (Xylocaine, etc.).
- reserpine (Ser-Ap-Es, etc.), causing sedation, depression, slowing of the heart rate, and lowering of blood pressure.
- verapamil (Calan, Isoptin), causing excessive depression of heart function; monitor this combination closely.

Timolol may *decrease* the effects of
- theophyllines (aminophylline, Theo-Dur, etc.), reducing their antiasthmatic effectiveness.

Timolol *taken concurrently* with
- clonidine (Catapres) requires close monitoring for rebound high blood pressure if clonidine is withdrawn while timolol is still being taken.
- epinephrine (Adrenalin, etc.) may cause a marked rise in blood pressure and slowing of the heart rate.
- insulin requires close monitoring to avoid undetected hypoglycemia.
- oral hypoglycemic agents such as acetohexamide (Dymelor) and glipizide (Glucotrol) may result in prolonged low blood sugar.
- venlafaxine (Effexor) may increase the risk of timolol toxicity.

The following drugs may *increase* the effects of timolol
- chlorpromazine (Thorazine, etc.).
- cimetidine (Tagamet).
- fluoxetine (Prozac) or fluvoxamine (Luvox).
- methimazole (Tapazole).
- propylthiouracil (Propacil).

The following drugs may *decrease* the effects of timolol
- barbiturates (phenobarbital, etc.).
- indomethacin (Indocin), and possibly other aspirin substitutes (NSAIDs); these may impair timolol's antihypertensive effect.
- rifampin (Rifadin, Rimactane)

Driving, Hazardous Activities: Use caution until the full extent of dizziness, lethargy, and blood pressure change have been determined.

Exposure to Heat: Caution is advised. Hot environments can lower blood pressure and exaggerate its effects.

Exposure to Cold: Caution is advised. Cold environments can enhance the circulatory deficiency in the extremities with this drug. The elderly should take precautions to prevent hypothermia.

Heavy Exercise or Exertion: Avoid exertion that produces lightheadedness, excessive fatigue, or muscle cramping. Use of this drug may intensify the hypertensive response to isometric exercise.

Occurrence of Unrelated Illness: The fever that accompanies systemic infections can lower blood pressure and require an adjustment of dosage. Illnesses that cause nausea or vomiting may interrupt the regular dosage schedule. Ask your doctor for guidance.

Discontinuation: Avoid sudden discontinuation of this drug in all situations, especially in the presence of coronary artery disease. If possible, gradual reduction of dose over a period of 2 to 3 weeks is recommended. Ask your doctor for specific guidance.

▷ **Saving Money When Using This Medicine:**
- Ask your doctor if this medicine offers the best balance of cost and outcome for you, how often your blood pressure should be checked, and about stress management and exercise programs available in your community.
- A generic form can be substituted for the brand name.
- Ask your doctor if taking aspirin every other day to help prevent a heart attack makes sense for you.

TOLAZAMIDE (tohl AZ a mide)

Prescription Needed: Yes   **Controlled Drug:** No   **Generic:** Yes

Brand Names: Ronase, Tolamide, Tolinase

Overview of BENEFITS versus RISKS	
Possible Benefits	*Possible Risks*
Helps regulate blood sugar in noninsulin-dependent diabetes (adjunctive to appropriate diet and weight control)	HYPOGLYCEMIA, severe and prolonged Drug-induced liver damage Bone marrow depression (rare) Hemolytic anemia

▷ **Illness This Medication Treats:**
Mild to moderately severe type II diabetes mellitus (adult, maturity-onset) that does not require insulin, but cannot be adequately controlled by diet alone.

▷ **Typical Dosage Range:** (Dosage or schedule must be determined by the doctor for each individual.)
Initially 100 to 250 mg daily with breakfast. At 4- to 6-day intervals the dose may be increased by increments of 100 to 250 mg daily as needed and tolerated. The total daily dosage should not exceed 1000 mg (1 g).

TOLBUTAMIDE (tohl BYU ta mide)

Prescription Needed: Yes   **Controlled Drug:** No   **Generic:** Yes

Brand Names: Oramide, Orinase, Sk-Tolbutamide

▷ **Warning:** The brand names Orinase, Ornade, and Ornex can be mistaken for each other, leading to serious medication errors. Orinase (a white tablet), the generic drug tolbutamide, is used to treat diabetes. Ornade (a red capsule containing colored beads), a combination of chlorpheniramine and phenylpropanolamine, is used to treat nasal and sinus congestion. Ornex (a blue caplet), a combination of acetaminophen and phenylpropanolamine, is used to treat head colds and sinus pain. Verify that you are taking the correct drug.

Overview of BENEFITS versus RISKS	
Possible Benefits	*Possible Risks*
Assistance in regulating blood sugar in noninsulin-dependent diabetes (adjunctive to appropriate diet and weight control)	HYPOGLYCEMIA, severe and prolonged
	Drug-induced liver damage
	Bone marrow depression (rare)
	Hemolytic anemia

▷ **Illness This Medication Treats:**
Mild to moderately severe type II diabetes mellitus (adult, maturity-onset) that does not require insulin, but cannot be adequately controlled by diet alone.

▷ **Typical Dosage Range:** (Dosage or schedule must be determined by the doctor for each individual.)
Initially 500 mg twice a day. The dose may be increased or decreased every 48 to 72 hours until the minimal amount required for satisfactory control is determined. The usual range is 500 to 2000 mg every 24 hours. Total daily dose should not exceed 3000 mg (3 g).

Author's note: The information in this profile has been abbreviated in order to make room for medicines more widely used.

TOLMETIN (TOHL met in)

Prescription Needed: Yes   **Controlled Drug:** No   **Generic:** No

Brand Names: Tolectin, Tolectin DS, Tolectin 600

```
┌─────────────────────────────────────────────────────────┐
│           Overview of BENEFITS versus RISKS              │
│     Possible Benefits            Possible Risks          │
│  EFFECTIVE RELIEF OF MILD     Increased blood pressure   │
│    TO MODERATE PAIN AND       Gastrointestinal pain,     │
│    INFLAMMATION                 ulceration, bleeding (rare)│
│                               Liver damage (rare)        │
│                               Kidney damage (rare)       │
│                               Blood cell disorders: hemolytic│
│                                 anemia, abnormally low   │
│                                 white blood cell and platelet│
│                                 counts (rare)            │
└─────────────────────────────────────────────────────────┘
```

See the acetic acids (NSAIDs) drug profile for further information.

TRAZODONE (TRAZ oh dohn)

Prescription Needed: Yes   **Controlled Drug:** No   **Generic:** Yes

Brand Names: Desyrel, Trialodine

```
┌─────────────────────────────────────────────────────────┐
│           Overview of BENEFITS versus RISKS              │
│     Possible Benefits            Possible Risks          │
│  EFFECTIVE TREATMENT          Adverse behavioral effects:│
│    FOR ALL TYPES OF             confusion, disorientation,│
│    DEPRESSIVE ILLNESS, with     delusions, hallucinations (all│
│    or without anxiety           infrequent)              │
│                               Potential for inducing heart│
│                                 rhythm disorders (in     │
│                                 individuals with heart   │
│                                 disease)                 │
└─────────────────────────────────────────────────────────┘
```

▷ **Illness This Medication Treats:**
  Symptomatic relief in all types of depression, with or without anxiety or agitation.

▷ **Typical Dosage Range:** (Dosage or schedule must be determined by the doctor for each individual.)
  Initially 50 mg three times daily. The dose may be increased by 50 mg daily at intervals of 3 or 4 days, as needed and tolerated. The total daily dosage should not exceed 400 mg.

▷ **Conditions Requiring Dosing Adjustments:**
  Liver function: Blood levels should be obtained to guide dosing. This drug is a rare cause of liver damage, and patients should be followed closely.

Kidney function: Metabolites of this drug are eliminated by the kidneys; however, dosage adjustment for patients with renal compromise is not defined.

▷ **How Best to Take This Medicine:** Best taken with food to improve absorption. The tablet may be crushed. If excessive drowsiness or dizziness occurs, take a larger portion of the total daily dose at bedtime and divide the remaining amount into two or three smaller doses to take during the day.

▷ **How Long This Medicine Is Usually Taken:** Regular use for 2 to 4 weeks determines the effectiveness of this drug in helping the symptoms of depression. Long-term use (weeks to months) requires supervision and periodic evaluation. See your doctor regularly.

▷ **Tell Your Doctor Before Taking This Medicine If You:**
- ever had an allergic reaction to it.
- are recovering from a recent heart attack (myocardial infarction).
- are taking, or have taken within the past 14 days, any MAO type A inhibitor.
- have a history of alcoholism, epilepsy, or heart disease (especially heart rhythm disorders).
- have impaired liver or kidney function.
- are taking any antihypertensives.
- plan to have surgery under general anesthesia soon.

▷ **Possible Side Effects:** Drowsiness, light-headedness, blurred vision, dry mouth, constipation, weight gain.

▷ **Possible Adverse Effects:**
If any of the following develop, call your doctor promptly for guidance.
Some Mild Problems Drug Can Cause
Allergic reaction: skin rash.
Headache, dizziness, fatigue, impaired concentration, tremors.
Rapid heart rate, palpitations.
Peculiar taste, cavities (dental caries), nausea, vomiting, diarrhea.
Muscular aches and pains.
Some Serious Problems Drug Can Cause
Behavioral effects: confusion, anger, hostility, disorientation, impaired memory, delusions, hallucinations, nightmares.
Irregular heart rhythms, low blood pressure, fainting.
Rare seizures or liver toxicity

▷ **Possible Effects on Sex Life:** Decreased male libido; increased female libido.
Inhibited ejaculation, impotence, priapism.
Altered timing and pattern of menstruation.

▷ *CAUTION*

1. If you experience a significant degree of mouth dryness, talk with your dentist about the risk of gum erosion or tooth decay. Ask for guidance on ways to keep your mouth comfortably moist.

2. Withhold treatment of this drug if electroconvulsive therapy is to be used for your depression.

3. Safety and effectiveness of this drug for those under 18 years old have not been established.

4. During the first 2 weeks of treatment for those over 60, observe for restlessness, agitation, excitement, forgetfulness, confusion, or disorientation. Be aware of possible unsteadiness and incoordination that may predispose to falling. This drug may enhance prostatism.

5. For patients with liver compromise, drug dosing should be guided by their drug levels.

Advisability of Use During Pregnancy or If Breast-Feeding:

Pregnancy Category: C. Avoid using this drug completely during the first 3 months. Otherwise use only if clearly needed. Ask your doctor for guidance. Present in breast milk; avoid taking this drug or refrain from nursing.

▷ **Overdose Symptoms:** Marked drowsiness, weakness, confusion, tremors, low blood pressure, rapid heart rate, stupor, coma, possible seizures.

▷ **Suggested Periodic Examinations While Taking This Drug:** (at doctor's discretion).

Complete blood cell counts (may cause slight reductions in white blood cell counts; should be monitored closely if infection, sore throat, or fever develops).

Serial blood pressure readings and electrocardiograms.

▷ **While Taking This Drug the Following Apply:**

Beverages: May be taken with milk.

Alcohol: Avoid completely. This drug can markedly increase the intoxicating effects of alcohol and accentuate its depressant action on brain functions.

Other Drugs:

Trazodone may *increase* the effects of

• antihypertensives, causing excessive lowering of blood pressure; dosage adjustments may be necessary.

• drugs with sedative effects, causing excessive sedation.

• phenytoin (Dilantin), by raising its blood level; observe for phenytoin toxicity.

Trazodone *taken concurrently* with

• clonidine will blunt clonidine's benefits.

• fluoxetine (Prozac) may result in increased trazodone levels and toxicity.

- monoamine oxidase inhibitors (MAOIs) (see Drug Classes) may result in undesirable side effects in some, and benefits in others.
- other medicines with central nervous system effects (see Drug Classes of benzodiazepines, opioids, and tranquilizers) may have additive effects.
- some phenothiazines (see Drug Classes) may excessively lower blood pressure.
- warfarin (Coumadin) may result in a decreased therapeutic benefit of warfarin. INR (prothrombin times) should be checked more frequently, and dosing adjusted to test results.

Driving, Hazardous Activities: May cause dizziness or drowsiness. Restrict your activities as necessary.

Discontinuation: Gradually discontinue taking this drug. Ask your doctor for guidance in dosage reduction over an appropriate period.

▷ **Saving Money When Using This Medicine:**
- Many new drugs are available to treat depression. Ask your doctor if this medicine offers the best balance of cost and outcome for you.
- A generic form can be substituted for the brand name.
- Depression has recently been associated with an increased risk of osteoporosis. Talk with your doctor about risk factors, exercise, calcium supplements, and need for bone mineral density testing.

TRIAMCINOLONE   (tri am SIN oh lohn)

Prescription Needed: Yes   **Controlled Drug:** No   **Generic:** No

Brand Names: Azmacort, Aristocort, Kenalog, Nasacort, Tristoject

Overview of BENEFITS versus RISKS	
Possible Benefits	*Possible Risks*
EFFECTIVE CONTROL OF SEVERE, CHRONIC BRONCHIAL ASTHMA	Yeast infections of mouth and throat
EFFECTIVE SUPPRESSION OF MANY INFLAMMATORY DISORDERS	Suppression of normal cortisone production
POSSIBLE REDUCTION OF SYSTEMIC STEROID USE	Euphoria and mental changes (long-term use)
EFFECTIVE TREATMENT OF SEASONAL OR PERENNIAL ALLERGIC RHINITIS IN ADULTS OR CHILDREN	Cushing's syndrome (moon face, obesity, buffalo hump)
	Osteoporosis or muscle wasting with long-term use

▷ **Illness This Medication Treats:**
(1) Chronic asthma in people who require cortisonelike drugs to control it (as an inhaler); (2) a variety of inflammatory disorders and combination therapy of childhood lymphocytic leukemia (in tablet form); (3) symptoms of seasonal or perennial allergic rhinitis in adults or children (in the nasal form).

▷ **Typical Dosage Range:** (Dosage or schedule must be determined by the doctor for each individual.)

Infants and Children: Up to 6 years old: Dosage not established.

6 to 12 years old: 0.1 to 0.2 mg (one or two metered sprays) three or four times a day. Adjust dosage as needed and tolerated. Limit total daily dosage to 1.2 mg (12 metered sprays).

12 to 60 Years of Age: Initially 0.2 mg (two metered sprays) three or four times a day.

For severe asthma: 1.2 to 1.6 mg (12 to 16 metered sprays) per day, in divided doses. Adjust dosage as needed and tolerated. Limit total daily dose to 1.6 mg (16 metered sprays).

Nasacort AQ and Nasacort may prove effective with 220 mcg per day.

For tablets: 4 to 48 mg daily for inflammatory conditions.

Cream: 0.025% applied to the affected area two to four times daily.

Over 60 Years of Age: Same as for 12 to 60 years of age.

▷ **Conditions Requiring Dosing Adjustments:**

Liver function: This drug is changed in the liver; however, dosing changes for patients with liver compromise are not defined.

Kidney function: Dosing adjustments do not appear warranted for patients with compromised kidneys.

▷ **How Best to Take This Medicine:**   May be used as needed without regard to eating. Shake the container well each time before using. Carefully follow the printed patient instructions provided with the unit. Rinse the mouth and throat (gargle) with water thoroughly after each inhalation; do not swallow the rinse water. The inhaler tends to give a more localized effect, avoiding many systemic problems. The Nasacort AQ form is a water-based form for treatment of allergic rhinitis that does not use chlorofluorocarbon propellants. Oral tablets: May lead to stomach upset, and can be taken with meals or snacks.

▷ **How Long This Medicine Is Usually Taken:**   Continual use on a regular schedule for 1 to 2 weeks is usually necessary to determine the effectiveness of this drug in controlling severe, chronic asthma. Long-term use requires your doctor's supervision.

▷ **Tell Your Doctor Before Taking This Medicine If You:**
• ever had an allergic reaction to it.
• are experiencing severe acute asthma or status asthmaticus that requires more intense treatment for prompt relief.

- have a form of nonallergic bronchitis with asthmatic features, or have chronic bronchitis or bronchiectasis.
- are now taking or have recently taken any cortisone-related drug (including ACTH by injection) for any reason.
- have a history of tuberculosis of the lungs.
- have diabetes, glaucoma, myasthenia gravis, or peptic ulcer disease.
- have an active infection of any kind, especially a respiratory infection.
- are taking warfarin, oral antidiabetic drugs, insulin, or digoxin.

▷ **Possible Side Effects:**   Yeast infections (thrush) of the mouth and throat.

Irritation of mouth, tongue, or throat.

▷ **Possible Adverse Effects:**

If any of the following develop, call your doctor promptly for guidance.

Some Mild Problems Drug Can Cause

Allergic reaction: skin rash.

Easy bruising (ecchymosis).

Swelling of face, hoarseness, voice change, cough.

Some Serious Problems Drug Can Cause

Allergic reaction: rare.

Long-term use may result in euphoria, depressive states, muscle wasting, Cushing's syndrome, or osteoporosis.

Rare toxic megacolon, pancreatitis, or decreased T lymphocytes.

Bronchospasm, asthmatic wheezing (rare).

▷ *CAUTION*

1. This drug does not act primarily as a brochodilator and should not be relied upon for the immediate relief of acute asthma.

2. If you were using any cortisone-related drugs for treatment of your asthma *before* transferring to this inhaler drug, you may need to resume their use if you experience injury or infection, or require surgery. Be sure to notify your doctor of your prior use by mouth or injection of cortisone-related drugs.

3. If severe asthma returns while using this drug, tell your doctor immediately so that additional supportive treatment with cortisone-related drugs can be provided as needed.

4. Carry a personal identification card noting (if applicable) that you have used cortisone-related drugs within the past year. During periods of stress it may be necessary to resume cortisone treatment in adequate dosage.

5. An interval of approximately 5 to 10 minutes should separate inhalant bronchodilators such as albuterol, epinephrine, or pirbuterol (which should be used first) and the inhaling of this drug. This sequence permits greater penetration of triamcinolone into

the bronchial tubes. The delay between inhalations also reduces the possibility of adverse effects from the propellants in the two inhalers.

6. Safety and effectiveness of the oral inhaler for those under 6 years old have not been established. To ensure adequate penetration and maximal benefit, the use of a spacer device is recommended for children.

7. People with chronic bronchitis or bronchiectasis should be observed closely for lung infections.

Advisability of Use During Pregnancy or If Breast-Feeding:

Pregnancy Category: C. Limit use of this drug for a very serious illness for which no satisfactory treatment alternatives are available. Presence in breast milk is unknown; avoid taking this drug or refrain from nursing.

▷ **Habit-Forming Potential:**   With the recommended dosage, a state of functional dependence is not likely to develop.

▷ **Overdose Symptoms:**   Indications of cortisone excess (due to systemic absorption)—fluid retention, flushing of the face, stomach irritation, nervousness.

▷ **Suggested Periodic Examinations While Taking This Drug:** (at doctor's discretion)

Inspection of mouth and throat for evidence of yeast infection.

Assessment of the status of adrenal gland function (cortisone production).

X-ray examination of the lungs of individuals with a prior history of tuberculosis.

▷ **While Taking This Drug the Following Apply:**

Foods: No specific restrictions beyond those advised by your doctor.

Tobacco Smoking: No interactions are expected. However, smoking can affect the condition under treatment and reduce the effectiveness of this drug.

Other Drugs:

The following drugs may **increase** the effects of triamcinolone

• inhalant bronchodilators (albuterol, bitolterol, epinephrine, pirbuterol, etc.).

• oral bronchodilators (aminophylline, ephedrine, terbutaline, theophylline, etc.).

The following drugs may **decrease** the effects of triamcinolone

• carbamazepine (Tegretol); increases triamcinolone metabolism and decreases its effectiveness.

• phenytoin (Dilantin); increases triamcinolone metabolism and decreases its effectiveness.

- primidone (Mysoline); increases steroid metabolism and decreases triamcinolone metabolism.
- rifampin (Rifadin).

Triamcinolone *taken concurrently* with

- aspirin may blunt aspirin's benefits.
- cyclosporine (Sandimmune) may change blood levels of both medicines.
- oral hypoglycemic agents or insulin may result in loss of blood sugar (glucose) control.
- thiazide diuretics (see Drug Classes) can lead to loss of glucose control.
- vaccines (flu, rabies, others) can result in a decreased protective response from the vaccine.
- warfarin (Coumadin) can change anticoagulation. Increased INR (prothrombin time) testing is needed, with dosing adjusted to test results.

Occurrence of Unrelated Illness: Acute infections, serious injuries, and surgical procedures can create an urgent need for additional supportive cortisone-related drugs given by mouth and/or injection. Tell your doctor immediately in the event of new illness or injury.

Discontinuation: If regular use has made it possible to reduce or discontinue maintenance doses of cortisonelike drugs by mouth, *do not* abruptly discontinue them. If you find it necessary to discontinue them for any reason, consult your doctor promptly. It may be necessary to resume cortisone preparations and institute other measures for satisfactory management.

Special Storage Instructions: Store at room temperature. Avoid exposure to temperatures above 120° F (49° C). Do not store or use inhaler near heat or open flame.

▷ **Saving Money When Using This Medicine:**
- Many new drugs are available to treat inflammation. Ask your doctor if this medicine offers the best balance of cost and outcome for you.
- Ask your doctor about using nebulized lidocaine to help treat your asthma.

TRIAMTERENE (tri AM ter cen)

Prescription Needed: Yes   **Controlled Drug:** No   **Generic:** No

Brand Names: Dyazide [CD], Dyrenium, Maxzide [CD], Maxzide-25 [CD]

```
┌─────────────────────────────────────────────────────────┐
│              Overview of BENEFITS versus RISKS            │
│     Possible Benefits              Possible Risks         │
│  EFFECTIVE PREVENTION OF      ABNORMALLY HIGH BLOOD       │
│     POTASSIUM LOSS               POTASSIUM LEVEL with     │
│     (adjunctively with other     excessive use           │
│     diuretics)                Blood cell disorders:       │
│  EFFECTIVE DIURETIC IN           megaloblastic anemia,    │
│     REFRACTORY CASES OF          abnormally low white blood│
│     FLUID RETENTION              cell and platelet counts (rare)│
│     (adjunctively with other  Rare kidney stones          │
│     diuretics)                                            │
└─────────────────────────────────────────────────────────┘
```

▷ **Illness This Medication Treats:**
  (1) Part of combination therapy of congestive heart failure or liver and kidney problems resulting in excessive fluid retention (edema); (2) in conjunction with other measures in treatment of high blood pressure; used primarily in situations where it is advisable to prevent potassium loss.

  As Combination Drug Product [CD]: In combination with hydrochlorothiazide, a diuretic that promotes potassium loss, triamterene counteracts the potassium-wasting effect of the thiazide diuretic.

▷ **Typical Dosage Range:** (Dosage or schedule must be determined by the doctor for each individual.)
  Initially 100 mg twice daily. The dose is then adjusted to individual response. The usual maintenance dose is 100 to 200 mg daily, divided into two doses. The total daily dosage should not exceed 300 mg.

▷ **Conditions Requiring Dosing Adjustments:**
  Liver function: Patients with liver disease should decrease dose and use with extreme caution. This drug is contraindicated for patients with severe liver disease.
  Kidney function: Patients with mild to moderate kidney failure may take the usual dose every 12 hours. Patients with severe or progressive kidney failure should NOT use this drug.

▷ **How Best to Take This Medicine:**   May be taken with or following meals to promote absorption and reduce stomach irritation. The capsule may be opened for administration. Intermittent or alternate-day use is recommended to minimize the possibility of sodium and potassium imbalance.

▷ **How Long This Medicine Is Usually Taken:**   Regular use for 3 to 5 days usually determines this drug's benefits in clearing edema, and for 2 to 3 weeks to determine its effect on hypertension. Long-term use (months to years) requires supervision and periodic evaluation by your doctor. See your doctor regularly.

▷ **Tell Your Doctor Before Taking This Medicine If You:**
- ever had an allergic reaction to it.
- have severely impaired liver or kidney function.
- have a history of liver or kidney disease.
- have diabetes or gout.
- are taking any antihypertensives, a digitalis preparation, another diuretic, lithium, or a potassium preparation.
- have a G6PD deficiency or a history of blood cell disorders.
- plan to have surgery under general anesthesia soon.

▷ **Possible Side Effects:** With excessive use: abnormally high blood potassium levels, abnormally low blood sodium levels, dehydration. Blue urine (of no significance). Excessive urination (SIADH). Rare liver toxicity or formation of kidney stones.

▷ **Possible Adverse Effects:**
If any of the following develop, call your doctor promptly for guidance.
Some Mild Problems Drug Can Cause
Allergic reactions: skin rash, itching.
Headache, dizziness, weakness, drowsiness, lethargy.
Dry mouth, nausea, vomiting, diarrhea.
Some Serious Problems Drug Can Cause
Allergic reaction: anaphylactic reaction.
Symptomatic potassium excess: confusion, numbness and tingling in lips and extremities, fatigue, weakness, shortness of breath, slow heart rate, low blood pressure.
Rare blood cell disorders: megaloblastic anemia, causing weakness and fatigue; abnormally low white blood cell count, causing infection, fever, or sore throat; abnormally low blood platelet count, causing abnormal bleeding or bruising.

▷ *CAUTION*
1. Do not take potassium supplements or increase your intake of potassium-rich foods while taking this drug.
2. Do not abruptly discontinue this drug unless abnormally high blood levels of potassium develop.
3. Avoid the liberal use of salt substitutes containing potassium; these are a potential cause of potassium excess.
4. This drug is not recommended for use in children.
5. The natural decline in kidney function may predispose to potassium retention for those over 60. Look for indications of potassium excess: slow heart rate, irregular heart rhythms, low blood pressure, confusion, or drowsiness. Excessive use of diuretics can cause harmful loss of body water, increase blood viscosity, and

increase the tendency for blood to clot, predisposing to stroke, heart attack, or thrombophlebitis.

6. Dose must be decreased for patients with liver or kidney compromise.

Advisability of Use During Pregnancy or If Breast-Feeding:

Pregnancy Category: B. This drug should not be used during pregnancy unless a very serious complication occurs for which it is significantly beneficial. Present in breast milk; avoid taking this drug or refrain from nursing.

▷ **Overdose Symptoms:** Thirst, drowsiness, fatigue, nausea, vomiting, confusion, irregular heart rhythm, low blood pressure.

▷ **Possible Effects of Long-Term Use:** Potassium accumulation to abnormally high blood levels.

▷ **Suggested Periodic Examinations While Taking This Drug:** (at doctor's discretion)

Complete blood cell counts.

Measurements of blood sodium, potassium, and chloride levels.

Kidney function tests.

▷ **While Taking This Drug the Following Apply:**

Foods: Avoid excessive salt restriction.

Beverages: May be taken with milk.

Alcohol: Use with caution until the combined effects have been determined. Alcohol may enhance drowsiness and this drug's blood pressure–lowering effect.

Other Drugs:

Triamterene may *increase* the effects of

- amantadine (Symmetrel).
- digoxin (Lanoxin).

Triamterene *taken concurrently* with

- captopril (Capoten) may cause excessively high blood potassium levels.
- histamine (H2) blockers (see Drug Classes) may blunt triamterene's benefits by decreasing the amount entering the body.
- indomethacin (Indocin) may increase the risk of kidney damage.
- lithium may cause lithium accumulation to toxic levels.
- NSAIDs (see Drug Classes) may blunt the blood pressure–lowering benefits of triamterene.
- potassium preparations may cause excessively high blood potassium levels.

Driving, Hazardous Activities: May cause dizziness and drowsiness. Restrict your activities as necessary.

Exposure to Sun: Use caution until your sensitivity has been determined. This drug may cause photosensitivity.

Discontinuation: With high dosage or prolonged use of this drug, withdraw gradually. Sudden discontinuation may cause rebound potassium excretion and resultant potassium deficiency. Ask your doctor for guidance.

▷ **Saving Money When Using This Medicine:**
- Many new drugs are available to treat high blood pressure. Ask your doctor if this medicine offers the best balance of cost and outcome for you. Ask if a magnesium level can be checked with your next laboratory work.
- The best outcomes ALWAYS come from keeping the blood pressure in the normal range most of the time.
- Ask your doctor if taking aspirin every other day to help prevent a heart attack makes sense for you.

TRIFLUOPERAZINE (tri floo oh PER a zeen)

Prescription Needed: Yes **Controlled Drug:** No **Generic:** Yes

Brand Names: Stelazine, Suprazine

Overview of BENEFITS versus RISKS	
Possible Benefits	*Possible Risks*
EFFECTIVE CONTROL OF ACUTE MENTAL DISORDERS	SERIOUS TOXIC EFFECTS ON BRAIN with long-term use
Beneficial effects on thinking, mood, and behavior	Liver damage with jaundice (infrequent)
	Blood cell disorders: abnormally low red and white blood cell and platelet counts (rare)

▷ **Illness This Medication Treats:**
(1) Thinking and behavior associated with acute psychoses of unknown nature, mania, paranoid states, and acute schizophrenia; most effective in withdrawn, apathetic individuals and those with agitation, delusions, and hallucinations. (2) Approved for anxiety disorders, but is not the first drug of choice.

▷ **Typical Dosage Range:** (Dosage or schedule must be determined by the doctor for each individual.)
Nonpsychotic anxiety: 1 or 2 mg twice daily. Dose may be increased by 1 or 2 mg at 3- to 4-day intervals to a maximum of 4 mg in patients not in the hospital. For psychosis: 2 to 5 mg twice daily. The dose may be increased every 3 or 4 days, as needed and tolerated. Usual

dosage range is 15 to 20 mg daily. The total daily dosage should not exceed 40 mg. Rare reports of uses of 100 mg daily have been made.

▷ **Conditions Requiring Dosing Adjustments:**
Liver function: Patients with liver compromise should use this drug with caution, and be closely monitored.
Kidney function: Patients with compromised kidneys should be closely followed.

▷ **How Best to Take This Medicine:**   May be taken with or following meals to reduce stomach irritation. The tablets may be crushed.

▷ **How Long This Medicine Is Usually Taken:**   Regular use determines the benefits of this drug in controlling psychotic disorders. If this drug is not beneficial within 6 weeks, discontinue its use. Long-term use (months to years) requires periodic evaluation of response, appropriate dosage adjustment, and consideration of continued need. See your doctor regularly.

▷ **Tell Your Doctor Before Taking This Medicine If You:**
- ever had an allergic reaction to it.
- have active liver disease or impaired liver or kidney function.
- have cancer of the breast.
- have a current blood cell or bone marrow disorder.
- are allergic or abnormally sensitive to any phenothiazine.
- have any type of seizure disorder.
- have diabetes, glaucoma, or heart disease.
- have a history of lupus erythematosus.
- are taking any drug with sedative effects.
- plan to have surgery under general or spinal anesthesia soon.

▷ **Possible Side Effects:**   Drowsiness (usually during the first 2 weeks), orthostatic hypotension, blurred vision, dry mouth, nasal congestion, constipation, impaired urination.
Pink or purple urine (of no significance).

▷ **Possible Adverse Effects:**
If any of the following develop, call your doctor promptly for guidance.
Some Mild Problems Drug Can Cause
Allergic reactions: skin rash, low-grade fever.
Lowering of body temperature, especially in the elderly.
Increased appetite and weight gain.
Dizziness, weakness, agitation, insomnia, impaired day and night vision.
Chronic constipation, fecal impaction.
Some Serious Problems Drug Can Cause
Allergic reactions: hepatitis with jaundice, severe skin reactions, anaphylactic reaction.
Idiosyncratic reactions: neuroleptic malignant syndrome.

Depression, disorientation, seizures, loss of peripheral vision.
Rapid heart rate, heart rhythm disorders.
Blood cell disorders: significant reduction in all cellular elements of the blood (reduced counts of red cells, white cells, and platelets).
Serious skin disorders: Stevens-Johnson syndrome (rare).
Rare drug-induced porphyria, pituitary tumors, or sudden death syndrome.
Nervous system reactions: Parkinson-like disorders, severe restlessness, muscle spasms of the face and neck, tardive dyskinesia.

▷ **Possible Effects on Sex Life:** Altered timing and pattern of menstruation.
Male breast enlargement and tenderness.
Female breast enlargement with milk production.
Spontaneous male orgasm, paradoxical (one case reported).
Inhibited ejaculation, painful ejaculation, priapism.
Delayed female orgasm.

▷ **Adverse Effects That May Mimic Natural Diseases or Disorders:**
Nervous system reactions may suggest true Parkinson's disease.
Liver reactions may suggest viral hepatitis.
Reactions resembling systemic lupus erythematosus may occur.

▷ *CAUTION*

1. Many over-the-counter medications for allergies, colds, and coughs contain drugs that can interact unfavorably with trifluoperazine. Ask your doctor or pharmacist for guidance before using any such medications.

2. Antacids that contain aluminum and/or magnesium may prevent this drug's absorption and reduce its effectiveness.

3. Obtain prompt evaluation of any change or disturbance of vision.

4. Use of this drug is not recommended in children under 6 years old. Do not use this drug in the presence of symptoms suggestive of Reye's syndrome. Children with acute infectious diseases (flu-like infections, chickenpox, measles, etc.) are more prone to develop muscular spasms of the face, back, and extremities.

5. Small doses are advisable for those over 60 until individual response has been determined. You may be more susceptible to drowsiness, lethargy, constipation, lowering of body temperature, and orthostatic hypotension. This drug may enhance existing prostatism. You may also be more susceptible to the development of Parkinson-like reactions and/or tardive dyskinesia. These reactions must be recognized early since they may become unresponsive to treatment and irreversible.

Advisability of Use During Pregnancy or If Breast-Feeding:
Pregnancy Category: C. Avoid using this drug during the first 3 months; avoid during the last month because of possible adverse effects on

the newborn infant. Present in breast milk in minute amounts. Monitor the nursing infant closely and discontinue drug or nursing if adverse effects develop.

▷ **Overdose Symptoms:**   Marked drowsiness, weakness, tremor, agitation, unsteadiness, deep sleep, coma, convulsions.

▷ **Suggested Periodic Examinations While Taking This Drug:** (at doctor's discretion)

Complete blood cell counts, especially between the fourth and tenth weeks of treatment.

Liver function tests, electrocardiograms.

Complete eye examinations—eye structures and vision.

Careful inspection of the tongue for early evidence of fine, involuntary, wavelike movements indicating the beginning of tardive dyskinesia.

▷ **While Taking This Drug the Following Apply:**

Nutritional Support: A riboflavin (vitamin B2) supplement should be taken with long-term use.

Beverages: Caffeine may blunt the calming effect of this medicine. Limit your caffeine intake.

Alcohol: Avoid completely. Alcohol can increase this drug's sedative action and accentuate its depressant effects on brain function and blood pressure. Phenothiazines can increase the intoxicating effects of alcohol.

Tobacco Smoking: Possible reduction of drowsiness from drug.

Marijuana Smoking: Moderate increase in drowsiness; accentuation of orthostatic hypotension; increased risk of precipitating latent psychoses, confusing the interpretation of mental status and drug responses.

Other Drugs:

Trifluoperazine may ***increase*** the effects of
- all sedative drugs, especially narcotic analgesics, causing excessive sedation.
- all atropinelike drugs, causing nervous system toxicity.

Trifluoperazine may ***decrease*** the effects of
- guanethidine (Ismelin, Esimil), reducing its effectiveness in lowering blood pressure.

Trifluoperazine ***taken concurrently*** with
- ascorbic acid (vitamin C) may blunt trifluoperazine's benefits.
- lithium (Lithobid, Lithotabs) may impair the effectiveness of lithium and cause nervous system toxicity.
- monoamine oxidase inhibitors (MAOIs) can increase the risk of extrapyramidal symptoms.
- oral hypoglycemic agents may blunt blood sugar control.

The following drugs may **decrease** the effects of trifluoperazine

- antacids containing aluminum and/or magnesium.
- barbiturates.
- benztropine (Cogentin).
- disulfiram (Antabuse).
- trihexyphenidyl (Artane).

Driving, Hazardous Activities: Can impair mental alertness, judgment, and physical coordination. Avoid hazardous activities.

Exposure to Sun: Use caution until your sensitivity has been determined. Some phenothiazines can cause photosensitivity.

Exposure to Heat: Use caution and avoid excessive heat as much as possible. This drug may impair body temperature regulation and increase the risk of heatstroke.

Exposure to Cold: Use caution and dress warmly. This drug can increase the risk of hypothermia in the elderly.

Discontinuation: After a period of long-term use, do not suddenly discontinue this drug. Gradual withdrawal over 2 to 3 weeks under your doctor's supervision is recommended. Do not stop taking this drug without your doctor's knowledge and approval.

▷ **Saving Money When Using This Medicine:**

- Many drugs are available to treat mental problems. Ask your doctor if this medicine offers the best balance of cost and outcome for you.
- A newly approved medicine appears to avoid the Parkinson-like problems of earlier antipsychotics.
- A generic form can be substituted for the brand name.

TRIMETHOPRIM (tri METH oh prim)

Prescription Needed: Yes   **Controlled Drug:** No   **Generic:** Yes

Brand Names: Bactrim [CD], Bactrim DS [CD], Bethaprim [CD], Comoxol [CD], Cotrim [CD], Proloprim, Septra [CD], Septra DS [CD], Trimpex, Uroplus DS [CD], Uroplus SS [CD]

Overview of BENEFITS versus RISKS

Possible Benefits	*Possible Risks*
EFFECTIVE TREATMENT OF INFECTIONS due to susceptible microorganisms	Rare blood cell disorders: megaloblastic anemia, methemoglobinemia, abnormally low white blood cell and platelet counts
Effective adjunctive prevention and treatment of *Pneumocystis carinii* pneumonia associated with AIDS	

▷ **Illness This Medication Treats:**
  (1) Certain urinary tract infections not complicated by the presence of kidney stones or urine flow obstructions. This drug is sometimes used to prevent the recurrence of such infections. (2) Some eye infections.

  Used in conjunction with dapsone (unlabeled) to treat *Pneumocystis carinii* pneumonia (PCP) in AIDS.

  As Combination Drug Product [CD]: This drug, available in combination with sulfamethoxazole—under the generic name co-trimoxazole in some countries—is very effective in treating certain urinary tract infections, middle ear infections, chronic bronchitis, acute enteritis, and pneumonia; also used as primary prevention and treatment of *Pneumocystis carinii* pneumonia associated with AIDS.

▷ **Typical Dosage Range:** (Dosage or schedule must be determined by the doctor for each individual.)
  Orally: 100 mg/12 hr for 10 days. For certain pneumonias, the same dose is given every 6 hours. The total daily dosage should not exceed 640 mg. Ophthalmic: One drop in the affected eye every 3 hours (up to six times daily) for 7 to 10 days.

▷ **Conditions Requiring Dosing Adjustments:**
  Liver function: Patients with both liver and renal compromise should use this drug with caution.
  Kidney function: Patients with mild kidney compromise can take the usual dose every 12 hours. Patients with moderate to severe kidney failure can take the usual dose every 18 hours. This drug is contraindicated for patients with severe or worsening kidney failure.

▷ **How Best to Take This Medicine:** May be taken without regard to meals. However, this drug may also be taken with or following food if necessary to reduce stomach irritation. The tablet may be crushed.

▷ **How Long This Medicine Is Usually Taken:** Continual use on a regular schedule for 7 to 14 days is usually necessary to determine the effectiveness of this drug in controlling responsive infections. The actual duration of use depends on the nature of the infection.

▷ **Tell Your Doctor Before Taking This Medicine If You:**
  • ever had an allergic reaction to it.
  • have an anemia due to folic acid deficiency or a history of folic acid deficiency.
  • have impaired liver or kidney function.
  • are pregnant or breast-feeding.

▷ **Possible Side Effects:** None with short-term use.

▷ **Possible Adverse Effects:**
  If any of the following develop, call your doctor promptly for guidance.

Author's note: Listed side effects are for oral or intravenous forms.

Some Mild Problems Drug Can Cause

Allergic reactions: skin rash, itching, drug fever.

Headache, abnormal taste, sore mouth or tongue, loss of appetite, nausea, vomiting, abdominal cramping, diarrhea.

Eye irritation (ophthalmic form).

Some Serious Problems Drug Can Cause

Allergic reactions: severe dermatitis with peeling of skin.

Blood cell disorders: megaloblastic anemia, methemoglobinemia, abnormally low white blood cell and platelet counts (all are rare).

Rare liver or kidney toxicity.

▷ *CAUTION*

1. Certain strains of bacteria that cause urinary tract infections can develop resistance to this drug. If you do not show significant improvement within 5 days, call your doctor.
2. Comply with your doctor's request for periodic blood counts during long-term therapy.
3. Safety and effectiveness of this drug for those under 2 months old have not been established.
4. The natural decline in liver and kidney function in those over 60 may require smaller doses. If you develop itching reactions in the genital or anal areas, tell your doctor promptly.
5. The dose must be decreased for patients with kidney compromise.

Advisability of Use During Pregnancy or If Breast-Feeding:

Pregnancy Category: C. Avoid use of this drug during the first 3 months and the last 2 weeks of pregnancy. Otherwise use only if clearly needed. Ask your doctor for guidance. Present in breast milk; avoid taking this drug or refrain from nursing.

▷ **Overdose Symptoms:** Headache, dizziness, confusion, depression, nausea, vomiting, bone marrow depression, possible liver toxicity with jaundice.

▷ **Possible Effects of Long-Term Use:** Impaired production of red and white blood cells and blood platelets.

▷ **Suggested Periodic Examinations While Taking This Drug:** (at doctor's discretion)

Complete blood cell counts.

▷ **While Taking This Drug the Following Apply:**

Beverages: May be taken with milk.

Other Drugs:

Trimethoprim may *increase* the effects of

- amantadine (Symmetrel), resulting in toxicity from both drugs.
- cyclosporine (Sandimmune), resulting in increased kidney toxicity.

- dapsone, resulting in toxicity from either drug.
- phenytoin (Dilantin), causing phenytoin toxicity.
- procainamide (Procan SR), resulting in procainamide toxicity.

The following drugs may **decrease** the effects of trimethoprim

- cholestyramine (Questran), and perhaps some other similar cholesterol-lowering medicines; may bind trimethoprim and blunt its therapeutic effects.
- rifampin (Rifadin, Rimactane).

▷ **Saving Money When Using This Medicine:**

- Many new drugs are available to treat infections. Ask your doctor if this medicine offers the best balance of cost and outcome for you.
- A generic form can be substituted for the brand name.
- Ask your doctor how soon your symptoms should improve, and what you should do if they don't. Treatment failures are more easily treated if addressed early.

VALPROIC ACID   (val PROH ik)

Prescription Needed: Yes   **Controlled Drug:** No   **Generic:** Yes

Brand Names: Depa, Depakene, Depakote (divalproex sodium), Deproic

---

Overview of BENEFITS versus RISKS

Possible Benefits	*Possible Risks*
EFFECTIVE CONTROL OF MULTIPLE SEIZURE TYPES: ABSENCE, TONIC-CLONIC, MYOCLONIC, PSYCHOMOTOR SEIZURES (adjunctively with other antiseizure drugs)	LIVER TOXICITY, infrequent but may be severe
	Rare lowered and impaired platelet function with risk of bleeding
HELPS CONTROL REFRACTORY MIGRAINES	Rare pancreatitis or liver toxicity
DIVALPROEX SODIUM HELPS MANIA	

▷ **Illness This Medication Treats:**

(1) Seizures: simple and complex absence (petit mal), tonic-clonic (grand mal), myoclonic, complex partial seizures (psychomotor, temporal lobe epilepsy); sometimes used adjunctively with other anticonvulsants as needed. (2) Divalproex sodium (Depakote) approved for use in treating mania.

▷ **Typical Dosage Range:** (Dosage or schedule must be determined by the doctor for each individual.)

Initially 15 mg per kilogram of body weight every 24 hours. The dose is increased cautiously by 5 to 10 mg per kilogram of body weight every 24 hours, every 7 days as needed and tolerated. *The usual daily dose is from 1000 to 1600 mg in divided doses.* The total daily dosage should not exceed 60 mg per kilogram of body weight.

▷ **Conditions Requiring Dosing Adjustments:**

Liver function: Blood levels should guide dosing. This drug can be a rare cause of fatal liver damage. This drug is not given to those with significant liver compromise.

Kidney function: No dosing changes are anticipated for patients with compromised kidneys.

▷ **How Best to Take This Medicine:** Best taken 1 hour before meals. However, it may be taken with or following food to prevent stomach irritation. Do not open regular capsule or crush tablet for administration. The sprinkle-capsule may be opened and the contents sprinkled on soft food. Do not administer the syrup in carbonated beverages; it may be diluted in water or milk.

▷ **How Long This Medicine Is Usually Taken:** Regular use for 2 weeks usually determines the effectiveness of this drug in reducing the frequency and severity of seizures. Long-term use (months to years) requires supervision and periodic evaluation. See your doctor regularly.

▷ **Tell Your Doctor Before Taking This Medicine If You:**

- ever had an allergic reaction to it.
- have active liver disease or a history of liver disease or impaired liver function.
- have an active bleeding disorder or a history of a bleeding disorder.
- are pregnant or planning pregnancy.
- have myasthenia gravis.
- are taking any anticoagulants; other anticonvulsants, or antidepressants, either tricyclics or MAO type A inhibitors (see Drug Classes).
- plan to have surgery or dental extraction soon.

▷ **Possible Side Effects:** Drowsiness and lethargy.

▷ **Possible Adverse Effects:**

If any of the following develop, call your doctor promptly for guidance.

Some Mild Problems Drug Can Cause

Allergic reaction: skin rash (rare).

Headache, dizziness, confusion, unsteadiness, slurred speech.

Nausea, diarrhea.

Temporary loss of scalp hair.

Some Serious Problems Drug Can Cause
Idiosyncratic reactions: bizarre behavior, hallucinations.
Drug-induced hepatitis with jaundice—children less than 2 years old have an increased risk of fatal liver toxicity.
Drug-induced pancreatitis.
Possible Reye's syndrome.
Reduced formation and impaired function of platelets, with increased risk of abnormal bleeding.
Rare pancreatitis, porphyria, or anemia.

▷ **Possible Effects on Sex Life:**   Altered timing and pattern of menstruation.
Female breast enlargement with milk production.
Decreased libido.
Decreased effectiveness of oral contraceptives.

▷ **Adverse Effects That May Mimic Natural Diseases or Disorders:**
Liver reactions may suggest viral hepatitis.

▷ *CAUTION*
1. The capsules and tablets should be swallowed whole without alteration, to avoid irritation of the mouth and throat.
2. This drug can impair normal blood clotting mechanisms. In the event of injury, dental extraction, or need for surgery, tell your doctor or dentist that you are taking this drug.
3. Because this drug can impair the normal function of blood platelets, avoid aspirin.
4. Over-the-counter drugs containing antihistamines (allergy and cold remedies, sleep aids) can enhance the sedative effects of this drug.
5. The concurrent use of aspirin with this drug can cause abnormal bleeding or bruising. Children with mental retardation, organic brain disease, or severe seizure disorders may be at increased risk for severe liver toxicity. Watch closely for development of fever that could indicate the onset of a drug-induced Reye's syndrome. Avoid concurrent use of clonazepam (Klonopin); the combined use could result in continuous petit mal episodes.
6. Those over 60 should start treatment with small doses and cautiously increase the dosage. Observe closely for excessive sedation, confusion, or unsteadiness that could predispose to falling and injury.
7. Dosing MUST be decreased for patients with liver compromise.

Advisability of Use During Pregnancy or If Breast-Feeding:
Pregnancy Category: D. Talk with your doctor about this drug's advantages and disadvantages. If it is used, keep the dose as low as possible. Present in breast milk in small amounts. Monitor the nursing

infant closely and discontinue taking this drug or nursing if adve
effects develop.

▷ **Overdose Symptoms:** Increased drowsiness, weakness, unsteadi
ness, confusion, stupor progressing to coma.

▷ **Suggested Periodic Examinations While Taking This Drug:** (at
doctor's discretion)
Complete blood cell counts and baseline liver function tests should be
done before treatment is started. During treatment, blood counts
should be repeated every month and liver function tests done every
2 months.

▷ **While Taking This Drug the Following Apply:**
Beverages: Do not administer the syrup in carbonated beverages; this
could liberate the valproic acid and irritate the mouth and throat.
This drug may be taken with milk.
Alcohol: Use extreme caution until the combined effects have been determined. Alcohol can increase the sedative effect of this drug. This
drug can increase the depressant effects of alcohol on brain function.
Other Drugs:
Valproic acid may *increase* the effects of
- anticoagulants (Coumadin, etc.), increasing the risk of bleeding.
More frequent INR (prothrombin time) tests are needed.
- antidepressants, both MAO type A inhibitors and tricyclics, causing
toxicity.
- phenobarbital, causing barbiturate intoxication.
- phenytoin (Dilantin), causing phenytoin toxicity.
Valproic acid *taken concurrently* with
- antacids (various) can blunt its therapeutic benefits. Separate the
doses by 2 hours.
- antiplatelet drugs—aspirin, dipyridamole (Persantine), sulfinpyrazone (Anturane)—may enhance inhibition of platelet function and
increase the risk of bleeding.
- carbamazepine (Tegretol) can change its blood levels. More fre
quent blood levels are needed.
- clonazepam (Klonopin) may result in repeat episodes of absence
seizures
- cyclosporine (Sandimmune) may increase the risk of liver toxicity.
- erythromycin (Ery-Tab, others) may increase the level of valproic
acid and result in toxicity.
- felbamate (Felbatol) can lead to increased valproic acid levels.
- isoniazid (INH) can cause valproic acid or isoniazid toxicity.
Driving, Hazardous Activities: May cause drowsiness, dizziness, or
confusion. Restrict your activities as necessary.

continuation: **Do not suddenly stop taking this drug.** Abrupt withdrawal can cause repetitive seizures that are difficult to control.

Saving Money When Using This Medicine:
- Many drugs are available to treat seizure disorders. Ask your doctor if this medicine offers the best balance of cost and outcome for you.
- A generic form can be substituted for the brand name.
- Blood levels are expensive. Make certain they are obtained at prudent, not excessive, intervals.

VANCOMYCIN (van koh MI sin)

Prescription Needed: Yes **Controlled Drug:** No **Generic:** No

Brand Names: Vancocin, Vancoled, Vancor

Overview of BENEFITS versus RISKS	
Possible Benefits	*Possible Risks*
HIGHLY EFFECTIVE IN TREATING ANTIBIOTIC-ASSOCIATED PSEUDOMEMBRANOUS COLITIS	Ringing in ears (tinnitus) Loss of hearing

▷ **Illness This Medication Treats:**
(1) Antibiotic-associated pseudomembranous colitis caused by *Clostridium difficile* when given in oral form; (2) enterocolitis caused by staphylococcal organisms; (3) a variety of serious infections, including methicillin-resistant *Staphylococcus aureus* (MRSA), when used in intravenous form.

▷ **Typical Dosage Range:** (Dosage or schedule must be determined by the doctor for each individual.)

Infants and Children: 10 mg per kilogram of body weight every 6 hours, for 5 to 10 days. The total daily dose should not exceed 2000 mg (2 g). Repeat course as necessary.

12 to 60 Years of Age: Pseudomembranous colitis: Oral: 125 mg every 6 hours, for 10 days. Repeat course as necessary.

Intravenously: Many clinicians use a loading dose of 15 mg per kilogram of body weight, and then calculate ongoing doses based on individual patient characteristics, the organism being treated, site of infection, and blood levels.

Over 60 Years of Age: Loading dose is the same as for 12 to 60 years of age and ongoing doses are adjusted to any age-related declines in kidney function.

▷ **Conditions Requiring Dosing Adjustments:**

Liver function: The liver is not involved in the elimination of vancomycin. Oral vancomycin is eliminated primarily in the feces.

Kidney function: Oral vancomycin is minimally absorbed, and dosing decreases are not needed. Intravenous dosing MUST be adjusted to any changes in kidney function, and laboratory tests for kidney function closely followed.

▷ **How Best to Take This Medicine:** Oral use: May be taken with or following food to reduce stomach irritation. Because of its unpleasant taste, the capsule should be swallowed whole without alteration. Use a measuring device to ensure accuracy of dose. Observe the expiration date.

Intravenous: The intravenous solution should be infused slowly in order to help avoid red man syndrome (see "Possible Adverse Effects," below).

▷ **How Long This Medicine Is Usually Taken:** Continual use on a regular schedule for 48 to 72 hours is usually necessary to determine the effectiveness of this drug in controlling colon infection. The course of oral treatment is 10 days. Intravenous use may depend on the site of infection. For example, bone infections may take 6 weeks to cure. See your doctor regularly.

▷ **Tell Your Doctor Before Taking This Medicine If You:**
- ever had an allergic reaction to it.
- have a history of Crohn's disease or ulcerative colitis.
- have impaired kidney function.
- have any degree of hearing loss.
- are taking cholestyramine (Questran) or colestipol (Colestid).

▷ **Possible Side Effects:** Bitter, unpleasant taste.

▷ **Possible Adverse Effects:**

If any of the following develop, call your doctor promptly **for guidance.**

Some Mild Problems Drug Can Cause

Allergic reactions: skin rash (with large doses or prolonged use). Nausea, vomiting.

Some Serious Problems Drug Can Cause

Allergic reactions: rare anaphylaxis. Serious skin changes, such as exfoliative dermatitis.

Ringing or buzzing in ears, sensation of ear fullness, loss of hearing.

Red man syndrome: excessive lowering of blood pressure, sudden rash on neck, chest, face, or extremities.

Dose- or nondose-dependent kidney toxicity.

CAUTION

1. Tell your doctor promptly about the development of fullness, ringing, or buzzing in either ear. This may indicate the onset of nerve damage that could lead to hearing loss.
2. Talking with your doctor before taking any medication to stop your diarrhea. The bacterial toxin that is causing your colitis is eliminated by diarrhea; arresting this could intensify and prolong your illness.
3. This drug is usually well tolerated in infants and children. Some cases may require doses up to 50 mg per kilogram of body weight daily.
4. Blood levels MUST be used to guide dosing for the intravenous forms, but are NOT needed for the oral form, as the oral form is not absorbed.
5. Those over 60 may be more susceptible to drug-induced hearing loss. Use the minimum course of treatment required.
6. Laboratory measures of kidney function should be routinely checked.

Advisability of Use During Pregnancy or If Breast-Feeding:

Pregnancy Category: B. Use this drug only if clearly needed. Ask your doctor for guidance. Present in breast milk; avoid taking this drug or refrain from nursing.

▷ **Overdose Symptoms:**   Possible nausea, vomiting, ringing in ears.

▷ **Suggested Periodic Examinations While Taking This Drug:** (at doctor's discretion)
Hearing tests, blood levels, and measures of kidney function. Complete blood counts.

▷ **While Taking This Drug the Following Apply:**

Beverages: May be taken with milk.

Alcohol: Use sparingly; alcohol may aggravate colitis.

Other Drugs:

The following drugs may ***decrease*** the effects of vancomycin

- cholestyramine (Questran).
- colestipol (Colestid).

Vancomycin ***taken concurrently*** with

- aminoglycoside antibiotics may increase the risk of toxicity to ears or kidneys.
- cyclosporine (Sandimmune) may increase toxicity risk.
- warfarin (Coumadin) may increase bleeding risk. Increased checks of INR (prothrombin time) are needed.

Discontinuation: To be determined by your doctor.

Special Storage Instructions: Refrigerate the oral solution.

Observe the Following Expiration Times: Provided on your prescription.

▷ **Saving Money When Using This Medicine:**
- Metronidazole, also used to treat *Clostridium difficile*, may be the drug of choice in early infections in people without multiple disease states. Ask your doctor if vancomycin offers the best balance of cost and outcome for you.
- Blood levels MUST be checked for the intravenous form.
- A generic form can be substituted for the brand name.
- Typically 10 days of therapy is needed for *Clostridium difficile* treatment. Ask your doctor how long your infection is usually treated.
- Ask your doctor about hearing tests if this medicine is to be combined with an aminoglycoside antibiotic.

VARICELLA VIRUS VACCINE (VAIR a cella)

Other Names: Chickenpox shot or chickenpox vaccine

Prescription Needed: Yes   **Controlled Drug:** No   **Generic:** No

Brand Names: Varivax

Overview of BENEFITS versus RISKS	
Possible Benefits	*Possible Risks*
PREVENTION OF VARICELLA (chickenpox)	Rare hypersensitivity Rash

▷ **Illness This Medication Treats:**
Prevention of chickenpox or varicella.

▷ **Typical Dosage Range:** (Dosage or schedule must be determined by the doctor for each individual.)
Infants and Children: Those 1 to 12 years old are given 0.5 ml.
Author's note: The Center for Disease Control's (CDC) Immunization Practices Committee has recommended that all children 12 to 18 months old should be given varicella vaccine if they have not had chickenpox. The vaccine is also recommended by the committee for children 19 months to 13 years old. Adults or adolescents who have not had chickenpox and are at risk for chickenpox exposure should also receive the vaccine.
12 to 55 Years of Age: Same as for infants and children, provided the patient has not had chickenpox.
Over 55 Years of Age: Not yet studied.

▷ **How Best to Take This Medicine: This vaccine is to be injected under the skin.** It may be given with measles, mumps, and rubella vaccine.

▷ **How Long This Medicine Is Usually Taken:** Exposure to chickenpox 5 years after vaccination may result in 20% of patients developing mild disease. More experience is needed before the question of repeat vaccination is answered.

Tell Your Doctor Before Taking This Medicine If You:
- had an allergic reaction to it.
- are allergic to eggs (the virus is grown on eggs).
- have a history of anaphylactic reaction to neomycin.
- have AIDS or an impaired immune system, leukemia, or a history of blood diseases.
- have untreated tuberculosis.
- are pregnant.
- have a condition that may require steroids.
- live with someone who has a depressed immune system (such as an AIDS patient), as you may be infectious to them.
- currently have an infection.

▷ **Possible Side Effects:** Pain at the vaccination site. Muscle aches, fever.

▷ **Possible Adverse Effects:**
If any of the following develop, call your doctor promptly for guidance.
Some Mild Problems This Drug Can Cause
Allergic reactions: swelling or redness.
Muscle aches or fever.
Varicella-like rash.
Chills or headache.
Rare joint pain.
Some Serious Problems This Drug Can Cause
Allergic reactions: rare anaphylactic reactions.
Very rare febrile seizures.
Herpes zoster.

▷ *CAUTION*
1. **DO NOT** give aspirin or other salicylates to patients who have received this vaccine for 6 weeks after the vaccination has been given. An increased risk of Reye's syndrome is associated with use of these medicines.
2. Safety and effectiveness of this vaccine for children less than 12 months old have not been established.

Advisability of Use During Pregnancy or If Breast-Feeding:
Pregnancy Category: C. The manufacturer says that the vaccine **should not** be given to pregnant women, and that pregnancy should be avoided for 3 months following vaccination. Presence in breast milk is expected. Avoid receiving this vaccine or refrain from nursing.

▷ **While Taking This Drug the Following Apply:**
Alcohol: An interaction is not expected, but excessive alcohol may blunt the immune response.

Other Drugs:

Varicella vaccine *taken concurrently* with

- acyclovir (Zovirax) may result in a blunted benefit from the vaccine.
- aspirin or other salicylates may increase the risk of Reye's syndrome. DO NOT take salicylates for 6 weeks following vaccination.
- corticosteroids may result in extreme reactions to the vaccine.
- immune globulins may result in a decreased beneficial response to the vaccine.
- immunosupressive agents (chemotherapy, corticosteroids, cyclosporine [Sandimmune]) may lead to extreme reactions to the vaccine.
- mesalamine (Asacol) may increase the risk of Reye's syndrome. DO NOT take salicylates for 6 weeks after receiving this vaccine.
- methotrexate can lead to extreme vaccine reactions.
- olsalazine (Dipentum) may increase the risk of Reye's syndrome. DO NOT take salicylates for 6 weeks after vaccination.
- valacyclovir (Valtrex) has not specifically been reported to blunt this vaccine's effect, but since it is converted into acyclovir in the body, this blunting effect is to be expected.

Author's note: There is now a Vaccine Adverse Event Reporting System (VAERS). The toll-free number is 1-800-822-7967.

Driving, Hazardous Activities: Caution: this medicine may make you feel lethargic for a few days.

▷ **Saving Money When Using This Medicine:**

- It is ALWAYS better to prevent a disease or condition than to have to treat it. Vaccination is clearly less expensive than the risk of complications or loss of work from a family wage-earner caring for a sick child. Additionally, avoiding chickenpox also avoids the risk of shingles (herpes zoster) in adults.

VENLAFAXINE (ven la FAX ene)

Prescription Needed: Yes   **Controlled Drug:** No   **Generic:** No

Brand Name: Effexor

Overview of BENEFITS versus RISKS	
Possible Benefits	*Possible Risks*
EFFECTIVE TREATMENT OF DEPRESSION	INCREASED BLOOD PRESSURE
BETTER SIDE EFFECT PROFILE THAN TRICYCLIC ANTIDEPRESSANTS	Seizures (rare)
	Constipation
	Increased heart rate
RAPID ONSET OF EFFECT	Increased serum lipids

▷ **Illness This Medication Treats:**
Depression.

▷ **Typical Dosage Range:** (Dosage or schedule must be determined by the doctor for each individual.)

Infants and Children: Safety and efficacy of this drug for those under 18 years old have not been established.

18 to 60 Years of Age: Therapy is started with 75 mg daily, given as 25-mg doses three times daily. If needed and tolerated, the dose may be increased at 4-day intervals up to a maximum of 225 mg/day. Some hospitalized patients have been given a maximum of 375 mg/day.

Over 60 Years of Age: Low starting doses and slow increases are indicated. Natural declines in kidney function may lead to drug accumulation at higher doses. This drug may worsen constipation.

▷ **Conditions Requiring Dosing Adjustments:**

Liver function: The total daily dose should be reduced by 50% for patients with moderate liver compromise. Further dose decreases and individualized dosing are indicated for patients with liver cirrhosis.

Kidney function: Patients with compromised kidneys (creatinine clearances of 10–70 ml/min) should take 75% of the usual daily dose.

▷ **How Best to Take This Medicine:** Food has no clinically significant effect on absorption.

▷ **How Long This Medicine Is Usually Taken:** Use on a regular schedule for 2 weeks usually determines the effectiveness of this drug in treating depression. Long-term use (months to years) requires your doctor's periodic evaluation of response and dosage adjustment.

▷ **Tell Your Doctor Before Taking This Medicine If You:**
- ever had an allergic reaction to it.
- are taking a monoamine oxidase inhibitor (MAOI).
- have a history of high blood pressure.
- have increased lipids or seizures.
- have a history of hypomania or mania.

▷ **Possible Side Effects:** Constipation or headache.

▷ **Possible Adverse Effects:**
If any of the following develop, call your doctor promptly for guidance.

Some Mild Problems Drug Can Cause
Palpitations.
Nausea or vomiting.
Dizziness (may ease over time).

Blurred vision.
Sweating or weight loss.
Some Serious Problems Drug Can Cause
Increased blood pressure.
Rare seizures.

▷ **Possible Effects on Sex Life:** Infrequent delayed orgasm, abnormal ejaculation, impotence, or erectile failure.

▷ **Possible Effects on Laboratory Tests:** Serum cholesterol: slight increases.

▷ *CAUTION*
1. This drug SHOULD NOT be taken within 14 days of the last dose of a monoamine oxidase (MAO) inhibitor drug (see Drug Classes).
2. The dose MUST be decreased for patients with kidney compromise. Ask your doctor if your dose has been decreased consistently with your degree of kidney compromise.

Advisability of Use During Pregnancy or If Breast-Feeding:
Pregnancy Category: C. Ask your doctor for guidance. Presence of this drug in breast milk is unknown. Monitor the nursing infant closely and discontinue taking this drug or nursing if adverse effects develop.

▷ **Overdose Symptoms:** Nausea, vomiting, constipation, or seizures.

▷ **Suggested Periodic Examinations While Taking This Drug:** (at doctor's discretion)
Blood pressure checks. A recent study found a relationship between depression and low bone mineral density. Periodic checks of bone mineral density are advised.

▷ **While Taking This Drug the Following Apply:**
Alcohol: May increase somnolence.
Marijuana Smoking: Additive somnolence.
Other Drugs:
Venlafaxine *taken concurrently* with
• beta-blockers (see Drug Classes) may increase this drug's effects. Dose changes may be needed for both medicines.
• calcium channel blockers (see Drug Classes) may lead to toxicity.
• cimetidine (Tagamet) may lead to venlafaxine toxicity.
• drugs with sedative properties will increase these effects.
• MAO inhibitors will lead to undesirable side effects, DO NOT combine.
• quinidine (Quinaglute, others) may lead to venlafaxine toxicity.
• tricyclic antidepressants (see Drug Classes) may lead to toxicity. Decreased doses may be needed.

- warfarin (Coumadin) may lead to bleeding. More frequent INR (prothrombin time) tests are needed.

Driving, Hazardous Activities: This medicine may cause somnolence; restrict your activities as needed.

Discontinuation: Talk to your doctor BEFORE discontinuing use of this medicine.

▷ **Saving Money When Using This Medicine:**

- Many new drugs are available to treat depression. Ask your doctor if this medicine offers the best balance of cost and outcome for you.
- Once your depression is under control, it may be possible to decrease the dose and gradually withdraw the medicine. Ask your doctor if he or she thinks this will be possible.
- Depression has recently been found to be associated with increased risk of osteoporosis. Talk with your doctor about exercise, risk factors, calcium supplements, and need for bone mineral density testing.

VERAPAMIL   (ver AP a mil)

Prescription Needed: Yes   **Controlled Drug:** No   **Generic:** Yes

Brand Names: Calan, Calan SR, Isoptin, Isoptin SR, Verelan

Controversies in Medicine: Results of several studies have indicated that medicines in this chemical family should NOT be used in some patients with extremely compromised hearts. Amlodipine (Norvasc) is the only calcium channel blocker that presently has data to show that it is SAFE, even in the most severely ill congestive heart failure patients. Amlodipine is the only calcium channel blocker to be FDA-approved as safe for use in treating hypertension or angina in patients who also have congestive heart failure. There have been several FDA hearings on calcium channel blockers in general.

One retrospective chart review yielded data showing that there was increased risk if nifedipine immediate-release forms were used for treating conditions other than angina in those over 71. There was a caution advised, but the form of nifedipine in question was not approved for uses other than angina. A recent FDA panel found medicines in this class to be safe and effective. A study of nearly 6,000 patients at Tel Aviv Medical Center found that there was no statistically significant risk of death in patients who took calcium channel blockers versus those who did not take these medicines.

```
┌─────────────────────────────────────────────────────────────┐
│              Overview of BENEFITS versus RISKS              │
│       Possible Benefits              Possible Risks         │
│  EFFECTIVE PREVENTION OF      Congestive heart failure      │
│    BOTH MAJOR TYPES OF        Low blood pressure            │
│    ANGINA                     Heart rhythm disturbance      │
│  EFFECTIVE CONTROL OF         Fluid retention               │
│    HEART RATE IN CHRONIC      Liver damage without jaundice │
│    ATRIAL FIBRILLATION AND      (very rare)                 │
│    FLUTTER                                                  │
│  EFFECTIVE PREVENTION OF                                    │
│    PAROXYSMAL ATRIAL                                        │
│    TACHYCARDIA (PAT)                                        │
│  EFFECTIVE TREATMENT OF                                     │
│    HYPERTENSION                                             │
└─────────────────────────────────────────────────────────────┘
```

▷ **Illness This Medication Treats:**

(1) Spontaneous angina pectoris due to coronary artery spasm (Prinz-metal's variant angina) not associated with exertion; (2) classical angina-of-effort (due to coronary atherosclerosis) not responding to other agents; (3) abnormally rapid heart rate due to chronic atrial fibrillation or flutter; (4) recurrent paroxysmal atrial tachycardia; and (5) primary hypertension.

▷ **Typical Dosage Range:** (Dosage or schedule must be determined by the doctor for each individual.)

Hypertension: Initially 80 mg three or four times daily. The dose may be increased gradually at 1- to 7-day intervals, as needed and toler-ated. The usual maintenance dose ranges from 240 mg to 480 mg daily, in three or four divided doses. The prolonged-action dosage forms permit once-a-day dosing. The total daily dosage should not exceed 360 mg.

Once-a-day treatment may be initiated with one prolonged-action capsule of 120 mg or one tablet of 180 mg.

▷ **Conditions Requiring Dosing Adjustments:**

Liver function: Blood levels should be obtained to guide dosing. For patients with liver compromise, the dose should be decreased to 20 to 50% of the usual dose and taken at the usual interval. Verapamil is a rare cause of liver damage, and patients should be monitored closely. EEG changes may provide an early indication of increasing blood levels.

Kidney function: For patients with severe compromise, decrease the dose by 50 to 75%. This drug should be used with caution by pa-tients with renal compromise.

▷ **How Best to Take This Medicine:**   Best taken with meals and with food at bedtime. The regular tablet may be crushed. The prolonged-action dosage forms (capsules and tablets) should be swallowed whole and not altered. Verelan capsules may be taken without regard to food intake.

▷ **How Long This Medicine Is Usually Taken:**   Regular use for 2 to 4 weeks usually determines the effectiveness of this drug in reducing the frequency and severity of angina. Reduction of elevated blood pressure may be apparent within the first 2 weeks. For long-term use (months to years), determine the smallest effective dose with your doctor's supervision and periodic evaluation. See your doctor regularly.

▷ **Tell Your Doctor Before Taking This Medicine If You:**
- ever had an allergic reaction to it.
- have active liver disease, impaired liver or kidney function, or a history of drug-induced liver damage.
- have a sick sinus syndrome and do not have an artificial pacemaker.
- have second- or third-degree heart block.
- have low blood pressure with systolic pressure below 90.
- ever had an unfavorable response to any calcium blocker.
- are currently taking any other drugs, especially digitalis or a beta-blocker.
- have had a recent stroke or heart attack, or a history of congestive heart failure or heart rhythm disorders.

▷ **Possible Side Effects:**   Low blood pressure, fluid retention. Numbness or coldness in the extremities.

▷ **Possible Adverse Effects:**
If any of the following develop, call your doctor promptly for guidance.
Some Mild Problems Drug Can Cause
Allergic reactions: skin rash, itching, aching joints.
Headache, dizziness, fatigue.
Nausea, indigestion, constipation.
Abnormal gum growth.
Some Serious Problems Drug Can Cause
Serious disturbances of heart rate and/or rhythm, congestive heart failure.
Drug-induced liver damage without jaundice (very rare).
Unmasking of parkinsonism.

▷ **Possible Effects on Sex Life:**   Altered timing and pattern of menstruation.
Male breast enlargement and tenderness (gynecomastia).
Impotence.

▷ *CAUTION*

1. Tell all doctors and dentists you visit that you are taking this drug. This medicine may have an antiplatelet effect and prolong bleeding. Note its use on your personal identification card.

2. You may use nitroglycerin and other nitrate drugs as needed to relieve acute episodes of angina pain. However, if your angina attacks are becoming more frequent or intense, notify your doctor promptly.

3. If this drug is used concurrently with a beta-blocker, you may develop excessively low blood pressure.

4. This drug may cause swelling of the feet and ankles; which may not be indicative of heart or kidney dysfunction.

5. Safety and effectiveness of this drug for those under 12 years old have not been established.

6. Those over 60 may be more susceptible to weakness, dizziness, fainting, and falling. Take the necessary precautions to prevent injury. Report promptly any changes in your pattern of thirst and urination.

7. The dose must be decreased for patients with liver or kidney compromise. Ask your doctor if your dose has been adjusted appropriately.

Advisability of Use During Pregnancy or If Breast-Feeding:
Pregnancy Category: C. Avoid using this drug during the first 3 months. Use verapamil during the last 6 months only if clearly needed. Ask your doctor for guidance. Probably present in breast milk; avoid taking this drug or refrain from nursing.

▷ **Overdose Symptoms:** Flushed and warm skin, sweating, light-headedness, irritability, rapid heart rate, low blood pressure, loss of consciousness.

▷ **Suggested Periodic Examinations While Taking This Drug:** (at doctor's discretion)
Evaluations of heart function, including electrocardiograms; liver and kidney function tests with long-term use.

▷ **While Taking This Drug the Following Apply:**
Foods: Avoid excessive salt intake.
Beverages: May be taken with milk.
Alcohol: Use with caution—alcohol may exaggerate the drop in blood pressure experienced by some people. Alcohol combined with verapamil may also cause abnormal alcohol elimination and prolong the blood level of alcohol.
Tobacco Smoking: Nicotine can reduce the effectiveness of this drug. Avoid all forms of tobacco.

Marijuana Smoking: Possible reduced effectiveness of this drug; mild to moderate increase in angina; changes in electrocardiogram, confusing interpretation.

Other Drugs:

Verapamil may *increase* the effects of

- carbamazepine (Tegretol), causing carbamazepine toxicity.
- digitoxin and digoxin, causing digitalis toxicity.

Verapamil *taken concurrently* with

- aspirin may result in bleeding.
- amiodarone (Cordarone) may result in cardiac arrest. DO NOT COMBINE.
- beta-blockers may adversely affect heart rate and rhythm. Careful monitoring by your doctor is necessary with concurrent use of these drugs.
- calcium supplements may blunt verapamil's therapeutic effects; take these drugs 2 hours apart.
- cyclosorine (Sandimmune) may result in cyclosporine toxicity and kidney compromise.
- dantrolene may depress the heart and cause increased potassium levels.
- disopyramide (Norpace) can lead to congestive heart failure.
- ethanol (alcohol) may result in abnormal elimination of ethanol and a prolonged blood level.
- lithium (Lithobid, others) may result in lithium toxicity and mania.
- NSAIDs (see Drug Classes) may blunt verapamil's therapeutic effect.
- phenytoin (Dilantin, others) may result in a decreased efficacy of verapamil.
- quinidine (Quinaglute, others) can result in quinidine toxicity.
- rifampin (Rifadin, others) may blunt verapamil's benefits.
- theophylline (Theo-Dur, others) can lead to theophylline toxicity.

The following drugs may *increase* the effects of verapamil

- cimetidine (Tagamet).
- tricyclic antidepressants (see Drug Classes).

Driving, Hazardous Activities: May cause dizziness. Restrict your activities as necessary.

Exposure to Sun: Use caution until your sensitivity has been determined. This drug may cause photosensitivity.

Exposure to Heat: Caution is advised. Hot environments can exaggerate the blood pressure–lowering effects of this drug. Observe for light-headedness or weakness.

Heavy Exercise or Exertion: This drug may allow you to be more active without resulting angina pain. Use caution and avoid excessive exercise that could impair heart function without warning pain.

Discontinuation: Do not abruptly discontinue taking this drug. Talk with your doctor about gradual withdrawal to prevent rebound angina.

▷ **Saving Money When Using This Medicine:**
- Many drugs are available to treat heart conditions and high blood pressure as well as calcium channel blockers,. Ask your doctor if this medicine offers the best balance of cost and outcome for you. Ask how often your blood pressure should be checked.
- A generic form can be substituted for the brand name.
- Ask your doctor about stress management and exercise programs available in your community.
- Ask your doctor if taking aspirin every other day to help prevent a heart attack makes sense for you.

WARFARIN (WAR far in)

Prescription Needed: Yes   **Controlled Drug:** No   **Generic:** Yes

Brand Names: Coumadin, Sofarin

Overview of BENEFITS versus RISKS

Possible Benefits	*Possible Risks*
EFFECTIVE PREVENTION OF BOTH ARTERIAL AND VENOUS THROMBOSIS	NARROW TREATMENT RANGE
EFFECTIVE PREVENTION OF EMBOLIZATION IN THROMBOEMBOLIC DISORDERS	Dose-related bleeding Rare skin and soft tissue hemorrhage with tissue death
HELPS PREVENT A REPEAT HEART ATTACK	
HELPS PREVENT STROKES IN PEOPLE WITH ATRIAL FIBRILLATION	

▷ **Illness This Medication Treats:**
(1) Acute thrombosis or thrombophlebitis of the deep veins; (2) acute pulmonary embolism resulting from blood clots that originate anywhere in the body; (3) atrial fibrillation, to prevent clotting inside the heart that could result in embolization of small clots to any part of the body; (4) acute myocardial infarction (heart attack), to prevent clotting and embolization and a repeat heart attack; (5) transient ischemic attack (TIA), to reduce the risk of repeated attacks or possible stroke; (6) mitral valve replacement; (7) prevents blood clots in the lung after hip replacement.

▷ **Typical Dosage Range:** (Dosage or schedule must be determined by the doctor for each individual.)

Initially 2 to 5 mg daily for 2 to 3 days. A large loading dose is inappropriate and may be hazardous. For maintenance, the dose is decided based on the INR (prothrombin time) response and the condition being treated or prevented. An INR of 2–3 is considered therapeutic for many situations.

▷ **Conditions Requiring Dosing Adjustments:**

Liver function: Blood testing (prothrombin times) should be obtained to guide dosing. This drug is contraindicated for patients with liver disease.

Kidney function: The kidneys are minimally involved in eliminating warfarin. This drug should be used with caution by patients with renal compromise, however, as it may cause microscopic kidney stones.

▷ **How Best to Take This Medicine:**   Preferably taken when the stomach is empty, and at the same time each day to ensure uniform results. The tablet may be crushed for administration.

▷ **How Long This Medicine Is Usually Taken:**   Continual use on a regular schedule for 3 to 5 days is usually necessary to determine the effectiveness of this drug in providing significant anticoagulation. An additional 10 to 14 days are required to determine the optimal maintenance dose for each individual. Long-term use (months to years) requires supervision and periodic evaluation. See your doctor regularly.

▷ **Tell Your Doctor Before Taking This Medicine If You:**
- ever had an allergic reaction to it.
- have an active peptic ulcer or ulcerative colitis.
- have had a recent stroke.
- are now taking *any other drugs*.
- are pregnant or planning pregnancy.
- have a history of a bleeding disorder.
- have high blood pressure.
- have abnormally heavy or prolonged menstrual bleeding.
- have diabetes.
- are using an indwelling catheter.
- have impaired liver or kidney function.
- plan to have surgery or dental extraction soon.

▷ **Possible Side Effects:**   Minor episodes of bleeding may occur even when dosage and INR (prothrombin times) are well within the recommended range.

▷ **Possible Adverse Effects:**
If any of the following develop, call your doctor promptly for guidance.
Some Mild Problems Drug Can Cause
Allergic reactions: skin rash, hives.
Loss of scalp hair.
Loss of appetite, nausea, vomiting, cramping, diarrhea.
Some Serious Problems Drug Can Cause
Allergic reaction: drug fever.
Idiosyncratic reactions: bleeding into skin and soft tissues causing gangrene of breast, toes, and localized areas anywhere (rare).
Abnormal bleeding from nose, gastrointestinal tract, urinary tract, or uterus.
Rare hemolytic anemia, sudden nerve damage, or kidney problems.

▷ **Adverse Effects That May Mimic Natural Diseases or Disorders:**
Drug-induced fever may suggest infection.

▷ **CAUTION**
1. Always carry a personal identification card that states *you are taking an anticoagulant drug.*
2. While taking this drug, always talk with your doctor *before* starting, changing the dosage schedule, or discontinuing any drug.
3. For those over 60, small doses are mandatory until individual sensitivity has been determined. Watch for indications of excessive drug effects: prolonged bleeding from shaving cuts, bleeding gums, bloody urine, rectal bleeding, excessive bruising.
4. This drug should NOT be used by people with liver disease.

Advisability of Use During Pregnancy or If Breast-Feeding:
Pregnancy Category: D. The manufacturers state this drug is contraindicated during entire pregnancy. Present in breast milk; avoid taking this drug or refrain from nursing.

▷ **Overdose Symptoms:** Episodes of bleeding from minor surface bleeding (nose, gums, small lacerations) to major internal bleeding: vomiting blood, bloody urine or stool.

▷ **Suggested Periodic Examinations While Taking This Drug:** (at doctor's discretion)
Regular determinations of INR (prothrombin time) is essential to safe dosage and proper control.
Urine analyses for blood.

▷ **While Taking This Drug the Following Apply:**
Foods: A larger intake than usual of foods rich in vitamin K may reduce this drug's effectiveness and make larger doses necessary. Foods rich in vitamin K include asparagus, bacon, beef liver, cab-

bage, cauliflower, fish, and green leafy vegetables, which should be avoided in large quantities.

Beverages: May be taken with milk.

Alcohol: Limit alcohol to one drink daily. Note: heavy drinkers with liver damage may be very sensitive to anticoagulants and require smaller than usual doses.

Tobacco Smoking: Heavy smokers may require relatively larger doses of this drug.

Other Drugs:

Warfarin may *increase* the effects of
- oral hypoglycemic agents (see Drug Classes).
- phenytoin (Dilantin).

The following drugs may *increase* the effects of warfarin
- acetaminophen (high dose).
- allopurinol (Zyloprim).
- amiodarone (Cordarone).
- androgens.
- aspirin and some other NSAIDs (see Drug Classes).
- carbamazepine (Tegretol).
- cephalosporins.
- chloral hydrate.
- cimetidine (Tagamet).
- ciprofloxacin and perhaps other quinolone antibiotics (see Drug Classes).
- clofibrate (Atromid-S).
- dextrothyroxine.
- disulfiram.
- erythromycins and other macrolides (see Drug Classes).
- fluconazole (Diflucan).
- fluvoxamine (Luvox).
- glucagon.
- influenza vaccine.
- itraconazole (Sporanox).
- ketoconazole (Nizoral).
- metronidazole (Flagyl).
- miconazole (Monistat).
- NSAIDs.
- omeprazole (Prilosec).
- pravastatin (Pravachol).
- quinidine.
- raniditine (Zantac).
- salicylates.
- sertraline (Zoloft).
- simvastatin (Zocor).

- sulfinpyrazone.
- sulfonamides.
- thyroid hormones.
- vancomycin (Vancoled).
- vitamin E.

The following drugs may *decrease* the effects of warfarin

- azathioprine (Imuran).
- barbiturates.
- carbamazepine (Tegretol).
- cholestyramine (Questran).
- ethchlorvynol.
- glutethimide.
- griseofulvin (Gris-PEG).
- oral contraceptives (birth control pills).
- phytonadione (vitamin K).
- rifampin.
- sucralfate (Carafate).

Discontinuation: Do not abruptly discontinue taking this drug unless abnormal bleeding occurs. Talk with your doctor about gradual reduction in dosage over a period of 3 to 4 weeks.

▷ **Saving Money When Using This Medicine:**

- Ask your doctor if this medicine offers the best balance of cost and outcome for you.
- A generic form can be substituted for the brand name.
- Ask your doctor how long this medicine is usually used to treat your condition.
- INR (prothrombin time) testing is expensive. Make certain that testing is performed at prudent, not excessive, intervals.
- Data for the Agency for Health Care Policy and Research have shown that expanded use of this medicine could cut in half the 80,000 strokes that occur each year in atrial fibrillation patients.

ZALCITABINE (zal SIT a been)

Other Names: Didcoxycytidine, DDC

Prescription Needed: Yes   **Controlled Drug:** No   **Generic:** No

Brand Names: HIVID

```
┌─────────────────────────────────────────────────────────────┐
│              Overview of BENEFITS versus RISKS               │
│      Possible Benefits              Possible Risks           │
│   DELAYED PROGRESSION OF       DRUG-INDUCED                  │
│     DISEASE IN HIV-INFECTED      PERIPHERAL NEURITIS         │
│     INDIVIDUALS WITH AIDS      Drug-induced pancreatitis     │
│     OR AIDS-RELATED              (rare)                      │
│     COMPLEX                    Drug-induced esophageal ulcers│
│                                 (rare)                       │
│                                Drug-induced                  │
│                                 cardiomyopathy/congestive    │
│                                 heart failure (rare)         │
│                                Drug-induced arthritis        │
└─────────────────────────────────────────────────────────────┘
```

▷ **Illness This Medication Treats:**
  Combination therapy (with zidovudine) of advanced (CD4 cell count less than or equal to 300 cells per cubic millimeter) HIV infection. This is not a cure for AIDS, and does not reduce the risk of transmitting HIV infection to others through sexual contact or contamination of body fluids, such as blood or urine.

▷ **Typical Dosage Range:** (Dosage or schedule must be determined by the doctor for each individual.)
  Infants and Children: Under investigation.
  12 to 60 Years of Age: The recommended combination regimen is one 0.75-mg tablet orally to be taken with 200 mg of zidovudine every 8 hours. The total daily dose for both drugs then becomes 2.25 mg of zalcitabine and 600 mg of zidovudine. The initial dose does not need to be reduced unless the patient weighs less than 30 kg (66 lb).

▷ **Conditions Requiring Dosing Adjustments:**
  Liver function: Liver toxicity may be more likely in people with a prior history of alcohol abuse or liver damage. The patient should be monitored closely, and the dosage reduced or the medication interrupted if toxicity occurs.
  Kidney function: People with moderate kidney failure can take 0.75 mg of zalcitabine every 12 hours. Patients with severe kidney failure can take 0.75 mg every 24 hours.

▷ **How Best to Take This Medicine:** For combination therapy dose adjustments must be based on the toxicity profiles for each drug. For example: if tingling and numbness of the hands (peripheral neuropathy) or severe mouth ulcers occur, the zalcitabine dose should be decreased or interrupted. Additionally, with anemia or low white blood cells (granulocytopenia), the zidovudine dose should be decreased or interrupted.
  If the zalcitabine is interrupted or stopped, the zidovudine dose should be changed from 200 mg/8 hr to 100 mg/4 hr. Zalcitabine is

not indicated alone. If zalcitabine is stopped, your doctor **must** consider other antiretroviral therapy. The largest peak concentration, the time it takes to achieve the peak, and the amount absorbed all change if this drug is taken with food. It is better to take it on an empty stomach.

▷ **How Long This Medicine Is Usually Taken:** Continual use on a regular schedule for several months is usually necessary to determine the effectiveness of this drug in slowing the progression of AIDS. Long-term use (months to years) requires your doctor's periodic evaluation.

▷ **Tell Your Doctor Before Taking This Medicine If You:**
- ever had an allergic reaction to it.
- have had pancreatitis recently.
- had allergic reactions to any drugs in the past.
- are currently taking any other drugs.
- have a history of pancreatitis or peripheral neuritis.
- have a history of alcoholism.
- have impaired liver or kidney function.

▷ **Possible Side Effects:** Mild and infrequent decreases in red blood cell, white blood cell, and platelet counts.

▷ **Possible Adverse Effects:**
If any of the following develop, call your doctor promptly for guidance.
Some Mild Problems Drug Can Cause
  Allergic reactions: skin rash and itching.
  Fever, joint pains.
  Mouth sores, nausea, vomiting, stomach pain.
Some Serious Problems Drug Can Cause
  Drug-induced peripheral neuritis, usually occurring after 7 to 18 weeks of treatment; more frequent and severe with high doses, and less frequent and mild with low doses.
  Drug-induced cardiomyopathy/congestive heart failure (rare).
  Drug-induced pancreatitis, usually within the first 6 months of treatment (rare).
  Rare electrolyte changes.
  Rare hearing toxicity.
  Worsening of preexisting liver disease or hepatoxicity in patients with a history of alcohol abuse.

▷ *CAUTION*
  1. This drug does not cure HIV infection or reduce the risk of transmitting infection to others through sexual contact or contamination of blood.
  2. Report promptly the development of stomach pain with nausea

and vomiting; this could indicate the onset of pancreatitis. It may be necessary to discontinue this drug.

3. Report promptly the development of pain, numbness, tingling, or burning in the hands or feet; this could indicate the onset of peripheral neuritis. It may be necessary to discontinue this drug.

4. Avoid all other drugs known to cause pancreatitis or peripheral neuritis; ask your doctor for guidance.

5. Safety and effectiveness of this drug in infants or children have not been established. Children may also be at risk for drug-induced pancreatitis and peripheral neuritis; monitor closely for significant symptoms.

6. The natural decline in kidney function in those over 60 may require dosage reduction.

7. Dosage of this drug must be decreased for people with compromised kidneys.

Advisability of Use During Pregnancy or If Breast-Feeding:
Pregnancy Category: C. Ask your doctor for specific guidance. Presence in breast milk is unknown; avoid taking this drug or refrain from nursing.
Note: HIV has been found in human breast milk. Breast-feeding may result in its transmission to the nursing infant.

▷ **Overdose Symptoms:** Nausea, vomiting, stomach pain, diarrhea, pain in hands and feet.

▷ **Suggested Periodic Examinations While Taking This Drug:** (at doctor's discretion)
Complete blood cell counts before starting treatment and weekly thereafter until tolerance is established.
Blood amylase levels, fractionated for salivary gland and pancreatic origin.
Triglyceride levels should be tested at baseline (before therapy is started) and periodically thereafter.
Assessment of CD4 counts.
Measurement of viral burden or load.

▷ **While Taking This Drug the Following Apply:**
Other Drugs:
Zalcitabine may *increase* the effects of
• zidovudine (Retrovir), enhancing its antiviral effect against HIV.
Zalcitabine *taken concurrently* with
• cimetidine (Tagamet) may lead to toxic zalcitabine levels.
• didanosine (Videx) may result in additive nerve toxicity.
• metoclopramide (Reglan) may decrease zalcitabine's benefits.
• other medicines toxic to nerves or the pancreas may lead to additive toxicity. These are best avoided.
• probenecid (Benemid) may lead to zalcitabine toxicity.

Driving, Hazardous Activities: May cause pain and weakness in the extremities. Restrict your activities as necessary.

Discontinuation: Do not stop taking this drug without your doctor's knowledge and guidance.

▷ **Saving Money When Using This Medicine:**
- Several new drugs are now available to treat AIDS. Ask your doctor if this medicine offers the best balance of cost and outcome for you.
- Ask your doctor about combination drug therapy, and use of viral load and CD4 counts to check the success of treatment.

ZIDOVUDINE (zi DOH vyoo deen)

Other Names: AZT, azidothymidine, Compound S, ZDV

Prescription Needed: Yes   **Controlled Drug:** No   **Generic:** No

Brand Names: Retrovir

Overview of BENEFITS versus RISKS	
Possible Benefits	*Possible Risks*
DELAYED PROGRESSION OF DISEASE IN HIV-INFECTED INDIVIDUALS	SERIOUS BONE MARROW DEPRESSION
DECREASED OCCURRENCE OF INFECTIONS IN HIV-POSITIVE PATIENTS WHEN USED AS PART OF COMBINATION THERAPY	Brain toxicity
HELPS AVOID MOTHER-TO-INFANT INFECTION DURING BIRTH	Lip, mouth, and tongue sores

▷ **Illness This Medication Treats:**
(1) AIDS or AIDS-related complex (ARC) caused by HIV. This is not a cure for AIDS, and does not reduce the risk of transmitting AIDS infection to others through sexual contact or contamination of body fluids such as blood or urine. (2) Prevention of transmission of HIV from mother to infant; (3) combination therapy with other antiretrovirals that work by other mechanisms.

▷ **Typical Dosage Range:** (Dosage or schedule must be determined by the doctor for each individual.)

For asymptomatic HIV infection: 100 mg/4 hr while awake (500 mg/day).

For symptomatic HIV infection: Initially 200 mg/4 hours five times a day or 200 mg every 8 hours; this is used unless HIV encephalopathy is present. Some clinicians suggest a maximum daily dose of 400 to 600 mg.

For prevention of mother-to-infant infection: 100 mg by mouth five times per day until the start of labor. During labor: intravenous AZT 2 mg per kilogram of body weight followed by 1 mg per kilogram of body weight per hour, continued until the umbilical cord is clamped. The infant then receives 1.5 mg per kilogram of body weight every 6 hours.

Author's note: Many clinicians now start therapy with combination treatment once the infection is diagnosed.

▷ **Conditions Requiring Dosing Adjustments:**

Liver function: The dose should be decreased by 50% or the dosing interval doubled for patients with significant liver compromise. This drug can be a rare cause of liver damage, and patients should be closely monitored.

Kidney function: No specific guidelines for dosage adjustments in patients with compromised kidneys are available. This drug should be used with caution by patients with renal compromise.

▷ **How Best to Take This Medicine:**   Preferably taken on an empty stomach, but this drug may be taken with or following food. Take this drug exactly as prescribed. The capsule may be opened and the contents mixed with food just prior to administration. It is best to take it with 120 ml of water and not lie down for half an hour to help avoid esophageal ulcers.

▷ **How Long This Medicine Is Usually Taken:**   Continual use on a regular schedule for 10 to 12 weeks is usually necessary to determine the effectiveness of this drug in improving the course of symptomatic AIDS infection. Long-term use requires periodic evaluation of response and dosage adjustment. Many clinicians now use CD4 and viral load to assess the success of treatment. See your doctor regularly.

▷ **Tell Your Doctor Before Taking This Medicine If You:**
- ever had an allergic reaction to it.
- have a serious degree of uncorrected bone marrow depression.
- have a history of either folic acid or vitamin B12 deficiency.
- have impaired liver or kidney function.

▷ **Possible Adverse Effects:**

If any of the following develop, call your doctor promptly for guidance.

Some Mild Problems Drug Can Cause

Allergic reactions: skin rash, hives, itching.

Headache, weakness, drowsiness, dizziness, nervousness, insomnia.

Nausea, diarrhea, loss of appetite and vomiting, altered taste, li sores, swollen mouth or tongue.

Muscle aches, fever, sweating.

Some Serious Problems Drug Can Cause

Loss of speech, twitching, tremors, seizures (representing brain toxicity).

Bone marrow depression: fatigue, weakness, fever, sore throat, abnormal bleeding or bruising. Anemia is most common after 4 to 6 weeks of treatment; abnormally low white blood cell counts occur after 6 to 8 weeks of treatment.

Esophageal ulcers or liver toxicity.

▷ **Possible Delayed Adverse Effects:** Significant anemia and deficient white blood cell counts may develop after discontinuation.

▷ **Adverse Effects That May Mimic Natural Diseases or Disorders:** Seizures may suggest the possibility of epilepsy.

▷ *CAUTION*

1. This drug is not a cure for AIDS or AIDS-related complex, nor does it protect completely against other infections or complications. Follow your doctor's instructions and take all medications exactly as prescribed.

2. This drug does not reduce the risk of transmitting AIDS to others through sexual contact or contamination of body fluids such as blood or urine. The use of an effective condom is mandatory. Needles for drug administration should not be shared.

3. Zidovudine syrup can be used in HIV-infected patients who are older than 3 months old. The usual dose is 180 mg per square meter of body surface.

4. The natural decline in kidney function in those over 60 requires dosage reduction.

5. Doses MUST be decreased for patients with liver compromise.

Advisability of Use During Pregnancy or If Breast-Feeding:

Pregnancy Category: C. Ask your doctor for specific guidance. If you are using zidovudine during pregnancy to prevent transmission from the mother to infant, it is best to call 1-800-722-9292, ext. 8465, to report your case. Presence of this drug in breast milk is unknown; avoid taking this drug or refrain from nursing.

▷ **Overdose Symptoms:** Nausea, vomiting, diarrhea, bone marrow depression.

▷ **Possible Effects of Long-Term Use:** Serious anemia and loss of white blood cells.

▷ **Suggested Periodic Examinations While Taking This Drug:** (at doctor's discretion)

Complete blood cell counts before starting treatment and weekly thereafter until tolerance is established. Continual monitoring for bone marrow depression is necessary during the entire course of treatment.

Periodic CD4 or viral load to check the success of therapy.

▷ **While Taking This Drug the Following Apply:**

Beverages: May be taken with milk.

Other Drugs:

The following drugs may *increase* the effects of zidovudine and enhance its toxicity:

- acetaminophen.
- acyclovir (Zovirax).
- aspirin.
- benzodiazepines.
- cimetidine (Tagamet).
- fluconazole (Diflucan).
- ganciclovir.
- indomethacin and other NSAIDs (see Drug Classes).
- interferon beta.
- morphine.
- probenecid.
- sulfonamides.

Zidovudine *taken concurrently* with

- didanosine may increase the risk of myelosuppression.
- filgrastim (Neupogen) may help maintain the white blood cell count.
- rifampin (Rifadin) can lead to decreased zidovudine blood levels and blunting of its therapeutic effect.
- trimetrexate can lead to additive blood toxicity.

Driving, Hazardous Activities: May cause dizziness or fainting. Restrict your activities as necessary.

Discontinuation: Do not stop taking this drug without your doctor's knowledge and guidance.

▷ **Saving Money When Using This Medicine:**

- Several new drugs are available to treat AIDS. Ask your doctor if this medicine offers the best balance of cost and outcome for you. Also ask about using viral load to check the continued success of treatment.
- Ask your doctor if combination therapy would be advisable.

ZOLPIDEM (ZOL pi dem)

Prescription Needed: Yes   **Controlled Drug:** C-IV*   Generic: No

Brand Names: Ambien

Overview of BENEFITS versus RISKS	
Possible Benefits	*Possible Risks*
SHORT-TERM RELIEF OF INSOMNIA WITH MINIMAL SLEEP DISRUPTION (REM)	Habit-forming potential with prolonged use Rebound insomnia upon withdrawal

▷ **Illness This Medication Treats:**
Short-term treatment of insomnia in adults.

▷ **Typical Dosage Range:** (Dosage or schedule must be determined by the doctor for each individual.)
Infants and Children: Safety and efficacy of this drug for those under 18 years old are not established.
18 to 60 Years of Age: 10 mg taken immediately before bedtime. Patients should be reevaluated after 10 days.
Over 60 Years of Age: Start with 5 mg taken at bedtime; cautiously increase dose to 10 mg at bedtime.

▷ **Conditions Requiring Dosing Adjustments:**
Liver function: The dose should be reduced by 50% for patients with liver compromise.
Kidney function: This drug may take twice as long as normal to be eliminated in people with compromised kidneys. The dose must be decreased.

▷ **How Best to Take This Medicine:** The tablet may be crushed and is best taken on an empty stomach. Do NOT abruptly discontinue this drug if taken for more than 7 days.

▷ **How Long This Medicine Is Usually Taken:** Use on a regular schedule for two nights usually determines the effectiveness of this drug in treating insomnia. Your doctor should assess the benefit after 10 days.

▷ **Tell Your Doctor Before Taking This Medicine If You:**
- ever had an allergic reaction to it.
- have abnormal liver or kidney function
- are pregnant or planning pregnancy.
- have a history of alcoholism or drug abuse.
- have a history of serious depression or mental disorder.

*See Controlled Drug Schedules inside this book's cover.

Possible Side Effects: Drowsiness and blurred vision; "hangover" effects following long-term use.

> **Possible Adverse Effects:**

If any of the following develop, call your doctor promptly for guidance.

Some Mild Problems Drug Can Cause
  Allergic reactions: skin rash.
  Drowsiness and dizziness.
  Nausea and diarrhea.
  Muscle tremors (infrequent).
  Blurred vision (infrequent).

Some Serious Problems Drug Can Cause
  Abnormal thoughts or hallucinations (infrequent).
  Rare elevation of liver function tests.
  Paradoxical aggression, agitation, or suicidal thoughts.

▷ **CAUTION**
  1. This drug works quickly. It is best to take it just before bedtime.
  2. Do NOT drink alcohol while taking this drug.
  3. Withdrawal may occur even if this drug is only taken for a week or two. Ask your doctor for advice before stopping zolpidem.
  4. You may experience trouble sleeping for one or two nights after stopping (rebound insomnia). This effect is usually short-term.
  5. Sleep disturbances may be a symptom of underlying psychological problems. Tell your doctor if unusual behaviors or odd thoughts occur.
  6. Drugs that depress the central nervous system may produce additive effects. Ask your doctor or pharmacist BEFORE combining other drugs with zolpidem.
  7. Safety and effectiveness of this drug for those under 18 years old are not established.
  8. For those over 60, the starting dose should be decreased to 5 mg. Since this drug works quickly, it is best taken immediately before going to bed. You may be at increased risk for falls if the drug remains in your system in the morning. Watch for lethargy, unsteadiness, nightmares, and paradoxical agitation and anger.
  9. The dose MUST be decreased for people with compromised livers or kidneys.

Advisability of Use During Pregnancy or If Breast-Feeding:
Pregnancy Category: B. Usage of this drug during pregnancy is NOT advisable. Ask your doctor for guidance. Present in breast milk; avoid taking this drug or refrain from nursing.

▷ **Habit-Forming Potential:**   May cause dependence.

▷ **Overdose Symptoms:** Marked change from lethargy to coma. diovascular and respiratory compromise were also repor Flumazenil may help reverse symptoms.

▷ **Suggested Periodic Examinations While Taking This Drug:** (doctor's discretion)
Liver function tests.

▷ **While Taking This Drug the Following Apply:**
Foods: Should NOT be taken with food.
Beverages: Avoid caffeine-containing beverages: coffee, tea, cola, chocolate.
Alcohol: This drug should NOT be combined with alcohol.
Tobacco Smoking: Nicotine is a stimulant and should be avoided.
Marijuana Smoking: May cause additive drowsiness.
Other Drugs:
Zolpidem may ***increase*** the effects of
- chlorpromazine (Thorazine).
- narcotics or other CNS depressants (see Drug Classes for benzodiazepines, opioids, and phenothiazines).

Driving, Hazardous Activities: May cause drowsiness and impair coordination. Restrict your activities as necessary.
Discontinuation: This drug should NOT be abruptly discontinued, even after a week of use. Ask your doctor for an appropriate withdrawal schedule.

▷ **Saving Money When Using This Medicine:**
- Many drugs are available to treat insomnia. Ask your doctor if this medicine offers the best balance of cost and outcome for you.
- This drug is indicated for SHORT-TERM therapy.
- Ask your doctor about the effects that diet; prescription, nonprescription, or herbal medicines; caffeine; late exercise; or stress may be having on your sleep. Ask if stress management and exercise programs available in your community are a good idea for you.

DRUG CLASSES

Many of the drug profiles refer to various drug classes. Medicines in a particular class are closely related in chemical composition. To prevent interactions it is important to know that *any* drug (or *all* drugs) within a given class may behave in a particular way.

Each class is organized with the broad drug class name followed by an alphabetic listing of its generic drugs. After each generic name (in parentheses) are some of its most common brand names. Some medications have so many brand names that a complete listing is not possible. If this happens with your medicine, call your pharmacist or doctor to get its generic name and check the master list to see if it is included.

ADRENOCORTICAL STEROIDS *(Cortisonelike Drugs)*

amcinonide (Cyclocort)
beclomethasone (Beclovent, Vanceril)
betamethasone (Celestone)
budesonide (Rhinocort)
cortisone (Cortone)
dexamethasone (Decadron)
fludrocortisone (Florinef)
flunisolide (AeroBid, Nasarel)
fluorometholone (FML)
fluticasone (Flonase)
halcinonide (Halog)
halobetasol (Ultravate)
hydrocortisone (Cortef)
medrysone (HMS ophthalmic suspension)
methylprednisolone (Medrol)
mometasone (Elocon)
paramethasone (Haldrone)
prednisolone (Delta-Cortef)
prednisone (Deltasone)
rimexalone (Vexol)
triamcinolone (Aristocort, Azmacort)

ALPHA GLUCOSIDASE INHIBITOR

acarbose (Precose)

AMEBICIDES *(Anti-Infectives)*

chloroquine (Aralen)
emetine (no brand name)
iodoquinol (Yodoxin)
metronidazole (Flagyl)
paromomycin (Humatin)

Drug Classes

AMINOGLYCOSIDES (*Anti-Infectives*)

amikacin (Amikin)
gentamicin (Garamycin)
kanamycin (Kantrex)
neomycin (Mycifradin,
  Neobiotic)

paromomycin (Humatin)
tobramycin (Nebcin)

AMPHETAMINELIKE DRUGS

amphetamine (no brand name)
benzphetamine (Didrex)
dextroamphetamine (Dexedrine)
diethylpropion (Tenuate,
  Tepanil)
methamphetamine (Desoxyn)
methylphenidate (Ritalin)

phendimetrazine (Anorex,
  Plegine)
phenmetrazine (Preludin)
phentermine (Fastin, Ionamin)
phenylpropanolamine
  (Dexatrim)

ANALGESICS, MILD

acetaminophen (Datril, Tylenol)
aspirin

lidocaine/prilocaine cream
  (Emla)

See Nonsteroidal Anti-Inflammatory Drugs (NSAIDs).

ANDROGENS (*Male Sex Hormones*)

fluoxymesterone (Halotestin)
methyltestosterone (Android,
  Metandren, Oreton)

testosterone (Depotest, Testone)

ANGIOTENSIN-CONVERTING ENZYME (ACE) INHIBITORS

benazepril (Lotensin)
captopril (Capoten)
enalapril (Vasotec)
fosinopril (Monopril)
lisinopril (Prinivil, Zestril)

moexipril (Univasc)
quinapril (Accupril)
ramipril (Altace)
spirapril (Renormax)

ANGIOTENSIN II RECEPTOR ANTAGONIST

losartan (Cozar)

ANOREXIANTS (*Appetite Suppressants*)

dexfenfluramine (Redux)
fenfluramine (Pondimin)

mazindol (Mazanor, Sanorex)

See also Amphetaminelike Drugs.

ANTI-ACNE DRUGS

benzoyl peroxide (Epi-Clear, others)

erythromycin (Eryderm)

isotretinoin (Accutane)

tetracycline (Achromycin V)

tretinoin (Retin-A)

ANTI-AIDS DRUGS

didanosine (DDI, Videx)

indinavir (Crixivan)

lamivudine (3TC)

nevirapine (Viramune)

saquinavir (Invirase)

stavudine (Zerit)

zalcitabine (dideoxycytidine, DDC, HIVID)

zidovudine (AZT, Retrovir)

ANTIALCOHOLISM DRUGS

disulfiram (Antabuse)

naltrexone (ReVia, Trexan)

ANTI-ALZHEIMER'S DRUGS

tacrine (Cognex)

ANTIANGINAL DRUGS

Beta-Adrenergic–Blocking Class

bepridil (Vascor)

Calcium-Channel–Blocking Class

diltiazem (Cardizem)

nicardipine (Cardene)

nifedipine (Adalat, Procardia)

nitrates

verapamil (Calan, Isoptin)

ANTIANXIETY DRUGS (*Minor Tranquilizers*)

buspirone (BuSpar)

chlormezanone (Trancopal)

hydroxyzine (Atarax, Vistaril)

lorazepam (Ativan)

meprobamate (Equanil, Miltown)

See also Benzodiazepines.

ANTIARRHYTHMIC DRUGS (*Heart Rhythm Regulators*)

acebutolol (Sectral)

amiodarone (Cordarone)

digitoxin (Crystodigin)

digoxin (Lanoxin)

disopyramide (Norpace)

flecainide (Tambocor)

mexiletine (Mexitil)

procainamide (Procan SR, Pronestyl)

propafenone (Rythmol)

propranolol (Inderal)
quinidine (Quinaglute,
  Quinidex, Quinora)

tocainide (Tonocard)
verapamil (Calan, Isoptin)

ANTIASTHMATIC DRUGS

Bronchodilators

albuterol (Proventil, Ventolin)
aminophylline (Phyllocontin)
bitolterol (Tornalate)
dyphylline (Lufyllin)
ephedrine (Efed II)
epinephrine (Adrenalin,
  Bronkaid Mist, Primatene
  Mist)
ipratropium
isoetharine (Bronkosol,
  Dey-Lute)

isoproterenol (Isuprel)
metaproterenol (Alupent,
  Metaprel)
oxtriphylline (Choledyl)
pirbuterol (Maxair)
salmeterol (Serevent)
terbutaline (Brethaire, Brethine,
  Bricanyl)
theophylline (Bronkodyl,
  Elixophyllin, Slo-Phyllin,
  others)

Mast Cell Stabilizing Agents

cromolyn sodium (Gastrocom,
  Intal)

nedocromil (Tilade)

Anti-Inflammatory Agents

corticosteroids

ANTIBIOTICS

See specific antibiotic class (Cephalosporins, Penicillins,
Tetracyclines, etc.).

ANTIBIOTICS, TOPICAL

mupirocin (Bactroban)

ANTICHOLINERGIC DRUGS *(Atropinelike Drugs)*

atropine
belladonna
hyoscyamine
scopolamine
antidepressants, tricyclic (see
  class below)
antihistamines, some (see class
  below)

antiparkinsonism drugs, some
  (see class below)
antispasmodics, synthetic, some
  (see class below)
muscle relaxants, some (see
  class below)

ANTICOAGULANT DRUGS

anisindione (Miradon)
dicumarol (no brand name)

warfarin (Coumadin)

ANTICONVULSANT DRUGS *(Antiepileptic Drugs)*

acetazolamide (Diamox)
carbamazepine (Tegretol)
clonazepam (Klonopin)
clorazepate (Tranxene)
diazepam (Valium)
ethosuximide (Zarontin)
ethotoin (Peganone)
felbamate (Felbatol)
gabapentin (Neurontin)
lamotrigine (Lamictal)

mephenytoin (Mesantoin)
methsuximide (Celontin)
paramethadione (Paradione)
phenacemide (Phenurone)
phenobarbital (Luminal)
phensuximide (Milontin)
phenytoin (Dilantin)
primidone (Mysoline)
trimethadione (Tridione)
valproic acid (Depakene)

ANTI-CYSTIC FIBROSIS AGENTS *(Recombinant DNase)*

dornase alfa (Pulmozyme)

ANTIDEPRESSANT DRUGS

Bicyclic Antidepressants

fluoxetine (Prozac)

venlafaxine (Effexor)

Tricyclic Antidepressants

amitriptyline (Elavil, Endep)
amoxapine (Asendin)
clomipramine (Anafranil)
desipramine (Norpramin,
  Pertofrane)

doxepin (Adapin, Sinequan)
imipramine (Janimine, Tofranil)
nortriptyline (Aventyl, Pamelor)
protriptyline (Vivactil)
trimipramine (Surmontil)

Tetracyclic Antidepressant

maprotiline (Ludiomil)

Other Antidepressants

bupropion (Wellbutrin)
fluvoxamine (Luvox)
nefazodone (Serzone)

paroxetine (Paxil)
sertraline (Zoloft)
trazodone (Desyrel)

Monoamine Oxidase (MAO) Inhibitors

See class below

...IEMETIC DRUGS *(Anti-Motion Sickness, Antinausea ...s)*

chlorpromazine (Thorazine)
cyclizine (Marezine)
dimenhydrinate (Dramamine)
diphenhydramine (Benadryl)
granisetron (Kytril)
hydroxyzine (Atarax, Vistaril)

meclizine (Antivert, Bonine)
ondansetron (Zofran)
prochlorperazine (Compazine)
promethazine (Phenergan)
scopolamine (Transderm Scop)
trimethobenzamide (Tigan)

ANTIFUNGAL DRUGS *(Anti-Infectives)*

amphotericin B (Fungizone)
amphotericin B, lipid-associated
    (Abelcet)
fluconazole (Diflucan)
flucytosine (Ancobon)
griseofulvin (Fulvicin, Grifulvin,

Grisactin)
itraconazole (Sporanox)
ketoconazole (Nizoral)
miconazole (Monistat)
nystatin (Mycostatin)

ANTI-GLAUCOMA DRUGS

acetazolamide (Diamox)
betaxolol (Betoptic)
epinephrine (Glaucon)

pilocarpine (Isopto-Carpine)
timolol (Timoptic)

ANTI-GOUT DRUGS

allopurinol (Zyloprim)
colchicine (no brand name)
diclofenac (Cataflam, Voltaren)
fenoprofen (Nalfon)
ibuprofen (Advil, Motrin,
    Nuprin, Rufen)
indomethacin (Indocin)
ketoprofen (Orudis)

mefenamic acid (Ponstel)
naproxen (Anaprox, Naprosyn)
oxaprozin (Daypro)
piroxicam (Feldene)
probenecid (Benemid)
sulfinpyrazone (Anturane)
sulindac (Clinoril)

ANTIHISTAMINES

astemizole (Hismanal)
azatadine (Optimine)
brompheniramine (Dimetane,
    others)
carbinoxamine (Clistin, Rondec)
cetirizine (Zyrtec)
chlorpheniramine
    (Chlor-Trimeton, Teldrin)
clemastine (Tavist)

cyclizine (Marezine)
cyproheptadine (Periactin)
dimenhydrinate (Dramamine)
diphenhydramine (Benadryl)
doxylamine (Unisom)
fexofenadine (Allegra)
loratadine (Claritin, Claritin
    Extra)
meclizine (Antivert, Bonine)

orphenadrine (Norflex)
pheniramine (component of Triaminic)
promethazine (Phenergan, others)
pyrilamine (component of Triaminic)

terfenadine (Seldane)
tripelennamine (Pyribenzamine, PBZ)
triprolidine (component of Actifed and Sudahist)

ANTIHYPERTENSIVE DRUGS

amlodipine/benazepril (Lotrel)
bisoprolol/hydrochlorothiazide (Ziac)
clonidine (Catapres)
doxazosin (Cardura)
guanabenz (Wytensin)
guanadrel (Hylorel)
guanethidine (Ismelin)

guanfacine (Tenex)
hydralazine (Apresoline)
methyldopa (Aldomet)
minoxidil (Loniten)
prazosin (Minipress)
reserpine (Serpasil)
terazosin (Hytrin)

See also the following drug classes: Angiotensin-Converting Enzyme (ACE) Inhibitors; Angiotensin II Receptor Antagonists; Beta-Adrenergic–Blocking Drugs; Calcium-Channel Blocking Drugs; Diuretics.

ANTI-INFECTIVE DRUGS

See specific anti-infective class: Amebicides; Aminoglycosides; Antifungal Drugs; Antileprosy Drugs; Antimalarial Drugs; Antituberculosis Drugs; Antiviral Drugs; Cephalosporins; Fluoroquinolones; Macrolide Antibiotics; Penicillins; Sulfonamides; Tetracyclines.

Miscellaneous Anti-Infective Drugs

atovaquone (Mepron)
chloramphenicol (Chloromycetin)
clindamycin (Cleocin)
colistin (Coly-Mycin S)
furazolidone (Furoxone)
lincomycin (Lincocin)
nalidixic acid (NegGram)

nitrofurantoin (Furadantin, Macrodantin)
novobiocin (Albamycin)
pentamidine (Pentam-300)
trimethoprim (Proloprim, Trimpex)
vancomycin (Vancocin)

ANTILEPROSY DRUGS (Anti-Infectives)

clofazimine (Lamprene)

dapsone (no brand name)

ANTIMALARIAL DRUGS *(Anti-Infectives)*

chloroquine (Aralen)
doxycycline (Vibramycin)
hydroxychloroquine (Plaquenil)
mefloquine (Lariam)
primaquine (no brand name)

pyrimethamine (Daraprim)
quinacrine (Atabrine)
quinine (no brand name)
sulfadoxine/pyrimethamine
  (Fansidar)

ANTI-MIGRAINE DRUGS

atenolol (Tenormin)
ergotamine (Ergostat)
methysergide (Sansert)
metoprolol (Lopressor)
nadolol (Corgard)

nifedipine (Procardia)
propranolol (Inderal)
sumatriptan (Imitrex)
timolol (Blocadren)
verapamil (Calan, Isoptin)

ANTIPARKINSONISM DRUGS

amantadine (Symmetrel)
benztropine (Cogentin)
bromocriptine (Parlodel)
diphenhydramine (Benadryl)
levodopa (Dopar, Larodopa)
levodopa/bensarazide (Prolopa)

levodopa/carbidopa (Sinemet,
  Sinemet CR)
pergolide (Permax)
selegiline (Eldepryl)
trihexyphenidyl (Artane)

ANTIPLATELET DRUGS *(Platelet Aggregation Inhibitors)*

aspirin (Bufferin, Ecotrin,
  others)
dipyridamole (Persantine)

sulfinpyrazone (Anturane)
ticlopidine (Ticlid)

ANTIPSYCHOTIC DRUGS *(Neuroleptics, Major Tranquilizers)*

chlorprothixene (Taractan)
clozapine (Clozaril)
haloperidol (Haldol)
loxapine (Loxitane)
molindone (Moban)

olanzapine (Zyprexa)
pimozide (Orap)
risperidone (Risperdal)
thiothixene (Navane)

See also Phenothiazines.

ANTIPYRETIC DRUGS *(Fever-Reducing Drugs)*

acetaminophen (Panadol,
  Tylenol, others)

aspirin (Bufferin, Ecotrin,
  others)

See also Nonsteroidal Anti-Inflammatory Drugs (NSAIDs).

ANTI-SICKLE CELL ANEMIA DRUG

hydroxyurea (Hydrea)

ANTISPASMODICS, SYNTHETIC

anisotropine (Valpin)
clidinium (Quarzan)
glycopyrrolate (Robinul)
hexocyclium (Tral)
isopropamide (Darbid)

mepenzolate (Cantil)
methantheline (Banthine)
methscopolamine (Pamine)
propantheline (Pro-BanthAne)
tridihexethyl (Pathilon)

ANTITUBERCULOSIS DRUGS

aminosalicylate sodium
  (Sodium P.A.S.)
capreomycin (Capastat)
cycloserine (Seromycin)
ethambutol (Myambutol)
ethionamide (Trecator-SC)

isoniazid (Laniazid, Nydrazid)
pyrazinamide (no brand name)
rifabutin (Mycobutin)
rifampin (Rifadin, Rimactane)
streptomycin (no brand name)

ANTITUSSIVE DRUGS *(Cough Suppressants)*

benzonatate (Tessalon)
codeine (no brand name)
dextromethorphan (Hold, DM,
  Suppress)

diphenhydramine (Benylin)
hydrocodone (Hycodan)
hydromorphone (Dilaudid)
promethazine (Phenergan)

ANTIVIRAL DRUGS *(Anti-Infectives)*

acyclovir (Zovirax)
amantadine (Symmetrel)
didanosine (Videx)
famciclovir (Famvir)
foscarnet (Foscavir)
ganciclovir (Cytovene)
indinavir (Crixivan)
lamivudine (Epivir)
nevirapine (Viramune)

ribavirin (Virazole)
rimantadine (Flumadine)
saquinavir (Invirase)
stavudine (Zerit)
valacyclovir (Valtrex)
vidarabine (Vira-A)
zalcitabine (HIVID)
zidovudine (Retrovir)

BARBITURATES

amobarbital (Amytal)
aprobarbital (Alurate)
butabarbital (Butisol)
mephobarbital (Mebaral)
metharbital (Gemonil)

pentobarbital (Nembutal)
phenobarbital (Luminal,
  Solfoton)
secobarbital (Seconal)
talbutal (Lotusate)

BENZODIAZEPINES

alprazolam (Xanax)
bromazepam (Lectopam)
chlordiazepoxide (Libritabs, Librium)
clonazepam (Klonopin)
clorazepate (Tranxene)
diazepam (Valium, Vazepam)
flurazepam (Dalmane)
halazepam (Paxipam)

ketazolam (Loftran)
lorazepam (Ativan)
midazolam (Versed)
nitrazepam (Mogadon)
oxazepam (Serax)
prazepam (Centrax)
quazepam (Doral)
temazepam (Restoril)
triazolam (Halcion)

BETA-ADRENERGIC–BLOCKING DRUGS
(Beta-Blockers)

acebutolol (Sectral)
atenolol (Tenormin)
betaxolol (Kerlone)
bisoprolol (Zebeta)
bisoprolol/hydrochlorothiazide (Ziac)
carteolol (Cartrol)
labetalol (Normodyne, Trandate)

metoprolol (Lopressor)
nadolol (Corgard)
penbutolol (Levatol)
pindolol (Visken)
propranolol (Inderal)
timolol (Blocadren)

BIGUANIDE

metformin (Glucophage)

BOWEL ANTI-INFLAMMATORY DRUGS
(Inflammatory Bowel Disease Suppressants)

azathioprine (Imuran)
mesalamine (Rowasa, Asacol)
metronidazole (Flagyl)

olsalazine (Dipentum)
sulfasalazine (Azulfidine)

CALCIUM-CHANNEL–BLOCKING DRUGS *(Calcium Blockers)*

amlodipine (Norvasc)
bepridil (Vascor)
diltiazem (Cardizem)
felodipine (Plendil)
isradipine (DynaCirc)

nicardipine (Cardene)
nifedipine (Adalat, Procardia)
nimodipine (Nimotop)
nisoldipine (Sular)
verapamil (Calan, Isoptin)

CEPHALOSPORINS *(Anti-Infectives)*

cefaclor (Ceclor)
cefadroxil (Duricef, Ultracef)
cefamandole (Mandol)
cefazolin (Ancef, Kefzol, Zolicef)
cefixime (Suprax)
cefmetazole (Zefazone)
cefonicid (Monocid)
cefoperazone (Cefobid)
ceforanide (Precef)
cefotaxime (Claforan)
cefotetan (Cefotan)
cefoxitin (Mefoxin)

cefprozil (Cefzil)
ceftazidime (Fortaz, Tazicef, Tazidime)
ceftizoxime (Cefizox)
ceftriaxone (Rocephin)
cefuroxime (Ceftin, Kefurox, Zinacef)
cephalexin (Keflex, Keftab)
cephalothin (Keflin)
cephapirin (Cefadyl)
cephradine (Anspor, Velosef)
moxalactam (Moxam)

CHOLESTEROL-REDUCING DRUGS

cholestyramine (Cholybar, Questran)
clofibrate (Atromid-S)
colestipol (Colestid)
dextrothyroxine (Choloxin)
fenofibrate (Lipidil)
fluvastatin (Lescol)

gemfibrozil (Lopid)
lovastatin (Mevacor)
niacin (Nicobid, Slo-Niacin, others)
pravastatin (Pravachol)
probucol (Lorelco)
simvastatin (Zocor)

DECONGESTANTS

ephedrine (Efedron, Ephedsol)
naphazoline (Naphcon, Vasocon)
oxymetazoline (Afrin, Duration, others)
phenylephrine (Neo-Synephrine, others)
phenylpropanolamine (Propadrine, Propagest, others)

pseudoephedrine (Afrinol, Sudafed, others)
tetrahydrozoline (Tyzine, Visine, others)
xylometazoline (Otrivin)

DIGITALIS PREPARATIONS

deslanoside (Cedilanid-D)
digitoxin (Crystodigin)

digoxin (Lanoxicaps, Lanoxin)

DIURETICS

acetazolamide (Diamox)
amiloride (Midamor)

bumetanide (Bumex)
chlorthalidone (Hygroton)

ethacrynic acid (Edecrin)
furosemide (Lasix)
indapamide (Lozol)

metolazone (Diulo, Zaroxolyn)
spironolactone (Aldactone)
triamterene (Dyrenium)

See also Thiazide Diuretics.

ESTROGENS *(Female Sex Hormones)*

chlorotrianisene (TACE)
diethylstilbestrol (DES, Stilphostrol)
estradiol (Estrace, Estraderm, others)
estrogens, conjugated (Premarin)

estrogens, esterified (Estratab, Menest)
estrone (Theelin, others)
estropipate (Ogen)
ethinyl estradiol (Estinyl)
quinestrol (Estrovis)

FLUOROQUINOLONES *(Anti-Infectives)*

ciprofloxacin (Cipro)
lomefloxacin (Maxaquin)

norfloxacin (Noroxin)
ofloxacin (Floxin)

GASTROINTESTINAL DRUGS

Miscellaneous

cisapride (Propulsid)

metoclopramide (Reglan)

HEMATOPOIETIC AGENT

filgrastim (Neupogen)

HISTAMINE (H_2) BLOCKING DRUGS

(H_2-Blockers)

cimetidine (Tagamet) (Tagamet HB-nonprescription)
famotidine (Pepcid) (Pepcid AC-nonprescription)

nizatidine (Axid) (Axid AR-nonprescription)
ranitidine (Zantac) (Zantac 75-nonprescription)

HYPNOTIC DRUGS *(Sedatives/Sleep Inducers)*

acetylcarbromal (Paxarel)
chloral hydrate (Aquachloral, Noctec)
estazolam (ProSom)
ethchlorvynol (Placidyl)

ethinamate (Valmid)
flurazepam (Dalmane)
glutethimide (Doriden)
methyprylon (Noludar)
paraldehyde (Paral)

propiomazine (Largon)
quazepam (Doral)
temazepam (Restoril)

triazolam (Halcion)
zolpidem (Ambien)

See also Barbiturates.

MACROLIDE ANTIBIOTICS *(Anti-Infectives)*

azithromycin (Zithromax)
clarithromycin (Biaxin)
dirithromycin (Dynabac)

erythromycin (E-Mycin, Ilosone,
Erythrocin, E.E.S.)
troleandomycin (Tao)

MONOAMINE OXIDASE (MAO) INHIBITOR DRUGS
(Type A: Antidepressants)

isocarboxazid (Marplan)
phenelzine (Nardil)

tranylcypromine (Parnate)

MUSCLE RELAXANTS *(Skeletal Muscle Relaxants)*

baclofen (Lioresal)
carisoprodol (Rela, Soma,
others)
chlorphenesin carbamate
(Maolate)
chlorzoxazone (Paraflex,
Parafon Forte)
cyclobenzaprine (Flexeril)
dantrolene (Dantrium)

diazepam (Valium)
meprobamate (Equanil,
Miltown, others)
metaxalone (Skelaxin)
methocarbamol (Robaxin,
others)
orphenadrine (Norflex,
others)

NITRATES

amyl nitrite (Amyl Nitrite
Vaporole, others)
erythrityl tetranitrate
(Cardilate)
isosorbide dinitrate (Isordil,
Sorbitrate, others)
isosorbide mononitrate (Ismo,
Imdur)

nitroglycerin (Nitrostat,
Nitrolingual, Nitrogard,
Nitrong, others)
pentaerythritol tetranitrate
(Duotrate, Peritrate)

NONNUCLEOSIDE REVERSE TRANSCRIPTASE INHIBITOR

nevirapine (Viramune)

NONSTEROIDAL ANTI-INFLAMMATORY DRUGS (NSAIDS) *(Aspirin Substitutes)*

Acetic Acids

diclofenac potassium (Cataflam)
diclofenac sodium (Voltaren)
etodolac (Lodine)
indomethacin (Indocin)
indomethacin, sustained-release
  (Indochron E-R, Indocin SR)

ketorolac (Toradol)
nabumetone (Relafen)
sulindac (Clinoril)
tolmetin (Tolectin, Tolectin DS)

Fenamates

meclofenamate (Meclomen)

mefenamic acid (Ponstel)

Oxicams

piroxicam (Feldene)

Propionic Acids

diflunisal (Dolobid)
fenoprofen (Nalfon)
flurbiprofen (Ansaid)
ibuprofen (Motrin, Nuprin,
  Rufen, Advil, Medipren,
  others)
ketoprofen (Orudis, Oruvail)

naproxen (Naprosyn)
naproxen sodium (Aleve,
  Anaprox, Anaprox DS)
oxaprozin (Daypro)
oxyphenbutazone (Oxalid)
suprofen (Profenal)

OPIOID DRUGS *(Narcotics)*

alfentanil (Alfenta)
codeine (no brand name)
fentanyl (Sublimaze, Duragesic)
hydrocodone (Hycodan)
hydromorphone (Dilaudid)
levorphanol (Levo-Dromoran)
meperidine (Demerol)
methadone (Dolophine)

morphine (Astramorph,
  Duramorph, MS Contin,
  Roxanol)
oxycodone (Roxicodone)
oxymorphone (Numorphan)
propoxyphene (Darvon)
sufentanil (Sufenta)

PENICILLINS *(Anti-Infectives)*

amoxicillin (Amoxil, Larotid,
  Polymox, Trimox, others)
amoxicillin/clavulanate
  (Augmentin)
ampicillin (Omnipen, Polycillin,
  Principen, Totacillin)
ampicillin/sulbactam (Unasyn)

bacampicillin (Spectrobid)
carbenicillin (Geocillin, Geopen,
  Pyopen)
cloxacillin (Cloxapen, Tegopen)
dicloxacillin (Dynapen, Pathocil,
  Veracillin)
methicillin (Staphcillin)

mezlocillin (Mezlin)
nafcillin (Nafcil, Unipen)
oxacillin (Prostaphlin)
penicillin G (Pentids, others)
penicillin V (Pen-Vee K, V-Cillin K, Veetids, others)

piperacillin (Pipracil)
ticarcillin (Ticar)
ticarcillin/clavulanate (Timentin)

PHENOTHIAZINES *(Antipsychotic Drugs)*

acetophenazine (Tindal)
chlorpromazine (Thorazine)
fluphenazine (Permitil, Prolixin)
mesoridazine (Serentil)
perphenazine (Trilafon)

prochlorperazine (Compazine)
promazine (Sparine)
thioridazine (Mellaril)
trifluoperazine (Stelazine)
triflupromazine (Vesprin)

PROGESTINS *(Female Sex Hormones)*

ethynodiol
hydroxyprogesterone (Duralutin, Gesterol L.A., others)
medroxyprogesterone (Amen, Curretab, Provera)

megestrol (Megace)
norethindrone (Micronor, Norlutate, Norlutin)
norgestrel (Ovrette)
progesterone (Gesterol 50, Progestaject)

PROTON PUMP INHIBITORS *(H/K ATPase Inhibitors)*

lansoprazole (Prevacid)
omeprazole (Prilosec)

pantoprazole (pending in U.S.)

RADIOPHARMACEUTICALS

strontium-89 (Metastron)

SALICYLATES

aspirin (A.S.A., Bufferin, Ecotrin, Empirin, others)
choline salicylate (Arthropan)
magnesium salicylate (Doan's, Magan, Mobidin)

salsalate (Amigesic, Disalcid, Salsitab)
sodium salicylate (no brand name)
sodium thiosalicylate (Rexolate, Tusal)

SMOKING DETERRENTS

nicotine (Habitrol, Nicoderm, Nicorette, Nicotrol, Prostep, others)

SULFONAMIDES *(Anti-Infectives)*

multiple sulfonamides (Triple Sulfa No. 2)
sulfacytine (Renoquid)
sulfadiazine (no brand name)
sulfamethizole (Thiosulfil)
sulfamethoxazole (Azo Gantanol)
sulfasalazine (Azulfidine)
sulfisoxazole (Gantrisin)

SULFONYLUREAS *(Oral Antidiabetic Drugs)*

acetohexamide (Dymelor)
chlorpropamide (Diabinese)
glimepiride (Amaryl)
glipizide (Glucotrol)
glyburide (DiaBeta, Micronase)
tolazamide (Ronase, Tolamide, Tolinase)
tolbutamide (Orinase)

TETRACYCLINES *(Anti-Infectives)*

demeclocycline (Declomycin)
doxycycline (Doryx, Doxychel, Vibramycin)
methacycline (Rondomycin)
minocycline (Minocin)
oxytetracycline (Terramycin)
tetracycline (Achromycin V, Panmycin, Sumycin)

THIAZIDE DIURETICS

bendroflumethiazide (Naturetin)
benzthiazide (Aquatag, Exna, Marazide)
chlorothiazide (Diuril)
cyclothiazide (Anhydron)
hydrochlorothiazide (Esidrix, Hydrodiuril, Oretic)
hydroflumethiazide (Diucardin, Saluron)
methyclothiazide (Enduron, Aquatensen)
polythiazide (Renese)
trichlormethiazide (Metahydrin, Naqua)

VACCINES

influenza vaccine (Fluogen, Flu-Shield, Fluzone)
varicella virus vaccine (Varivax)

VASODILATORS *(Peripheral Vasodilators)*

cyclandelate (Cyclospasmol)
ethaverine (Ethaquin, Isovex)
isoxsuprine (Vasodilan)
nylidrin (Arlidin)
papaverine (Cerespan, Pavabid)

XANTHINES *(Bronchodilators)*

aminophylline (Phyllocontin, Truphylline)

dyphylline (Dilor, Lufyllin)

oxtriphylline (Choledyl)

theophylline (Bronkodyl, Slo-Phyllin, Theolair, others)

SECTION FIVE

GLOSSARY

Addiction Addiction is a state of intense drug dependence characterized by uncontrollable drug-seeking behavior, *tolerance* for the drug's pleasure-giving effects, and *withdrawal* manifestations when the drug is withheld. This *physical dependence* involves physical incorporation of the drug into the fundamental biochemistry of specific brain activities. (See DEPENDENCE and TOLERANCE.)

Adverse Effect or Reaction An abnormal, unexpected, and usually unpredictable harmful response to a drug. In this restrictive sense the term does *not* include undesirable and unintended drug effects that are normally a part of its pharmacologic action. (See SIDE EFFECT.) Adverse reactions include drug *allergy,* individual *idiosyncrasy,* and *toxic* effects on tissue structure and function (see ALLERGY, IDIOSYNCRASY, and TOXICITY).

Allergy (Drug) An abnormal drug response in people who make antibodies* to a specific drug or chemical features of the drug or drug class. People who are allergic by nature and have a history of hay fever, asthma, hives, or eczema are more likely to develop drug allergies. Forms include: skin eruptions, fever, swollen glands, painful joints, jaundice, breathing problems, and acute collapse of circulation. They may develop gradually or suddenly, requiring emergency medical help.

Alternative Delivery System (ADS) A term that describes a variety of health care forums other than the traditional fee-for-service model. Examples include HMOs and PPOs.

Analgesic A drug that relieves pain. (1) Nonnarcotic analgesics relieve pain by blocking production of prostaglandins and related chemicals. Examples are acetaminophen, aspirin, and drugs known as aspirin substitutes (Motrin, Advil, Naprosyn, etc.). (2) Narcotic analgesics or opioids (such as opium derivatives) relieve pain by blocking its perception in the brain. Examples are morphine, codeine, and hydrocodone (natural derivatives of opium), and meperidine or pentazocine (synthetic drugs). (3) Local anes-

---

*Antibodies are special proteins that attack substances foreign to the body. Protective antibodies destroy bacteria and neutralize toxins. Injurious antibodies, reacting with foreign substances, cause the release of histamine.

thetics prevent or relieve pain by making sensory nerve endings insensitive to painful stimulation; e.g. phenazopyridine (Pyridium).

Current pain theory supports the use of scheduled pain medicines versus as-needed or PRN dosing. Effective pain control is one hallmark of quality care.

Anaphylactic (Anaphylactoid) Reaction Symptoms that represent (or resemble) an overwhelming and dangerous allergic reaction, often involving several body systems due to extreme hypersensitivity to a drug. Mild symptoms: itching, hives, nasal congestion, nausea, abdominal cramping, diarrhea. Severe symptoms: choking, shortness of breath, sudden loss of consciousness (anaphylactic shock).

An anaphylactic reaction develops suddenly, sometimes from a very small dose, usually within a few minutes after taking the drug. This reaction can rapidly progress and lead to fatal collapse in a short time if not reversed by appropriate treatment. A developing anaphylactic reaction is a true medical emergency. Any adverse effect that appears within 20 minutes after taking a drug should be considered the early phase of a possible anaphylactic reaction. Get medical help immediately! (See ALLERGY and HYPERSENSITIVITY.)

Antihypertensive A drug used to lower high blood pressure. *Hypertension* is blood pressure above the normal range. *Antihypertensive* is sometimes used erroneously as if it had the same meaning as *antianxiety* (or tranquilizing) drug action.

Of the more than 100 drugs used for hypertension, the most frequently prescribed for long-term use fall into three major groups: drugs that increase urine production (the diuretics), drugs that relax blood vessel walls, or drugs that reduce the activity of the sympathetic nervous system.

All share an ability to lower the blood pressure. Many drugs can interact with antihypertensive medicines adding to their effect or reducing their benefits.

Antipyretic A drug that lowers increased body temperature, relieving fever through its effects on the temperature-regulating center in the hypothalamus. An antipyretic drug may also be analgesic (acetaminophen), or analgesic and anti-inflammatory (aspirin).

Aplastic Anemia A form of bone marrow failure where production of all three types of blood cells is seriously impaired (also known as pancytopenia). About one-half of reported cases are induced by drugs or chemicals, which may be difficult to identify because a 1- to 6-month delay may occur between their use and the detection of anemia. The symptoms include deficiency of red blood cells (anemia), fatigue, weakness, and pallor; predisposition to infections from deficiency of white blood cells (leukopenia); deficiency of blood platelets (thrombocytopenia); and spontaneous bruising and hemorrhage. Treatment is difficult and the outcome unpredictable. Even with the best of care, approximately 50% of cases end fatally.

Although aplastic anemia is a rare consequence of drug treatment (3 in 100,000 users of quinacrine, for example), anyone taking a drug capable of causing this reaction should periodically have complete blood cell counts if the drug is to be used over an extended period of time. For a listing of causative drugs, see Table 4, "Drugs That May Cause Blood Problems," Section Six.

Bioavailability Usually applied to a tablet or capsule; refers to how rapidly the active drug ingredient is absorbed into the bloodstream and the extent of absorption. Two types of measurements—(1) blood levels of the drug at certain time intervals after administration and (2) the duration of the drug's presence in the blood—tell how much of the drug is available for biological activity and for how long. Another method is to measure (1) the cumulative amount of the drug (or any breakdown product after transformation) excreted in the urine and (2) the rate of accumulation in the urine.

Two major factors that govern a drug product's bioavailability are the chemical and physical characteristics (the formulation) of the dosage form, and how well the patient's digestive system works. Specially designed laboratory tests are now available to evaluate a drug's potential bioavailability in the average person.

Bioequivalence The ability of a drug to produce its intended therapeutic effect is directly related to its bioavailability. When a particular drug is made by several manufacturers, often in a variety of dosage forms, substantial variations occur in their formulations. Although the principal drug ingredient of products from different makers may be chemically identical, it cannot be assumed that these products possess equal bioavailability and are therefore therapeutically equal.

The bioavailability of any drug product is governed to a large extent by its physical characteristics. Drug products that contain the same principal drug ingredient but are combined with different inert additives, coated with different substances, or enclosed in different capsules may not have the same bioavailability. Those that do are said to be bioequivalent, and can be relied upon to be equally effective in achieving therapeutic results. If you are considering filling your prescription with the generic equivalent of a brand-name drug product, ask your doctor *and* pharmacist for help.

Blood Platelets The smallest of the three types of blood cells made by the bone marrow. Normally present in large numbers, they help blood to clot. If enough are present and they work correctly, platelets preserve the retaining power of the walls of the smaller blood vessels; preventing bleeding to death from a small cut.

Some drugs or chemicals reduce the available platelets to abnormally low levels, suppressing their formation or hastening their destruction. When the functioning platelets fall below a critical level, blood begins to leak through the thin walls of smaller vessels. This first shows as scattered bruises of the thighs and legs, referred to as purpura. Bleeding may also occur anywhere in the body, internally as well as superficially into the tissues immediately beneath the skin.

Bone Marrow Depression A serious decrease in the ability of the bone marrow to make critical blood cells. This can be caused by an adverse reaction to certain drugs and chemicals of bone marrow components. The bone marrow produces the majority of the body's blood cells. The red blood cells, white blood cells, and platelets each perform specific indispensable functions.

Drugs that depress bone marrow activity can block production of all types of blood cells or only one type selectively. Periodic blood examinations can reveal significant changes in the structure and number of the blood cells that indicate a possible drug effect on bone marrow activity.

Anemia, a condition of abnormally low red cells and hemoglobin, results in weakness, lack of energy or stamina, and intolerance of cold environments or physical exertion. A reduction in the formation of white blood cells can limit immunity and lower resistance to infection, resulting in fever, sore throat, or pneumonia. Platelet suppression to abnormally low levels reduces the blood's ability to quickly seal small points of leakage in blood vessel walls, producing spontaneous bruising or prolonged bleeding.

These symptoms should alert both patient and physician to the need for prompt studies of blood and bone marrow (see Table 4, "Drugs That May Cause Blood Problems," Section Six).

Brand Name The registered trade name given to a drug product by its manufacturer. Many drugs are marketed by more than one manufacturer or distributor. The brand name designates a proprietary drug—one that is protected by patent or copyright.

Capitation A health care system where a fixed amount of money is paid to a health care provider on a negotiated per-person rate. Ask if your HMO negotiates capitated payment. If it does, ask how outcomes are compared among providers of care.

Cause-and-Effect Relationship A possible causative association between a drug and an observed biological event, most commonly a side effect or adverse effect. In an evaluation of a cause-and-effect relationship, therefore, meticulous consideration must be given to such factors as the time sequence of drug administration and possible reaction, the use of multiple drugs, possible interactions among these drugs, the effects of the disease under treatment, the physiological and psychological characteristics of the patient, and the possible influence of unrecognized disorders and malfunctions.

The majority of adverse drug reactions occur sporadically, unpredictably, and infrequently in the general population. A *definite* cause-and-effect relationship between drug and reaction is established when (1) the adverse effect immediately follows administration of the drug; or (2) the adverse effect disappears after the drug is discontinued (dechallenge) and promptly reappears when the drug is used again (rechallenge); or (3) the adverse effects are clearly the expected and predictable toxic consequences of drug overdoses. A large gray area of probable, possible, and coincidental associations often apply to drug reactions that require a relatively long time to develop, are rare, and have causal mechanisms that are not very clear-cut.

Clarification of cause-and-effect relationships in uncertain groups requires carefully designed observation over a long period of time, followed by sophisticated statistical analysis. The most competent techniques have been devised by the Division of Tissue Reactions to Drugs, a research unit of the Armed Forces Institute of Pathology. Based upon a highly critical examination of all available evidence, the Division's study of 2,800 drug-related deaths yielded the following levels of certainty regarding cause-and-effect relationship.

No association	5.0%
Coincidental	14.5%
Possible	33.0%

Probable	30.0%
Causative	17.5%

It is significant that this expert evaluation substantiated only 47.5% cases as definitely or probably causative.

Contraindication A condition or disease that precludes the use of a particular drug. Some contraindications are *absolute*, meaning that the use of the drug would expose the patient to extreme hazard and cannot be justified. Others are *relative*, meaning that the condition or disease does not entirely exclude the use of the drug but requires special consideration be given to factors which could aggravate existing disease, interfere with current treatment, or produce new injury.

Critical or Clinical Path An assortment of coordinated measures taken by individual physicians or practitioners to organize, standardize, coordinate, and obtain the best outcomes from available evaluations, diagnostic tests, and treatments available to address a particular disease or condition.

Dependence A term used to identify the drug-dependent states of *psychological dependence* (or *habituation*), *physical dependence* (or *addiction*), and *functional dependence*.

Psychological dependence is a form of neurotic behavior. A common form in today's culture is the increasing reliance upon drugs to help in coping with the everyday problems of living: pills for frustration, disappointment, nervous stomach, tension headache, and insomnia. This compulsive drug abuse is characterized by little or no tendency to increase the dose (see TOLERANCE) and no or only minor physical manifestations upon withdrawal. Some authorities choose to broaden the definition of addiction to include psychological dependence.

Physical dependence, which is true addiction, includes *tolerance* and *withdrawal*. Addicting drugs provide relief from anguish and pain and cause a physiological tolerance that requires increasing doses or repeated use to remain effective. The drug becomes a functioning component in the biochemistry of the brain, assuming an essential role in ongoing chemical processes. (Thus some authorities prefer the term *chemical dependence.*) Sudden removal of the drug causes a withdrawal syndrome—the intense mental and physical pain—that is the hallmark of addiction.

Functional dependence occurs when a drug relieves an annoying or distressing condition and the body function involved becomes increasingly dependent upon the drug to provide a sense of well-being. Drugs that are capable of inducing functional dependence are used primarily for the relief of symptoms. They do not act on the brain to produce alteration of mood or consciousness. The most familiar example of functional dependence is the laxative habit. Some types of constipation are actually worsened by laxatives, and natural bowel function gradually fades with increased dependence.

Disease Management A concept in health care where specific approaches appropriate to address a given condition are developed to insure the best use of health care dollars and result in the best outcomes or results, from laboratory tests to drug therapy.

Disulfiramlike (Antabuse-like) Reaction The symptoms that result from the interaction of alcohol and any drug. The interacting drug interrupts the metabolism of alcohol by the liver and permits accumulation of a toxic by-product. Symptoms include flushing and warming of the face, a severe throbbing headache, shortness of breath, chest pains, nausea, repeated vomiting, sweating, and weakness. If the amount of alcohol ingested has been large enough, the reaction may progress to blurred vision, vertigo, confusion, a marked drop in blood pressure, and loss of consciousness. Severe reactions may lead to convulsions and death. The reaction can last from 30 minutes to several hours, depending upon the amount of alcohol in the body. As the symptoms subside, the person is exhausted and usually sleeps for several hours.

Diuretic A drug that increases the volume of urine. Diuretics use several different ways to increase urine volume, and have different effects on body chemistry. Diuretics are used to (1) remove excess water from the body (as in congestive heart failure and some types of liver and kidney disease), and (2) treat hypertension by promoting the excretion of sodium from the body.

Divided Doses The total daily dose of a medicine is split into smaller individual doses over the course of a day. For example: a 1500 mg/day dose of ciprofloxacin is taken in divided doses of 750 mg/12 hr.

Drug, Drug Product Terms often used interchangeably to designate a medicine (in any of its dosage forms) used in medical practice. The term *drug* refers to a chemical entity that provokes a specific response when placed within a biological system—the active ingredient. A *drug product* is the manufactured dosage form—tablet, capsule, elixir, etc.—that contains the active drug mixed with inactive ingredients to provide convenient administration. Drug products with only one active ingredient are single-entity drugs. Drug products with two or more active ingredients are combination drugs (designed [CD] in the lists of brand names in the drug profiles).

Drug Class A group of medicines that are similar in chemistry, method of action, and use in treatment. Many drugs within a class will cause the same side effects and have similar potential for provoking adverse reactions and interactions. However, significant variations among members within a drug class can occur. This may allow the physician important latitude in choosing a drug in order to increase certain benefits or avoid a particular side effect. Examples: Antihistamines, phenothiazines, tetracyclines.

Drug Fever Elevated temperature that is caused by a drug. Drugs can cause fever by allergic reaction; drug-induced tissue damage; acceleration of tissue metabolism; constriction of blood vessels in the skin, which decreases body heat loss; and direct action on the temperature-regulating center in the brain.

The most common form is associated with allergic reactions. The fever usually appears about 7 to 10 days after starting the drug and may vary from low-grade to alarmingly high levels. It may be sustained or intermittent, but usually persists for as long as the drug is taken. In people who have taken the drug previously, drug fever may occur within 1 or 2 hours after taking the first dose.

Following are the most commonly responsible drugs:

allopurinol
antihistamines
atropinelike drugs
barbiturates
coumarin anticoagulants
hydralazine
iodides
isoniazid
methyldopa
nadolol
novobiocin
para-aminosalicylic acid
penicillin
pentazocine
phenytoin
procainamide
propylthiouracil
quinidine
rifampin
sulfonamides

Extension Effect An unwanted but predictable drug response that is a consequence of mild to moderate overdose. An extension effect is an exaggeration of a drug's pharmacologic action (what it normally does). An extension effect can be thought of as a mild form of dose-related toxicity (see OVERDOSAGE and TOXICITY).

Examples: The "hangover" of drowsiness and sluggishness that persists in the morning is a common extension effect of a long-acting sleep-inducing drug (hypnotic or sleeping pill). Persistent intestinal cramping and diarrhea caused by too generous a dose of laxative are extension effects of the drug's action.

FDA Approvable A stage in the FDA approval process wherein a medicine has been reviewed by an appropriate panel, and has been found to meet current criteria. At this point only final details need to be resolved before the drug becomes FDA-approved and widely available to the public.

Generic Name The official name used to designate an active drug entity, whether in pure form or in dosage form. Generic names are coined by committees of officially appointed drug experts and are approved by governmental agencies for national and international use. Many drug products are marketed under the generic name of the principal active ingredient and bear no brand name of the manufacturer.

Genetic Therapy One of today's most promising approaches to diseases with a genetic basis. Healthy genetic material is isolated and inserted into appropriate, but diseased, cells. For example, normal lung genes are given to a person with cystic fibrosis. This approach is still experimental, but may allow people with genetically based diseases to receive therapy that actually changes the affected genes and cures the underlying condition.

Habituation A form of drug dependence based upon strong psychological gratification rather than the physical (chemical) dependence of addiction. The habitual use of drugs that alter mood or relieve minor discomforts results from a compulsive need to feel pleasure and satisfaction or escape emotional distress. If these drugs are stopped suddenly, a withdrawal syndrome does not happen. Habituation is a *psychological dependence*.

Hemolytic Anemia A form of anemia (decreased red blood cells and hemoglobin) resulting from premature destruction (hemolysis) of red blood cells. This happens in several ways; among these is the action of certain drugs and chemicals. Some people are susceptible to hemolytic anemia because of a genetic deficiency in the makeup of their red blood cells. If such people are given certain antimalarial drugs, sulfa drugs, or numerous other drugs, some of their red cells will disintegrate on contact with the drug. (About 10% of American blacks have this genetic trait.)

Many drugs in wide use (including quinidine, methyldopa, levodopa, and chlorpromazine) cause hemolytic destruction of red cells as a hypersensitivity (allergic) reaction.

Hemolytic anemia can occur abruptly (with evident symptoms) or silently. The acute form lasts about 7 days and is characterized by fever, pallor, weakness, dark-colored urine, and varying degrees of jaundice (yellow coloration of eyes and skin). When drug-induced hemolytic anemia is mild, there may be no symptoms. Such episodes are detected only by means of laboratory studies (see IDIOSYNCRASY and ALLERGY).

For listings of causative drugs, see Table 4, "Drugs That May Cause Blood Problems," Section Six.

Hepatitislike Reaction Changes in the liver caused by some drugs, which resemble changes seen in viral hepatitis. The correct cause cannot be established without precise laboratory studies.

Hepatitis due to drugs may be a form of drug allergy (as in a reaction to many of the phenothiazines), or it may be a toxic adverse effect (as in a reaction to some MAO inhibitors). Liver reactions of significance usually cause jaundice and represent serious adverse effects (see JAUNDICE). See Table 6, "Drugs That May Cause Liver Damage or Dysfunction," Section Six.

HMO Health Maintenance Organization: An HMO is a health care delivery system that provides a broad spectrum of medical therapies and services by a collective group of medical practitioners. When considering an HMO, you should make sure to ask: (1) how their outcomes of treatment compare to other HMOs available in your area; (2) whether you will have to use a mail-order pharmacy; (3) whether they have a closed formulary (this restricts the use of some medicines); (4) what incentives their doctors are paid for achieving the best results (outcomes) versus merely cutting costs.

Hypersensitivity Overresponsiveness to drug action, that is, intolerance to even small doses. The nature of the response is appropriate but the degree is exaggerated.

The term is more widely used today to identify a state of allergy to a drug (see ALLERGY).

Some people develop cross-hypersensitivity. This means that once a person has developed an allergy to a certain drug, they will have an allergic reaction to other drugs that are closely related.

Hypnotic A drug used to cause sleep. Several drug classes have hypnotic effects: antihistamines, barbiturates, benzodiazepines, and several unrelated compounds. Within the past 15 years the benzodiazepines, because of their relative safety and lower potential for inducing dependence, have largely replaced the barbiturates. To maintain their effectiveness, hypnotics should be used intermittently for short periods.

Hypoglycemia A condition caused by below normal blood glucose (a sugar). Since the brain requires glucose to work, reducing the level of glucose in the blood below a critical point will cause serious impairment of brain activity. The symptoms are characteristic of the hypoglycemic state.

Early signs of hypoglycemia are headache, a sensation resembling mild drunkenness, and inability to think clearly. These may be accompanied by hunger. As the level of blood glucose continues to fall, nervousness and confusion develop. Varying degrees of weakness, numbness, trembling, sweating, and rapid heart action follow. If sugar is not provided and the blood glucose level drops further, impaired speech, incoordination, and unconsciousness, with or without convulsions, will follow. Hypoglycemia in any stage requires prompt recognition and treatment.

Hypothermia An unexpected decline of internal body temperature to levels significantly below 98.6° F, or 37° C. By definition, hypothermia means a body temperature of less than 95° F, or 35° C. The elderly and debilitated are more prone to develop hypothermia if clothed inadequately and exposed to cool environments. Most episodes are initiated by room temperatures below 65° F or 18.3° C. The condition often develops suddenly, can mimic a stroke, and has a mortality rate of 50%. Some drugs, such as phenothiazines, barbiturates, and benzodiazepines, are conducive to its development in susceptible people.

Idiosyncrasy An abnormal drug response that happens in people who have a defect in their body chemistry (often hereditary), producing a symptom totally unrelated to the drug's normal pharmacologic action. Idiosyncrasy is not a form of allergy.

Example: Approximately 100 million people in the world (including 10% of American blacks) have a specific red blood cell defect that causes these cells to disintegrate when exposed to drugs such as sulfonamides, nitrofurantoin, probenecid, quinine, and quinidine, causing a significant anemia. Approximately 5% of the U.S. population is susceptible to glaucoma from prolonged use of cortisone-related drugs.

Immunosuppressive A drug that suppresses the immune system. In some cases immunosuppression is an intended drug effect. Cyclosporine helps prevent rejection of a transplanted heart or kidney. In other instances it is an unwanted side effect, as in long-term use of cortisonelike drugs.

Interaction A change in the body's response to a drug which results when a second drug that can alter its action is given at the same time. Some drug interactions enhance the effect of either drug, producing an overresponse similar to overdose. Other interactions reduce drug effectiveness and cause inadequate therapy. A third type of interaction causes a seemingly unrelated toxic response with no associated increase or decrease in the pharmacologic actions of the interacting drugs.

Theoretically many drugs can interact with one another, but in reality, interactions are comparatively infrequent. Many interactions can be anticipated, and the physician can make appropriate adjustments in dosage.

Jaundice A yellow coloration of the skin (and the white portion of the eyes) occurring when excessive bile pigments accumulate in the blood as a result of impaired liver function. Jaundice is produced by several mechanisms, including a wide variety of diseases or an adverse drug reaction.

Drug-induced jaundice is always a serious adverse effect. Anyone taking a drug that can cause jaundice should watch closely for any significant change in the color of urine or feces. Dark discoloration of the urine and paleness (lack of color) of the stool may be early signs of a developing jaundice. If this happens, stop taking the drug and call the prescribing physician promptly. See Table 6, "Drugs That May Cause Liver Damage or Dysfunction," Section Six.

Lupus Erythematosus (LE) A serious disease of unknown cause that occurs in two forms, one limited to the skin (discoid LE) and the other involving several body systems (systemic LE). Both forms occur mainly in young women. About 5% of cases of the discoid form convert to the systemic form, a disorder of the body's immune system that may result in chronic, progressive inflammation and destruction of the connective tissue framework of the skin, blood vessels, joints, brain, heart muscle, lungs, and kidneys. Altered proteins in the blood lead to the formation of antibodies that react with organ tissues. White blood cell and platelet numbers are often reduced. The course is usually protracted and unpredictable. Although no cure is known, satisfactory management may be achieved by the judicious use of cortisonelike drugs.

Several drugs are capable of causing systemic LE, including procainamide. Symptoms may appear as early as 2 weeks or as late as 8 years after starting the responsible drug. The initial symptoms usually consist of low-grade fever, skin rashes, aching muscles, and multiple joint pains. Chest pains (pleurisy) are fairly common. Enlargement of the lymph glands occurs less frequently. Symptoms usually subside when the drug is stopped, but laboratory evidence of the reaction may persist for many months.

Neuroleptic Malignant Syndrome (NMS) A rare, serious, sometimes fatal idiosyncratic reaction to the use of neuroleptic (antipsychotic) drugs. Hyperthermia (temperatures of 102 to 104° F), marked muscle rigidity, and coma result. Other symptoms include rapid heart rate and breathing, profuse sweating, tremors, and seizures. Two-thirds of reported cases occurred in men. The mortality rate is 15 to 20%.

The following drugs have a potential for inducing this reaction:

amitriptyline + perphenazine (Triavil)
amoxapine (Asendin)
chlorpromazine (Thorazine)
chlorprothixene (Taractan)
clomipramine (Anafranil)
fluphenazine (Permitil, Prolixin)
haloperidol (Haldol)
imipramine (Tofranil, etc.)
levodopa + carbidopa (Sinemet)
loxapine (Loxitane)
metoclopramide (Reglan, Octamide)
molindone (Moban)
olanzapine (Zyprexa)
perphenazine (Etrafon, Trilafon)
pimozide (Orap)
prochlorperazine (Compazine)
thioridazine (Mellaril)
thiothixene (Navane)
trifluoperazine (Stelazine)
trimeprazine (Temaril)

Orthostatic Hypotension A type of low blood pressure related to body position or posture (also called postural hypotension). People subject to orthostatic hypotension may have a normal blood pressure while lying down, but on sitting upright or standing experience sudden light-headedness, dizziness, and a feeling of impending faintness. These symptoms are caused by inadequate blood flow (oxygen supply) to the brain.

Many drugs (especially antihypertensives) cause orthostatic hypotension. Failure to correct or compensate for these sudden drops in blood pressure can lead to severe falls and injury.

The tendency to orthostatic hypotension can be reduced by avoiding sudden standing, prolonged standing, vigorous exercise, and exposure to hot environments. Alcoholic beverages should be used cautiously until their combined effect with the drug in use has been determined.

Outcomes Research A health care concept that considers the comparative benefits (gauged by a variety of techniques) of one medicine over another in treating a specific disease or condition. This concept should also be expanded to check how well physicians in your area treat illness versus simple cutting costs and also how well your HMO measures against other HMOs in getting the best results.

Overdosage This term is not limited to doses that clearly exceed the normal dosage range. The ideal dose of many drugs varies greatly from person to person. An average dose for some people may be an overdose for some and an underdose for others. Numerous factors, such as age, body size, nutritional status, and liver and kidney function significantly influence dosage requirements. Drugs with narrow safety margins often produce signs of overdose if something delays their elimination. In this case, overdosage results from accumulation of prescribed daily doses. Massive overdosage—as occurs with accidental ingestion of drugs by children or with suicidal intention by adults—is referred to as poisoning.

Over-the-Counter (OTC) Drugs Drug products that can be purchased without prescription. Because of their unrestricted availability, many people do not regard OTC medicines as drugs. They are capable of causing a wide variety of actions and are clearly important medicines. Recently regulations requiring more specific information about OTC medicines were presented to the FDA.

Within the last 30 years many OTC drugs have assumed greater importance because of potential drug-drug interactions. Serious problems in drug therapy can arise when (1) the patient fails to inform the physician of the OTC drug(s) he or she is taking and (2) the physician fails to specify that medicines being taken currently *include all OTC drugs.* During any course of treatment, whether medical or surgical, the patient should consult with the physician regarding any OTC drug that he or she wishes to take.

Paradoxical Reaction An unexpected drug response not consistent with known pharmacology of a drug; it may be the opposite of the intended and anticipated response. Such reactions are due to individual sensitivity or variability and can occur in any age group. They are seen more commonly, however, in children and the elderly.

Example: An 80-year-old man admitted to a nursing home following the death of his wife had difficulty adjusting to his new environment. He was given a trial of the tranquilizer diazepam (Valium) to relax him. On the second day of medication he became confused and when the dose was increased on the third, he began to wander aimlessly, talked in a loud voice, and became hostile when attempts were made to help him. All behavioral disturbances subsided within 3 days when the drug was stopped.

Parkinson-Like Disorders (Parkinsonism) A group of symptoms like those caused by Parkinson's disease. The characteristic features include a fixed, emotionless facial expression (masklike); trembling of the hands, arms, or legs; and stiffness of the extremities that limits movement and produces a rigid posture and gait.

Parkinsonism is a fairly common adverse effect with large doses of strong tranquilizers (notably the phenothiazines) or their use over an extended period. If recognized early, it lessens or disappears with reduced dosage or change in medication. In some instances, however, Parkinson-like changes may become permanent.

Peripheral Neuritis (Peripheral Neuropathy) A group of symptoms resulting from nerve tissue injury. A variety of drugs and chemicals can cause changes in nerve structure or function. Symptoms include a sensation of numbness and tingling that starts in the fingers and toes, accompanied by altered sensation to touch and vague discomfort ranging from aching to burning pain. Severe forms may include loss of muscular strength and coordination.

A relatively common form is seen with the long-term use of isoniazid treatment of tuberculosis when vitamin B_6 (pyridoxine) is not given with isoniazid.

Since peripheral neuritis can also occur as a late complication of many viral infections, care must be taken to avoid assigning a cause-and-effect relationship to a drug (see CAUSE-AND-EFFECT RE-

LATIONSHIP). See Table 8, "Drugs That May Cause Nerve Damage or Dysfunction," Section Six.

Peyronie's Disease A permanent deformity of the penis caused by dense fibrous (scarlike) tissue within the system of penile vessels that become engorged with blood during erection. During sexual arousal, this inelastic fibrous tissue causes a painful downward bowing of the penis that hampers or precludes satisfactory intercourse. This condition has been associated with the use of phenytoin (Dilantin, etc.) and most beta-blockers (see Drug Classes and Table 1, "Drugs That May Adversely Affect Sexuality," Section Six).

Pharmacoeconomics The study of the issues involved in costs versus benefits using a variety of measures such as material and personnel costs, treatment outcomes, and quality of life. Study results help decide where and how health care resources should be utilized.

Pharmacology The medical science of development and use of medicinal drugs, and their composition and action. Used in its broadest sense, pharmacology embraces the related sciences of medicinal chemistry, experimental therapeutics, and toxicology.

Example: Investigation of the mechanisms of action (*pharmacology*) of widely used sulfonylurea drugs revealed that they stimulate the pancreas to release insulin. *Pharmacologic* studies on another group of sulfa-related drugs, the thiazide diuretics, revealed that they could cause the kidney to excrete more water and salt in the urine. This drug action is of great value in treating high blood pressure and heart failure.

Photosensitivity A drug-induced change in the skin that results in a rash or exaggerated sunburn on exposure to the sun or ultraviolet lamps.

Porphyria The porphyrias are a group of hereditary disorders characterized by excessive production of prophyrins, essential respiratory pigments of the body. One porphyrin is a component of hemoglobin, the pigment of red blood cells. Certain drugs activate two forms of porphyria: acute intermittent porphyria and cutaneous porphyria.

Acute intermittent porphyria involves damage to the nervous system; an acute attack can include fever, rapid heart rate, vomiting, pain in the abdomen and legs, hallucinations, seizures, paralysis, and coma. Twenty-three drugs (or drug classes) can induce an acute attack, including the barbiturates, sulfa drugs, chlordiazepoxide (Librium), chlorpropamide (Diabinese), methyldopa

(Aldomet), and phenytoin (Dilantin). Cutaneous porphyria involves damage to the skin and liver. An episode can include reddening and blistering of the skin, followed by crust formation, scarring, and excessive hair growth; repeated liver damage can lead to cirrhosis. This form is precipitated by chloroquine, estrogen, oral contraceptives, and excessive iron.

Priapism Prolonged, painful erection of the penis usually unassociated with sexual arousal or stimulation. It is caused by obstruction to drainage of blood through the veins at the root of the penis. Erection may persist for 30 minutes to a few hours and then subside spontaneously, or up to 30 hours, requiring surgical drainage of blood from the penis. More than half of the drug-induced episodes result in permanent impotence. Sickle cell anemia (or trait) may predispose to priapism.

Drugs reported to induce priapism include the following:

anabolic steroids
chlorpromazine (Thorazine)
cocaine
guanethidine (Ismelin)
haloperidol (Haldol)
heparin
levodopa (Sinemet)
molindone (Moban)
prazosin (Minipress)
prochlorperazine (Compazine)
trazodone (Desyrel)
trifluoperazine (Stelazine)
warfarin (Coumadin)

Prostatism Difficulties associated with an enlarged prostate gland. As the prostate enlarges (a natural development in aging men), it constricts the urethra (outflow passage) and impedes urination. This causes a reduction in the size and force of the urine stream, hesitancy in starting the flow of urine, interruption of urination, and incomplete emptying of the bladder. Atropine and drugs with atropinelike effects can intensify all of these symptoms.

Raynaud's Phenomenon Intermittent episodes of reduced blood flow into the fingers or toes, with resulting paleness, discomfort, numbness, and tingling due to an exaggerated constriction of the small arteries that supply blood to fingers. Attacks are often precipitated by emotional stress or exposure to cold, part of a systemic disorder (lupus erythematosus, scleroderma), or without apparent cause (Raynaud's disease). Some widely used drugs, notably beta-adrenergic–blockers and products that contain ergotamine, are conducive to the development of Raynaud-like symptoms in predisposed individuals.

Reye (Reye's) Syndrome An acute, often fatal childhood illness characterized by swelling of the brain and toxic degeneration of the liver. It usually develops during recovery from a flu-like infection, measles, or chickenpox. Symptoms include fever, headache, delirium, loss of consciousness, and seizures. It is one of the 10 major causes of death in children 1 to 10 years old.

Evidence suggests that it may be due to the combined effects of viral infection and chemical toxins (possibly drugs) in a genetically predisposed child. Drugs that have been used just prior to the onset of symptoms include acetaminophen, aspirin, antibiotics, and antiemetics. Current recommendations are to avoid the use of such drugs in children with flu-like infections, chickenpox, or measles.

Secondary Effect A by-product or complication of drug use that does not occur as part of the drug's primary pharmacologic activity. Secondary effects are unwanted and adverse effects.

Examples: Reactivation of dormant tuberculosis can be a *secondary effect* of long-term cortisone administration for arthritis. The cramping of leg muscles can be a *secondary effect* of diuretic (urine-producing) drug treatment for high blood pressure.

Side Effect A normal, expected, and predictable response to a drug that accompanies the principal (intended) response. Side effects are part of a drug's pharmacologic activity and thus unavoidable. Most are undesirable. The majority cause minor annoyance and inconvenience; some may cause serious problems; a few can be hazardous.

Superinfection (Suprainfection) A second infection that happens at the same time as the initial infection under treatment. The superinfection is caused by organisms that are not susceptible to the killing action of the drug(s) used to treat the original (primary) infection. Superinfections usually occur during or immediately following treatment with a broad-spectrum antibiotic, which alters the customary balance of bacterial populations in the body. This permits the overgrowth of organisms that normally exist in numbers too small to cause disease. The superinfection may also require treatment.

Example: Repeated courses of treatment of recurrent infections of the kidney and bladder with a variety of anti-infective drugs can suppress the normally dominant bacteria in the colon and rectum, encouraging the overgrowth of yeast organisms.

Tardive Dyskinesia A late-developing, drug-induced disorder of the nervous system characterized by involuntary bizarre movements of the eyelids, jaws, lips, tongue, neck, and fingers. It occurs after long-term treatment with drugs used to manage serious mental illness. It may occur in any age group, but is more common in the middle-aged and the elderly, particularly older, chronically ill women.

Once developed, the pattern of uncontrollable chewing, lip puckering, and repetitive tongue protruding (fly-catching movement) appears to be irreversible. To date, there is no way of identifying beforehand the individual who may develop this reaction to treatment, and there is no known prevention. Fortunately the persistent dyskinesia (abnormal movement) is not accompanied by further impairment of mental function or deterioration of intelligence.

Tolerance An adaptation by the body that lessens its responsiveness to a drug on continuous administration. It can be beneficial or harmful.

Examples: Beneficial tolerance occurs when drowsiness gradually disappears after 4 or 5 days of continuous use of antihistamines. Harmful tolerance occurs when the usual dose of codeine is no longer sufficient to relieve pain of shingles.

Toxicity The capacity of a drug to dangerously impair body functions or damage body tissues. Most drug toxicity is related to total dosage: the larger the overdose, the greater the toxic effects. Some drugs, however, produce toxic reactions in normal doses. Such adverse effects are not due to allergy or idiosyncrasy; in many instances their mechanisms are not fully understood.

Toxic effects due to overdosage are generally a harmful extension of the drug's normal pharmacologic actions and, to some extent, predictable and preventable. Toxic reactions with normal dosage are unrelated to the drug's known pharmacology and, for the most part, unpredictable and unexplainable.

Tyramine A chemical present in many foods and beverages that usually does not cause problems. The main pharmacologic action is to raise the blood pressure, but enzymes in many body tissues normally neutralize this action. The principal neutralizing enzyme is monoamine oxidase (MAO) type A, which helps balance several of the chemical processes in the body that control certain activities of the nervous system. If its action is blocked, chemical substances such as tyramine function unopposed, and relatively small amounts can cause alarming and dangerous elevations of blood pressure.

Several drugs can block the action of monoamine oxidase type A. These type A inhibitors (see Drug Classes) may produce a sudden increase in blood pressure in an individual whose diet includes a significant amount of tyramine.

Any protein-containing food that has undergone partial decomposition may present a hazard because of its increased tyramine content. The following foods and beverages have been reported to contain varying amounts of tyramine. Unless their tyramine content is known to be insignificant, they should be avoided altogether while taking an MAO type A inhibitor.

FOODS
Aged cheeses of all kinds*
Avocado
Banana skins
Bean curd
Bologna
Bovril extract
Broad bean pods
Chicken liver (unless fresh
    and used at once)
Chocolate
Figs, canned
Fish, canned
Fish, dried and salted
Herring, pickled
Liver, if not very fresh
Marmite extract
Meat extracts
Meat tenderizers
Pepperoni
Raisins
Raspberries
Salami
Shrimp paste
Sour cream
Soy sauce
Yeast extracts

BEVERAGES
Beer (unpasteurized)
Chianti wine
Sherry wine
Vermouth

*Cottage cheese, cream cheese, and processed cheese are safe.

Note: *Any* high-protein food that is aged or has undergone breakdown by putrefaction probably contains tyramine.

Viral Load or Burden A term used in reference to AIDS patients to describe the amount of HIV present in the body at any given time. Many clinicians use this test to help ensure that the present therapy is working, and also may use an increasing viral load as an indication that therapy must be changed.

WHO Pain Ladder A therapeutic model developed by the World Health Organization that organizes medicines available to treat pain on a three-step ladder. The medicines included are: NSAIDs, opiates, and adjuvant-control pain drugs. The concept lets the prescriber increase or decrease combinations of medicines appropriately to effectively control pain.

TABLES OF DRUG AND HEALTH CARE INFORMATION

TABLE 1

Drugs That May Adversely Affect Sexuality

Many medicines change sexual function in a variety of ways. Often, patients are not aware that problems in their sex life may actually be caused by the medicines they are taking to help an unrelated disease or condition, or they are embarrassed to discuss the problem with their doctor.

Sexual dysfunction may also be a natural consequence of the disorder under treatment or a concurrent and undetected disorder. Diabetes, kidney failure, hypertension, depression, and alcoholism may reduce libido and cause failure of erection. In addition, many of the drugs commonly used to treat these conditions may worsen a subclinical sexual dysfunction through unavoidable pharmacologic activity. These situations require the closest cooperation between doctor and patient to assess the possible cause-and-effect relationships and change the therapy.

Possible Drug Effects on Male Sexuality

Increased sex drive (libido)

androgens
(replacement
therapy in
deficiency states)
baclofen (Lioresal)

chlordiazepoxide
(Librium)
(antianxiety effect)
diazepam (Valium)
(antianxiety effect)

haloperidol (Haldol)
levodopa (Larodopa,
Sinemet) (may be
an indirect effect
due to improved
sense of well-being)

Decreased sex drive (libido)

antihistamines
barbiturates
chlordiazepoxide
(Librium) (sedative
effect)

chlorpromazine
(Thorazine) 10 to
20% of users
cimetidine (Tagamet)

clofibrate
(Atromid-S)
clonidine (Catapres)
10 to 20% of users
danazol (Danocrine)

Possible Drug Effects on Male Sexuality (cont.)

diazepam (Valium)
(sedative effect)

disulfiram
(Antabuse)

estrogens (therapy
for prostatic
cancer)

fenfluramine
(Pondimin)

heroin

licorice

medroxyprogesterone
(Provera)

methyldopa
(Aldomet) 10 to
15% of users

metoclopramide
(Reglan) 80% of
users

perhexiline (Pexid)

prazosin (Minipress)
15% of users

propranolol (Inderal)
rarely

reserpine (Serpasil,
Ser-Ap-Es)

spironolactone
(Aldactone)

tricyclic
antidepressants
(TCAs)

Erection problems (impotence)

anticholinergics

antihistamines

baclofen (Lioresal)

barbiturates (when
abused)

beta-blockers

chlordiazepoxide
(Librium) (in high
dosages)

chlorpromazine
(Thorazine)

cimetidine (Tagamet)

clofibrate
(Atromid-S)

clonidine (Catapres)
10 to 20% of users

cocaine

diazepam (Valium)
(in high dosage)

digitalis and its
glycosides

disopyramide
(Norpace)

disulfiram
(Antabuse)
(uncertain)

estrogens (therapy
for prostatic
cancer)

ethacrynic acid
(Edecrin) 5% of
users

ethionamide
(Trecator-SC)

fenfluramine
(Pondimin)

finasteride (Proscar)

furosemide (Lasix)
5% of users

guanethidine
(Ismelin)

haloperidol (Haldol)
10 to 20% of users

heroin

hydroxyprogesterone
(therapy for
prostatic cancer)

licorice

lithium (Lithonate)

marijuana

mesoridazine
(Serentil)

methantheline
(Banthine)

methyldopa
(Aldomet) 10 to
15% of users

metoclopramide
(Reglan) 60% of
users

monoamine oxidase
(MAO) type A
inhibitors, 10 to
15% of users

perhexiline (Pexid)

prazosin (Minipress)
infrequently

reserpine (Serpasil,
Ser-Ap-Es)

spironolactone
(Aldactone)

thiazide diuretics, 5%
of users

thioridazine
(Mellaril)

tricyclic
antidepressants
(TCAs)

Impaired ejaculation

anticholinergics

barbiturates (when
abused)

chlorpromazine
(Thorazine)

clonidine (Catapres)

estrogens (therapy
for prostatic
cancer)

Possible Drug Effects on Male Sexuality (cont.)

finasteride (Proscar)
(decreased volume)
guanethidine
(Ismelin)
heroin
mesoridazine
(Serentil)
methyldopa
(Aldomet)

monoamine oxidase
(MAO) type A
inhibitors
phenoxybenzamine
(Dibenzyline)
phentolamine
(Regitine)

reserpine (Serpasil,
Ser-Ap-Es)
thiazide diuretics
thioridazine
(Mellaril)
tricyclic
antidepressants
(TCAs)

Decreased male sex hormone (testosterone)

adrenocorticotropic
hormone (ACTH)
barbiturates
digoxin (Lanoxin)
haloperidol (Haldol)
(increased
testosterone with
low dosage;

decreased
testosterone with
high dosage)
lithium (Lithonate)
marijuana
medroxyprogesterone
(Provera)

monoamine oxidase
(MAO) type A
inhibitors
spironolactone
(Aldactone)

Reduced fertility (Decreased sperm formation)

adrenocorticosteroids
(prednisone, etc.)
androgens (moderate
to high dosage,
extended use)
antimalarials
aspirin (abusive,
chronic use)
chlorambucil
(Leukeran)
cimetidine (Tagamet)
colchicine
co-trimoxazole
(Bactrim, Septra)

cyclophosphamide
(Cytoxan)
estrogens (therapy
for prostatic
cancer)
marijuana
medroxyprogesterone
(Provera)
methotrexate
metoclopramide
(Reglan)
monoamine oxidase
(MAO) type A
inhibitors

niridazole (Ambilhar)
nitrofurantoin
(Furadantin)
spironolactone
(Aldactone)
sulfasalazine
(Azulfidine)
testosterone
(moderate to high
dosage, extended
use)
vitamin C (in doses of
1 g or more)

Testicular problems

Swelling
tricyclic
antidepressants
(TCAs)

Inflammation
oxyphenbutazone
(Tandearil)

Atrophy
androgens
(moderate to high
dosage, extended
use)

Possible Drug Effects on Male Sexuality (cont.)

chlorpromazine
(Thorazine)

cyclophosphamide
(Cytoxan) (in
prepubescent boys)

spironolactone
(Aldactone)

Penis problems

Priapism
  anabolic steroids
  (male hormonelike
  drugs)
  chlorpromazine
  (Thorazine)
  cocaine
  guanethidine
  (Ismelin)
  haloperidol
  (Haldol)

heparin
levodopa (Sinemet)
molindone
  (Moban)
prazosin
  (Minipress)
prochlorperazine
  (Compazine)
trazodone (Desyrel)

trifluoperazine
  (Stelazine)
warfarin
  (Coumadin)

Peyronie's disease
  beta-blockers
  phenytoin
  (Dilantin, etc.)

Male breast enlargement (gynecomastia)

androgens (partial
  conversion to
  estrogen)
busulfan (Myleran)
carmustine (BiCNU)
chlormadinone
chlorpromazine
  (Thorazine)
chlortetracycline
  (Aureomycin)
cimetidine (Tagamet)
clonidine (Catapres)
  (infrequently)
diethylstilbestrol
  (DES)
digitalis and its
  glycosides

estrogens (therapy
  for prostatic
  cancer)
ethionamide
  (Trecator-SC)
finasteride (Proscar)
griseofulvin
  (Fulvicin, etc.)
haloperidol (Haldol)
heroin
human chorionic
  gonadotropin
isoniazid (INH,
  Nydrazid)
marijuana
mestranol

methyldopa
  (Aldomet)
metoclopramide
  (Reglan)
phenelzine (Nardil)
reserpine (Serpasil,
  Ser-Ap-Es)
spironolactone
  (Aldactone)
thioridazine
  (Mellaril)
tricyclic
  antidepressants
  (TCAs)
vincristine (Oncovin)

Feminization (loss of libido, impotence, gynecomastia, testicular atrophy)

conjugated estrogens
  (Premarin, etc.)

Precocious puberty

anabolic steroids	androgens	isoniazid (INH)

Possible Drug Effects on Female Sexuality

Increased sex drive (libido)

androgens	diazepam (Valium)	oral contraceptives
chlordiazepoxide	(antianxiety effect)	(freedom from fear
(Librium)	mazindol (Sanorex)	of pregnancy)
(antianxiety effect)		

Decreased sex drive (libido)

See list of drug effects on male sexuality, above. Some of these *may* have potential for reducing libido in females. The literature is sparse on this subject.

Impaired arousal and orgasm

anticholinergics	monoamine oxidase	tricyclic
clonidine (Catapres)	inhibitors (MAOIs)	antidepressants
methyldopa		(TCAs)
(Aldomet)		

Breast enlargement

penicillamine	tricyclic
	antidepressants
	(TCAs)

Spontaneous milk flow (galactorrhea)

amphetamines	methyldopa	reserpine (Serpasil,
chlorpromazine	(Aldomet)	Ser-Ap-Es)
(Thorazine)	metoclopramide	sulpiride (Equilid)
cimetidine (Tagamet)	(Reglan)	tricyclic
haloperidol (Haldol)	oral contraceptives	antidepressants
heroin	phenothiazines	(TCAs)

Decreased fertility (ovarian failure)

anesthetic gases	cyclophosphamide	danazol (Danocrine)
(operating room	(Cytoxan)	medroxyprogesterone
staff)	cytostatic drugs	(Provera)

Menstrual disorders (altered menstruation)

adrenocorticosteroids (prednisone, etc.)
androgens
barbiturates (when abused)
chlorambucil (Leukeran)
chlorpromazine (Thorazine)
cyclophosphamide (Cytoxan)
danazol (Danocrine)
estrogens

ethionamide (Trecator-SC)
haloperidol (Haldol)
heroin
isoniazid (INH, Nydrazid)
marijuana
medroxyprogesterone (Provera)
metoclopramide (Reglan)
oral contraceptives

phenothiazines
progestins
radioisotopes
rifampin (Rifadin, Rifamate, Rimactane)
spironolactone (Aldactone)
testosterone
thioridazine (Mellaril)
vitamin A (in excessive dosage)

Virilization (acne, hirsutism, lowering of voice, enlargement of clitoris)

anabolic drugs
androgens

haloperidol (Haldol)

oral contraceptives (lowering of voice)

Precocious puberty

estrogens (in hair lotions)

isoniazid (INH, Nydrazid)

TABLE 2

Drugs That May Adversely Affect Behavior

Some drugs have side effects that alter mood and disturb emotional stability, as well as causing unexpected and unpredictable patterns of abnormal thinking and behavior. These effects are infrequent, but the nature and degree of mental disturbance is alarming and potentially dangerous for both patient and family. It is now well recognized that such paradoxical responses are often idiosyncratic. People with a history of serious mental or emotional disorders are more likely to experience bizarre reactions.

It is often difficult to judge whether a particular aberration is a feature of the disorder under treatment or of one (or more) drugs the patient is taking. If in doubt, it is best to stop taking any drug with the potential for such side effects and watch for changes during a drug-free period.

Drugs reported to impair *concentration* and/or *memory*

antihistamines*
antiparkinsonism
    drugs*
barbiturates*

benzodiazepines*
isoniazid
monoamine oxidase
    (MAO) inhibitors*

phenytoin
primidone
scopolamine

Drugs reported to cause *confusion, delirium,* or *disorientation*

acetazolamide
aminophylline
amphotericin B
antidepressants*
antihistamines*
atropinelike drugs*
barbiturates*
benzodiazepines*
bromides
carbamazepine
chloroquine
cimetidine
clonidine
cortisonelike drugs*
cycloserine
digitalis
digitoxin

digoxin
disulfiram
diuretics
ethchlorvynol
ethinamate
fenfluramine
glutethimide
histamine (H_2)
    receptor
    antagonists
isoniazid
levodopa
meprobamate
metoclopramide
narcotic pain
    relievers

para-aminosalicylic
    acid
phenelzine
phenothiazines*
phenytoin
piperazine
primidone
propranolol
quinolone antibiotics
ranitidine
reserpine
scopolamine
theophylline
tricyclic
    antidepressants
    (TCAs)

Drugs reported to cause *paranoid thinking*

bromides
cortisonelike drugs*

diphenhydramine
disulfiram

isoniazid
levodopa

Drugs reported to cause *schizophreniclike behavior*

amphetamines*
ephedrine

fenfluramine
phenmetrazine

phenylpropanolamine

Drugs reported to cause *maniclike behavior*

antidepressants*
cortisonelike drugs*
levodopa

monoamine oxidase
    inhibitor (MAOI)
    drugs*

*See Drug Classes.

Less apparent, but no less important, are mood-altering *side effects*. Emotional and behavioral effects may be quite unpredictable from person to person. The following experiences have been observed with sufficient frequency to establish recognizable patterns.

Drugs reported to cause *nervousness* (anxiety and irritability)

amantadine
amphetaminelike
  drugs* (appetite
  suppressants)
antihistamines*
caffeine
chlorphenesin
cortisonelike drugs*
ephedrine

epinephrine
isoproterenol
levodopa
liothyronine (in
  excessive dosage)
methylphenidate
methysergide
monoamine oxidase
  inhibitors
  (MAOIs)*

nylidrin
oral contraceptives
theophylline
thyroid (in excessive
  dosage)
thyroxine (in
  excessive dosage)

Drugs reported to cause *emotional depression*

amantadine
amphetamines* (on
  withdrawal)
benzodiazepines*
carbamazepine
chloramphenicol
cortisonelike drugs*
cycloserine
digitalis
digitoxin
digoxin
diphenoxylate

estrogens
ethionamide
fenfluramine (on
  withdrawal)
fluphenazine
guanethidine
haloperidol
indomethacin
isoniazid
levodopa
methsuximide
methyldopa

methysergide
metoprolol
oral contraceptives
phenylbutazone
procainamide
progesterones
propranolol
reserpine
sulfonamides*
vitamin D (in
  excessive dosage)

Drugs reported to cause *euphoria*

amantadine
aminophylline
amphetamines
antihistamines*
  (some)
antispasmodics,
  synthetic*

aspirin
barbiturates*
benzphetamine
chloral hydrate
clorazepate
codeine
cortisonelike drugs*

diethylpropion
diphenoxylate
ethosuximide
flurazepam
haloperidol
levodopa
meprobamate

*See Drug Classes.

Drugs reported to cause *euphoria* (cont.)

methysergide
monoamine oxidase
    inhibitors
    (MAOIs)*

morphine
pargyline
pentazocine
phenmetrazine

propoxyphene
scopolamine
tybamate

Drugs reported to cause *excitement*

acetazolamide
amantadine
amphetaminelike
    drugs*
antidepressants*
antihistamines*
atropinelike drugs*
barbiturates*
    (paradoxical
    response)
benzodiazepines*
    (paradoxical
    response)
cortisonelike drugs

cycloserine
diethylpropion
digitalis
ephedrine
epinephrine
ethinamate
    (paradoxical
    response)
ethionamide
glutethimide
    (paradoxical
    response)
isoniazid
isoproterenol

levodopa
meperidine and MAO
    inhibitors*
methyldopa and
    MAO inhibitors*
methyprylon
    (paradoxical
    response)
nalidixic acid
orphenadrine
quinine
scopolamine

TABLE 3

Drugs That May Adversely Affect Vision

Many adverse drug effects involve vision problems or frank damage to structures of the eye. Some effects (blurring of vision, double vision) may happen quickly after starting a drug and rapidly disappear with adjustment of dosage. More subtle and serious effects, such as development of cataracts or damage to the retina or optic nerve, may not happen until a drug has been used for an extended period of time and may not be reversible. Call your doctor immediately if eye discomfort or a change in vision occurs.

Drugs reported to cause *blurring of vision*

acetazolamide
antiarthritic/anti-infl-
    ammatory drugs
antidepressants*

antihistamines*
atropinelike drugs*
chlorthalidone
ciprofloxacin

cortisonelike drugs*
diethylstilbestrol
etretinate
fenfluramine

*See Drug Classes.

Drugs reported to cause *blurring of vision* (cont.)

norfloxacin
oral contraceptives

phenytoin
sulfonamides*

tetracyclines*
thiazide diuretics*

Drugs reported to cause *double vision*

antidepressants*
antidiabetic drugs*
antihistamines*
aspirin
barbiturates*
benzodiazepines*
bromides
carbamazepine
carisoprodol
chloroquine
chlorprothixene
ciprofloxacin
clomiphene
colchicine
colistin
cortisonelike drugs*
digitalis

digitoxin
digoxin
ethionamide
ethosuximide
etretinate
guanethidine
hydroxychloroquine
indomethacin
isoniazid
levodopa
mephenesin
methocarbamol
methsuximide
morphine
nalidixic acid
nitrofurantoin
norfloxacin

oral contraceptives
orphenadrine
oxyphenbutazone
pentazocine
phenothiazines*
phensuximide
phenylbutazone
phenytoin
primidone
propranolol
quinidine
sedatives/sleep
  inducers*
thiothixene
tranquilizers*

Drugs reported to cause *farsightedness*

ergot derivatives
penicillamine

sulfonamides*
  (possibly)

tolbutamide
  (possibly)

Drugs reported to cause *nearsightedness*

acetazolamide
aspirin
carbachol
chlorthalidone
codeine
cortisonelike drugs*

ethosuximide
methsuximide
morphine
oral contraceptives
penicillamine
phenothiazines*

phensuximide
spironolactone
sulfonamides*
tetracyclines*
thiazide diuretics*

Drugs reported to *alter color vision*

acetaminophen
amodiaquine

amyl nitrite
aspirin

atropine
barbiturates*

*See Drug Classes.

Drugs reported to *alter color vision* (cont.)

belladonna
chloramphenicol
chloroquine
chlorpromazine
chlortetracycline
ciprofloxacin
cortisonelike drugs*
digitalis
digitoxin
digoxin
disulfiram
epinephrine
ergotamine
erythromycin
ethchlorvynol
ethionamide
fluphenazine
furosemide

hydroxychloroquine
indomethacin
isocarboxazid
isoniazid
mefenamic acid
mesoridazine
methysergide
nalidixic acid
norfloxacin
oral contraceptives
oxyphenbutazone
paramethadione
pargyline
penicillamine
pentylenetetrazol
perphenazine
phenacetin
phenylbutazone

primidone
prochlorperazine
promazine
promethazine
quinacrine
quinidine
quinine
reserpine
sodium salicylate
streptomycin
sulfonamides*
thioridazine
tranylcypromine
trifluoperazine
triflupromazine
trimeprazine
trimethadione

Drugs reported to cause *sensitivity to light* (photophobia)

antidiabetic drugs*
atropinelike drugs*
bromides
chloroquine
ciprofloxacin
clomiphene
digitoxin
doxepin
ethambutol

ethionamide
ethosuximide
etretinate
hydroxychloroquine
mephenytoin
methsuximide
monoamine oxidase
   inhibitors
   (MAOIs)*

nalidixic acid
norfloxacin
oral contraceptives
paramethadione
phenothiazines*
quinidine
quinine
tetracyclines*
trimethadione

Drugs reported to cause *halos around lights*

amyl nitrite
chloroquine
cortisonelike drugs*
digitalis
digitoxin

digoxin
hydroxychloroquine
nitroglycerin
norfloxacin
oral contraceptives

paramethadione
phenothiazines*
quinacrine
trimethadione

*See Drug Classes.

Drugs reported to cause *visual hallucinations*

amantadine
amphetaminelike
    drugs*
amyl nitrite
antihistamines*
aspirin
atropinelike drugs*
barbiturates*
benzodiazepines*
bromides
carbamazepine
cephalexin
cephaloglycin
chloroquine
cycloserine

digitalis
digoxin
disulfiram
ephedrine
furosemide
griseofulvin
haloperidol
hydroxychloroquine
indomethacin
isosorbide
levodopa
nialamide
oxyphenbutazone
pargyline
pentazocine

phenothiazines*
phenylbutazone
phenytoin
primidone
propranolol
quinine
sedatives/sleep
    inducers*
sulfonamides*
tetracyclines*
tricyclic
    antidepressants
    (TCAs)*
tripelennamine

Drugs reported to impair the use of *contact lenses*

brompheniramine
carbinoxamine
chlorpheniramine
cyclizine
cyproheptadine

dexbrompheniramine
dexchlorpheniramine
dimethindene
diphenhydramine
diphenylpyraline

furosemide
oral contraceptives
terfenadine
tripelennamine

Drugs reported to cause *cataracts* or *lens deposits*

allopurinol
busulfan
chlorpromazine
chlorprothixene
cortisonelike drugs*
fluphenazine
mesoridazine

methotrimeprazine
perphenazine
phenmetrazine
pilocarpine
prochlorperazine
promazine
promethazine

thioridazine
thiothixene
trifluoperazine
triflupromazine
trimeprazine

TABLE 4

Drugs That May Cause Blood Problems

All blood cells originate and mature in the bone marrow. They come from self-renewing stem cells that change into specific cell lines. These cells produce fully developed, distinctive blood cell

*See Drug Classes.

forms: erythrocytes (red blood cells), leukocytes (white blood cells), and thrombocytes (blood platelets). The leukocytes include three varieties: granulocytes, monocytes (macrophages), and lymphocytes. Drugs that adversely affect formation and development of blood cells can (1) act on any stage of cell production; (2) impair the production of one cell line; (3) influence the production of all cell lines.

Through a variety of mechanisms, mature cells in the bloodstream can be disrupted.

Drugs that cause inevitable (dose-dependent) *aplastic anemia*

actinomycin D	cytarabine	mercaptopurine
azathioprine	doxorubicin	methotrexate
busulfan	epirubicin	mitomycin
carboplatin	etoposide	mitoxantrone
carmustine	fluorouracil	plicamycin
chlorambucil	hydroxyurea	procarbazine
cisplatin	lomustine	thioguanine
cyclophosphamide	melphalan	thiotepa

Drugs that may cause idiosyncratic (dose-independent) *aplastic anemia*

amodiaquine	mepacrine	pyrimethamine
benoxaprofen	oxyphenbutazone	sulfonamides*
carbimazole	penicillamine	sulindac
chloramphenicol	phenylbutazone	thiouracils
chlorpromazine	phenytoin	trimethoprim/sulfam-
gold	piroxicam	ethoxazole
indomethacin	prothiaden	

Drugs that may *impair red blood cell production* (only)

azathioprine	halothane	phenytoin
carbamazepine	isoniazid	pyrimethamine
chloramphenicol	methyldopa	stavudine
chlorpropamide	penicillin	sulfasalazine
dapsone	pentachlorophenol	sulfathiazide
fenoprofen	phenobarbital	sulfonamides*
gold	phenylbutazone	sulfonylureas*

*See Drug Classes.

Drugs that may *impair red blood cell production* (only) (cont.)

thiamphenicol
tolbutamide

trimethoprim/sulfam-
    ethoxazole

zidovudine

Drugs that may significantly *reduce granulocyte cell counts* (various mechanisms)

acetaminophen
acetazolamide
allopurinol
amitriptyline
amodiaquine
benzodiazepines*
captopril
carbamazepine
carbimazole
cephalosporins*
chloramphenicol
chloroquine
chlorothiazide
chlorpromazine
chlorpropamide
chlorthalidone
cimetidine
clindamycin
dapsone
desipramine
disopyramide

ethacrynic acid
gentamicin
gold
hydralazine
hydrochlorothiazide
imipramine
indomethacin
isoniazid
levamisole
meprobamate
methimazole
methyldopa
oxyphenbutazone
penicillamine
penicillins*
pentazocine
phenacetin
phenothiazines*
phenylbutazone
phenytoin
procainamide

propranolol
propylthiouracil
pyrimethamine
quinidine
quinine
ranitidine
rifampin
sodium
    aminosalicylate
streptomycin
sulfadoxine
sulfonamides*
tetracyclines*
tocainide
tolbutamide
trimethoprim/
    sulfamethoxazole
vancomycin
zalcitabine
zidovudine

Drugs that may significantly *reduce blood platelet counts*

acetazolamide
actinomycin
allopurinol
alpha-interferon
amiodarone
ampicillin
aspirin
carbamazepine
carbenicillin

cephalosporins*
chenodeoxycholic
    acid
chloroquine
chlorothiazide
chlorpheniramine
chlorpropamide
chlorthalidone
cimetidine

cyclophosphamide
danazol
desferrioxamine
diazepam
diazoxide
diclofenac
didanosine
digoxin
diltiazem

*See Drug Classes.

Drugs that may significantly *reduce blood platelet counts* (cont.)

furosemide
gentamicin
gold
hydrochlorothiazide
imipramine
isoniazid
isotretinoin
levamisole
meprobamate
methyldopa
mianserin
minoxidil
morphine

nitrofurantoin
oxprenolol
oxyphenbutazone
penicillamine
penicillins
phenylbutazone
phenytoin
piroxicam
procainamide
quinidine
quinine
ranitidine
rifampin

sodium
  aminosalicylate
sulfasalazine
sulfonamides*
thioguanine
trimethoprim/
  sulfamethoxazole
valproate
vancomycin
zalcitabine
zidovudine

Drugs that cause significant *hemolytic anemia* due to red cell glucose-6-phosphate dehydrogenase (G6PD) deficiency

acetanilid
methylene blue
nalidixic acid
naphthalene
niridazole
nitrofurantoin

pamaquine
phenazopyridine
phenylhydrazine
primaquine
sulfacetamide
sulfamethoxazole

sulfanilamide
sulfapyridine
thiazolsulfone
toluidine blue

Drugs that may cause *hemolytic anemia* by other mechanisms

antimony
chlorpropamide
cisplatin
mephenesin
methotrexate

para-aminosalicylic
  acid
penicillamine
phenazopyridine
quinidine

quinine
rifampin
sulfasalazine

Drugs that may cause *megaloblastic anemia*

acyclovir
alcohol
aminopterin
azathioprine

colchicine
cycloserine
cytarabine
floxuridine

fluorouracil
hydroxyurea
mercaptopurine
metformin

*See Drug Classes.

Drugs that may cause *megaloblastic anemia* (cont.)

methotrexate
neomycin
nitrofurantoin
nitrous oxide
oral contraceptives
para-aminosalicylic acid
pentamidine

phenformin
phenobarbital
phenytoin
primidone
pyrimethamine
sulfasalazine
tetracyclines*
thioguanine

triamterene
trimethoprim
vinblastine
vitamin A
vitamin C (large doses)
zidovudine

Drugs that may cause *sideroblastic anemia*

alcohol
chloramphenicol
cycloserine

isoniazid
penicillamine
phenacetin

pyrazinamide

TABLE 5

Drugs That May Cause Heart Damage or Dysfunction

Drugs can adversely affect the function and structure of the heart. Heart disorders that require drug therapy often determine the nature of adverse drug effects. Some are due to direct drug actions on the heart tissues (antiarrhythmics); others are indirect from altered chemical balances that change heart function (potassium loss from diuretics, causing abnormal heart rhythms and digitalis toxicity).

Drugs that may cause or contribute to *abnormal heart rhythms* (arrhythmias)

aminophylline
amiodarone
amitriptyline
antiarrhythmic drugs*
bepridil
beta-adrenergic–blocking drugs*
beta-adrenergic bronchodilators*
carbamazepine
chlorpromazine

cimetidine
digitoxin
digoxin
diltiazem
disopyramide
diuretics*
doxepin
encainide
fentolterol
flecainide
isoproterenol
ketanserin

lidocaine
maprotiline
methyldopa
mexiletine
milrinone
phenothiazines*
prenylamine
procainamide
quinidine
ranitidine
sotalol
terbutaline

*See Drug Classes.

Drugs that may cause or contribute to *abnormal heart rhythms* (arrhythmias) (cont.)

theophylline
thiazide diuretics*
thioridazine

trazodone
tricyclic
  antidepressants
  (TCAs)*

verapamil

Drugs that may *depress heart function* (reduce pumping efficiency)

beta-adrenergic
  blockers*
cocaine
daunorubicin
diltiazem

disopyramide
doxorubicin
epinephrine
flecainide
fluorouracil

isoproterenol
nifedipine
verapamil

Drugs that may *reduce coronary artery blood flow* (reduce oxygen supply to heart muscle)

amphetamines*
beta-adrenergic
  blockers* (abrupt
  withdrawal)
cocaine

ergotamine
fluorouracil
nifedipine
oral contraceptives
ritodrine

vasopressin
vinblastine
vincristine

Drugs that may *impair healing of heart muscle* following a heart attack (myocardial infarction)

adrenocortical
  steroids*

nonsteroidal
  anti-inflammatory

drugs (NSAIDs)*

Drugs that may cause *heart valve damage*

ergotamine
methysergide

minocycline
  (blue-black
  pigmentation)

Drugs that may cause *pericardial disease*

actinomycin D
anthracyclines
bleomycin
cisplatin
cyclophosphamide

cytarabine
fluorouracil
hydralazine
methysergide
minoxidil

phenylbutazone
practolol
procainamide
sulfasalazine

*See Drug Classes.

TABLE 6

Drugs That May Cause Liver Damage or Dysfunction

The liver changes drugs into forms that are readily eliminated from the body. A broad spectrum of adverse drug effects on liver function and structures has been documented, from mild increases in liver function tests to complete liver failure and death. Liver function tests MUST be carefully followed during the entire course of drug treatment.

Drugs that may cause *acute dose-dependent liver damage* (resembling acute viral hepatitis)

acetaminophen   salicylates* (doses
  (overdosage)   over 2 g daily)

Drugs that may cause *acute dose-independent liver damage* (resembling acute viral hepatitis)

acebutolol   isoniazid   phenytoin
allopurinol   ketoconazole   piroxicam
atenolol   labetalol   probenecid
carbamazepine   maprotiline   pyrazinamide
cimetidine   metoprolol   quinidine
dantrolene   mianserin   quinine
diclofenac   naproxen   ranitidine
diltiazem   nifedipine   rifampin
disulfiram   para-aminosalicylic sulfonamides*
enflurane   acid   sulindac
ethambutol   penicillins*   tricyclic
ethionamide   phenelzine   antidepressants
halothane   phenindione   (TCAs)*
ibuprofen   phenobarbital   valproic acid
indomethacin   phenylbutazone   verapamil

Drugs that may cause *acute fatty infiltration of the liver*

adrenocortical   methotrexate   sulfonamides*
  steroids*   phenothiazines*   tetracyclines*
antithyroid drugs   phenytoin   valproic acid
isoniazid   salicylates*

*See Drug Classes.

Drugs that may cause *cholestatic jaundice*

actinomycin D
amoxicillin/
   clavulanate
azathioprine
captopril
carbamazepine
carbimazole
cephalosporins*
chlordiazepoxide
chlorpropamide
cloxacillin
cyclophosphamide
cyclosporine
danazol
diazepam
disopyramide
enalapril

erythromycin
flecainide
flurazepam
flutamide
glyburide
gold
griseofulvin
haloperidol
ketoconazole
mercaptopurine
methyltestosterone
nifedipine
nitrofurantoin
nonsteroidal
   anti-inflammatory
   drugs*
norethandrolone

oral contraceptives
oxacillin
penicillamine
phenothiazines*
phenytoin
propoxyphene
propylthiouracil
sulfonamides*
tamoxifen
thiabendazole
tolbutamide
tricyclic
   antidepressants
   (TCAs)*
troleandomycin
verapamil

Drugs that may cause *liver granulomas* (chronic inflammatory nodules)

allopurinol
aspirin
carbamazepine
chlorpromazine
chlorpropamide
diltiazem
disopyramide

gold
hydralazine
isoniazid
methyldopa
nitrofurantoin
penicillins
phenylbutazone

phenytoin
procainamide
quinidine
ranitidine
sulfonamides*
tolbutamide

Drugs that may cause *chronic liver disease*

Active chronic hepatitis

acetaminophen
   (chronic use, large
   doses)

dantrolene
isoniazid
methyldopa

nitrofurantoin

Liver cirrhosis or fibrosis (scarring)

methotrexate

nicotinic acid

*See Drug Classes.

Chronic cholestasis (resembling primary biliary cirrhosis)

chlorpromazine/
   valproic acid
   (combination)
chlorpropamide/

erythromycin
   (combination)
imipramine
phenothiazines*

phenytoin
thiabendazole
tolbutamide

Drugs that may cause *liver tumors* (benign and malignant)

anabolic steroids
danazol

oral contraceptives
testosterone

thorotrast

Drugs that may cause *damage to liver blood vessels*

anabolic steroids
azathioprine
carmustine
cyclophosphamide/
   cyclosporine
   (combination)

dacarbazine
doxorubicin
mercaptopurine
methotrexate
mitomycin
oral contraceptives

thioguanine
vincristine
vitamin A (excessive
   doses)

TABLE 7

Drugs That May Cause Kidney Damage or Dysfunction

The kidneys play a minor role in changing a drug's chemical structure to help medicine removal, but they have a major role in eliminating the drug in the urine. Many drugs adversely affect the kidneys in several ways. The kidneys are very sensitive to toxic drug effects.

Drugs that may primarily *impair kidney function* (without damage)

amphotericin
angiotensin-
   converting enzyme
   (ACE) inhibitors*
   (with renal artery
   stenosis; congestive
   heart failure)

beta-adrenergic
   blockers*
colchicine
demeclocycline
diuretics/NSAIDs*
   (avoid this
   combination)

glyburide
isofosfamide
lithium/tricyclic
   antidepressants
   (TCAs)* (avoid this
   combination)
methoxyflurane

*See Drug Classes.

Drugs that may primarily *impair kidney function* (without damage) (cont.)

nifedipine
nitroprusside

nonsteroidal
anti-inflammatory
drugs*

rifampin
vinblastine

Drugs that may cause *acute kidney failure* (due to kidney damage)

Drugs that may damage the kidney filtration unit (the nephron)

acetaminophen
(excessive dosage)
allopurinol
aminoglycoside
antibiotics*
amphotericin
bismuth thiosulfate
carbamazepine

cisplatin
cyclosporine
enalapril
ergometrine
hydralazine
metronidazole
mitomycin
oral contraceptives

penicillamine
phenytoin
quinidine
rifampin
streptokinase
sulfonamides*
thiazide diuretics*

Drugs that may cause acute interstitial nephritis

allopurinol
amoxicillin
ampicillin
aspirin
azathioprine
aztreonam
captopril
carbamazepine
carbenicillin
cefaclor
cefoxitin
cephalexin
cephalothin
cephapirin
cephradine
cimetidine
ciprofloxacin
clofibrate
cloxacillin
diazepam

diclofenac
diflunisal
fenoprofen
foscarnet
furosemide
gentamicin
glafenine
ibuprofen
indomethacin
ketoprofen
meclofenamate
methicillin
methyldopa
mezlocillin
minocycline
nafcillin
naproxen
oxacillin
penicillamine
penicillins*

phenindione
phenobarbital
phenylbutazone
phenytoin
piroxicam
pirprofen
pyrazinamide
rifampin
sulfamethoxazole
sulfinpyrazone
sulfonamides*
sulindac
thiazide diuretics*
tolmetin
trimethoprim
valproate
vancomycin
warfarin

*See Drug Classes.

Muscle destruction and associated acute kidney failure

adrenocortical steroids*
alcohol
amphetamines*
amphotericin
carbenoxolone
chlorthalidone
clofibrate
cocaine
cytarabine
fenofibrate
haloperidol
halothane
heroin
lovastatin
opioid analgesics*
pentamidine
phenothiazines*
streptokinase
suxamethonium

Drugs that may cause *kidney damage resembling glomerulonephritis or nephrosis*

captopril
fenoprofen
gold
ketoprofen
lithium
mesalamine
penicillamine
phenytoin
practolol
probenecid
quinidine

Drugs (all with long-term use) that may cause *chronic interstitial nephritis and papillary necrosis* (analgesic kidney damage)

acetaminophen   aspirin   phenacetin

Drugs that may cause or contribute to *urinary tract crystal or stone formation*

acetazolamide
acyclovir
cytotoxic drugs
dihydroxyadenine
magnesium trisilicate
mercaptopurine
methotrexate
methoxyflurane
phenylbutazone
probenecid
salicylates*
sulfonamides*
thiazide diuretics*
triamterene
uricosuric drugs
vitamin A
vitamin C
vitamin D
warfarin
zoxazolamine

TABLE 8

Drugs That May Cause Nerve Damage or Dysfunction

Medications can damage the nervous system from the brain to peripheral nerves in the fingers. This table groups drugs according to the familiar clinical syndromes that are actually drug-induced neurological disorders.

*See Drug Classes.

Drugs that may cause *significant headache*

amyl nitrite
bromocriptine
clonidine
ergotamine
  (prolonged use)
etretinate
hydralazine
ibuprofen

indomethacin
labetalol
naproxen
nifedipine
nitrofurantoin
nitroglycerin
perhexiline
propranolol

sulindac
terbutaline
tetracyclines*
theophylline
tolmetin
trimethoprim/
  sulfamethoxazole

Drugs that may cause *seizures* (convulsions)

ampicillin
atenolol
carbenicillin
cephalosporins*
chloroquine
cimetidine
ciprofloxacin
cycloserine
disopyramide
ether

halothane
indomethacin
isoniazid
lidocaine
lithium
mefenamic acid
nalidixic acid
norfloxacin
oxacillin

penicillins*
  (synthetic)
phenothiazines*
pyrimethamine
terbutaline
theophylline
ticarcillin
tricyclic
  antidepressants
  (TCAs)*
vincristine

Drugs that may cause *stroke*

anabolic steroids
cocaine

oral contraceptives
phenylpropanolamine

Drugs that may cause features of *parkinsonism*

amitriptyline
amodiaquine
chloroquine
chlorprothixene
desipramine
diazoxide

diphenhydramine
droperidol
haloperidol
imipramine
levodopa
lithium

methyldopa
metoclopramide
phenothiazines*
reserpine
thiothixene
trifluperidol

Drugs that may cause *acute dystonias* (acute involuntary movement syndromes)

carbamazepine
chlorzoxazone
haloperidol
metoclopramide

phenothiazines*
phenytoin
propranolol

tricyclic
  antidepressants
  (TCAs)*

*See Drug Classes.

Drugs that may cause *tardive dyskinesia*

haloperidol   phenothiazines*   thiothixene

See also NEUROLEPTIC MALIGNANT SYNDROME (NMS) in Glossary.

Drugs that may cause *peripheral neuritis*

amiodarone
amitriptyline
amphetamines*
amphotericin
anticoagulants*
carbutamide
chlorambucil
chloramphenicol
chloroquine
chlorpropamide
cimetidine
clioquinol
clofibrate
colchicine
colistin
cytarabine
dapsone
disopyramide

disulfiram
ergotamine
ethambutol
glutethimide
gold
hydralazine
imipramine
indomethacin
isoniazid
methaqualone
methimazole
methysergide
metronidazole
nalidixic acid
nitrofurantoin
nitrofurazone
penicillamine
penicillins*

perhexiline
phenelzine
phenylbutazone
phenytoin
podophyllin
procarbazine
propranolol
propylthiouracil
stavudine
streptomycin
sulfonamides*
sulfoxone
thalidomide
tolbutamide
vinblastine
vincristine

Drugs that may cause *myasthenia gravis* syndrome

aminoglycoside
    antibiotics*
beta-adrenergic

blockers*
penicillamine
phenytoin

polymyxin B
trihexyphenidyl

TABLE 9

Drugs That May Adversely Affect the Fetus and Newborn Infant

In 1961, when thalidomide was prescribed to help pregnant women sleep, it caused major birth defects. Since then many studies have increased the understanding of adverse drug effects on the developing fetus and newborn infant and have helped identify medicines that cause significant harm to the unborn and newborn child.

*See Drug Classes.

Many drugs cause (or contribute to) malformations, retarded growth, functional disorders, and death of the fetus or newborn. It is strongly recommended that only those drugs that offer clear and essential benefits be used during pregnancy.

Drugs that *probably* cause adverse effects during the first 3 months (first trimester)

aminopterin
anticonvulsants*
antithyroid drugs
cytarabine
danazol
diethylstilbestrol
etretinate

fluorouracil
iodides
isotretinoin
kanamycin
mercaptopurine
methotrexate
misoprostol

opioid analgesics*
progestins*
quinine
streptomycin
testosterone
warfarin

Drugs that *possibly* cause adverse effects during the first trimester

angiotensin-
   converting enzyme
   (ACE) inhibitors*
busulfan
chlorambucil

estrogens*
lithium
mebendazole
monoamine oxidase
   inhibitors
   (MAOIs)*

oral contraceptives
piperazine
rifampin
tetracyclines*

Drugs that *probably* cause adverse effects during the second and third trimesters

amiodarone
androgens*
angiotensin-
   converting enzyme
   (ACE) inhibitors*
antithyroid drugs
aspirin
benzodiazepines*
chloramphenicol
estrogens*

iodides
kanamycin
lithium
nonsteroidal
   anti-inflammatory
   drugs (NSAIDs)*
opioid analgesics*
phenothiazines*
progestins*
rifampin

streptomycin
sulfonamides*
sulfonylureas*
tetracyclines*
thiazide diuretics*
tricyclic
   antidepressants
   (TCAs)*
warfarin

*See Drug Classes.

Drugs that *possibly* cause adverse effects during the *second and third trimesters*

acetazolamide	ethacrynic acid	hydroxyzine
clemastine	fluoroquinolones*	promethazine
diphenhydramine	haloperidol	

TABLE 10

Drugs That May Interact With Alcohol

Alcohol is a drug, though we tend not to think of it as such. Beverages containing alcohol may interact unfavorably with a wide variety of medicines. Most people are familiar with the possible increased effect of sedatives, sleep-inducing drugs, tranquilizers, and narcotics combined with alcohol. Alcohol also reduces the effectiveness of some drugs, and causes toxic effects. Some drugs worsen the intoxicating effects of alcohol, further impairing mental alertness, judgment, physical coordination, and reaction time.

Drug interactions with alcohol are usually predictable; however, their intensity and significance vary greatly because many factors influence the interaction. These factors include individual variations in sensitivity to drugs, the chemistry and quantity of the drug, the type and amount of alcohol consumed, and the sequence in which the drug and alcohol are taken. If you need to use any of the drugs listed in the following tables, you should ask your doctor for guidance concerning the use of alcohol.

Drugs with which it is advisable to avoid alcohol completely

Drug Name or Class	Possible Interaction With Alcohol
amphetamines	excessive rise in blood pressure with alcoholic beverages containing tyramine**
antidepressants*	excessive sedation, increased intoxication
barbiturates*	excessive sedation
bromides	confusion, delirium, increased intoxication
calcium carbimide	disulfiramlike reaction**
carbamazepine	excessive sedation
chlorprothixene	excessive sedation
chlorzoxazone	excessive sedation
disulfiram	disulfiram reaction**
ergotamine	reduced effectiveness of ergotamine

*See Drug Classes.
**See Glossary.

Drug Name or Class	Possible Interaction With Alcohol
fenfluramine	excessive stimulation of nervous system with some beers and wines
furazolidone	disulfiramlike reaction**
haloperidol	excessive sedation
MAO inhibitors*	excessive rise in blood pressure with alcoholic beverages containing tyramine**
meperidine	excessive sedation
meprobamate	excessive sedation
methotrexate	increased liver toxicity and excessive sedation
metronidazole	disulfiramlike reaction**
narcotic drugs	excessive sedation
oxyphenbutazone	increased stomach irritation and/or bleeding
pentazocine	excessive sedation
pethidine	excessive sedation
phenothiazines*	excessive sedation
phenylbutazone	increased stomach irritation and/or bleeding
procarbazine	disulfiramlike reaction**
propoxyphene	excessive sedation
reserpine	excessive sedation, orthostatic hypotension**
sleep-inducing drugs (hypnotics)	excessive sedation
carbromal	
chloral hydrate	
ethchlorvynol	
ethinamate	
glutethimide	
flurazepam	
methaqualone	
methyprylon	
temazepam	
triazolam	
thiothixene	excessive sedation
tricyclic antidepressants (TCAs)*	excessive sedation, increased intoxication
trimethobenzamide	excessive sedation

Drugs with which alcohol should be used only in small amounts (until combined effects are determined)

Drug Name or Class	Possible Interaction With Alcohol
acetaminophen (Tylenol, etc.)	increased liver toxicity

*See Drug Classes.
**See Glossary.

Drug Name or Class	Possible Interaction With Alcohol
amantadine	excessive lowering of blood pressure
antiarthritic/anti-inflammatory drugs	increased stomach irritation and/or bleeding
anticoagulants (coumarins)*	increased anticoagulant effect
antidiabetic drugs (sulfonylureas)*	increased antidiabetic effect, excessive hypoglycemia**
antihistamines*	excessive sedation
antihypertensives*	excessive orthostatic hypotension**
aspirin (large doses or continuous use)	increased stomach irritation and/or bleeding
benzodiazepines*	excessive sedation
carisoprodol	increased alcoholic intoxication
diethylpropion	excessive nervous system stimulation with alcoholic beverages containing tyramine**
dihydroergotoxine	excessive lowering of blood pressure
diphenoxylate	excessive sedation
dipyridamole	excessive lowering of blood pressure
diuretics*	excessive orthostatic hypotension**
ethionamide	confusion, delirium, psychotic behavior
fenoprofen	increased stomach irritation and/or bleeding
griseofulvin	flushing and rapid heart action
ibuprofen	increased stomach irritation and/or bleeding
indomethacin	increased stomach irritation and/or bleeding
insulin	excessive hypoglycemia**
iron	excessive absorption of iron
isoniazid	decreased effectiveness of isoniazid, increased incidence of hepatitis
lithium	increased confusion and delirium (avoid all alcohol if any indication of lithium overdosage)
methocarbamol	excessive sedation
methotrimeprazine	excessive sedation
methylphenidate	excessive nervous system stimulation with alcoholic beverages containing tyramine**
metoprolol	excessive orthostatic hypotension**
nalidixic acid	increased alcoholic intoxication
naproxen	increased stomach irritation and/or bleeding
nicotinic acid	possible orthostatic hypotension**
nitrates* (vasodilators)	possible orthostatic hypotension**
nylidrin	increased stomach irritation

*See Drug Classes.
**See Glossary.

Drug Name or Class	*Possible Interaction With Alcohol*
orphenadrine	excessive sedation
phenelzine	increased alcoholic intoxication
phentermine	excessive nervous system stimulation with alcoholic beverages containing tyramine**
phenytoin	decreased effect of phenytoin
pilocarpine	prolongation of alcohol effect
prazosin	excessive lowering of blood pressure
primidone	excessive sedation
propranolol	excessive orthostatic hypotension**
sulfonamides*	increased alcoholic intoxication
sulindac	increased stomach irritation and/or bleeding
tolmetin	increased stomach irritation and/or bleeding
tranquilizers (mild)	excessive sedation
chlordiazepoxide	
clorazepate	
diazepam	
hydroxyzine	
meprobamate	
oxazepam	
phenaglycodol	
tybamate	
tranylcypromine	increased alcoholic intoxication

Drugs capable of producing a disulfiramlike reaction** when used concurrently with alcohol

antidiabetic drugs (sulfonylureas)*	disulfiram	procarbazine
calcium carbimide	furazolidone	quinacrine
chloral hydrate	metronidazole	sulfonamides*
chloramphenicol	nifuroxime	tinidazole
	nitrofurantoin	tolazoline

TABLE 11

High-Potassium Foods

Drugs such as diuretics cause potassium loss, but also treat conditions that require reduced sodium intake. The high-potassium foods listed here have been selected for their compatibility with a sodium-restricted diet (500 to 1000 mg of sodium daily).

*See Drug Classes.
**See Glossary.

Beverages

orange juice	skim milk	tomato juice
prune juice	tea	whole milk

Breads and Cereals

brown rice	muffins	waffles
cornbread	oatmeal	
griddle cakes	shredded wheat	

Fruits

apricot	fig	orange
avocado	honeydew melon	papaya
banana	mango	prune

Meats

beef	haddock	rockfish
chicken	halibut	salmon
codfish	liver	turkey
flounder	pork	veal

Vegetables

baked beans	parsnips	tomato
lima beans	radishes	white potato
mushrooms	squash	
navy beans	sweet potato	

TABLE 12

Medications That Cause Hair Loss

Medicines can change a person's physical appearance dramatically by causing hair loss. This is usually an undesirable side effect of a particular drug and may be confusing and disturbing to the person taking the medicine.

auranofin (Ridaura)	cyclophosphamide	etoposide (VePesid)
cancer chemotherapy in general	(Cytoxan)	etretinate (Tegison)
chloroquine (Aralen)	dacarbazine (DTIC-Dome)	fluorouracil
cimetidine (Tagamet)	doxorubicin (Adriamycin)	heparin
colchicine (ColBenemid)	ethambutol (Myambutol)	indomethacin (Indocin)

isotretinoin
   (Accutane)
levodopa (Dopar)
lithium (Lithobid)
methotrexate

(Mexate)
methyldopa
   (Aldomet)
oral contraceptives
propranolol (Inderal)

radiation therapy
thallium
valproic acid
   (Depakote)

TABLE 13

Incubation Times of Contagious Diseases

Specific symptoms of a contagious disease usually appear within a given time after exposure, referred to as the *incubation time* or *incubation period*.

Disease: Acquired Immunodeficiency Syndrome (AIDS)

Incubation time: Up to 12 years.

How long it is usually contagious: No cure; remains contagious for the entire course.

Treatment: Multiple medicines available; many infectious disease specialists suggest combination therapy.

Disease: Gonorrhea, Clap

Incubation time: Some people may never have symptoms. In men, it takes from 3 to 14 days or longer to develop symptoms. Some women never have symptoms.

How long it is usually contagious: May result in meningitis or endocarditis; length of infectivity depends on the place and duration of infection prior to therapy. Ask your doctor for help.

Treatment: The most widely used drugs now are ceftriaxone (Rocephin) or spectinomycin, because of widespread resistant organisms.

Disease: Hepatitis, Hep B

Incubation time: From 5 weeks to 6 months.

How long it is usually contagious: 2 weeks before onset and may persist for years.

Treatment: Prevention is the best treatment. Hepatitis B vaccine is effective and recommended for those at risk. Once the disease is contracted, treatment is supportive.

Disease: Meningitis, Meningococcus

Incubation time: 1 to 14 days or longer.

How long it is usually contagious: Any time prior to onset and up to 48 hours after antibiotics are started.

Treatment: Drug of choice is penicillin G; second drug of choice is ceftriaxone (Rocephin).

Disease: Mononucleosis, Mono
Incubation time: 1 to 7 weeks.
How long it is usually contagious: Up to 3 months.
Treatment: Supportive care only.

Disease: Mumps
Incubation time: 12 to 28 days.
How long it is usually contagious: 5 days before and 10 days after onset.
Treatment: Supportive therapy only.

Disease: Rubella, German Measles
Incubation time: 14 to 21 days.
How long it is usually contagious: 7 days before the rash, until 5 days after the full rash appears.
Treatment: Prevention is best treatment. Once the disease is present, therapy is only supportive.

Disease: Rubella, Measles
Incubation time: 8 to 15 days in children and 10 to 21 days in adults.
How long it is usually contagious: Usually when the cough starts, about 5 days after exposure; contagiousness continues until 5 days after the rash appears.
Treatment: Supportive only.

Disease: Streptococcal Pharyngitis, Strep Throat
Incubation time: 2 to 7 days.
How long it is usually contagious: Up to 48 hours after antibiotics are started.
Treatment: The drug of choice is penicillin. The second drug of choice is erythromycin.

Disease: Syphilis, Bad Blood, Old Joe, Siph
Incubation time: 10 to 60 days.
How long it is usually contagious: This disease can be passed via the blood within a few hours after the person is infected. Length of infectivity depends on the stage of the disease. Ask your doctor for help.

Treatment: Depends on the stage of the disease. Primary syphilis, which is relatively early in the infection, or the secondary stage of this disease can be treated with penicillin G benzathine or tetracycline. Latent disease or neurosyphilis may involve the heart or blood vessels and require more involved therapy.

Disease: Varicella, Chickenpox
Incubation time: This disease may be "given" to someone 4 days before the rash appears and until 7 days after ALL the lesions have crusted.

How long it is usually contagious: Until ALL the lesions have crusted over.

Treatment: Prevention via a vaccine is the best course, and the vaccine is now available. Once the disease is contracted, supportive therapy is usually the standard; however, acyclovir (Zovirax) has been used in some immunosuppressed children.

Disease: Venereal Warts
Incubation time: 6 to 8 weeks.

How long it is usually contagious: Highly contagious until removed.

Treatment: Surgical removal, podophyllin resins, or fluorouracil.

TABLE 14

Poison Control Centers

Many medications have a very narrow blood level range that separates the therapeutic effects from the toxic effects. Accidental poisoning with prescription and nonprescription medications can be life-threatening; immediate medical help is critical.

Please call the toll-free information number in your state *today*, and get the current toll-free number of the nearest Poison Control Center in your state. Keep the number posted by each phone at all times.

SOURCES

The following sources were consulted in compiling this book:

AMA Department of Drugs. *AMA Drug Evaluations.* Chicago: American Medical Association, 1992.

Andreoli, T.E., C.C.J. Carpenter, F. Plum, and L.H. Smith, eds. *Cecil Essentials of Medicine.* Philadelphia: W.B. Saunders, 1986.

Annals of Pharmacotherapy, The. Cincinnati, OH: Harvey Whitney Books, 1996.

Bartlett, J. *Medical Management of HIV.* 1996. Glenview, I.L.: Physicians & Scientists Publishing Co., Inc.

Berkow, R., ed. *The Merck Manual.* 15th ed. Rahway, N.J.: Merck Sharp & Dohme Research Laboratories, 1996.

Billups, N.F., ed. *American Drug Index 1992.* 36th ed. St. Louis: Facts and Comparisons, 1992.

Briggs, G.G., T.W. Bodendorfer, R.K. Freeman, and S.J. Yaffee. *Drugs in Pregnancy and Lactation.* Baltimore: Williams & Wilkins, 1983.

Canadian Pharmaceutical Association. *Compendium of Pharmaceuticals and Specialties.* 26th ed. Ottawa: Canadian Pharmaceutical Association, 1991.

Clin-Alert. Medford, N.J.: Clin-Alert, 1992—1994.

Clinical Abstracts: Current Therapeutic Findings. Edited by D.J. Thordsen and H.A. Barenholtz. Cincinnati, O.H.: Harvey Whitney Books, 1996.

Clinisphere, Facts and Comparisons 1.0. St. Louis, M.O.: Facts & Comparisons, Inc.

Davies, D.M., ed. *Adverse Drug Reaction Bulletin.* Weybridge, Surrey, U.K.: Meditext, 1992.

Davies, D.M., ed. *Textbook of Adverse Drug Reactions.* 4th ed. New York: Oxford University Press, 1991.

DiGregorio, J.G., et. al. *Handbook of Pain Management.* Westchester, N.Y.: Medical Surveillance, 1991.

Drug Information Journal. Ambler, P.A.: Drug Information Association, 1996.

Drug Interactions Newsletter. Edited by P.D. Hansten and J.R. Horn. Spokane, W.A.: Applied Therapeutics, 1992.

Drugs & Therapy Perspectives. Auckland, New Zealand: Adis International, 1996.

Drug Therapy: Physicians' Prescribing Update. Lawrenceville, N.J.: Excerpta Medica, 1992.

Dukes, M.N.G., ed. *Meyler's Side Effects of Drugs.* 11th ed. Amsterdam: Excerpta Medica, 1988.

Electronic Library of Medicine, The. Boston: Little, Brown, 1996.

Facts and Comparisons Drug Newsletter. Edited by B.R. Olin. St. Louis: Facts and Comparisons Division, J.B. Lippincott, 1996.

F.D.A. Drug Bulletin. Rockville, M.D.: Department of Health and Human Services, Food and Drug Administration, 1996.

Fraunfelder, F.T. *Drug-Induced Ocular Side Effects and Drug Interactions.* 3rd ed. Philadelphia: Lea & Febiger, 1989.

Goodman, L.S., and A. Gilman, eds. *The Pharmacological Basis of Therapeutics.* 9th ed. New York: Macmillan, 1996.

Greenberger, N.J., C. Arvanitakis, and A. Hurwitz. *Drug Treatment of Gastrointestinal Disorders.* New York: Churchill Livingstone, 1978.

Hansten, P.D. *Drug Interactions.* 6th ed. Philadelphia: Lea & Febiger, 1992.

Heinonen, O.P., D. Slone, and S. Shapiro. *Birth Defects and Drugs in Pregnancy.* Littleton, M.A.: PSG Publishing, 1977.

Hollister, L.E. *Clinical Pharmacology of Psychotherapeutic Drugs.* 2d ed. New York: Churchill Livingstone, 1983.

Huff, B.B., ed. *The Physicians' Desk Reference.* Montvale, N.J.: Medical Economics Company, 1996.

International Drug Therapy Newsletter. Edited by F.J. Ayd. Baltimore: Ayd Medical Communications, 1996.

Jefferson, J.W., and J.H. Greist. *Primer of Lithium Therapy.* Baltimore: Williams & Wilkins, 1977.

Journal of the American Medical Association. Edited by G.D. Lundberg. Chicago: American Medical Association, 1996.

Klippel, J.H., ed. "Systemic Lupus Erythematosus." *Rheumatic Disease Clinics of North America* 14, no. 1 (April 1988).

Koda-Kimble (Lloyd Yee Young). *Applied Therapeutics, The Clinical Use of Drugs.* 6th ed. Vancouver, W.A.: Applied Therapeutics, Inc., 1995

Kolodny, R.C., W.H. Masters, and V.E. Johnson. *Textbook of Sexual Medicine.* Boston: Little, Brown, 1979.

Lawrence, R.A. *Breast-Feeding.* St. Louis: Mosby, 1980.

Lieberman, M.L. *The Sexual Pharmacy.* New York: New American Library, 1988.

Long, J.W. *Clinical Management of Prescription Drugs.* Philadelphia: Harper & Row, 1984.

Maddin, S., ed. *Current Dermatologic Therapy.* Philadelphia: W.B. Saunders, 1982.

McEvoy, G.K., ed. *American Hospital Formulary Service, Drug Information 1996.* Bethesda, M.D.: American Society of Hospital Pharmacists, 1996.

Medical Letter on Drugs and Therapeutics, The. Edited by H. Aaron. New Rochelle, N.Y.: The Medical Letter, 1996.

Messerli, F.H., ed. *Current Clinical Practice.* Philadelphia: W.B. Saunders, 1992.

Micromedex: DRUGDEX. Computerized Clinical Information Systems, 1996.

New England Journal of Medicine. Edited by J.P. Kassirer. Boston: The Massachusetts Medical Society, 1996.

Patient Drug Facts. Edited by B.R. Olin. St. Louis: Facts and Comparisons Division, St. Louis: J.B. Lippincott, 1992.

Physicians GenRx, version 96.1a. St. Louis, M.O.: Mosby.

Postgraduate Medicine, The Journal of Applied Medicine for the Primary Care Physician. Minneapolis: McGraw-Hill, 1992.

Rakel, R.E., ed. *Conn's Current Therapy 1992.* Philadelphia: W.B. Saunders, 1992.

Rational Drug Therapy, Pharmacology for Physicians. Bethesda, M.D.: American Society for Pharmacology and Experimental Therapeutics, 1990.

Reynolds, J.E.F., ed. *Martindale, The Extra Pharmacopoeia.* London: The Pharmaceutical Press, 1996.

Rogers, C.S., and J.D. McCue, eds. *Managing Chronic Disease.* Oradell, N.J.: Medical Economics Books, 1987.

Schardein, J.L. *Drugs as Teratogens.* Cleveland: CRC Press, 1976.

Scientific American Medicine. CD-ROM. New York: Enigma Information Systems.

Shepard, T.H. *Catalog of Teratogenic Agents.* 6th ed. Baltimore: Johns Hopkins University Press, 1989.

Smith, L.H., and S.O. Thier. *Pathophysiology, The Biological Principles of Disease.* 2d ed. Philadelphia: W.B. Saunders, 1985.

Speight, T.M., ed. *Avery's Drug Treatment.* 3rd ed. Auckland: ADIS Press, 1987.

Tatro, D.S., ed. *Drug Interaction Facts.* St. Louis: Facts and Comparisons Division, J.B. Lippincott, 1992.

Tuchmann-Duplessis, H. *Drug Effects on the Fetus.* Sydney: ADIS Press, 1975.

USP Dispensing Information 1996. 12th ed. Vol. 1, *Drug Information for the Health Care Provider.* Rockville, M.D.: United States Pharmacopeia Convention, 1996.

Wallach, J. *Interpretation of Diagnostic Tests.* 6th ed. Boston: Little, Brown, 1996.

Wartak, J. *Drug Dosage and Administration.* Baltimore: University Park Press, 1983.

Worley, R.J., ed. "Menopause," *Clinical Obstetrics and Gynecology* 24, no. 1 (1981).

Young, D.S. *Effects of Drugs on Clinical Laboratory Tests.* 1991 Supplement. Washington, D.C.: AACC Press, 1991.

INDEX

NOTE: In the text the symbol [CD] indicates that the brand name given is a combination drug consisting of the generic drug components in the drug profile section of this book. To be fully familiar with any combination drug, read the profile of each of the components listed. When an asterisk but no page number appears, it indicates an active component for which there is no profile in this book. It appears here to alert you to its presence, should you wish to consult your doctor regarding its significance for you.

*See note at beginning of Index.

*See note at beginning of Index.

*See note at beginning of Index.

*See note at beginning of Index.

*See note at beginning of Index.

*See note at beginning of Index.

*See note at beginning of Index.

*See note at beginning of Index.

*See note at beginning of Index.

*See note at beginning of Index.

ABOUT THE AUTHOR

James J. Rybacki, Pharm. D., was born in Oneonta, New York. He received his prepharmacy education at Creighton University, and his doctor of pharmacy degree from the College of Pharmacy at the University of Nebraska Medical Center in Omaha. His more than 24 years of hospital and clinical experience include early efforts in gas-liquid chromatography research characterizing human drug metabolites, and data collection for the College of American Pathologists establishing normal values for laboratory studies. He is a member of the clinical faculty at the University of Maryland School of Pharmacy and has provided clinical rounding and hospital experience for undergraduate and pharmacy doctoral students at Dorchester General Hospital. A resident of Easton, Maryland, he presently teaches a drug information rotation at The Clearwater Group. He is board certified in pain management at the Diplomat level by the American Academy of Pain Management, and provides ongoing pain management and outcomes research consulting as part of the Pain Center at Advantage Orthopedics. Dr. Rybacki is actively involved in the postmarketing monitoring of medicines via The Drug Surveillance Network, a nationwide association of clinical pharmacists, and he is an approved external new drug application reviewer for the Canadian Drug Ministry.

Dr. Rybacki's efforts in drug information and clinical pharmacy include eight years of active practice provided at Dorchester General Hospital in Cambridge, Maryland, providing infectious disease, pharmacokinetic, nutrition support, pain management, and pharmacologic consultations. He offered independent pain management and pharmacologic consultations nationwide through the Occupational Health Unit, and now continues these in independent practice. He has advised the World Health Organization's Expert Committee regarding revisions as well as selection of drugs to be listed in the 1995 edition of *The Use of Essential Drugs* and is an assistant editor for the Drugdex drug information system. His past hospital-based role as vice president of clinical services has brought him added expertise in overseeing occupational health, physical medicines, laboratory services, imaging, cardiology, respiratory therapy, cancer programs, and continuing medical education. He has served as conference coordinator for the first and second annual Dorchester General Hospital Pain conferences, and served as seminar coordinator for the Eastern Shore of Maryland for the "Take Control" physician and public pain education programs with Johns Hopkins Medical School.

Dr. Rybacki is president of The Clearwater Group, and provides clinical pharmacy consults on drug information and therapeutics to physician groups and employers; holds seminars on medical cost containment, infectious disease, pain management and therapeutics, and medical editing and writing; and conducts independent pharmacologic evaluations. He provides clinical consultations on osteoporosis as a certified clinical densitometrist, and is a board-certified forensic examiner. He provides ongoing pain management consultations, has been selected for full membership in the American College of Clinical Pharmacy, and is a lifetime member of Who's Who in Global Business.

Dr. Rybacki has been a guest and guest host on numerous radio and television shows, and participates in many speakers bureaus including Miles, Dupont Pharma, Glaxo, and Lederle's Distinguished Speakers in Medicine. He is also a member of the Bristol-Myers Distinguished Faculty in HIV. He has co-authored several articles in professional journals on the use of medicines in critical care, therapeutics, and cost containment. *The Essential Guide to Prescription Drugs*, first published in 1977, was co-authored by Dr. Rybacki since 1994 before he assumed full authorship in 1996.

He is a member of The International Society of Clinical Densitometry, and became the first doctor of pharmacy in the world to be a certified clinical densitometrist. In 1995 he produced and hosted *The Medicine Man*, a nationally broadcast call-in live radio show on medication use. Subsequently Dr. Rybacki wrote and hosted "The Pharmacist Minute," a nationally and then internationally syndicated radio program of The American Pharmaceutical Association, sponsored by a grant from Pepcid AC™. He believes that the new art of prescribing medicines lies in cost containment without sacrifice of clinical outcomes.

MY PERSONAL DRUG PROFILE

This table is a medication profile, which gathers all of the important disease information and information about prescription and nonprescription medicines into a valuable and logical form. Use this form when you see a new doctor or pharmacy, and for organizing your health care information for use in emergencies.

Name:

Age:

Weight in kilograms: (pounds divided by 2.2)

Height in inches:

Prescription drug allergies:

Nonprescription drug allergies:

Food allergies:

My kidneys* are: normal_____

mildly_____ moderately_____ severely ____ compromised.

My liver* is: normal_____

mildly_____ moderately_____ severely_____ compromised.

*Make certain your dose is decreased if the drug is eliminated by an organ (such as the liver or kidneys) with which you have a problem. To determine which organs are involved, refer to the drug profile and "Conditions Requiring Dosing Adjustments" section for each medication you are taking.

Conditions or diseases that I have or have had:

Prescription and nonprescription medications I take regularly:

Prescription and nonprescription medications I take periodically:

I find it very difficult_____

I find it very easy_____ to remember to take medicines.

I become constipated

rarely_____ occasionally_____ never_____.

Urination is usually

easy_____ rather difficult_____ difficult_____.

The phone number of the nearest Poison Control Center is

_____.

I sleep well_____ OK_____ poorly_____ little_____ on most nights.

I have_____ have never_____ had blood problems in the past.

I am considering becoming_____ might be_____ am_____ pregnant.

I want the medications that offer the best balance of **price** and **outcome** for my specific medical history and present conditions.

At least once a year, but ideally every 6 months, schedule an appointment with your doctor or pharmacist to review all prescription, nonprescription, nutritional, homeopathic, herbal, or nutritional products you currently take.